Cancer
SOURCEBOOK

Seventh Edition

Health Reference Series

Seventh Edition

Cancer
SOURCEBOOK

Basic Consumer Health Information about Major Forms and Stages of Cancer, Featuring Facts about Head and Neck Cancers, Lung Cancers, Gastrointestinal Cancers, Genito-Urinary Cancers, Lymphomas, Blood Cell Cancers, Endocrine Cancers, Skin Cancers, Bone Cancers, Metastatic Cancers, and More.

Along with Facts about Cancer Treatments, Cancer Risks and Prevention, a Glossary of Related Terms, Statistical Data, and a Directory of Resources for Additional Information.

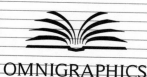

OMNIGRAPHICS

155 W. Congress, Suite 200 Detroit, MI 48226

Bibliographic Note

Because this page cannot legibly accommodate all the copyright notices, the Bibliographic Note portion of the Preface constitutes an extension of the copyright notice.

* * *

Omnigraphics, Inc.

Editorial Services provided by Omnigraphics, Inc.,
a division of Relevant Information, Inc.

Keith Jones, *Managing Editor*

* * *

Table of Contents

Part IV: Cancer Detection and Diagnosis

Part IX: Additional Help and Information

Preface

About This Book

Every year, nearly 1.5 million Americans receive a diagnosis of cancer. Cancer is not a single disease, however. It is many different diseases that all share one common characteristic: Some of the body's cells do not die when they should. Instead they continue to grow and divide. Through this process, cancer cells can damage the body's tissues and organs, leading to a broad array of symptoms and even death. The cellular changes that lead to the development of cancer are sometimes inherited but they may also result from environmental or lifestyle factors. Although the survival rates for many types of cancer have improved in recent years and innovative treatment protocols are being developed, cancer remains the second leading cause of death in the United States.

Cancer Sourcebook, Seventh Edition provides updated information about common types of cancer affecting the head, neck, central nervous system, endocrine system, lungs, digestive and urinary tracts, blood cells, immune system, skin, bones, and other body systems. It explains how people can reduce their risk of cancer by adopting a healthy lifestyle, addressing issues related to cancer risk, and taking advantage of screening exams. Various treatment choices—including surgery, chemotherapy, radiation therapy, and biological therapies—are discussed. The book concludes with a glossary of related terms, a directory of national cancer organizations, and suggestions for finding community-based resources.

How to Use This Book

This book is divided into parts and chapters. Parts focus on broad areas of interest. Chapters are devoted to single topics within a part.

Part I: Cancer Overview defines what cancer is and gives brief insight into its classification. It also focuses on general signs and symptoms of cancer, metastatic cancer and cancer clusters.

Part II: Risk Factors and Cancer Prevention offers an overview of the factors that are known to increase the risk of cancer (cigarette smoking, "light" cigarettes, cigar smoking, secondhand smoke, and smokeless tobacco). It also includes details of risks caused by asbestos exposure, diethylstilbestrol, HIV infection, HPV, Helicobacter Pylori, cell phones, magnetic field exposure, accidents at nuclear power plants, and radon. Cancer risks associated with pregnancy, contraceptives, menopausal hormones and psychological stress are also discussed. Besides risk factors, it also focuses on prevention of cancer, especially pertaining to diet factors. The part concludes with a description about the necessity of early screening.

Part III: Cancer Types includes a head-to-toe list of the most frequently occurring types of cancer. Individual chapters describe the development, identification, and treatment of cancers that affect the various components of the body, including the brain and central nervous system, endocrine system, respiratory system, blood and immune system, digestive and urinary tracts, and reproductive organs, as well as the bones and skin.

Part IV: Cancer Detection and Diagnosis describes the stages of cancer, screening methods to detect cancer at early stages, and commonly-used procedures in cancer diagnosis. Diagnostic methods such as CT scan, mammograms, genetic testing, PAP and HPV testing, PSA test, Sentinel Lymph node biopsy, tumor grade, tumor markers and understanding laboratory tests are described.

Part V: Cancer Treatment extensively covers general treatment options including chemotherapy, radiation therapy, biological therapy, targeted cancer therapies, laser treatment, and photodynamic therapy. It also highlights complementary and alternative medicine (CAM) practices in cancer care. It briefly makes a reference to creating awareness on cancer treatment scams.

Part VI: Coping with Cancer discusses side effects, cardiopulmonary syndromes, oral complications of chemotherapy and radiation. It includes advice from experts on nutrition care.

Part VII: Research and Clinical Trials focuses on the importance of biorepositories and emphasizes on the participation of cancer patients in this research method. Further, it also outlines the benefits of bio-specimens in clinical research.

Part VIII: Trends and Statistics includes an overview of cancer statistics, statistical information on common cancer types, and statistics based on age, gender and ethnicity. It also discusses cancer health disparities and the programs undertaken to address these concerns.

Part IX: Additional Help and Information includes a glossary of terms and a directory of national cancer organizations that provide information about specific cancers.

Bibliographic Note

This volume contains documents and excerpts from publications issued by the following U.S. government agencies: National Cancer Institute (NCI), Surveillance, Epidemiology and End Results Program (SEER), and U.S. Food and Drug Administration (FDA).

About the Health Reference Series

The *Health Reference Series* is designed to provide basic medical information for patients, families, caregivers, and the general public. Each volume takes a particular topic and provides comprehensive coverage. This is especially important for people who may be dealing with a newly diagnosed disease or a chronic disorder in themselves or in a family member. People looking for preventive guidance, information about disease warning signs, medical statistics, and risk factors for health problems will also find answers to their questions in the *Health Reference Series*. The *Series*, however, is not intended to serve as a tool for diagnosing illness, in prescribing treatments, or as a substitute for the physician/patient relationship. All people concerned about medical symptoms or the possibility of disease are encouraged to seek professional care from an appropriate health care provider.

A Note about Spelling and Style

Health Reference Series editors use *Stedman's Medical Dictionary* as an authority for questions related to the spelling of medical terms and the *Chicago Manual of Style* for questions related to grammatical structures, punctuation, and other editorial concerns. Consistent adherence is not always possible, however, because the individual volumes within the *Series* include many documents from a wide variety of different producers, and the editor's primary goal is to present material from each source as accurately as is possible. This sometimes means that information in different chapters or sections may follow other guidelines and alternate spelling authorities.

Our Advisory Board

We would like to thank the following board members for providing guidance to the development of this Series:

- Dr. Lynda Baker, Associate Professor of Library and Information Science, Wayne State University, Detroit, MI

- Nancy Bulgarelli, William Beaumont Hospital Library, Royal Oak, MI

- Karen Imarisio, Bloomfield Township Public Library, Bloomfield Township, MI

- Karen Morgan, Mardigian Library, University of Michigan-Dearborn, Dearborn, MI

- Rosemary Orlando, St. Clair Shores Public Library, St. Clair Shores, MI

Health Reference Series Update Policy

The inaugural book in the *Health Reference Series* was the first edition of Cancer Sourcebook published in 1989. Since then, the *Series* has been enthusiastically received by librarians and in the medical community. In order to maintain the standard of providing high-quality health information for the layperson, the editorial staff at Omnigraphics felt it was necessary to implement a policy of updating volumes when warranted.

Medical researchers have been making tremendous strides, and it is the purpose of the *Health Reference Series* to stay current with the most recent advances. Each decision to update a volume is made on an individual basis. Some of the considerations include how much new information is available and the feedback we receive from people who use the books. If there is a topic you would like to see added to the update list, or an area of medical concern you feel has not been adequately addressed, please write to:

Managing Editor
Health Reference Series
Omnigraphics, Inc.
155 W. Congress, Suite 200
Detroit, MI 48226

Part One

Cancer Overview

Chapter 1

Cancer Defined

What is Cancer?

There are many texts and references that attempt to define cancer. The simplest definition is from the American Cancer Society (ACS). According to the ACS, cancer is a group of diseases characterized by uncontrolled growth and spread of abnormal cells. If the spread is not controlled, it can result in death.

A group of diseases

Although cancer is often referred to as a single condition, it actually consists of more than 100 different diseases. These diseases are characterized by uncontrolled growth and spread of abnormal cells. Cancer can arise in many sites and behave differently depending on its organ of origin. Breast cancer, for example, has different characteristics than those of lung cancer. It is important to understand that cancer originating in one body organ takes its characteristics with it even if it spreads to another part of the body. For example, metastatic breast cancer in the lungs continues to behave like breast cancer when viewed under a microscope, and it continues to look like a cancer that originated in the breast.

This chapter includes excerpts from "What is Cancer; Cancer Terms; and Cell Biology of Cancer," National Cancer Institute at the National Institutes of Health (NIH).

Characteristics of Cancer

Abnormality

Cells are the structural units of all living things. Each of us has trillions of cells, as does a growing tree. Cells make it possible for us to carry out all kinds of functions of life: the beating of the heart, breathing, digesting food, thinking, walking, and so on. However, all of these functions can only be carried out by normal healthy cells. Some cells stop functioning or behaving as they should, serving no useful purpose in the body at all, and become cancerous cells.

Uncontrollability

The most fundamental characteristic of cells is their ability to reproduce themselves. They do this simply by dividing: one cell becomes two, the two become four, and so on. The division of normal and healthy cells occurs in a regulated and systematic fashion. In most parts of the body, the cells continually divide and form new cells to supply the material for growth or to replace worn-out or injured cells. For example, when you cut your finger, certain cells divide rapidly until the tissue is healed and the skin is repaired. They will then go back to their normal rate of division. In contrast, cancer cells divide in a haphazard manner. The result is that they typically pile up into a non-structured mass or tumor.

Invasiveness

Sometimes tumors do not stay harmlessly in one place. They destroy the part of the body in which they originate and then spread to other parts where they start new growth and cause more destruction. This characteristic distinguishes cancer from benign growths, which remain in the part of the body in which they start. Although benign tumors may grow quite large and press on neighboring structures, they do not spread to other parts of the body. Frequently, they are completely enclosed in a protective capsule of tissue and they typically do not pose danger to human life like malignant tumors (cancer) do.

Cancer Terms

Cancer, Neoplasia, Tumor, Neoplasm

The word cancer comes from the Latin (originally Greek) derived term for crab, because of the way a cancer adheres to any part that it seizes upon in an obstinate manner like the crab. Hippocrates first described cancer as having a central body with the tendency to reach out and spread like "the arms of a crab." Besides the popular, generic term "cancer" used by most people, there is another more technical term: neoplasia. Neoplasia (neo = new, plasia = tissue or cells) or neoplasm literally means new tissue in Greek. This indicates that cancers are actually new growths of cells in the body.

Another term for cancer is "malignant." Tumor literally means "swelling" or "mass." In this case, it refers to a mass of non-structured new cells, which have no known purpose in the physiological function of the body.

There are two general types of tumors: benign (non-cancerous) tumors and malignant (cancerous) tumors. A benign tumor is composed of cells that will not invade other unrelated tissues or organs of the body, although it may continue to grow in size abnormally. A malignant tumor is composed of cells that invade the basement membrane and invade or spread to other parts of the body. This occurs either by direct extension to neighboring organs and/or tissues or by metastasizing to distant sites by means of the vascular system (the blood stream), the lymphatic system, or by seeding or implantation of cancer cells in body cavities.

Terms such as "mass" and "lump" are used to describe any overgrowth of tissue. However, these terms may not necessarily mean that such growths contain cancer cells.

Types of Abnormal Cell Growth

In addition to neoplasia, there are several other terms referring to abnormal cell growth. These include the following:

Hyperplasia refers to an abnormal increase in the number of cells, which are in a normal component of that tissue and are arranged in a normal fashion with subsequent enlargement of the affected part. One example is thyroid hyperplasia, an enlargement of the thyroid gland caused by an abnormal rapid growth of the epithelial cells lining the follicles. Another example is: Guitar strumming leads to hyperplasia of the cells on the thumb (a callus is formed). The callus on the thumb is a hyperplastic growth.

Hypertrophy refers to an abnormal increase in the size of each cell, for example, the increase in cell size of cardiac muscle.

Metaplasia refers to the replacement of one mature cell type with another mature cell type: for example, squamous metaplasia of the respiratory columnar epithelium—as evidenced by the metaplastic cough of a smoker.

Dysplasia refers to the replacement of one mature cell type with a less mature cell type: for example, dysplasia of the cervix epithelium.

Hyperplasia, metaplasia, and dysplasia are reversible because they are results of a stimulus. Neoplasia is irreversible because it is autonomous.

Tumor Terminology Generalizations

Names of benign tumors usually end with "oma" regardless of their cell type. For example, a benign glandular tumor (epithelium tissue) is called adenoma and a benign bone tumor is called osteoma, while a

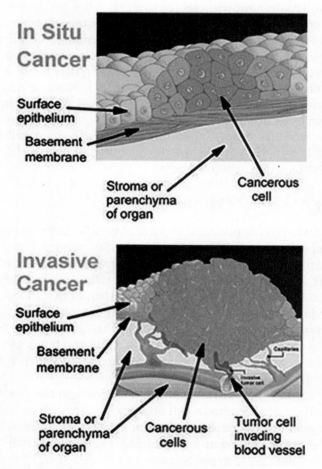

Figure 1.1. *Representation of In Situ and Invasive cancer*

malignant glandular tumor is called adenocarcinoma and a malignant bone tumor is called osteosarcoma.

In addition to benign tumors, there are in situ tumors and invasive tumors. In situ tumors do not invade the basement membrane, whereas invasive tumors do invade the basement membrane.

Cell Biology of Cancer

The cell is the fundamental unit of life. It is the smallest structure of the body capable of performing all of the processes that define life. Each of the organs in the body, such as the lung, breast, colon, and brain, consists of specialized cells that carry out the organ's functions such as the transportation of oxygen, digestion of nutrients, excretion of waste materials, locomotion, reproduction, thinking, etc.

To assure the proper performance of each organ, worn out or injured cells must be replaced, and particular types of cells must increase in response to environmental changes. For example, the bone marrow increases its production of oxygen-carrying red blood cells sevenfold or greater in response to bleeding or high altitude. Certain white blood cells are produced more rapidly during an infection. Similarly, the liver or endocrine organs frequently respond to injury by regenerating damaged cells.

As stated in the previous section, reproduction of cells is a process of cell division. The division of normal cells is a highly regulated process. The cell growth, inheritance and containment is controlled by its DNA (deoxyribonucleic acid).

DNA is a highly complex molecule manufactured in the cell nucleus and serves as the cell's "brain." DNA is the blueprint for everything the cell does. In a human cell, the DNA is arranged in 46 distinct sections called chromosomes. They are arranged in pairs, 23 chromosomes from each biological parent.

Together, the 46 chromosomes contain more than 100,000 genes. A gene is a segment of DNA that determines the structure of a protein, which is needed for development and growth as well as carrying out vital chemical functions in the body. Like the chromosomes, genes are arranged in pairs—one gene from the mother and one from the father.

Each gene occupies a specific location on a chromosome. Through a number of biochemical steps, each gene tells a cell to make a different protein. Some genes instruct the cell to manufacture structural proteins, which serve as building blocks. Other genes tell the cell to produce hormones, growth factors or cytokines, which exit the cell and communicate with other cells. Still other genes tell the cell to produce regulatory proteins that control the function of other proteins or tell other genes when to turn "on" or "off." When a gene is turned on, it manufactures another complex molecule called ribonucleic acid (RNA), which contains all the information the cell needs to make new proteins.

Cells divide only when they receive the proper signals from growth factors that circulate in the bloodstream or from a cell they directly contact. For example, if a person loses blood, a growth factor called erythropoietin, which is produced in the kidneys, circulates in the bloodstream and tells the bone marrow to manufacture more blood cells.

When a cell receives the message to divide, it goes through the cell cycle, which includes several phases for the division to be completed. Checkpoints along each step of the process make sure that everything goes the way it should.

Many processes are involved in cell reproduction and all these processes have to take place correctly for a cell to divide properly. If anything goes wrong during this complicated process, a cell may become cancerous.

A cancer cell is a cell that grows out of control. Unlike normal cells, cancer cells ignore signals to stop dividing, to specialize, or to die and be shed. Growing in an uncontrollable manner and unable to recognize its own natural boundary, the cancer cells may spread to areas of the body where they do not belong.

In a cancer cell, several genes change (mutate) and the cell becomes defective. There are two general types of gene mutations. One type, dominant mutation, is caused by an abnormality in one gene in a pair. An example is a mutated gene that produces a defective protein that causes the growth-factor receptor on a cell's surface to be constantly "on" when, in fact, no growth factor is present. The result is that the cell receives a constant message to divide. This dominant "gain of function gene" is often called an oncogene (onco = cancer).

The second general type of mutation, recessive mutation, is characterized by both genes in the pair being damaged. For example, a normal gene called p53 produces a protein that turns "off" the cell cycle and thus helps to control cell growth. The primary function of the p53 gene is to repair or destroy defective cells, thereby controlling potential cancerous cells. This type of gene is called an anti-oncogene or tumor suppressor gene. If only one p53 gene in the pair is mutated, the other gene will still be able to control the cell cycle. However, if both genes are mutated, the "off" switch is lost, and the cell division is no longer under control.

Abnormal cell division can occur either when active oncogenes are expressed or when tumor suppressor genes are lost. In fact, for a cell to become malignant, numerous mutations are necessary. In some cases, both types of mutations—dominant and recessive—may occur.

A gene mutation may allow an already abnormal cell to invade the normal tissue where the cancer started or to travel in the bloodstream (metastasize) to remote parts of the body, where it continues to divide.

A normal cell can become damaged in different ways. A cell can become abnormal when part of a gene is lost (deleted), when part of a chromosome is rearranged and ends up in the wrong place (translocation), or when an extremely small defect occurs in the DNA, which results in an abnormal DNA "blueprint" and production of a defective protein occurs.

Abnormal cell division can also be caused by viruses. In this case, genes may be normal, but the protein may not function normally because the cell contains a cancer-producing virus.

How a specific cancer cell behaves depends on which processes are not functioning properly. Some cancer cells simply divide and produce more cancer cells, and the tumor mass stays where it began. Other cancer cells are able to invade normal tissue, enter the bloodstream, and metastasize to a remote site in the body.

In summary, cancer cells have defects in normal cellular functions that allow them to divide, invade the surrounding tissue, and spread by way of vascular and/or lymphatic systems. These defects are the result of gene mutations sometimes caused by infectious viruses.

Chapter 2

Cancer Classification

Cancers are classified in two ways: by the type of tissue in which the cancer originates (histological type) and by primary site, or the location in the body where the cancer first developed. This section introduces you to the first method: cancer classification based on histological type.

From a histological standpoint there are hundreds of different cancers, which are grouped into six major categories:

- Carcinoma
- Sarcoma
- Myeloma
- Leukemia
- Lymphoma
- Mixed Types

Carcinoma

Carcinoma refers to a malignant neoplasm of epithelial origin or cancer of the internal or external lining of the body. Carcinomas, malignancies of epithelial tissue, account for 80 to 90 percent of all cancer cases.

Epithelial tissue is found throughout the body. It is present in the skin, as well as the covering and lining of organs and internal passageways, such as the gastrointestinal tract.

Text in this chapter is excerpted from "Cancer Classification," National Cancer Institute at the National Institutes of Health (NIH).

Carcinomas are divided into two major subtypes: adenocarcinoma, which develops in an organ or gland, and squamous cell carcinoma, which originates in the squamous epithelium.

Adenocarcinomas generally occur in mucus membranes and are first seen as a thickened plaque-like white mucosa. They often spread easily through the soft tissue where they occur. Squamous cell carcinomas occur in many areas of the body.

Most carcinomas affect organs or glands capable of secretion, such as the breasts, which produce milk, or the lungs, which secrete mucus, or colon or prostate or bladder.

Sarcoma

Sarcoma refers to cancer that originates in supportive and connective tissues such as bones, tendons, cartilage, muscle, and fat. Generally occurring in young adults, the most common sarcoma often develops as a painful mass on the bone. Sarcoma tumors usually resemble the tissue in which they grow.

Examples of sarcomas are:

- Osteosarcoma or osteogenic sarcoma (bone)
- Chondrosarcoma (cartilage)
- Leiomyosarcoma (smooth muscle)
- Rhabdomyosarcoma (skeletal muscle)
- Mesothelial sarcoma or mesothelioma (membranous lining of body cavities)
- Fibrosarcoma (fibrous tissue)
- Angiosarcoma or hemangioendothelioma (blood vessels)
- Liposarcoma (adipose tissue)
- Glioma or astrocytoma (neurogenic connective tissue found in the brain)
- Myxosarcoma (primitive embryonic connective tissue)
- Mesenchymous or mixed mesodermal tumor (mixed connective tissue types)

Myeloma

Myeloma is cancer that originates in the plasma cells of bone marrow. The plasma cells produce some of the proteins found in blood.

Leukemia

Leukemias ("liquid cancers" or "blood cancers") are cancers of the bone marrow (the site of blood cell production). The word leukemia means "white blood" in Greek. The disease is often associated with the overproduction of immature white blood cells. These immature white blood cells do not perform as well as they should, therefore the patient is often prone to infection. Leukemia also affects red blood cells and can cause poor blood clotting and fatigue due to anemia. Examples of leukemia include:

- Myelogenous or granulocytic leukemia (malignancy of the myeloid and granulocytic white blood cell series)

- Lymphatic, lymphocytic, or lymphoblastic leukemia (malignancy of the lymphoid and lymphocytic blood cell series)

- Polycythemia vera or erythremia (malignancy of various blood cell products, but with red cells predominating)

Lymphoma

Lymphomas develop in the glands or nodes of the lymphatic system, a network of vessels, nodes, and organs (specifically the spleen, tonsils, and thymus) that purify bodily fluids and produce infection-fighting white blood cells, or lymphocytes. Unlike the leukemias which are sometimes called "liquid cancers," lymphomas are "solid cancers." Lymphomas may also occur in specific organs such as the stomach, breast or brain. These lymphomas are referred to as extranodal lymphomas. The lymphomas are sub-classified into two categories: Hodgkin lymphoma and Non-Hodgkin lymphoma. The presence of Reed-Sternberg cells in Hodgkin lymphoma diagnostically distinguishes Hodgkin lymphoma from Non-Hodgkin lymphoma.

Mixed Types

The type components may be within one category or from different categories. Some examples are:

- adenosquamous carcinoma
- mixed mesodermal tumor
- carcinosarcoma
- teratocarcinoma

13

Chapter 3

Cancer Symptoms

Cancer can cause many different symptoms. These are some of them:

- Skin changes, such as:
  - A new mole or a change in an existing mole
  - A sore that does not heal
- Breast changes, such as:
  - Change in size or shape of the breast or nipple
  - Change in texture of breast skin
- A thickening or lump on or under the skin
- Hoarseness or cough that does not go away
- Changes in bowel habits
- Difficult or painful urination
- Problems with eating, such as:
  - Discomfort after eating
  - A hard time swallowing
  - Changes in appetite

Text in this chapter is excerpted from " Symptoms," National Cancer Institute at the National Institutes of Health (NIH), March 5, 2015.

- Weight gain or loss with no known reason
- Abdominal pain
- Unexplained night sweats
- Unusual bleeding or discharge, including:
  - Blood in the urine
  - Vaginal bleeding
  - Blood in the stool
- Feeling weak or very tired

Most often, these symptoms are not due to cancer. They may also be caused by benign tumors or other problems. If you have symptoms that last for a couple of weeks, it is important to see a doctor so that problems can be diagnosed and treated as early as possible.

Usually, early cancer does not cause pain. If you have symptoms, do not wait to feel pain before seeing a doctor.

Chapter 4

Metastatic Cancer

What is metastatic cancer?

Metastatic cancer is cancer that has spread from the place where it first started to another place in the body. A tumor formed by metastatic cancer cells is called a metastatic tumor or a metastasis. The process by which cancer cells spread to other parts of the body is also called metastasis.

Metastatic cancer has the same name and the same type of cancer cells as the original, or primary, cancer. For example, breast cancer that spreads to the lung and forms a metastatic tumor is metastatic breast cancer, not lung cancer.

Under a microscope, metastatic cancer cells generally look the same as cells of the original cancer. Moreover, metastatic cancer cells and cells of the original cancer usually have some molecular features in common, such as the expression of certain proteins or the presence of specific chromosome changes.

Although some types of metastatic cancer can be cured with current treatments, most cannot. Nevertheless, treatments are available for all patients with metastatic cancer. In general, the primary goal of these treatments is to control the growth of the cancer or to relieve symptoms caused by it. In some cases, metastatic cancer treatments may help prolong life. However, most people who die of cancer die of metastatic disease.

Text in this chapter is excerpted from "Metastatic Cancer," National Cancer Institute at the National Institutes of Health (NIH), March 28, 2013.

17

Can any type of cancer form a metastatic tumor?

Virtually all cancers, including cancers of the blood and the lymphatic system (leukemia, multiple myeloma, and lymphoma), can form metastatic tumors. Although rare, the metastasis of blood and lymphatic system cancers to the lung, heart, central nervous system, and other tissues has been reported.

Where does cancer spread?

The most common sites of cancer metastasis are, in alphabetical order, the bone, liver, and lung. Although most cancers have the ability to spread to many different parts of the body, they usually spread to one site more often than others. The following table shows the most common sites of metastasis, excluding the lymph nodes, for several types of cancer:

Table 4.1. Common sites of metastasis.

Cancer type	Main sites of metastasis*
Bladder	Bone, liver, lung
Breast	Bone, brain, liver, lung
Colorectal	Liver, lung, peritoneum
Kidney	Adrenal gland, bone, brain, liver, lung
Lung	Adrenal gland, bone, brain, liver, other lung
Melanoma	Bone, brain, liver, lung, skin/muscle
Ovary	Liver, lung, peritoneum
Pancreas	Liver, lung, peritoneum
Prostate	Adrenal gland, bone, liver, lung
Stomach	Liver, lung, peritoneum
Thyroid	Bone, liver, lung
Uterus	Bone, liver, lung, peritoneum, vagina

In alphabetical order. Brain includes the neural tissue of the brain (parenchyma) and the leptomeninges (the two innermost membranes—arachnoid mater and pia mater—of the three membranes known as the meninges that surround the brain and spinal cord; the space between the arachnoid mater and the pia mater contains cerebrospinal fluid). Lung includes the main part of the lung (parenchyma) as well as the pleura (the membrane that covers the lungs and lines the chest cavity).

How does cancer spread?

Cancer cell metastasis usually involves the following steps:

- **Local invasion**: Cancer cells invade nearby normal tissue.
- **Intravasation**: Cancer cells invade and move through the walls of nearby lymph vessels or blood vessels.
- **Circulation**: Cancer cells move through the lymphatic system and the bloodstream to other parts of the body.
- **Arrest and extravasation**: Cancer cells arrest, or stop moving, in small blood vessels called capillaries at a distant location. They then invade the walls of the capillaries and migrate into the surrounding tissue (extravasation).
- **Proliferation**: Cancer cells multiply at the distant location to form small tumors known as micrometastases.
- **Angiogenesis**: Micrometastases stimulate the growth of new blood vessels to obtain a blood supply. A blood supply is needed to obtain the oxygen and nutrients necessary for continued tumor growth.

Because cancers of the lymphatic system or the blood system are already present inside lymph vessels, lymph nodes, or blood vessels, not all of these steps are needed for their metastasis. Also, the lymphatic system drains into the blood system at two locations in the neck.

The ability of a cancer cell to metastasize successfully depends on its individual properties; the properties of the noncancerous cells, including immune system cells, present at the original location; and the properties of the cells it encounters in the lymphatic system or the bloodstream and at the final destination in another part of the body. Not all cancer cells, by themselves, have the ability to metastasize. In addition, the noncancerous cells at the original location may be able to block cancer cell metastasis. Furthermore, successfully reaching another location in the body does not guarantee that a metastatic tumor will form. Metastatic cancer cells can lie dormant (not grow) at a distant site for many years before they begin to grow again, if at all.

Does metastatic cancer have symptoms?

Some people with metastatic tumors do not have symptoms. Their metastases are found by x-rays or other tests.

When symptoms of metastatic cancer occur, the type and frequency of the symptoms will depend on the size and location of the metastasis.

For example, cancer that spreads to the bone is likely to cause pain and can lead to bone fractures. Cancer that spreads to the brain can cause a variety of symptoms, including headaches, seizures, and unsteadiness. Shortness of breath may be a sign of lung metastasis. Abdominal swelling or jaundice (yellowing of the skin) can indicate that cancer has spread to the liver.

Sometimes a person's original cancer is discovered only after a metastatic tumor causes symptoms. For example, a man whose prostate cancer has spread to the bones in his pelvis may have lower back pain (caused by the cancer in his bones) before he experiences any symptoms from the original tumor in his prostate.

Can someone have a metastatic tumor without having a primary cancer?

No. A metastatic tumor is always caused by cancer cells from another part of the body.

In most cases, when a metastatic tumor is found first, the primary cancer can also be found. The search for the primary cancer may involve lab tests, x-rays, computed tomography (CT) scans, magnetic resonance imaging (MRI) scans, positron emission tomography (PET) scans, and other procedures.

However, in some patients, a metastatic tumor is diagnosed but the primary tumor cannot be found, despite extensive tests, because it either is too small or has completely regressed. The pathologist knows that the diagnosed tumor is a metastasis because the cells do not look like those of the organ or tissue in which the tumor was found. Doctors refer to the primary cancer as unknown or occult (hidden), and the patient is said to have cancer of unknown primary origin (CUP). Because diagnostic techniques are constantly improving, the number of cases of CUP is going down.

If a person who was previously treated for cancer gets diagnosed with cancer a second time, is the new cancer a new primary cancer or metastatic cancer?

The cancer may be a new primary cancer, but, in most cases, it is metastatic cancer.

What treatments are used for metastatic cancer?

Metastatic cancer may be treated with systemic therapy (chemotherapy, biological therapy, targeted therapy, hormonal therapy), local therapy (surgery, radiation therapy), or a combination of these treatments. The choice of treatment generally depends on the type of primary cancer; the size, location, and number of metastatic tumors; the patient's age and general health; and the types of treatment the patient has had in the past. In patients with CUP, it is possible to treat the disease even though the primary cancer has not been found.

Are new treatments for metastatic cancer being developed?

Yes, researchers are studying new ways to kill or stop the growth of primary cancer cells and metastatic cancer cells, including new ways to boost the strength of immune responses against tumors. In addition, researchers are trying to find ways to disrupt individual steps in the metastatic process.

Before any new treatment can be made widely available to patients, it must be studied in clinical trials (research studies) and found to be safe and effective in treating disease. NCI and many other organizations sponsor clinical trials that take place at hospitals, universities, medical schools, and cancer centers around the country. Clinical trials are a critical step in improving cancer care. The results of previous clinical trials have led to progress not only in the treatment of cancer but also in the detection, diagnosis, and prevention of the disease. Patients interested in taking part in a clinical trial should talk with their doctor.

Chapter 5

Cancer Clusters

What is a cancer cluster?

A cancer cluster is the occurrence of a greater than expected number of cancer cases among a group of people in a defined geographic area over a specific time period. A cancer cluster may be suspected when people report that several family members, friends, neighbors, or coworkers have been diagnosed with the same or related types of cancer.

Cancer clusters can help scientists identify cancer-causing substances in the environment. For example, in the early 1970s, a cluster of cases of angiosarcoma of the liver, a rare cancer, was detected among workers in a chemical plant. Further investigation showed that the workers were all exposed to vinyl chloride and that workers in other plants that used vinyl chloride also had an increased rate of angiosarcoma of the liver. Exposure to vinyl chloride is now known to be a major risk factor for angiosarcoma of the liver.

However, most suspected cancer clusters turn out, on detailed investigation, not to be true cancer clusters. That is, no cause can be identified, and the clustering of cases turns out to be a random occurrence.

Text in this chapter is excerpted from "Cancer Clusters," National Cancer Institute at the National Institutes of Health (NIH), March 18, 2014.

Where can someone report a suspected cancer cluster or find out if one is being investigated?

Concerned individuals can contact their local or state health department to report a suspected cancer cluster or to find out if one is being investigated. Health departments provide the first response to questions about cancer clusters because they, together with state cancer registries, will have the most up-to-date data on cancer incidence in the area. If additional resources are needed to investigate a suspected cancer cluster, the state health department may request assistance from federal agencies, including the Centers for Disease Control and Prevention (CDC) and the Agency for Toxic Substances and Disease Registry (ATSDR), which is part of the CDC.

The CDC website provides links to state and local health departments. These agencies may also be listed in the blue pages of government listings in telephone books. Although NCI does not lead investigations of individual cancer clusters, NCI researchers and staff may provide assistance to other investigative agencies as needed. In addition, scientists at NCI and researchers who are funded by NCI analyze variations in cancer trends, including the frequency, distribution, and patterns of cancer in groups of people. These analyses can detect patterns of cancer in specific populations. For example, NCI's Cancer Mortality Maps website uses data on deaths from the National Center for Health Statistics, which is part of the CDC, and population estimates from the U.S. Census Bureau to provide dynamically generated maps that show geographic patterns of cancer death rates throughout the United States.

How are suspected cancer clusters investigated?

Health departments use established criteria to investigate reports of cancer clusters. The Centers for Disease Control and the Council of State and Territorial Epidemiologists have released updated guidelines for investigating suspected cancer clusters and responding to community concerns.

As a first step, the investigating agency gathers information from the person who reported the suspected cancer cluster. The investigators ask for details about the suspected cluster, such as the types of cancer and number of cases of each type, the age of the people with cancer, and the area and time period over which the cancers were diagnosed. They also ask about specific environmental hazards or concerns in the affected area.

If the review of the findings from this initial investigation suggests the need for further evaluation, investigators then compare information about cases in the suspected cluster with records in the state cancer registry and census data.

If the second step reveals a statistically significant excess of cancer cases, the third step is to determine whether an epidemiologic study can be carried out to investigate whether the cluster is associated with risk factors in the local environment. Sometimes, even if there is a clear excess of cancer cases, it is not feasible to carry out further study—for example, if the total number of cases is very small.

Finally, if an epidemiologic study is feasible, the fourth step is to determine whether the cluster of cancer cases is associated with a suspect contaminant in the environment. Even if a possible association with an environmental contaminant is found, however, further studies would be needed to confirm that the environmental contaminant did cause the cluster.

What are the challenges in investigating suspected cancer clusters?

Investigators face several challenges when determining whether a greater than expected number of cancer cases represents a cancer cluster.

Understanding the kind of cancers involved

To assess a suspected cancer cluster accurately, investigators must determine whether the type of cancer involved is a primary cancer (a cancer that is located in the original organ or tissue where the cancer started) or a cancer that has metastasized (spread) to another site in the body from the original tissue or organ where the cancer began (also called a secondary cancer). Investigators consider only the primary cancer when they investigate a suspected cancer cluster. A confirmed cancer cluster is more likely if it involves one type of cancer than if it involves multiple different cancer types. This is because most carcinogens in the environment cause only a specific cancer type rather than causing cancer in general.

Ascertaining the number of cancer cases in the suspected cluster

Many reported clusters include too few cancer cases for investigators to determine whether the number of cancer cases is statistically significantly greater than the expected number.

Determining statistical significance

To confirm the existence of a cluster, investigators must show that the number of cancer cases in the cluster is statistically significantly greater than the number of cancer cases expected given the age, sex, and racial distribution of the group of people who developed the disease. If the difference between the actual and expected number of cancer cases is statistically significant, the finding is unlikely to be the result of chance alone. However, it is important to keep in mind that even a statistically significant difference between actual and expected numbers of cases can arise by chance.

Determining the relevant population and geographic area

An important challenge in confirming a cancer cluster is accurately defining the group of people who should be considered potentially at risk of developing the specific cancer (typically the total number of people who live in a specific geographic area). When defining a cancer cluster, there can be a tendency to expand the geographic borders as additional cases of the suspected disease are discovered. However, if investigators define the borders of a cluster based on where they find cancer cases, they may alarm people about cancers that are not related to the suspected cluster. Instead, investigators first define the population and geographic area that is "at risk" and then identify cancer cases within those parameters.

Identifying a cause for a cluster

A confirmed cancer cluster—that is, a finding of a statistically significant excess of cancers—may not be the result of any single external cause or hazard (also called an exposure). A cancer cluster could be the result of chance, an error in the calculation of the expected number of cancer cases, differences in how cancer cases were classified, or a known cause of cancer, such as smoking. Even if a cluster is confirmed, it can be very difficult to identify the cause. People move in and out of a geographic area over time, which can make it difficult for investigators to identify hazards or potential carcinogens to which they may have been exposed and to obtain medical records to confirm the diagnosis of cancer. Also, it typically takes a long time for cancer to develop, and any relevant exposure may have occurred in the past or in a different geographic area from where the cancer was diagnosed.

Part Two

Risk Factors and Cancer Prevention

Chapter 6

Factors That Are Known to Increase the Risk of Cancer

Chapter Contents

29

Factors That Are Known to Increase the Risk of Cancer

Scientists study risk factors and protective factors to find ways to prevent new cancers from starting. Anything that increases your chance of developing cancer is called a cancer risk factor; anything that decreases your chance of developing cancer is called a cancer protective factor.

Some risk factors for cancer can be avoided, but many cannot. For example, both smoking and inheriting certain genes are risk factors for some types of cancer, but only smoking can be avoided. Risk factors that a person can control are called modifiable risk factors. Many other factors in our environment, diet, and lifestyle may cause or prevent cancer.

Section 6.1

Cigarette Smoking

This section includes excerpts from "Risk Factors—Cancer Prevention Overview," National Cancer Institute at the National Institutes of Health (NIH), April 17, 2014; and from "18 Ways Smoking Affects Your Health," smokefree.gov at the NIH.

Cigarette Smoking and Tobacco Use

Tobacco use is strongly linked to an increased risk for many kinds of cancer. Smoking cigarettes is the leading cause of the following types of cancer:

- Acute myelogenous leukemia (AML).
- Bladder cancer.
- Esophageal cancer.
- Kidney cancer.
- Lung cancer.
- Oral cavity cancer.
- Pancreatic cancer.
- Stomach cancer.

Not smoking or quitting smoking lowers the risk of getting cancer and dying from cancer. Scientists believe that cigarette smoking causes about 30% of all cancer deaths in the United States.

Smoking harms nearly every organ of the body. Some of these harmful effects are immediate.

Brain

Become addicted

Nicotine from cigarettes is as addictive as heroin. Nicotine addiction is hard to beat because it changes your brain. The brain develops extra nicotine receptors to accommodate the large doses of nicotine from tobacco. When the brain stops getting the nicotine it's used to, the result is nicotine withdrawal. You may feel anxious, irritable, and have strong cravings for nicotine.

Head and Face

Ears

Hearing loss. Smoking reduces the oxygen supply to the cochlea, a snail-shaped organ in the inner ear. This may result in permanent damage to the cochlea and mild to moderate hearing loss.

Eyes

Blindness and night vision. Smoking causes physical changes in the eyes that can threaten your eyesight. Nicotine from cigarettes restricts the production of a chemical necessary for you to be able to see at night. Also, smoking increases your risk of developing cataracts and macular degeneration (both can lead to blindness).

Mouth

Cavities. Smoking takes a toll on your mouth. Smokers have more oral health problems than nonsmokers, like mouth sores, ulcers and gum disease. You are more likely to have cavities and lose your teeth at a younger age. You are also more likely to get cancers of the mouth and throat.

Face

Smoker's face. Smoking can cause your skin to be dry and lose elasticity, leading to wrinkles and stretch marks. Your skin tone may

31

become dull and grayish. By your early 30s, wrinkles can begin to appear around your mouth and eyes, adding years to your face.

Heart

Stressed heart

Smoking raises your blood pressure and puts stress on your heart. Over time, stress on the heart can weaken it, making it less able to pump blood to other parts of your body. Carbon monoxide from inhaled cigarette smoke also contributes to a lack of oxygen, making the heart work even harder. This increases the risk of heart disease, including heart attacks.

Sticky blood

Smoking makes your blood thick and sticky. The stickier the blood, the harder your heart must work to move it around your body. Sticky blood is also more likely to form blood clots that block blood flow to your heart, brain, and legs. Over time, thick, sticky blood damages the delicate lining of your blood vessels. This damage can increase your risk for a heart attack or stroke.

Fatty deposits

Smoking increases the amount of cholesterol and unhealthy fats circulating in the bloods, leading to unhealthy fatty deposits. Over time, cholesterol, fats, and other debris build up on the walls of your arteries. This buildup narrows the arteries and blocks normal blood flow to the heart, brain, and legs. Blocked blood flow to the heart or brain can cause a heart attack or stroke. Blockage in the blood vessels of your legs could result in the amputation of your toes or feet.

Lungs

Scarred Lungs

Smoking causes inflammation in the small airways and tissues of your lungs. This can make your chest feel tight or cause you to wheeze or feel short of breath. Continued inflammation builds up scar tissue, which leads to physical changes to your lungs and airways that can make breathing hard. Years of lung irritation can give you a chronic cough with mucus.

Emphysema

Smoking destroys the tiny air sacs, or alveoli, in the lungs that allow oxygen exchange. When you smoke, you are damaging some of those air sacs. Alveoli don't grow back, so when you destroy them, you have permanently destroyed part of your lungs. When enough alveoli are destroyed, the disease emphysema develops. Emphysema causes severe shortness of breath and can lead to death.

Cilia

Respiratory infections. Your airways are lined with tiny brush like hairs, called cilia. The cilia sweep out mucus and dirt so your lungs stay clear. Smoking temporarily paralyzes and even kills cilia. This makes you more at risk for infection. Smokers get more colds and respiratory infections than nonsmokers.

DNA

Cancer

Your body is made up of cells that contain genetic material, or DNA, that acts as an "instruction manual" for cell growth and function. Every single puff of a cigarette causes damages to your DNA. When DNA is damaged, the "instruction manual" gets messed up, and the cell can begin growing out of control and create a cancer tumor. Your body tries to repair the damage that smoking does to your DNA, but over time, smoking can wear down this repair system and lead to cancer (like lung cancer). One-third of all cancer deaths are caused by tobacco.

Stomach and Hormones

Belly

Bigger belly. Smokers have bigger bellies and less muscle than nonsmokers. They are more likely to develop type 2 diabetes, even if they don't smoke every day. Smoking also makes it harder to control diabetes once you already have it. Diabetes is a serious disease that can lead to blindness, heart disease, kidney failure, and amputations.

Lower estrogen levels

Smoking lowers a female's level of estrogen. Low estrogen levels can cause dry skin, thinning hair, and memory problems. Women who smoke have a harder time getting pregnant and having a healthy baby. Smoking can also lead to early menopause, which increases your risk of developing certain diseases (like heart disease).

Erectile Dysfunction

Failure to launch

Smoking increases the risk of erectile dysfunction—the inability to get or an keep an erection. Toxins from cigarette smoke can also damage the genetic material in sperm, which can cause infertility or genetic defects in your children.

Blood and the Immune System

High white blood cell count

When you smoke, the number of white blood cells (the cells that defend your body from infections) stays high. This is a sign that your body is under stress—constantly fighting against the inflammation and damage caused by tobacco. A high white blood cell count is like a signal from your body, letting you know you've been injured. White blood cell counts that stay elevated for a long time are linked with an increased risk of heart attacks, strokes, and cancer.

Longer to heal

Nutrients, minerals, and oxygen are all supplied to the tissue through the blood stream. Nicotine causes blood vessels to tighten, which decreases levels of nutrients supplied to wounds. As a result, wounds take longer to heal. Slow wound healing increases the risk of infection after an injury or surgery and painful skin ulcers can develop, causing the tissue to slowly die.

Weakened immune system

Cigarette smoke contains high levels of tar and other chemicals, which can make your immune system less effective at fighting off infections. This means you're more likely to get sick. Continued weakening of the immune system can make you more vulnerable to auto-immune diseases like rheumatoid arthritis and multiple sclerosis. It also decreases your body's ability to fight off cancer!

Muscles and Bones

Tired muscles

Muscle deterioration. When you smoke, less blood and oxygen flow to your muscles, making it harder to build muscle. The lack of oxygen also makes muscles tire more easily. Smokers have more muscle aches and pains than nonsmokers.

More Broken Bones

Ingredients in cigarette smoke disrupt the natural cycle of bone health. Your body is less able to form healthy new bone tissue, and it breaks down existing bone tissue more rapidly. Over time, smoking leads to a thinning of bone tissue and loss of bone density. This causes bones to become weak and brittle. Compared to nonsmokers, smokers have a higher risk of bone fractures, and their broken bones take longer to heal.

Section 6.2

"Light" Cigarettes and Cancer Risk

Text in this section is excerpted from "Light Cigarettes and Cancer Risk," National Cancer Institute at the National Institutes of Health (NIH), October 28, 2010.

What is a so-called light cigarette?

Tobacco manufacturers have been redesigning cigarettes since the 1950s. Certain redesigned cigarettes with the following features were marketed as "light" cigarettes:

- Cellulose acetate filters (to trap tar).

- Highly porous cigarette paper (to allow toxic chemicals to escape).

- Ventilation holes in the filter tip (to dilute smoke with air).

- Different blends of tobacco.

When analyzed by a smoking machine, the smoke from a so-called light cigarette has a lower yield of tar than the smoke from a regular cigarette. However, a machine cannot predict how much tar a smoker inhales. Also, studies have shown that changes in cigarette design have not lowered the risk of disease caused by cigarettes.

On June 22, 2009, President Barack Obama signed into law the Family Smoking Prevention and Tobacco Control Act, which granted the U.S. Food and Drug Administration the authority to regulate tobacco products. One provision of the new law bans tobacco manufacturers from using the terms "light," "low," and "mild" in product labeling and advertisements. This provision went into effect on June 22, 2010. However, some tobacco manufacturers are using color-coded packaging (such as gold or silver packaging) on previously marketed products and selling them to consumers who may continue to believe that these cigarettes are not as harmful as other cigarettes.

Are light cigarettes less hazardous than regular cigarettes?

No. Many smokers chose so-called low-tar, mild, light, or ultra-light cigarettes because they thought these cigarettes would expose them to less tar and would be less harmful to their health than regular or full-flavor cigarettes. However, light cigarettes are no safer than regular cigarettes. Tar exposure from a light cigarette can be just as high as that from a regular cigarette if the smoker takes long, deep, or frequent puffs. The bottom line is that light cigarettes do not reduce the health risks of smoking.

Moreover, there is no such thing as a safe cigarette. The only guaranteed way to reduce the risk to your health, as well as the risk to others, is to stop smoking completely.

Because all tobacco products are harmful and cause cancer, the use of these products is strongly discouraged. There is no safe level of tobacco use. People who use any type of tobacco product should quit.

Do light cigarettes cause cancer?

Yes. People who smoke any kind of cigarette are at much greater risk of lung cancer than people who do not smoke. Smoking harms nearly every organ of the body and diminishes a person's overall health.

People who switched to light cigarettes from regular cigarettes are likely to have inhaled the same amount of toxic chemicals, and they remain at high risk of developing smoking-related cancers and other disease. Smoking causes cancers of the lung, esophagus, larynx (voice box), mouth, throat, kidney, bladder, pancreas, stomach, and cervix, as well as acute myeloid leukemia.

Regardless of their age, smokers can substantially reduce their risk of disease, including cancer, by quitting.

What were the tar yield ratings used by the tobacco industry for light cigarettes?

Although no Federal agency formally defined the range of tar yield for light or ultra-light cigarettes, the tobacco industry used the ranges shown in the table below. (*See* Table 6.1)

These ratings were not an accurate indicator of how much tar a smoker might have been exposed to, because people do not smoke cigarettes the same way the machines do and no two people smoke the same way.

Ultra-light and light cigarettes are no safer than full-flavor cigarettes. There is no such thing as a safe cigarette.

Are machine-measured tar yields misleading?

Yes. The ratings cannot be used to predict how much tar a smoker will actually get because the way the machine smokes a cigarette is not the way a person smokes a cigarette. A rating of 7 milligrams does not mean that you will get only 7 milligrams of tar. You can get just as much tar from a light cigarette as from a full-flavor cigarette. It all depends on how you smoke. Taking deeper, longer, and more frequent puffs will lead to greater tar exposure. Also, a smoker's lips or fingers may block the air ventilation holes in the filter, leading to greater tar exposure.

Table 6.1. Range of tar yield

Industry Terms on Packages	Machine-measured Tar Yield (in milligrams)
Ultralight or Ultralow tar	Usually 7 or less
Light or Low tar	Usually 8–14
Full flavor or Regular	Usually 15 or more

Why would someone smoking a light cigarette take bigger puffs than with a regular cigarette?

Cigarette features that reduce the yield of machine-measured tar also reduce the yield of nicotine. Because smokers crave nicotine, they may inhale more deeply; take larger, more rapid, or more frequent puffs; or smoke extra cigarettes each day to get enough nicotine to satisfy their craving. As a result, smokers end up inhaling more tar, nicotine, and other harmful chemicals than the machine-based numbers suggest.

Tobacco industry documents show that companies were aware that smokers of light cigarettes compensated by taking bigger puffs. Industry documents also show that the companies were aware of the difference between machine-measured yields of tar and nicotine and what the smoker actually inhaled.

Section 6.3

Cigar Smoking and Cancer

Text in this section is excerpted from "Cigar Smoking and Cancer," National Cancer Institute at the National Institutes of Health (NIH), October 27, 2010.

How are cigars different from cigarettes?

Cigarettes usually differ from cigars in size and in the type of tobacco used. Moreover, in contrast with cigarette smoke, cigar smoke is often not inhaled.

The main features of these tobacco products are:

- **Cigarettes**: Cigarettes are uniform in size and contain less than 1 gram of tobacco each. U.S. cigarettes are made from different blends of tobaccos, which are never fermented, and they are wrapped with paper. Most U.S. cigarettes take less than 10 minutes to smoke.

- **Cigars**: Most cigars are composed primarily of a single type of tobacco (air-cured and fermented), and they have a tobacco wrapper. They can vary in size and shape and contain between 1 gram and 20 grams of tobacco. Three cigar sizes are sold in the United States:

  - **Large cigars** can measure more than 7 inches in length, and they typically contain between 5 and 20 grams of tobacco. Some premium cigars contain the tobacco equivalent of an entire pack of cigarettes. Large cigars can take between 1 and 2 hours to smoke.

  - **Cigarillos** are a type of smaller cigar. They are a little bigger than little cigars and cigarettes and contain about 3 grams of tobacco.

  - **Little cigars** are the same size and shape as cigarettes, are often packaged like cigarettes (20 little cigars in a package), and contain about 1 gram of tobacco. Also, unlike large cigars, some little cigars have a filter, which makes it seem they are designed to be smoked like cigarettes (that is, for the smoke to be inhaled).

Are there harmful chemicals in cigar smoke?

Yes. Cigar smoke, like cigarette smoke, contains toxic and cancer-causing chemicals that are harmful to both smokers and nonsmokers. Cigar smoke is possibly more toxic than cigarette smoke. Cigar smoke has:

- **A higher level of cancer-causing substances**: During the fermentation process for cigar tobacco, high concentrations of cancer-causing nitrosamines are produced. These compounds are released when a cigar is smoked. Nitrosamines are found at higher levels in cigar smoke than in cigarette smoke.

- **More tar**: For every gram of tobacco smoked, there is more cancer-causing tar in cigars than in cigarettes.

- **A higher level of toxins**: Cigar wrappers are less porous than cigarette wrappers. The nonporous cigar wrapper makes the burning of cigar tobacco less complete than the burning of cigarette tobacco. As a result, cigar smoke has higher concentrations of toxins than cigarette smoke.

Furthermore, the larger size of most cigars (more tobacco) and longer smoking time result in higher exposure to many toxic substances (including carbon monoxide, hydrocarbons, ammonia, cadmium, and other substances).

Cigar smoke can be a major source of indoor air pollution. There is no safe level of exposure to tobacco smoke. If you want to reduce the health risk to yourself and others, stop smoking.

Do cigars cause cancer and other diseases?

Yes. Cigar smoking causes cancer of the oral cavity, larynx, esophagus, and lung. It may also cause cancer of the pancreas. Moreover, daily cigar smokers, particularly those who inhale, are at increased risk for developing heart disease and other types of lung disease. Regular cigar smokers and cigarette smokers have similar levels of risk for oral cavity and esophageal cancers. The more you smoke, the greater the risk of disease.

What if I don't inhale the cigar smoke?

Unlike nearly all cigarette smokers, most cigar smokers do not inhale. Although cigar smokers have lower rates of lung cancer, coronary heart disease, and lung disease than cigarette smokers, they have higher rates of these diseases than those who do not smoke cigars.

All cigar and cigarette smokers, whether or not they inhale, directly expose their lips, mouth, tongue, throat, and larynx to smoke and its toxic and cancer-causing chemicals. In addition, when saliva containing the chemicals in tobacco smoke is swallowed, the esophagus is exposed to carcinogens. These exposures probably account for the similar oral and esophageal cancer risks seen among cigar smokers and cigarette smokers.

Are cigars addictive?

Yes. Even if the smoke is not inhaled, high levels of nicotine (the chemical that causes addiction) can still be absorbed into the body. A cigar smoker can get nicotine by two routes: by inhalation into the lungs and by absorption through the lining of the mouth. Either way, the smoker becomes addicted to the nicotine that gets into the body. A single cigar can potentially provide as much nicotine as a pack of cigarettes.

40

Are cigars less hazardous than cigarettes?

Because all tobacco products are harmful and cause cancer, the use of these products is strongly discouraged. There is no safe level of tobacco use. People who use any type of tobacco product should be encouraged to quit.

Do nicotine replacement products help cigar smokers to quit?

Nicotine replacement products, or nicotine replacement therapy (NRT), deliver measured doses of nicotine into the body, which helps to relieve the cravings and withdrawal symptoms often felt by people trying to quit smoking. Strong and consistent evidence shows that NRT can help people quit smoking cigarettes. Limited research has been completed to determine the usefulness of NRT for people who smoke cigars. For help with quitting cigar smoking, ask your doctor or pharmacist about NRT, as well as about individual or group counseling, telephone quit lines, or other methods.

Section 6.4

Secondhand Smoke and Cancer

Text in this section is excerpted from "Secondhand Smoke and Cancer," National Cancer Institute at the National Institutes of Health (NIH), January 12, 2011.

What is secondhand smoke?

Secondhand smoke (also called environmental tobacco smoke, involuntary smoke, and passive smoke) is the combination of "side-stream" smoke (the smoke given off by a burning tobacco product) and "mainstream" smoke (the smoke exhaled by a smoker).

People can be exposed to secondhand smoke in homes, cars, the workplace, and public places, such as bars, restaurants, and recreational settings. In the United States, the source of most secondhand smoke is from cigarettes, followed by pipes, cigars, and other tobacco products.

The amount of smoke created by a tobacco product depends on the amount of tobacco available for burning. The amount of secondhand smoke emitted by smoking one large cigar is similar to that emitted by smoking an entire pack of cigarettes.

How is secondhand smoke exposure measured?

Secondhand smoke exposure can be measured by testing indoor air for nicotine or other chemicals in tobacco smoke. Exposure to secondhand smoke can also be tested by measuring the level of cotinine (a by-product of the breakdown of nicotine) in a nonsmoker's blood, saliva, or urine. Nicotine, cotinine, carbon monoxide, and other smoke-related chemicals have been found in the body fluids of nonsmokers exposed to secondhand smoke.

Does secondhand smoke contain harmful chemicals?

Yes. Among the more than 7,000 chemicals that have been identified in secondhand tobacco smoke, at least 250 are known to be harmful, for example, hydrogen cyanide, carbon monoxide, and ammonia.

At least 69 of the toxic chemicals in secondhand tobacco smoke cause cancer. These include the following:

- Arsenic

- Benzene

- Beryllium (a toxic metal)

- 1,3–Butadiene (a hazardous gas)

- Cadmium

- Chromium (a metallic element)

- Ethylene oxide

- Nickel (a metallic element)

- Polonium-210 (a radioactive chemical element)

- Vinyl chloride

Other toxic chemicals in secondhand smoke are suspected to cause cancer, including:

- Formaldehyde

- Benzo[α]pyrene

- Toluene

Many factors affect which chemicals are found in secondhand smoke, such as the type of tobacco, the chemicals added to the tobacco, the way the tobacco product is smoked, and, for cigarettes and cigars, the material in which the tobacco is wrapped.

Does exposure to secondhand smoke cause cancer?

Yes. The U.S. Environmental Protection Agency, the U.S. National Toxicology Program, the U.S. Surgeon General, and the International Agency for Research on Cancer have all classified secondhand smoke as a known human carcinogen (a cancer-causing agent).

Inhaling secondhand smoke causes lung cancer in nonsmoking adults. Approximately 3,000 lung cancer deaths occur each year among adult nonsmokers in the United States as a result of exposure to secondhand smoke. The U.S. Surgeon General estimates that living with a smoker increases a nonsmoker's chances of developing lung cancer by 20 to 30 percent.

Some research also suggests that secondhand smoke may increase the risk of breast cancer, nasal sinus cavity cancer, and nasopharyngeal cancer in adults and the risk of leukemia, lymphoma, and brain tumors in children. Additional research is needed to learn whether a link exists between secondhand smoke exposure and these cancers.

What are the other health effects of exposure to secondhand smoke?

Secondhand smoke is associated with disease and premature death in nonsmoking adults and children. Exposure to secondhand smoke irritates the airways and has immediate harmful effects on a person's heart and blood vessels. It may increase the risk of heart disease by an estimated 25 to 30 percent. In the United States, secondhand smoke is thought to cause about 46,000 heart disease deaths each year. There may also be a link between exposure to secondhand smoke and the risk of stroke and hardening of the arteries; however, additional research is needed to confirm this link.

Children exposed to secondhand smoke are at increased risk of sudden infant death syndrome, ear infections, colds, pneumonia, bronchitis, and more severe asthma. Being exposed to secondhand smoke slows the growth of children's lungs and can cause them to cough, wheeze, and feel breathless.

What is a safe level of secondhand smoke?

There is no safe level of exposure to secondhand smoke. Even low levels of secondhand smoke can be harmful. The only way to fully protect nonsmokers from secondhand smoke is to completely eliminate smoking in indoor spaces. Separating smokers from nonsmokers, cleaning the air, and ventilating buildings cannot completely eliminate exposure to secondhand smoke.

What is being done to reduce nonsmokers' exposure to secondhand smoke?

On the national level, several laws restricting smoking in public places have been passed. Federal law bans smoking on domestic airline flights, nearly all flights between the United States and foreign destinations, interstate buses, and most trains. Smoking is also banned in most federally owned buildings. The Pro-Children Act of 1994 prohibits smoking in facilities that routinely provide federally funded services to children.

Many state and local governments have passed laws prohibiting smoking in public facilities, such as schools, hospitals, airports, bus terminals, parks, and beaches, as well as private workplaces, including restaurants and bars. Some states have passed laws regulating smoking in multiunit housing and cars. More than half of the states have enacted statewide bans on workplace smoking.

To highlight the health risks from secondhand smoke, the National Cancer Institute, a component of the National Institutes of Health, holds meetings and conferences in states, counties, cities, or towns that are smoke free, unless specific circumstances justify an exception to this policy.

The U.S. Department of Health and Human Services Healthy People 2020, a comprehensive, nationwide health promotion and disease prevention agenda, includes the goal of reducing illness, disability, and death related to tobacco use and secondhand smoke exposure. Currently, most Americans are exposed to secondhand smoke, and children are at greatest risk. For 2020, the goal is to reduce the proportion of people exposed to secondhand smoke by 10 percent. To assist with achieving this goal, Healthy People 2020 includes ideas for community interventions, such as encouraging the introduction of smoke-free policies in workplaces and other public areas. Internationally, a growing number of nations, including France, Ireland, New Zealand, Norway, and Uruguay, require all workplaces, including bars and restaurants, to be smoke free.

Section 6.5

Smokeless Tobacco and Cancer

Text in this section is excerpted from "Smokeless Tobacco and Cancer," National Cancer Institute at the National Institutes of Health (NIH), October 25, 2010.

What is smokeless tobacco?

Smokeless tobacco is tobacco that is not burned. It is also known as chewing tobacco, oral tobacco, spit or spitting tobacco, dip, chew, and snuff. Most people chew or suck (dip) the tobacco in their mouth and spit out the tobacco juices that build up, although "spit less" smokeless tobacco has also been developed. Nicotine in the tobacco is absorbed through the lining of the mouth.

People in many regions and countries, including North America, northern Europe, India and other Asian countries, and parts of Africa, have a long history of using smokeless tobacco products.

There are two main types of smokeless tobacco:

- **Chewing tobacco**, which is available as loose leaves, plugs (bricks), or twists of rope. A piece of tobacco is placed between the cheek and lower lip, typically toward the back of the mouth. It is either chewed or held in place. Saliva is spit or swallowed.

- **Snuff**, which is finely cut or powdered tobacco. It may be sold in different scents and flavors. It is packaged moist or dry; most American snuff is moist. It is available loose, in dissolvable lozenges or strips, or in small pouches similar to tea bags. The user places a pinch or pouch of moist snuff between the cheek and gums or behind the upper or lower lip. Another name for moist snuff is snus (pronounced "snoose"). Some people inhale dry snuff into the nose.

Are there harmful chemicals in smokeless tobacco?

Yes. There is no safe form of tobacco. At least 28 chemicals in smokeless tobacco have been found to cause cancer. The most harmful

45

chemicals in smokeless tobacco are tobacco-specific nitrosamines, which are formed during the growing, curing, fermenting, and aging of tobacco. The level of tobacco-specific nitrosamines varies by product. Scientists have found that the nitrosamine level is directly related to the risk of cancer.

In addition to a variety of nitrosamines, other cancer-causing substances in smokeless tobacco include polonium–210 (a radioactive element found in tobacco fertilizer) and poly-nuclear aromatic hydrocarbons (also known as polycyclic aromatic hydrocarbons).

Does smokeless tobacco cause cancer?

Yes. Smokeless tobacco causes oral cancer, esophageal cancer, and pancreatic cancer.

Does smokeless tobacco cause other diseases?

Yes. Using smokeless tobacco may also cause heart disease, gum disease, and oral lesions other than cancer, such as leukoplakia (precancerous white patches in the mouth).

Can a user get addicted to smokeless tobacco?

Yes. All tobacco products, including smokeless tobacco, contain nicotine, which is addictive. Users of smokeless tobacco and users of cigarettes have comparable levels of nicotine in the blood. In users of smokeless tobacco, nicotine is absorbed through the mouth tissues directly into the blood, where it goes to the brain. Even after the tobacco is removed from the mouth, nicotine continues to be absorbed into the bloodstream. Also, the nicotine stays in the blood longer for users of smokeless tobacco than for smokers.

The level of nicotine in the blood depends on the amount of nicotine in the smokeless tobacco product, the tobacco cut size, the product's pH (a measure of its acidity or basicity), and other factors.

A Centers for Disease Control and Prevention study of the 40 most widely used popular brands of moist snuff showed that the amount of nicotine per gram of tobacco ranged from 4.4 milligrams to 25.0 milligrams. Other studies have shown that moist snuff had between 4.7 and 24.3 milligrams per gram of tobacco, dry snuff had between 10.5 and 24.8 milligrams per gram of tobacco, and chewing tobacco had between 3.4 and 39.7 milligrams per gram of tobacco.

Is using smokeless tobacco less hazardous than smoking cigarettes?

Because all tobacco products are harmful and cause cancer, the use of all of these products should be strongly discouraged. There is no safe level of tobacco use. People who use any type of tobacco product should be urged to quit.

As long ago as 1986, the advisory committee to the Surgeon General concluded that the use of smokeless tobacco "is not a safe substitute for smoking cigarettes. It can cause cancer and a number of noncancerous oral conditions and can lead to nicotine addiction and dependence". Furthermore, a panel of experts convened by the National Institutes of Health (NIH) in 2006 stated that the "range of risks, including nicotine addiction, from smokeless tobacco products may vary extensively because of differing levels of nicotine, carcinogens, and other toxins in different products."

Should smokeless tobacco be used to help a person quit smoking?

No. There is no scientific evidence that using smokeless tobacco can help a person quit smoking. Because all tobacco products are harmful and cause cancer, the use of all tobacco products is strongly discouraged. There is no safe level of tobacco use. People who use any type of tobacco product should be urged to quit. For help with quitting, ask your doctor about individual or group counseling, telephone quit lines, or other methods.

Chapter 7

Asbestos Exposure and Cancer

What is asbestos?

Asbestos is the name given to a group of naturally occurring fibrous minerals that are resistant to heat and corrosion. Because of these properties, asbestos has been used in commercial products such as insulation and fireproofing materials, automotive brakes, and wallboard materials.

How are people exposed to asbestos?

If products containing asbestos are disturbed, tiny asbestos fibers are released into the air. When asbestos fibers are breathed in, they may get trapped in the lungs and remain there for a long time. Over time, accumulated asbestos fibers can cause tissue inflammation and scarring, which can affect breathing and lead to serious health problems.

Low levels of asbestos fibers are present in the air, water, and soil. Most people, however, do not become ill from this type of exposure. People who become ill from asbestos usually have been exposed to it on a regular basis, most often in a job where they have worked directly with the material or through substantial environmental contact.

Most heavy exposures to asbestos occurred in the past. The heaviest exposures today tend to occur in the construction industry and in ship

---

Text in this chapter is excerpted from "Asbestos," National Cancer Institute at the National Institutes of Health (NIH), March 20, 2015 repair, particularly during the removal of asbestos-containing materials due to renovation, repairs, or demolition. Workers may also be exposed during the manufacture of asbestos-containing products, such as textiles, friction products, insulation, and other building materials.

Which cancers are associated with exposure to asbestos?

Exposure to asbestos is associated with an increased risk of lung cancer and mesothelioma, which is a cancer of the thin membranes that line the chest and abdomen. Mesothelioma is the most common form of cancer associated with asbestos exposure, although the disease is relatively rare.

What can be done to reduce the hazards of asbestos?

The use of asbestos is now highly regulated in the United States. The Occupational Safety and Health Administration has issued standards for the construction industry, general industry, and shipyard employment sectors.

How does smoking tobacco affect the risk of asbestos-associated cancers?

Many studies have shown that the combination of tobacco smoking and asbestos exposure is particularly hazardous. However, there is also evidence that quitting smoking reduces the risk of lung cancer among asbestos-exposed workers.

Chapter 8

Cancer Risks Associated with Pregnancy, Contraceptives, and Menopausal Hormones

Chapter Contents

Section 8.1

Reproductive History and Breast Cancer Risk

Text in this section is excerpted from "Reproductive History and
Breast Cancer Risk," National Cancer Institute at the National
Institutes of Health (NIH), May 10, 2011.

Is there a relationship between pregnancy and breast cancer risk?

Studies have shown that a woman's risk of developing breast cancer
is related to her exposure to hormones that are produced by her ovaries
(endogenous estrogen and progesterone). Reproductive factors that
increase the duration and/or levels of exposure to ovarian hormones,
which stimulate cell growth, have been associated with an increase
in breast cancer risk. These factors include early onset of menstruation, late onset of menopause, later age at first pregnancy, and never
having given birth.

Pregnancy and breastfeeding both reduce a woman's lifetime number of menstrual cycles, and thus her cumulative exposure to endogenous hormones. In addition, pregnancy and breastfeeding have direct
effects on breast cells, causing them to differentiate, or mature, so they
can produce milk. Some researchers hypothesize that these differentiated cells are more resistant to becoming transformed into cancer
cells than cells that have not undergone differentiation.

Are any pregnancy-related factors associated with a lower risk of breast cancer?

Some pregnancy-related factors have been associated with a reduced
risk of developing breast cancer later in life. These factors include the
following:

- **Early age at first full-term pregnancy:** Women who have
  their first full-term pregnancy at an early age have a decreased
  risk of developing breast cancer later in life. For example, in
  women who have a first full-term pregnancy before age 20, the
  risk of developing breast cancer is about half that of women

whose first full-term pregnancy occurs after the age of 30. This risk reduction is limited to hormone receptor-positive breast cancer; age at first full-term pregnancy does not appear to affect the risk of hormone receptor-negative breast cancer.

- **Increasing number of births:** The risk of breast cancer declines with the number of children borne. Women who have given birth to five or more children have half the risk of women who have not given birth. Some evidence indicates that the reduced risk associated with an increased number of births may be limited to hormone receptor-positive breast cancer.

- **History of preeclampsia:** Women who have had preeclampsia may have a decreased risk of developing breast cancer. Preeclampsia is a complication of pregnancy in which a woman develops high blood pressure and excess amounts of protein in her urine. Scientists are studying whether certain hormones and proteins associated with preeclampsia may affect breast cancer risk.

- **Longer duration of breastfeeding:** Breastfeeding for an extended period (at least a year) is associated with a decreased risk of both hormone receptor-positive and hormone receptor-negative breast cancer.

Are any pregnancy-related factors associated with an increase in breast cancer risk?

Some factors related to pregnancy may increase the risk of breast cancer. These factors include the following:

- **Older age at birth of first child:** The older a woman is when she has her first full-term pregnancy, the higher her risk of breast cancer. Women who are older than 30 when they give birth to their first child have a higher risk of breast cancer than women who have never given birth.

- **Recent childbirth:** Women who have recently given birth have a short-term increase in risk that declines after about 10 years. The reason for this temporary increase is not known, but some researchers believe that it may be due to the effect of high levels of hormones on microscopic cancers or to the rapid growth of breast cells during pregnancy.

- **Taking diethylstilbestrol (DES) during pregnancy:** Women who took DES during pregnancy have a slightly higher risk of developing breast cancer than women who did not take DES during pregnancy. Daughters of women who took DES during pregnancy may also have a slightly higher risk of developing breast cancer after age 40 than women who were not exposed to DES while in the womb. DES is a synthetic form of estrogen that was used between the early 1940s and 1971 to prevent miscarriages and other pregnancy problems.

Is abortion linked to breast cancer risk?

A few retrospective (case-control) studies reported in the mid-1990s suggested that induced abortion (the deliberate ending of a pregnancy) was associated with an increased risk of breast cancer. However, these studies had important design limitations that could have affected the results. A key limitation was their reliance on self-reporting of medical history information by the study participants, which can introduce bias. Prospective studies, which are more rigorous in design and unaffected by such bias, have consistently shown no association between induced abortion and breast cancer risk. Moreover, in 2009, the Committee on Gynecologic Practice of the American College of Obstetricians and Gynecologists concluded that "more rigorous recent studies demonstrate no causal relationship between induced abortion and a subsequent increase in breast cancer risk". Major findings from these recent studies include the following:

- Women who have had an induced abortion have the same risk of breast cancer as other women.

- Women who have had a spontaneous abortion (miscarriage) have the same risk of breast cancer as other women.

- Cancers other than breast cancer also appear to be unrelated to a history of induced or spontaneous abortion.

Does pregnancy affect the risk of other cancers?

Research has shown the following with regard to pregnancy and the risk of other cancers:

- Women who have had a full-term pregnancy have reduced risks of ovarian and endometrial cancer. Furthermore, the risks of these cancers decline with each additional full-term pregnancy.

- Pregnancy also plays a role in an extremely rare type of tumor called a gestational trophoblastic tumor. In this type of tumor, which starts in the uterus, cancer cells grow in the tissues that are formed following conception.

- There is some evidence that pregnancy-related factors may affect the risk of other cancer types, but these relationships have not been as well studied as those for breast and gynecologic cancers. The associations require further study to clarify the exact relationships.

As in the development of breast cancer, exposures to hormones are thought to explain the role of pregnancy in the development of ovarian, endometrial, and other cancers. Changes in the levels of hormones during pregnancy may contribute to the variation in risk of these tumors after pregnancy.

Section 8.2

Oral Contraceptives and Cancer Risk

Text in this section is excerpted from "Oral Contraceptives and Cancer Risk," National Cancer Institute at the National Institutes of Health (NIH), March 21, 2012.

What types of oral contraceptives are available in the United States today?

Two types of oral contraceptives (birth control pills) are currently available in the United States. The most commonly prescribed type of oral contraceptive contains man-made versions of the natural female hormones estrogen and progesterone. This type of birth control pill is often called a "combined oral contraceptive." The second type is called the mini pill. It contains only progestin, which is the man-made version of progesterone that is used in oral contraceptives.

How could oral contraceptives influence cancer risk?

Naturally occurring estrogen and progesterone have been found to influence the development and growth of some cancers. Because birth control pills contain female hormones, researchers have been interested in determining whether there is any link between these widely used contraceptives and cancer risk.

The results of population studies to examine associations between oral contraceptive use and cancer risk have not always been consistent. Overall, however, the risks of endometrial and ovarian cancer appear to be reduced with the use of oral contraceptives, whereas the risks of breast, cervical, and liver cancer appear to be increased.

How do oral contraceptives affect breast cancer risk?

A woman's risk of developing breast cancer depends on several factors, some of which are related to her natural hormones. Hormonal and reproductive history factors that increase the risk of breast cancer include factors that may allow breast tissue to be exposed to high levels of hormones for longer periods of time, such as the following:

- Beginning menstruation at an early age
- Experiencing menopause at a late age
- Later age at first pregnancy
- Not having children at all

A 1996 analysis of epidemiologic data from more than 50 studies worldwide by the Collaborative Group on Hormonal Factors in Breast Cancer found that women who were current or recent users of birth control pills had a slightly higher risk of developing breast cancer than women who had never used the pill. The risk was highest for women who started using oral contraceptives as teenagers. However, 10 or more years after women stopped using oral contraceptives, their risk of developing breast cancer had returned to the same level as if they had never used birth control pills, regardless of family history of breast cancer, reproductive history, geographic area of residence, ethnic background, differences in study design, dose and type of hormone(s) used, or duration of use. In addition, breast cancers diagnosed in women who had stopped using oral contraceptives for 10 or more years were less advanced than breast cancers diagnosed in women who had never used oral contraceptives.

A recent analysis of data from the Nurses' Health Study, which has been following more than 116,000 female nurses who were 24 to 43 years old when they enrolled in the study in 1989, found that the participants who used oral contraceptives had a slight increase in breast cancer risk. However, nearly all of the increased risk was seen among women who took a specific type of oral contraceptive, a "triphasic" pill, in which the dose of hormones is changed in three stages over the course of a woman's monthly cycle.

Because the association with the triphasic formulation was unexpected, more research will be needed to confirm the findings from the Nurses' Health Study.

How do oral contraceptives affect ovarian cancer risk?

Oral contraceptive use has consistently been found to be associated with a reduced risk of ovarian cancer. In a 1992 analysis of 20 studies, researchers found that the longer a woman used oral contraceptives the more her risk of ovarian cancer decreased. The risk decreased by 10 to 12 percent after 1 year of use and by approximately 50 percent after 5 years of use.

Researchers have studied how the amount or type of hormones in oral contraceptives affects ovarian cancer risk. One study, the Cancer and Steroid Hormone (CASH) study, found that the reduction in ovarian cancer risk was the same regardless of the type or amount of estrogen or progestin in the pill. A more recent analysis of data from the CASH study, however, indicated that oral contraceptive formulations with high levels of progestin were associated with a lower risk of ovarian cancer than formulations with low progestin levels. In another study, the Steroid Hormones and Reproductions (SHARE) Study, researchers investigated new, lower-dose progestins that have varying androgenic (testosterone-like) effects. They found no difference in ovarian cancer risk between androgenic and non-androgenic pills.

Oral contraceptive use by women at increased risk of ovarian cancer due to a genetic mutation in the BRCA1 or BRCA2 gene has been studied. One study showed a reduction in risk among BRCA1- or BRCA2-mutation carriers who took oral contraceptives, whereas another study showed no effect. A third study, published in 2009, found that women with BRCA1 mutations who took oral contraceptives had about half the risk of ovarian cancer as those who did not.

How do oral contraceptives affect endometrial cancer risk?

Women who use oral contraceptives have been shown to have a reduced risk of endometrial cancer. This protective effect increases with the length of time oral contraceptives are used and continues for many years after a woman stops using oral contraceptives.

How do oral contraceptives affect cervical cancer risk?

Long-term use of oral contraceptives (5 or more years) is associated with an increased risk of cervical cancer. An analysis of 24 epidemiologic studies found that the longer a woman used oral contraceptives, the higher her risk of cervical cancer. However, among women who stopped taking oral contraceptives, the risk tended to decline over time, regardless of how long they had used oral contraceptives before stopping.

In a 2002 report by the International Agency for Research on Cancer, which is part of the World Health Organization, data from eight studies were combined to assess the association between oral contraceptive use and cervical cancer risk among women infected with the human papillomavirus (HPV). Researchers found a nearly threefold increase in risk among women who had used oral contraceptives for 5 to 9 years compared with women who had never used oral contraceptives. Among women who had used oral contraceptives for 10 years or longer, the risk of cervical cancer was four times higher.

Virtually all cervical cancers are caused by persistent infection with high-risk, or oncogenic, types of HPV, and the association of cervical cancer with oral contraceptive use is likely to be indirect. The hormones in oral contraceptives may change the susceptibility of cervical cells to HPV infection, affect their ability to clear the infection, or make it easier for HPV infection to cause changes that progress to cervical cancer. Questions about how oral contraceptives may increase the risk of cervical cancer will be addressed through ongoing research.

How do oral contraceptives affect liver cancer risk?

Oral contraceptive use is associated with an increase in the risk of benign liver tumors, such as hepatocellular adenomas. Benign tumors can form as lumps in different areas of the liver, and they have a high risk of bleeding or rupturing. However, these tumors rarely become malignant.

Whether oral contraceptive use increases the risk of malignant liver tumors, also known as hepatocellular carcinomas, is less clear. Some studies have found that women who take oral contraceptives for more than 5 years have an increased risk of hepatocellular carcinoma, but others have not.

Section 8.3

Menopausal Hormone Use

Text in this section is excerpted from "Menopausal Hormone Therapy and Cancer," National Cancer Institute at the National Institutes of Health (NIH), December 5, 2011.

What is menopausal hormone therapy?

Menopausal hormone therapy (MHT) is a treatment that doctors may recommend to relieve common symptoms of menopause and to address long-term biological changes, such as bone loss, that result from declining levels of the natural hormones estrogen and progesterone in a woman's body during and after the completion of menopause.

MHT usually involves treatment with estrogen alone, estrogen plus progesterone, or estrogen plus progestin, which is a synthetic hormone with effects similar to those of progesterone. Women who have had a hysterectomy are generally prescribed estrogen alone. Women who have not had this surgery are prescribed estrogen plus progestin, because estrogen alone is associated with an increased risk of endometrial cancer, whereas research has suggested that estrogen plus progestin may not be.

How do the hormones used in MHT differ from the hormones produced by a woman's body?

The hormones used in MHT come from a variety of plants and animals, or they can be made in a laboratory. The chemical structure of these hormones is similar, although usually not identical, to those of hormones produced by women's bodies.

The U.S. Food and Drug Administration (FDA) has approved many hormone products for use in MHT. FDA-approved products have undergone extensive testing and are produced under standardized conditions to ensure that every dose—whether in a pill, a skin patch, or a cream—contains the proper amount of the appropriate hormones. These FDA-approved products are available only with a

59

doctor's prescription. The FDA has more information about MHT in Menopause—Medicines to Help You.

Non-FDA-approved hormone products, sometimes referred to as "bio-identical hormones," are widely promoted and sold without a prescription on the Internet. Claims that these products are "safer" or more "natural" than FDA-approved hormonal products are not supported by credible scientific evidence. The FDA provides more information about these products in Menopausal Hormone Therapy and "Bio-identical" Hormones.

Where does evidence about risks and benefits of MHT come from?

The most comprehensive evidence about risks and benefits of MHT comes from two randomized clinical trials that were sponsored by the National Institutes of Health as part of the Women's Health Initiative (WHI):

- The **WHI Estrogen-plus-Progestin Study**, in which women with a uterus were randomly assigned to receive either a hormone medication containing both estrogen and progestin (Prempro™) or a placebo.

- The **WHI Estrogen-Alone Study**, in which women without a uterus were randomly assigned to receive either a hormone medication containing estrogen alone (Premarin™) or a placebo.

More than 27,000 healthy women who were 50 to 79 years of age at the time of enrollment took part in the two trials. Although both trials were stopped early (in 2002 and 2004, respectively) when it was determined that both types of therapy were associated with specific health risks, longer-term follow-up of the participants continues to provide new information about the health effects of MHT.

What are the benefits of menopausal hormone therapy?

Research from the WHI Estrogen-plus-Progestin study has shown that women taking combined hormone therapy had the following benefits:

- One-third fewer hip and vertebral fractures than women taking the placebo. In absolute terms, this meant 10 fractures per 10,000 women per year who took hormone therapy compared with 15 fractures per 10,000 women per year who took the placebo.

- One-third lower risk of colorectal cancer than women taking the placebo. In absolute terms, this meant 10 cases of colorectal cancer per 10,000 women per year who took hormone therapy compared with 16 cases of colorectal cancer per 10,000 women per year who took the placebo.

However, a follow-up study found that neither benefit persisted after the study participants stopped taking combined hormone therapy medication.

Women taking estrogen alone experienced the following benefits:

- One-third lower risk for hip and vertebral fractures than women taking the placebo. In absolute terms, this meant 11 hip and 11 vertebral fractures per 10,000 women per year who took estrogen compared with 17 hip and 17 vertebral fractures per 10,000 women per year who took the placebo.

- A 23 percent reduced risk of breast cancer than women taking the placebo. In absolute terms, this meant 26 cases of invasive breast cancer per 10,000 women per year who took estrogen compared with 33 cases of invasive breast cancer per 10,000 women per year who took the placebo.

After 10.7 years of follow-up, however, the risk of hip fractures was slightly higher in the estrogen-alone group, but the risk of breast cancer remained lower than that among women who took the placebo.

What are the health risks of MHT?

Before the WHI studies began, it was known that MHT with estrogen alone increased the risk of endometrial cancer in women with an intact uterus. It was for this reason that, in the WHI trials, women randomly assigned to receive hormone therapy took estrogen plus progestin if they had a uterus and estrogen alone if they didn't have one.

Research from the WHI studies has shown that MHT is associated with the following harms:

- **Urinary incontinence.** Use of estrogen plus progestin increased the risk of urinary incontinence.

- **Dementia.** Use of estrogen plus progestin doubled the risk of developing dementia among postmenopausal women age 65 and older.

- **Stroke, blood clots, and heart attack.** Women who took either combined hormone therapy or estrogen alone had an increased risk of stroke, blood clots, and heart attack. For women in both groups, however, this risk returned to normal levels after they stopped taking the medication.

- **Breast cancer.** Women who took estrogen plus progestin were more likely to be diagnosed with breast cancer. The breast cancers in these women were larger and more likely to have spread to the lymph nodes by the time they were diagnosed. The number of breast cancers in this group of women increased with the length of time that they took the hormones and decreased after they stopped taking the hormones.

These studies also showed that both combination and estrogen-alone hormone use made mammography less effective for the early detection of breast cancer. Women taking hormones had more repeat mammograms to check on abnormalities found in a screening mammogram and more breast biopsies to determine whether abnormalities detected in mammograms were cancer.

The rate of death from breast cancer among those taking estrogen plus progestin was 2.6 per 10,000 women per year, compared with 1.3 per 10,000 women per year among those taking the placebo. The rate of death from any cause after a diagnosis of breast cancer was 5.3 per 10,000 women per year among women taking combined hormone therapy, compared with 3.4 per 10,000 women per year among those taking the placebo.

- **Lung cancer.** Women who took combined hormone therapy had the same risk of lung cancer as women who took the placebo. However, among those who were diagnosed with lung cancer, women who took estrogen plus progestin were more likely to die of the disease than those who took the placebo.

There were no differences in the number of cases or the number of deaths from lung cancer among women who took estrogen alone compared with those among women who took the placebo.

- **Colorectal cancer.** In the initial study report, women taking combined hormone therapy had a lower risk of colorectal cancer than women who took the placebo. However, the colorectal tumors that arose in the combined hormone therapy group were more advanced at detection than those in the placebo group. There was no difference in either the risk of colorectal cancer or the stage of disease at diagnosis between women who took estrogen alone and those who took the placebo.

- However, a subsequent analysis of the WHI trials found no strong evidence that either estrogen alone or estrogen plus progestin had any effect on the risk of colorectal cancer, tumor stage at diagnosis, or death from colorectal cancer.

Does hysterectomy affect the cancer risks associated with MHT?

Women who had a hysterectomy and who are prescribed MHT generally take estrogen alone.

In 2004, when the WHI Estrogen-Alone Study was stopped early, women taking estrogen alone had a 23 percent reduced risk of breast cancer compared with those who took the placebo. An analysis conducted after study participants had been followed for an average of 10.7 years found that women who had taken estrogen alone still had a lower risk of breast cancer than women who had taken the placebo.

Do the cancer risks from MHT change over time?

Women who have had a hysterectomy and who use estrogen-alone MHT have a reduced risk of breast cancer that continues for at least 5 years after they stop taking MHT.

Women who take combined hormone therapy have an increased risk of breast cancer that continues after they stop taking the medication. In the WHI study, where women took the combined hormone therapy for an average of 5.6 years, this increased risk persisted after an average follow-up period of 11 years. Breast cancers diagnosed in this group of women were larger and more likely to have spread to the lymph nodes (a sign of more advanced disease).

Studies have documented a decline in breast cancer diagnoses in the United States after the sharp reduction in the use of MHT that followed publication of the initial results of the Estrogen-plus-Progestin Study in July 2002. Additional factors, such as a reduction in the use of mammography, may also have contributed to this decline.

Is it safe for women who have had a cancer diagnosis to take MHT?

One of the roles of naturally occurring estrogen is to promote the normal growth of cells in the breast and uterus. For this reason, it is generally believed that MHT may promote further tumor growth in women who have already been diagnosed with breast cancer. However, studies of hormone use to treat menopausal symptoms in breast cancer survivors have produced conflicting results, with some showing an increased risk of breast cancer recurrence and others showing no increased risk of recurrence.

What should women do if they have symptoms of menopause but are concerned about taking MHT?

Although MHT provides short-term benefits, such as relief from hot flashes and vaginal dryness, several health concerns are associated with its use. Women should discuss whether to take MHT and what alternatives may be appropriate for them with their health care provider. The FDA currently advises women to use MHT for the shortest time and at the lowest dose possible to control menopausal symptoms. The FDA publication Menopause and Hormones provides additional information about the risks and benefits of MHT use for the symptoms of menopause.

Are there alternatives for women who choose not to take menopausal hormone therapy?

Women who are concerned about the health effects that occur naturally with the decline in hormone production that occurs during menopause can make changes in their lifestyle and diet to reduce certain risks. For example, eating foods that are rich in calcium and vitamin D or taking dietary supplements containing these nutrients may help to prevent osteoporosis. FDA-approved drugs such as alendronate (Fosamax®), raloxifene (Evista®), and risedronate (Actonel®) have been shown in randomized trials to prevent bone loss.

Medications approved by the FDA for treating depression and seizures may help to relieve menopausal symptoms such as hot flashes. Those that have been shown in randomized clinical trials to be effective in treating hot flashes include the following:

- Venlafaxine (Effexor®)

- Desvenlafaxine (Pristiq®)

- Paroxetine (Paxil®)

- Fluoxetine (Prozac®)

- Citalopram (Celexa®)

- Gabapentin (Neurontin®)

- Pregabalin (Lyrica®)

Some women seek relief from the symptoms of menopause with over-the-counter complementary and alternative therapies. Some of these remedies contain estrogen-like compounds derived from sources such as soy products, whole-grain cereals, oilseeds (primarily flaxseed), legumes, or the plant black cohosh. To date, however, randomized clinical trials have not shown that any of these remedies is superior to a placebo in relieving hot flashes. Trials of other herbal remedies, such as evening primrose oil, ginseng, and wild yam, have also not shown that they effectively reduce menopausal symptoms.

The National Institute on Aging (NIA), which is part of the National Institutes of Health (NIH), has more information about how to manage the symptoms of menopause on the Menopause AgePage.

What questions remain in this area of research?

The WHI trials were landmark studies that have transformed our understanding of the health effects of MHT. Follow-up studies have expanded and refined the original findings of these two trials. Many questions, however, remain to be answered, such as the following:

- Are different forms of hormones, lower doses, different hormones, or different methods of administration safer or more effective than those tested in the WHI trials?

- Does hormone use present different risks and benefits for women younger than those studied in the WHI trials?

- Is there an optimal age at which to initiate MHT or an optimal duration of therapy that maximizes benefits and minimizes risks?

It's important to note that women who were enrolled in the WHI trials were, on average, 63 years old, although about 5,000 of them were under age 60, so the results of the study may also apply to younger women. However, women in the study were not using MHT to relieve symptoms of menopause. In addition, the WHI trials tested single-dose strengths of one estrogen-only medication (Premarin) and one estrogen-plus-progestin medication (Prempro).

Chapter 9

Diethylstilbestrol (DES) and Cancer

What is DES?

Diethylstilbestrol (DES) is a synthetic form of the female hormone estrogen. It was prescribed to pregnant women between 1940 and 1971 to prevent miscarriage, premature labor, and related complications of pregnancy. The use of DES declined after studies in the 1950s showed that it was not effective in preventing these problems.

In 1971, researchers linked prenatal (before birth) DES exposure to a type of cancer of the cervix and vagina called clear cell adenocarcinoma in a small group of women. Soon after, the Food and Drug Administration (FDA) notified physicians throughout the country that DES should not be prescribed to pregnant women. The drug continued to be prescribed to pregnant women in Europe until 1978.

DES is now known to be an endocrine-disrupting chemical, one of a number of substances that interfere with the endocrine system to cause cancer, birth defects, and other developmental abnormalities. The effects of endocrine-disrupting chemicals are most severe when exposure occurs during fetal development.

Text in this chapter is excerpted from "Diethylstilbestrol (DES) and Cancer," National Cancer Institute at the National Institutes of Health (NIH), October 5, 2011.

What is the cancer risk of women who were exposed to DES before birth?

The daughters of women who used DES while pregnant—commonly called DES daughters—have about 40 times the risk of developing clear cell adenocarcinoma of the lower genital tract than unexposed women. However, this type of cancer is still rare; approximately 1 in 1,000 DES daughters develops it.

The first DES daughters who were diagnosed with clear cell adenocarcinoma were very young at the time of their diagnoses. Subsequent research has shown that the risk of developing this disease remains elevated as women age into their 40s.

DES daughters have an increased risk of developing abnormal cells in the cervix and the vagina that are precursors of cancer (dysplasia, cervical intraepithelial neoplasia, and squamous intraepithelial lesions). These abnormal cells resemble cancer cells, but they do not invade nearby healthy tissue and are not cancer. They may develop into cancer, however, if left untreated. Scientists estimated that DES-exposed daughters were 2.2 times more likely to have these abnormal cell changes in the cervix than unexposed women. Approximately 4 percent of DES daughters developed these conditions because of their exposure. It has been recommended that DES daughters have a yearly Pap test and pelvic exam to check for abnormal cells.

DES daughters may also have a slightly increased risk of breast cancer after age 40. A 2006 study from the United States suggested that, overall, breast cancer risk is not increased in DES daughters, but that, after age 40, DES daughters have approximately twice the risk of breast cancer as unexposed women of the same age and with similar risk factors. However, a 2010 study from Europe found no difference in breast cancer risk between DES daughters and unexposed women and no difference in overall cancer risk. A 2011 study found that about 2 percent of a large cohort of DES daughters has developed breast cancer due to their exposure.

DES daughters should be aware of these health risks, share their medical history with their doctors, and get regular physical examinations.

Do DES daughters have problems with fertility and pregnancy?

Several studies have found increased risks of premature birth, miscarriage, and ectopic pregnancy associated with DES exposure. An analysis of updated data published in 2011 is outlined in the table below.

Table 9.1. Fertility Problems in DES Daughters

Fertility Problems in DES Daughters			
Fertility Complication	Hazard Ratio	Percent Cumulative Risk* to Age 45, DES-exposed Women	Percent Cumulative Risk* to Age 45, Unexposed Women
Premature delivery	4.68	53.3	17.8
Stillbirth	2.45	8.9	2.6
Neonatal death	8.12	7.8	0.6
Ectopic pregnancy	3.72	14.6	2.9
Miscarriage (second trimester)	3.77	16.4	1.7
Preeclampsia	1.42	26.4	13.7
Infertility	2.37	33.3	15.5

The total risk (probability) that a certain problem will occur.

Some studies suggest that the increased risk of infertility is mainly due to uterine or fallopian tube problems.

What other health problems might DES daughters have?

Concerns have been raised that DES daughters may have problems with their immune system. However, research thus far suggests that DES daughters do not have an increased risk of autoimmune diseases. Researchers found no difference in the rates of lupus, rheumatoid arthritis, optic neuritis, and idiopathic thrombocytopenia purpura between DES-exposed and unexposed women.

Studies examining the risk of depression among DES daughters have had conflicting results. One study found a 40 percent increase in risk of depression, whereas another found no increased risk for these women. A study published in 2003 found little support for the possibility that prenatal exposure to DES influences certain psychological and sexual characteristics of adult men and women, such as the likelihood of ever having been married, age at first sexual intercourse, number of sexual partners, and having had a same-sex sexual partner in adulthood.

DES daughters have more than twice the risk of early menopause (menopause that begins before age 45) as unexposed women. Scientists estimate that 3 percent of DES-exposed women have experienced early menopause due to their exposure to DES.

What health problems might DES-exposed sons have?

Some studies have found that men whose mothers used DES during pregnancy have an increased risk of testicular abnormalities, including undescended testicles or development of cysts in the epididymis. There is also some evidence of increased risks of inflammation or infection of the testicles.

Whether DES-exposed sons have increased risks of testicular or prostate cancer is unclear; studies to date have produced mixed results. As the cohort of these men gets older, more data will be available to help answer this question.

Research has shown that men who were exposed to DES through their mothers do not have an increased risk of infertility, even when they have genital abnormalities.

What health problems might women who took DES during pregnancy have?

Women who used DES themselves have a slightly increased risk of breast cancer—approximately 30 percent higher than that of women who did not take DES. Women who used DES also have a 30 percent higher risk of death from breast cancer than unexposed women. This risk has been found to be stable over time—that is, it does not increase as the mothers become older. No evidence exists to suggest that women who took DES are at higher risk for any other type of cancer.

What health problems might DES-exposed grandchildren have?

Researchers are also studying possible health effects among women and men who are the children of DES daughters. These groups are called DES granddaughters and DES grandsons, or the third generation. Researchers are studying these groups because studies in animal models suggest that DES may cause DNA changes (i.e., altered patterns of methylation) in mice exposed to the chemical during early development. These changes can be heritable and have the potential to affect subsequent generations.

A comparison of the results of DES granddaughters' pelvic exams with those of their mothers' first pelvic exams found none of the changes that had been associated with prenatal DES exposure in their mothers. However, another analysis showed that DES granddaughters began their menstrual periods later and were more likely to have menstrual irregularities than other women of the same age. The data also suggested that infertility was greater among DES granddaughters, and that they tended to have fewer live birth. However, this association is based on small numbers of events and was not statistically significant. Researchers will continue to follow these women to study the risk of infertility.

Recent studies have found that DES granddaughters and DES grandsons may have a slightly higher risk of cancer and birth defects, including hypospadias in DES grandsons. However, because each of these associations is based on small numbers of events, researchers will continue to study these groups to clarify the findings.

How can people find out if they took DES during pregnancy or were exposed to DES in utero?

It is estimated that 5 to 10 million Americans—pregnant women and the children born to them—were exposed to DES between 1940 and 1971. DES was given widely to pregnant women between 1940 and 1971 to prevent complications during pregnancy. DES was provided under many different product names and also in various forms, such as pills, creams, and vaginal suppositories. The table below includes examples of products that contained DES.

DES Product Names

Nonsteroidal Estrogens		
Benzestrol	Gynben	Stil-Rol
Chlorotrianisene	Gyneben	Stilbal
Comestrol	Hexestrol	Stilbestrol
Cyren A.	Hexoestrol	Stilbestronate
Cyren B.	Hi-Bestrol	Stilbetin
Delvinal	Menocrin	Stilbinol
DES	Meprane	Stilboestroform
Desplex	Mestilbol	Silboestrol
Dibestil	Microest	Stilboestrol DP
Diestryl	Methallenestril	Stilestrate
Dienostrol	Mikarol	Stilpalmitate
Dienoestrol	Mikarol forti	Stilphostrol
Diethylsteilbestrol	Milestrol	Stilronate
dipalmitate	Monomestrol	Stilrone

Nonsteroidal Estrogens		
Diethylstilbestrol diphosphate	Neo-Oestranol I	Stils
Diethylstilbestrol dipropionate	Neo-Oestranol II	Synestrin
	Nulabort	Synestrol
Diethylstilbenediol	Oestrogenine	Synthosestrin
Digestil	Oestromenin	Tace
Dinestrol	Oestromon	Vallestril
Domestrol	Orestol	Willestrol
Estilben	Pabestrol D	
Estrobene	Palestrol	
Estrobene DP	Restrol	
Estrosyn		
Fonatol		
Nonsteroidal Estrogen-Androgen Combinations		
Amperone	Teserene	
Di-Erone	Tylandril	
Estan	Tylostereone	
Metystil		
Nonsteroidal Estrogen-Progesterone Combinations		
Progravidium		
Vaginal Cream Suppositories with Nonsteroidal Estrogens		
AVC Cream with Dienestrol		
Dienestrol Cream		

Women who think they used DES during pregnancy, or people who think that their mother used DES during pregnancy, can try contacting the physician or institution where they received their care to request a review of their medical records. If any pills were taken during pregnancy, [obstetrical] records could be checked to determine the name of the drug.

However, finding medical records after a long period of time can be difficult. If the doctor has retired or died, another doctor may have taken over the practice as well as the records. The county medical society or health department may know where the records have been stored. Some pharmacies keep records for a long time and can be contacted regarding prescription dispensing information. Military medical records are kept for 25 years. In most cases, however, it may be impossible to determine whether DES was used.

What should DES-exposed daughters do?

Women who know or believe they were exposed to DES before birth should be aware of the health effects of DES and inform their doctor about their possible exposure. It has been recommended that exposed women have an annual medical examination to check for the adverse health effects of DES. A thorough examination may include the following:

- Pelvic examination
- Pap test and colposcopy: A routine cervical Pap test is not adequate for DES daughters. The Pap test must gather cells from the cervix and the vagina. It is also good for a clinician to see the cervix and vaginal walls. They may use a colposcope to follow-up if there are any abnormal findings.
- Biopsy
- Breast examinations—It is recommended that DES daughters continue to rigorously follow the routine breast cancer screening recommendations for their age group.

What should DES-exposed mothers do?

A woman who took DES while pregnant or who suspects she may have taken it should inform her doctor. She should try to learn the dosage, when the medication was started, and how it was used. She also should inform her children who were exposed before birth so that this information can be included in their medical records.

It is recommended that DES-exposed mothers have regular breast cancer screenings and yearly medical checkups that include a pelvic examination and a Pap test.

What should DES-exposed sons do?

Men whose mothers took DES while pregnant should inform their physician of their exposure and be examined periodically. Although the risk of developing testicular cancer among DES-exposed sons is unclear, males with undescended or unusually small testicles have an increased risk of testicular cancer whether or not they were exposed to DES.

73

Is it safe for DES daughters to use hormone replacement therapy?

Each woman should discuss this question with her doctor. Studies have not shown that hormone replacement therapy is unsafe for DES daughters. However, some doctors believe that DES daughters should avoid these medications because they contain estrogen.

Chapter 10

HIV Infection and Cancer

Do people infected with human immunodeficiency virus (HIV) have an increased risk of cancer?

Yes. People infected with HIV have a substantially higher risk of some types of cancer compared with uninfected people of the same age. Three of these cancers are known as "acquired immunodeficiency syndrome (AIDS)-defining cancers" or "AIDS-defining malignancies": Kaposi sarcoma, non-Hodgkin lymphoma, and cervical cancer. A diagnosis of any one of these cancers marks the point at which HIV infection has progressed to AIDS.

People infected with HIV are several thousand times more likely than uninfected people to be diagnosed with Kaposi sarcoma, at least 70 times more likely to be diagnosed with non-Hodgkin lymphoma, and, among women, at least 5 times more likely to be diagnosed with cervical cancer.

In addition, people infected with HIV are at higher risk of several other types of cancer. These other malignancies include anal, liver, and lung cancer, and Hodgkin lymphoma.

People infected with HIV are at least 25 times more likely to be diagnosed with anal cancer than uninfected people, 5 times as likely to be diagnosed with liver cancer, 3 times as likely to be diagnosed with lung cancer, and at least 10 times more likely to be diagnosed with Hodgkin lymphoma.

Text in this chapter is excerpted from "HIV Infection and Cancer Risk," National Cancer Institute at the National Institutes of Health (NIH), May 16, 2011.

People infected with HIV do not have increased risks of breast, colorectal, prostate, or many other common types of cancer. Screening for these cancers in HIV-infected people should follow current guidelines for the general population.

Why do people infected with HIV have a higher risk of cancer?

Infection with HIV weakens the immune system and reduces the body's ability to fight infections that may lead to cancer. Many people infected with HIV are also infected with other viruses that cause certain cancers. The following are the most important of these cancer-related viruses:

- Human herpes virus 8 (HHV-8), also known as Kaposi sarcoma-associated herpes virus (KSHV), is the cause of Kaposi sarcoma.

- Epstein Barr virus (EBV) causes some subtypes of non-Hodgkin and Hodgkin lymphoma.

- Human papillomavirus (HPV) causes cervical cancer and some types of anal, penile, vaginal, vulvar, and head and neck cancer.

- Hepatitis B virus (HBV) and hepatitis C virus (HCV) both can cause liver cancer.

Infection with most of these viruses is more common among people infected with HIV than among uninfected people.

In addition, the prevalence of some traditional risk factors for cancer, especially smoking (a known cause of lung cancer) and heavy alcohol use (which can increase the risk of liver cancer), is higher among people infected with HIV.

Has the introduction of antiretroviral therapy changed the cancer risk of people infected with HIV?

The introduction of highly active antiretroviral therapy (HAART) in the mid-1990s greatly reduced the incidence of Kaposi sarcoma and non-Hodgkin lymphoma among people infected with HIV. HAART lowers the amount of HIV circulating in the blood, thereby allowing partial restoration of immune system function.

Although lower than before, the risk of these two cancers is still much higher among people infected with HIV than among people in the general population. This persistently high risk may be due, at least in part, to the fact that immune system function remains substantially impaired in people treated with HAART. In addition, over time HIV can develop resistance to the drugs used in HAART. Many people infected with HIV have had difficulty in accessing medical care or taking their medication as prescribed.

Although HAART has led to reductions in the incidence of Kaposi sarcoma and non-Hodgkin lymphoma among HIV-infected individuals, it has not reduced the incidence of cervical cancer, which has essentially remained unchanged. Moreover, the incidence of several other cancers, particularly Hodgkin lymphoma and anal cancer, has been increasing among HIV-infected individuals since the introduction of HAART. The influence of HAART on the risk of these other cancer types is not well understood.

As HAART has reduced the number of deaths from AIDS, the HIV-infected population has grown in size and become older. The fastest growing proportion of HIV-infected individuals is the over-40 age group. These individuals are now developing cancers common in older age. In 2003, the proportion of these other cancers exceeded the number of AIDS-defining malignancies. However, HIV-infected people do not develop most cancers at a younger age than is typically seen in the general population.

What can people infected with HIV do to reduce their risk of cancer or to find cancer early?

Taking HAART as indicated based on current HIV treatment guidelines lowers the risk of Kaposi sarcoma and non-Hodgkin lymphoma and increases overall survival.

The risk of lung cancer can be reduced by quitting smoking. Because HIV-infected people have a higher risk of lung cancer, it is especially important that they do not smoke. Help with quitting smoking is available through the National Cancer Institute's (NCI) smoking quitline at 1–877–448–7848 (1–877–44U–QUIT) and in other NCI resources.

The higher incidence of liver cancer among HIV-infected people appears to be related to more frequent infection with hepatitis virus (particularly HCV) and alcohol abuse or dependence than among uninfected people. Therefore, HIV-infected individuals should know their hepatitis status. If blood tests show that they have previously been infected with HBV or HCV, they should consider reducing their alcohol consumption.

In addition, if they currently have viral hepatitis, they should discuss with their health care provider whether HBV- or HCV-suppressing therapy is an option for them. Some drugs may be used for both HBV-suppressing therapy and HAART.

Because HIV-infected women have a higher risk of cervical cancer, it is important that they be screened regularly for this disease. Studies have suggested that Pap test abnormalities are more common among HIV-infected women and that HPV DNA tests may not be as effective as Pap tests in screening these women for cervical cancer.

Some researchers recommend anal Pap test screening to detect and treat early lesions before they progress to anal cancer. This type of screening may be most beneficial for men who have had sexual intercourse with other men. HIV-infected patients should discuss such screening with their medical providers.

Chapter 11

HPV and Cancer

What are HPVs?

HPVs, also called human papillomaviruses, are a group of more than 150 related viruses. More than 40 of these viruses can be easily spread through direct skin-to-skin contact during vaginal, anal, and oral sex.

HPV infections are the most common sexually transmitted infections in the United States. In fact, more than half of sexually active people are infected with one or more HPV types at some point in their lives. Recent research indicates that, at any point in time, 42.5 percent of women have genital HPV infections, whereas less than 7 percent of adults have oral HPV infections.

Sexually transmitted HPVs fall into two categories:

- Low-risk HPVs, which do not cause cancer but can cause skin warts (technically known as condylomata acuminata) on or around the genitals or anus. For example, HPV types 6 and 11 cause 90 percent of all genital warts.

- High-risk or oncogenic HPVs, which can cause cancer. At least a dozen high-risk HPV types have been identified. Two of these, HPV types 16 and 18, are responsible for the majority of HPV-caused cancers.

Text in this chapter is excerpted from "HPV and Cancer," National Cancer Institute at the National Institutes of Health (NIH), March 15, 2012.

What is the association between HPV infection and cancer?

High-risk HPV infection accounts for approximately 5 percent of all cancers worldwide. However, most high-risk HPV infections occur without any symptoms, go away within 1 to 2 years, and do not cause cancer. These transient infections may cause cytologic abnormalities, or abnormal cell changes, that go away on their own.

Some HPV infections, however, can persist for many years. Persistent infections with high-risk HPV types can lead to more serious cytologic abnormalities or lesions that, if untreated, may progress to cancer.

Which cancers are caused by HPVs?

Virtually all cervical cancers are caused by HPV infections, with just two HPV types, 16 and 18, responsible for about 70 percent of all cases. HPV also causes anal cancer, with about 85 percent of all cases caused by HPV-16. HPV types 16 and 18 have also been found to cause close to half of vaginal, vulvar, and penile cancers.

Most recently, HPV infections have been found to cause cancer of the oropharynx, which is the middle part of the throat including the soft palate, the base of the tongue, and the tonsils. In the United States, more than half of the cancers diagnosed in the oropharynx are linked to HPV-16.

The incidence of HPV-associated oropharyngeal cancer has increased during the past 20 years, especially among men. It has been estimated that, by 2020, HPV will cause more oropharyngeal cancers than cervical cancers in the United States.

Other factors may increase the risk of developing cancer following a high-risk HPV infection. These other factors include the following:

- Smoking

- Having a weakened immune system

- Having many children (for increased risk of cervical cancer)

- Long-term oral contraceptive use (for increased risk of cervical cancer)

- Poor oral hygiene (for increased risk of oropharyngeal cancer)

- Chronic inflammation

Can HPV infection be prevented?

The most reliable way to prevent infection with either a high-risk or a low-risk HPV is to avoid any skin-to-skin oral, anal, or genital contact with another person. For those who are sexually active, a long-term, mutually monogamous relationship with an uninfected partner is the strategy most likely to prevent HPV infection. However, because of the lack of symptoms it is hard to know whether a partner who has been sexually active in the past is currently infected with HPV.

Research has shown that correct and consistent use of condoms can reduce the transmission of HPVs between sexual partners. Areas not covered by a condom can be infected with the virus, though, so condoms are unlikely to provide complete protection against virus spread.

The Food and Drug Administration (FDA) has approved two HPV vaccines: Gardasil® for the prevention of cervical, anal, vulvar, and vaginal cancer, as well as precancerous lesions in these tissues and genital warts caused by HPV infection; and Cervarix® for the prevention of cervical cancer and precancerous cervical lesions caused by HPV infection. Both vaccines are highly effective in preventing infections with HPV types 16 and 18. Gardasil also prevents infection with HPV types 6 and 11. These vaccines have not been approved for prevention of penile or oropharyngeal cancer.

More information about HPV vaccines is available in the NCI fact sheet Human Papillomavirus (HPV) Vaccines.

How are HPV infections detected?

HPV infections can be detected by testing a sample of cells to see if they contain viral DNA or RNA.

The most common test detects DNA from several high-risk HPV types, but it cannot identify the type(s) that are present. Another test is specific for DNA from HPV types 16 and 18, the two types that cause most HPV-associated cancers. A third test can detect DNA from several high-risk HPV types and can indicate whether HPV-16 or HPV-18 is present. A fourth test detects RNA from the most common high-risk HPV types. These tests can detect HPV infections before cell abnormalities are evident.

Theoretically, the HPV DNA and RNA tests could be used to identify HPV infections in cells taken from any part of the body. However, the tests are approved by the FDA for only two indications: for follow-up testing of women who seem to have abnormal Pap test results and for cervical cancer screening in combination with a Pap test among women over age 30.

There are no FDA-approved tests to detect HPV infections in men. There are also no currently recommended screening methods similar to a Pap test for detecting cell changes caused by HPV infection in anal, vulvar, vaginal, penile, or oropharyngeal tissues. However, this is an area of ongoing research.

What are treatment options for HPV-infected individuals?

There is currently no medical treatment for HPV infections. However, the genital warts and precancerous lesions resulting from HPV infections can be treated.

Methods commonly used to treat precancerous cervical lesions include cryosurgery (freezing that destroys tissue), LEEP (loop elec- trosurgical excision procedure, or the removal of cervical tissue using a hot wire loop), surgical conization (surgery with a scalpel, a laser, or both to remove a cone-shaped piece of tissue from the cervix and cervical canal), and laser vaporization conization (use of a laser to destroy cervical tissue).

Treatments for other types of precancerous lesions caused by HPV (vaginal, vulvar, penile, and anal lesions) and genital warts include topical chemicals or drugs, excisional surgery, cryosurgery, electro- surgery, and laser surgery.

HPV-infected individuals who develop cancer generally receive the same treatment as patients whose tumors do not harbor HPV infections, according to the type and stage of their tumors. However, people who are diagnosed with HPV-positive oropharyngeal cancer may be treated differently than people with oropharyngeal cancers that are HPV-negative. Recent research has shown that patients with HPV-positive oropharyngeal tumors have a better prognosis and may do just as well on less intense treatment. An ongoing clinical trial is investigating this question.

How do high-risk HPVs cause cancer?

HPVs infect epithelial cells. These cells, which are organized in layers, cover the inside and outside surfaces of the body, including the skin, the throat, the genital tract, and the anus. Because HPVs are not thought to enter the blood stream, having an HPV infection in one part of the body should not cause an infection in another part of the body.

Once an HPV enters an epithelial cell, the virus begins to make proteins. Two of the proteins made by high-risk HPVs interfere with normal functions in the cell, enabling the cell to grow in an uncontrolled manner and to avoid cell death.

Many times these infected cells are recognized by the immune system and eliminated. Sometimes, however, these infected cells are not destroyed, and a persistent infection results. As the persistently infected cells continue to grow, they may develop mutations that promote even more cell growth, leading to the formation of a high-grade lesion and ultimately, a tumor.

Researchers believe that it can take between 10 and 20 years from the time of an initial HPV infection until a tumor forms. However, even high-grade lesions do not always lead to cancer. The percentage of high-grade cervical lesions that progress to invasive cervical cancer has been estimated to be 50 percent or less.

Chapter 12

Helicobacter Pylori and Cancer

What is Helicobacter pylori?

Helicobacter pylori, or H. pylori, is a spiral-shaped bacterium that grows in the mucus layer that coats the inside of the human stomach.

To survive in the harsh, acidic environment of the stomach, H. pylori secretes an enzyme called urease, which converts the chemical urea to ammonia. The production of ammonia around H. pylori neutralizes the acidity of the stomach, making it more hospitable for the bacterium. In addition, the helical shape of H. pylori allows it to burrow into the mucus layer, which is less acidic than the inside space, or lumen, of the stomach. H. pylori can also attach to the cells that line the inner surface of the stomach.

Although immune cells that normally recognize and attack invading bacteria accumulate near sites of H. pylori infection, they are unable to reach the stomach lining. In addition, H. pylori has developed ways of interfering with local immune responses, making them ineffective in eliminating this bacterium.

H. pylori has coexisted with humans for many thousands of years, and infection with this bacterium is common. The Centers for Disease Control and Prevention (CDC) estimates that approximately two-thirds

Text in this chapter is excerpted from "Helicobacter Pylori and Cancer," National Cancer Institute at the National Institutes of Health (NIH), September 5, 2013.

of the world's population harbors the bacterium, with infection rates much higher in developing countries than in developed nations.

Although H. pylori infection does not cause illness in most infected people, it is a major risk factor for peptic ulcer disease and is responsible for the majority of ulcers of the stomach and upper small intestine.

In 1994, the International Agency for Research on Cancer classified H. pylori as a carcinogen, or cancer-causing agent, in humans, despite conflicting results at the time. Since then, it has been increasingly accepted that colonization of the stomach with H. pylori is an important cause of gastric cancer and of gastric mucosa-associated lymphoid tissue (MALT) lymphoma. Infection with H. pylori is also associated with a reduced risk of esophageal adenocarcinoma.

H. pylori is thought to spread through contaminated food and water and through direct mouth-to-mouth contact. In most populations, the bacterium is first acquired during childhood. Infection is more likely in children living in poverty, in crowded conditions, and in areas with poor sanitation.

What is gastric cancer?

Gastric cancer, or cancer of the stomach, was once considered a single entity. Now, scientists divide this cancer into two main classes: gastric cardia cancer (cancer of the top inch of the stomach, where it meets the esophagus) and non-cardia gastric cancer (cancer in all other areas of the stomach).

According to NCI's Surveillance, Epidemiology, and End Results (SEER) Program, an estimated 21,600 people in the United States will be diagnosed with gastric cancer and 10,990 people will die of this cancer during 2013. Gastric cancer is the second most common cause of cancer-related deaths in the world, killing approximately 738,000 people in 2008. Gastric cancer is less common in the United States and other Western countries than in countries in Asia and South America.

Overall gastric cancer incidence is decreasing. However, this decline is mainly in the rates of non-cardia gastric cancer. Gastric cardia cancer, which was once very uncommon, has risen in incidence in recent decades.

Infection with H. pylori is the primary identified cause of gastric cancer. Other risk factors for gastric cancer include chronic gastritis; older age; male sex; a diet high in salted, smoked, or poorly preserved foods and low in fruits and vegetables; tobacco smoking; pernicious anemia; a history of stomach surgery for benign conditions; and a family history of stomach cancer.

H. pylori has different associations with the two main classes of gastric cancer. Whereas people infected with H. pylori have an increased risk of non-cardia gastric cancer, their risk of gastric cardia cancer is not increased and may even be decreased.

What evidence shows that H. pylori infection causes non-cardia gastric cancer?

Epidemiologic studies have shown that individuals infected with H. pylori have an increased risk of gastric adenocarcinoma. The risk increase appears to be restricted to non-cardia gastric cancer. For example, a 2001 combined analysis of 12 case-control studies of H. pylori and gastric cancer estimated that the risk of non-cardia gastric cancer was nearly six times higher for H. pylori-infected people than for uninfected people).

Additional evidence for an association between H. pylori infection and the risk of non-cardia gastric cancer comes from prospective cohort studies such as the Alpha-Tocopherol, Beta-Carotene (ATBC) Cancer Prevention Study in Finland. Comparing subjects who developed non-cardia gastric cancer with cancer-free control subjects, the researchers found that H. pylori-infected individuals had a nearly eightfold increased risk for non-cardia gastric cancer.

What is the evidence that H. pylori infection may reduce the risk of some cancers?

Several studies have detected an inverse relationship between H. pylori infection and gastric cardia cancer, although the evidence is not entirely consistent. The possibility of an inverse relationship between the bacterium and gastric cardia cancer is supported by the corresponding decrease in H. pylori infection rates in Western countries during the past century—the result of improved hygiene and widespread antibiotic use—and the increase in rates of gastric cardia cancer in these same regions.

Similar epidemiologic evidence suggests that H. pylori infection may be associated with a lower risk of esophageal adenocarcinoma. For example, a large case-control study in Sweden showed that the risk of esophageal adenocarcinoma in H. pylori-infected individuals was one-third that of uninfected individuals. A meta-analysis of 13 studies, including the Swedish study, found a 45 percent reduction in risk of esophageal adenocarcinoma with H. pylori infection. Moreover, as with gastric cardia cancer, dramatic increases in esophageal adenocarcinoma rates in several Western countries parallel the declines in H. pylori infection rates.

How might H. pylori infection decrease the risk of some cancers but increase the risk of other cancers?

Although it is not known for certain how H. pylori infection increases the risk of non-cardia gastric cancer, some researchers speculate that the long-term presence of an inflammatory response predisposes cells in the stomach lining to become cancerous. This idea is supported by the finding that increased expression of a single cytokine (interleukin-1-beta) in the stomach of transgenic mice causes sporadic gastric inflammation and cancer. The increased cell turnover resulting from ongoing cellular damage could increase the likelihood that cells will develop harmful mutations.

One hypothesis that may explain reduced risks of gastric cardia cancer and esophageal adenocarcinoma in H. pylori-infected individuals relates to the decline in stomach acidity that is often seen after decades of H. pylori colonization. This decline would reduce acid reflux into the esophagus, a major risk factor for adenocarcinomas affecting the upper stomach and esophagus.

What is cagA-positive H. pylori and how does it affect the risk of gastric and esophageal cancers?

Some H. pylori bacteria use a needle-like appendage to inject a toxin produced by a gene called cytotoxin-associated gene A (cagA) into the junctions where cells of the stomach lining meet. This toxin (known as CagA) alters the structure of stomach cells and allows the bacteria to attach to them more easily. Long-term exposure to the toxin causes chronic inflammation. However, not all strains of H. pylori carry the cagA gene; those that do are classified as cagA-positive.

Epidemiologic evidence suggests that infection with cagA-positive strains is especially associated with an increased risk of non-cardia gastric cancer and with reduced risks of gastric cardia cancer and esophageal adenocarcinoma. For example, a meta-analysis of 16 case-control studies conducted around the world showed that individuals infected with cagA-positive H. pylori had twice the risk of non-cardia gastric cancer than individuals infected with cagA-negative H. pylori. Conversely, a case-control study conducted in Sweden found that people infected with cagA-positive H. pylori had a statistically significantly reduced risk of esophageal adenocarcinoma. Similarly, another case-control study conducted in the United States found that infection with cagA-positive H. pylori was associated with a reduced risk of esophageal adenocarcinoma and gastric cardia cancer combined, but that infection with cagA-negative strains was not associated with risk.

Recent research has suggested a potential mechanism by which CagA could contribute to gastric carcinogenesis. In three studies, infection with CagA-positive H. pylori was associated with inactivation of tumor suppressor proteins, including p53.

What is gastric mucosa-associated lymphoid tissue (MALT) lymphoma, and what is the evidence that it can be caused by H. pylori infection?

Gastric MALT lymphoma is a rare type of non-Hodgkin lymphoma that is characterized by the slow multiplication of B lymphocytes, a type of immune cell, in the stomach lining. This cancer represents approximately 12 percent of the extranodal (outside of lymph nodes) non-Hodgkin lymphoma that occurs among men and approximately 18 percent of extranodal non-Hodgkin lymphoma among women. During the period 1999–2003, the annual incidence of gastric MALT lymphoma in the United States was about one case for every 100,000 persons in the population.

Normally, the lining of the stomach lacks lymphoid (immune system) tissue, but development of this tissue is often stimulated in response to colonization of the lining by H. pylori. Only in rare cases does this tissue give rise to MALT lymphoma. However, nearly all patients with gastric MALT lymphoma show signs of H. pylori infection, and the risk of developing this tumor is more than six times higher in infected people than in uninfected people.

Is H. pylori infection associated with any other cancer?

Whether H. pylori infection is associated with risk of other cancers remains unclear. Some studies have found a possible association between H. pylori infection and pancreatic cancer, but the evidence is conflicting. Studies investigating the possibility that H. pylori is a risk factor for colorectal adenocarcinoma or lung cancer have found no evidence that it is associated with the risk of either type of cancer.

Can treatment to eradicate H. pylori infection reduce gastric cancer rates?

Long-term follow-up of data from a randomized clinical trial carried out in Shandong, China—an area where rates of gastric cancer are very high—found that short-term treatment with antibiotics to eradicate H. pylori reduced the incidence of gastric cancer. During a nearly 15-year period after treatment, gastric cancer incidence was reduced by almost 40 percent. When the results of this trial were pooled with those of several smaller trials examining the effects on gastric cancer incidence of antimicrobial treatment to eradicate H. pylori, a similar reduction was seen.

Who should seek diagnosis and treatment of an H. pylori infection?

According to the Centers for Disease Control and Prevention (CDC), people who have active gastric or duodenal ulcers or a documented history of ulcers should be tested for H. pylori, and if they are infected, should be treated. Testing for and treating H. pylori infection is also recommended after resection of early gastric cancer and for low-grade gastric MALT lymphoma. However, most experts agree that the available evidence does not support widespread testing for and eradication of H. pylori infection.

Chapter 13

Cell Phones and Cancer Risk

Why is there concern that cell phones may cause cancer or other health problems?

There are three main reasons why people are concerned that cell phones (also known as "wireless" or "mobile" telephones) might have the potential to cause certain types of cancer or other health problems:

- Cell phones emit radiofrequency energy (radio waves), a form of non-ionizing radiation. Tissues nearest to where the phone is held can absorb this energy.

- The number of cell phone users has increased rapidly. As of 2010, there were more than 303 million subscribers to cell phone service in the United States, according to the Cellular Telecommunications and Internet Association. This is a nearly threefold increase from the 110 million users in 2000. Globally, the number of cell phone subscriptions is estimated by the International Telecommunications Union to be 5 billion.

- Over time, the number of cell phone calls per day, the length of each call, and the amount of time people use cell phones have increased. Cell phone technology has also undergone substantial changes.

Text in this chapter is excerpted from "Cell Phones and Cancer Risk," National Cancer Institute at the National Institutes of Health (NIH), June 24, 2013.

What is radiofrequency energy and how does it affect the body?

Radiofrequency energy is a form of electromagnetic radiation. Electromagnetic radiation can be categorized into two types: ionizing (e.g., x-rays, radon, and cosmic rays) and non-ionizing (e.g., radiofrequency and extremely low-frequency or power frequency).

Exposure to ionizing radiation, such as from radiation therapy, is known to increase the risk of cancer. However, although many studies have examined the potential health effects of non-ionizing radiation from radar, microwave ovens, and other sources, there is currently no consistent evidence that non-ionizing radiation increases cancer risk.

The only known biological effect of radiofrequency energy is heating. The ability of microwave ovens to heat food is one example of this effect of radiofrequency energy. Radiofrequency exposure from cell phone use does cause heating; however, it is not sufficient to measurably increase body temperature.

A recent study showed that when people used a cell phone for 50 minutes, brain tissues on the same side of the head as the phone's antenna metabolized more glucose than did tissues on the opposite side of the brain. The researchers noted that the results are preliminary, and possible health outcomes from this increase in glucose metabolism are still unknown.

How is radiofrequency energy exposure measured in epidemiologic studies?

Levels of radiofrequency exposure are indirectly estimated using information from interviews or questionnaires. These measures include the following:

- How "regularly" study participants use cell phones (the minimum number of calls per week or month)

- The age and the year when study participants first used a cell phone and the age and the year of last use (allows calculation of the duration of use and time since the start of use)

- The average number of cell phone calls per day, week, or month (frequency)

- The average length of a typical cell phone call

- The total hours of lifetime use, calculated from the length of typical call times, the frequency of use, and the duration of use

What has research shown about the possible cancer-causing effects of radiofrequency energy?

Although there have been some concerns that radiofrequency energy from cell phones held closely to the head may affect the brain and other tissues, to date there is no evidence from studies of cells, animals, or humans that radiofrequency energy can cause cancer.

It is generally accepted that damage to DNA is necessary for cancer to develop. However, radiofrequency energy, unlike ionizing radiation, does not cause DNA damage in cells, and it has not been found to cause cancer in animals or to enhance the cancer-causing effects of known chemical carcinogens in animals.

Researchers have carried out several types of epidemiologic studies to investigate the possibility of a relationship between cell phone use and the risk of malignant (cancerous) brain tumors, such as gliomas, as well as benign (noncancerous) tumors, such as acoustic neuromas (tumors in the cells of the nerve responsible for hearing), most meningiomas (tumors in the meninges, membranes that cover and protect the brain and spinal cord), and parotid gland tumors (tumors in the salivary glands).

In one type of study, called a case-control study, cell phone use is compared between people with these types of tumors and people without them. In another type of study, called a cohort study, a large group of people is followed over time and the rate of these tumors in people who did and didn't use cell phones is compared. Cancer incidence data can also be analyzed over time to see if the rates of cancer changed in large populations during the time that cell phone use increased dramatically. The results of these studies have generally not provided clear evidence of a relationship between cell phone use and cancer, but there have been some statistically significant findings in certain subgroups of people.

Findings from specific research studies are summarized below:

- The Interphone Study, conducted by a consortium of researchers from 13 countries, is the largest health-related case-control study of use of cell phones and head and neck tumors. Most published analyses from this study have shown no statistically significant increases in brain or central nervous system cancers related to higher amounts of cell phone use. One recent analysis showed a statistically significant, albeit modest, increase in the risk of glioma among the small proportion of study participants who spent the most total time on cell phone calls. However, the researchers considered this finding inconclusive because they felt that the amount of use reported by some respondents was unlikely and because the participants who reported lower levels of use appeared to have a slightly reduced risk of brain cancer compared with people who did not use cell phones regularly. Another recent study from the group found no relationship between brain tumor locations and regions of the brain that were exposed to the highest level of radiofrequency energy from cell phones.

- A cohort study in Denmark linked billing information from more than 358,000 cell phone subscribers with brain tumor incidence data from the Danish Cancer Registry. The analyses found no association between cell phone use and the incidence of glioma, meningioma, or acoustic neuroma, even among people who had been cell phone subscribers for 13 or more years.

- The prospective Million Women Study in the United Kingdom found that self-reported cell phone use was not associated with an increased risk of glioma, meningioma, or non-central nervous system tumors. The researchers did find that the use of cell phones for more than 5 years was associated with an increased risk of acoustic neuroma, and that the risk of acoustic neuroma increased with increasing duration of cell phone use. However, the incidence of these tumors among men and women in the United Kingdom did not increase during 1998 to 2008, even though cell phone use increased dramatically over that decade.

- An early case-control study in the United States was unable to demonstrate a relationship between cell phone use and glioma or meningioma.

- Some case-control studies in Sweden found statistically significant trends of increasing brain cancer risk for the total amount of cell phone use and the years of use among people who began using cell phones before age 20. However, another large, case-control study in Sweden did not find an increased risk of brain cancer among people between the ages of 20 and 69. In addition, the international CEFALO study, which compared children who were diagnosed with brain cancer between ages 7 and 19 with similar children who were not, found no relationship between their cell phone use and risk for brain cancer.

- NCI's Surveillance, Epidemiology, and End Results (SEER) Program, which tracks cancer incidence in the United States over time, found no increase in the incidence of brain or other central nervous system cancers between 1987 and 2007, despite the dramatic increase in cell phone use in this country during that time. Similarly, incidence data from Denmark, Finland, Norway, and Sweden for the period 1974–2008 revealed no increase in age-adjusted incidence of brain tumors. A 2012 study by NCI researchers, which compared observed glioma incidence rates in SEER with projected rates based on risks observed in the Interphone study, found that the projected rates were consistent with observed U.S. rates. The researchers also compared the SEER rates with projected rates based on a Swedish study published in 2011. They determined that the projected rates were at least 40 percent higher than, and incompatible with, the actual U.S. rates.

- Studies of workers exposed to radiofrequency energy have shown no evidence of increased risk of brain tumors among U.S. Navy electronics technicians, aviation technicians, or fire control technicians, those working in an electromagnetic pulse test program, plastic-ware workers, cellular phone manufacturing workers, or Navy personnel with a high probability of exposure to radar.

Why are the findings from different studies of cell phone use and cancer risk inconsistent?

A limited number of studies have shown some evidence of statistical association of cell phone use and brain tumor risks, but most studies have found no association. Reasons for these discrepancies include the following:

- **Recall bias,** which may happen when a study collects data about prior habits and exposures using questionnaires administered after disease has been diagnosed in some of the study participants. It is possible that study participants who have brain tumors may remember their cell phone use differently than individuals without brain tumors. Many epidemiologic studies of cell phone use and brain cancer risk lack verifiable data about the total amount of cell phone use over time. In addition, people who develop a brain tumor may have a tendency to recall using their cell phone mostly on the same side of their head where the tumor was found, regardless of whether they actually used their phone on that side of their head a lot or only a little.

95

- **Inaccurate reporting**, which may happen when people say that something has happened more or less often than it actually did. People may not remember how much they used cell phones in a given time period.

- **Morbidity and mortality** among study participants who have brain cancer. Gliomas are particularly difficult to study, for example, because of their high death rate and the short survival of people who develop these tumors. Patients who survive initial treatment are often impaired, which may affect their responses to questions. Furthermore, for people who have died, next-of-kin are often less familiar with the cell phone use patterns of their deceased family member and may not accurately describe their patterns of use to an interviewer.

- **Participation bias**, which can happen when people who are diagnosed with brain tumors are more likely than healthy people (known as controls) to enroll in a research study. Also, controls who did not or rarely used cell phones were less likely to participate in the Interphone study than controls who used cell phones regularly. For example, the Interphone study reported participation rates of 78 percent for meningioma patients (range 56–92 percent for the individual studies), 64 percent for the glioma patients (range 36–92 percent), and 53 percent for control subjects (range 42–74 percent). One series of Swedish studies reported participation rates of 85 percent in people with brain cancer and 84 percent in control subjects.

- **Changing technology and methods of use**. Older studies evaluated radiofrequency energy exposure from analog cell phones. However, most cell phones today use digital technology, which operates at a different frequency and a lower power level than analog phones. Digital cell phones have been in use for more than a decade in the United States, and cellular technology continues to change. Texting, for example, has become a popular way of using a cell phone to communicate that does not require bringing the phone close to the head. Furthermore, the use of hands-free technology, such as wired and wireless headsets, is increasing and may decrease radiofrequency energy exposure to the head and brain.

What do expert organizations conclude?

The International Agency for Research on Cancer (IARC), a component of the World Health Organization, has recently classified

96

radiofrequency fields as "possibly carcinogenic to humans," based on limited evidence from human studies, limited evidence from studies of radiofrequency energy and cancer in rodents, and weak mechanistic evidence (from studies of genotoxicity, effects on immune system function, gene and protein expression, cell signaling, oxidative stress, and apoptosis, along with studies of the possible effects of radiofrequency energy on the blood-brain barrier).

The American Cancer Society (ACS) states that the IARC classification means that there could be some risk associated with cancer, but the evidence is not strong enough to be considered causal and needs to be investigated further. Individuals who are concerned about radiofrequency exposure can limit their exposure, including using an ear piece and limiting cell phone use, particularly among children.

The National Institute of Environmental Health Sciences (NIEHS) states that the weight of the current scientific evidence has not conclusively linked cell phone use with any adverse health problems, but more research is needed.

The U.S. Food and Drug Administration (FDA), which is responsible for regulating the safety of machines and devices that emit radiation (including cell phones), notes that studies reporting biological changes associated with radiofrequency energy have failed to be replicated and that the majority of human epidemiologic studies have failed to show a relationship between exposure to radiofrequency energy from cell phones and health problems.

The U.S. Centers for Disease Control and Prevention (CDC) states that, although some studies have raised concerns about the possible risks of cell phone use, scientific research as a whole does not support a statistically significant association between cell phone use and health effects.

The Federal Communications Commission (FCC) concludes that there is no scientific evidence that proves that wireless phone use can lead to cancer or to other health problems, including headaches, dizziness, or memory loss.

Do children have a higher risk of developing cancer due to cell phone use than adults?

In theory, children have the potential to be at greater risk than adults for developing brain cancer from cell phones. Their nervous systems are still developing and therefore more vulnerable to factors that may cause cancer. Their heads are smaller than those of adults and therefore have a greater proportional exposure to the field of radiofrequency radiation that is emitted by cell phones. And children have the potential of accumulating more years of cell phone exposure than adults do.

So far, the data from studies in children with cancer do not support this theory. The first published analysis came from a large case-control study called CEFALO, which was conducted in Denmark, Sweden, Norway, and Switzerland. The study included children who were diagnosed with brain tumors between 2004 and 2008, when their ages ranged from 7 to 19. Researchers did not find an association between cell phone use and brain tumor risk in this group of children. However, they noted that their results did not rule out the possibility of a slight increase in brain cancer risk among children who use cell phones, and that data gathered through prospective studies and objective measurements, rather than participant surveys and recollections, will be key in clarifying whether there is an increased risk.

Researchers from the Centre for Research in Environmental Epidemiology in Spain are conducting another international study— Mobi-Kids —to evaluate the risk associated with new communications technologies (including cell phones) and other environmental factors in young people newly diagnosed with brain tumors at ages 10 to 24 years.

What can cell phone users do to reduce their exposure to radiofrequency energy?

The FDA and FCC have suggested some steps that concerned cell phone users can take to reduce their exposure to radiofrequency energy:

- Reserve the use of cell phones for shorter conversations or for times when a landline phone is not available.

- Use a hands-free device, which places more distance between the phone and the head of the user.

Hands-free kits reduce the amount of radiofrequency energy exposure to the head because the antenna, which is the source of energy, is not placed against the head.

Where can I find more information about radiofrequency energy from my cell phone?

The FCC provides information about the specific absorption rate (SAR) of cell phones produced and marketed within the last 1 to 2 years. The SAR corresponds with the relative amount of radiofrequency energy absorbed by the head of a cell phone user. [Consumers can access this information using the phone's FCC ID number, which is usually located on the case of the phone, and the FCC's ID search form.]

What are other sources of radiofrequency energy?

The most common exposures to radiofrequency energy are from telecommunications devices and equipment. In the United States, cell phones currently operate in a frequency range of about 1,800 to 2,200 megahertz (MHz). In this range, the electromagnetic radiation produced is in the form of non-ionizing radiofrequency energy.

Cordless phones (phones that have a base unit connected to the telephone wiring in a house) often operate at radio frequencies similar to those of cell phones; however, since cordless phones have a limited range and require a nearby base, their signals are generally much less powerful than those of cell phones.

Among other radiofrequency energy sources, AM/FM radios and VHF/UHF televisions operate at lower radio frequencies than cell phones, whereas sources such as radar, satellite stations, magnetic resonance imaging (MRI) devices, industrial equipment, and microwave ovens operate at somewhat higher radio frequencies.

How common is brain cancer? Has the incidence of brain cancer changed over time?

Brain cancer incidence and mortality (death) rates have changed little in the past decade. In the United States, 23,130 new diagnoses and 14,080 deaths from brain cancer are estimated for 2013.

The 5-year relative survival for brain cancers diagnosed from 2003 through 2009 was 35 percent. This is the percentage of people diagnosed with brain cancer who will still be alive 5 years after diagnosis compared with the survival of a person of the same age and sex who does not have cancer.

The risk of developing brain cancer increases with age. From 2006 through 2010, there were fewer than 5 brain cancer cases for every 100,000 people in the United States under age 65, compared with approximately 19 cases for every 100,000 people in the United States who were ages 65 or older.

Chapter 14

Magnetic Field Exposure and Cancer

What are electric and magnetic fields?

Electric and magnetic fields are invisible areas of energy that are produced by electricity, which is the movement of electrons, or current, through a wire.

An electric field is produced by voltage, which is the pressure used to push the electrons through the wire, much like water being pushed through a pipe. As the voltage increases, the electric field increases in strength.

A magnetic field results from the flow of current through wires or electrical devices and increases in strength as the current increases. The strength of a magnetic field decreases rapidly with increased distance from its source.

Electric fields are produced whether or not a device is turned on, but magnetic fields are produced only when current is flowing, which usually requires a device to be turned on. Power lines produce magnetic fields continuously because current is always flowing through them.

Electric and magnetic fields together are referred to as electromagnetic fields, or EMFs. There are both natural and human-made sources of EMFs. The earth's magnetic field, which causes a compass to

Text in this chapter is excerpted from "Magnetic Field Exposure and Cancer," National Cancer Institute at the National Institutes of Health (NIH), November 3, 2014.

point North, is an example of a naturally occurring EMF. Power lines, wiring, and electrical appliances, such as electric shavers, hair dryers, computers, televisions, and electric blankets produce what are called extremely low frequency (ELF) EMFs. ELF-EMFs have frequencies of up to 300 cycles per second, or Hertz (Hz); for example, the frequency of alternating current in power lines is 50 or 60 Hz. Cell phones produce radiofrequency EMFs above the ELF range.

Electric fields are easily shielded or weakened by walls and other objects, whereas magnetic fields can pass through buildings, living things, and most other materials. Consequently, magnetic fields are the component of ELF-EMFs that are usually studied in relation to their possible health effects.

Why are ELF-EMFs studied in relation to cancer?

Any possible health effects of ELF-EMFs would be of concern because power lines and electrical appliances are present everywhere in modern life, and people are constantly encountering these fields, both in their homes and in certain workplaces. Also, the presence of ELF-EMFs in homes means that children are exposed. Even if ELF-EMFs were to increase an individual's risk of disease only slightly, widespread exposure to ELF-EMFs could translate to meaningful increased risks at the population level.

Several early epidemiologic studies raised the possibility of an association between certain cancers, especially childhood cancers, and ELF-EMFs. Most subsequent studies have not shown such an association, but scientists have continued to investigate the possibility that one exists.

No mechanism by which ELF-EMFs could cause cancer has been identified. Unlike high-energy (ionizing) radiation, ELF-EMFs are low energy and non-ionizing and cannot damage DNA or cells directly. Some scientists have speculated that ELF-EMFs could cause cancer through other mechanisms, such as by reducing levels of the hormone melatonin. (There is some evidence that melatonin may suppress the development of certain tumors.) However, studies of animals exposed to ELF-EMFs have not provided any indications that ELF-EMF exposure is associated with cancer.

What is the evidence for an association between magnetic field exposure and cancer in children?

Numerous epidemiologic studies and comprehensive reviews of the scientific literature have evaluated possible associations between exposure to ELF magnetic fields and risk of cancer in children. Most of the research has focused on leukemia and brain tumors, the two most common cancers in children. Studies have examined associations of these cancers with living near power lines, with magnetic fields in the home, and with exposure of parents to high levels of magnetic fields in the workplace.

Exposure from power lines

Although a study in 1979 pointed to a possible association between living near electric power lines and childhood leukemia, more recent studies have had mixed findings. Currently, researchers conclude that there is little evidence that exposure to ELF-EMFs from power lines causes leukemia, brain tumors, or any other cancers in children.

Exposure in homes

Many studies have also looked for possible associations between magnetic fields measured in homes and residences and the risk of childhood cancers, especially leukemia. Individual studies have had varying results, but most have not found an association or have found it only for those children who lived in homes with very high levels of magnetic fields, which are present in few residences.

To develop the most accurate estimates of the risks of leukemia in children from magnetic fields in the home, researchers have analyzed the combined data from many studies. In one such analysis that combined data from nine studies done in several countries, leukemia risk was increased only in those children with the highest exposure (a category that included less than 1 percent of the children); these children had a twofold excess risk of childhood leukemia. In another analysis that combined data from 15 individual studies, a similar increase in risk was seen in children with the highest exposure level. A more recent analysis of seven studies published after 2000 found a similar trend, but the increase was not statistically significant.

Overall, these analyses suggest that if there is any increase in leukemia risk from magnetic fields, it is restricted to children with the very highest exposure levels. But it is possible that this increase is not real, because if magnetic fields caused childhood leukemia, certain patterns would have been found, such as increasing risk with increasing levels of magnetic field exposure. Such patterns were not seen.

Another way that people can be exposed to magnetic fields in the home is from household electrical appliances. Although magnetic fields near many electrical appliances are higher than those near power lines, appliances contribute less to a person's total exposure to magnetic fields because most appliances are used only for short periods of time. Again, studies have not found consistent evidence for an association between the use of household electrical appliances and risk of childhood leukemia.

Parental exposure and risk in children

Several studies have examined possible associations between maternal or paternal exposure to high levels of magnetic fields before conception and/or during pregnancy and the risk of cancer in their future children. The results to date have been inconsistent. Studies are ongoing to evaluate this question.

Exposure and cancer survival

A few studies have investigated whether magnetic field exposure is associated with prognosis or survival of children with leukemia. Several small retrospective studies of this question have yielded inconsistent results. An analysis that combined prospective data for more than 3000 children with acute lymphoid leukemia from eight countries showed that ELF magnetic field exposure was not associated with their survival or risk of relapse.

What is the evidence that magnetic field exposure is linked to cancer in adults?

Although some studies have reported associations between ELF-EMF exposure and cancer in adults, other studies have not found evidence for such associations.

The majority of epidemiologic studies have shown no relationship between breast cancer in women and exposure to ELF-EMFs in the home, although several individual studies have shown hints of an association.

Several studies conducted in the 1980s and early 1990s reported that people who worked in some electrical occupations (such as power station operators and phone line workers) had higher-than-expected rates of some types of cancer, particularly leukemia, brain tumors, and male breast cancer. Some occupational studies showed very small increases in the risks of leukemia and brain cancer, but these results were based on participants' job titles and not on actual measurements of their exposures. More recent studies, including some that considered the participant's job title as well as measurements of their exposures, have not shown consistent findings of an increasing risk of leukemia, brain tumors, or female breast cancer with increasing exposure to magnetic fields at work.

Chapter 15

Accidents at Nuclear Power Plants and Cancer Risk

What is ionizing radiation?

Ionizing radiation consists of subatomic particles (that is, particles that are smaller than an atom, such as protons, neutrons, and electrons) and electromagnetic waves. These particles and waves have enough energy to strip electrons from, or ionize, atoms in molecules that they strike. Ionizing radiation can arise in a number of ways, including the following:

- From the spontaneous decay (breakdown) of unstable isotopes. Unstable isotopes, which are also called radioactive isotopes, give off, or emit, ionizing radiation as part of the decay process. Radioactive isotopes occur naturally in the Earth's crust, soil, atmosphere, and oceans. These isotopes are also produced in nuclear reactors and nuclear weapons explosions.

- From cosmic rays originating in the sun and other extraterrestrial sources and from technological devices ranging from dental and medical x-ray machines to the picture tubes of old-style televisions.

Text in this chapter is excerpted from "Accidents at Nuclear Power Plants and Cancer Risk," National Cancer Institute at the National Institutes of Health (NIH), April 19, 2011.

107

Everyone on Earth is exposed to low levels of ionizing radiation from natural and technological sources in varying proportions, depending on their geographic location, diet, occupation, and lifestyle.

At high doses, ionizing radiation can cause immediate damage to a person's body, including radiation sickness and death. Ionizing radiation is also a carcinogen, even at low doses; it causes cancer primarily because it damages DNA. However, the lower the dose of ionizing radiation, the lower the chances of harm.

Children and adolescents are more sensitive to the cancer-causing effects of ionizing radiation than adults because their bodies are still growing and developing. In addition, children and adolescents usually have more years of life following radiation exposure during which cancer may develop.

What cancer risks are associated with nuclear power plant accidents?

Nuclear power plants use energy released by the decay of certain radioactive isotopes to produce electricity. Additional radioactive isotopes are produced during this process. In nuclear power plants, specially designed fuel rods and containment structures enclose the radioactive materials to prevent them, and the ionizing radiation they produce, from contaminating the environment. If the fuel and surrounding containment structures are severely damaged, radioactive materials and ionizing radiation may be released, potentially posing a health risk for people. The actual risk depends on several factors:

- The specific radioactive materials, or isotopes, released, and the quantities released.

- How a person comes into contact with the released radioactive materials (such as through contaminated food, water, air, or on the skin).

- The person's age (those exposed at younger ages are generally at higher risk).

- The duration and amount of the exposure.

The radioactive isotopes released in nuclear power plant accidents include I-131 and Cs-137. In the most severe kinds of accidents, such as the Chernobyl accident in 1986, other dangerous radioactive isotopes, such as strontium-90 (Sr-90) and plutonium-239, may also be released.

Human exposure to I-131 released from nuclear power plant accidents comes mainly from consuming contaminated water, milk, or foods. People may also be exposed by breathing dust particles in the air that are contaminated with I-131.

Inside the body, I-131 accumulates in the thyroid gland, which is an organ in the neck. The thyroid gland uses iodine to produce hormones that control how quickly the body uses energy. Because the thyroid does not distinguish between I-131 and nonradioactive iodine, the thyroid gland will accumulate either form. Exposure to radioactive iodine may increase the risk of thyroid cancer many years later, especially for children and adolescents.

Exposure to Cs-137 can be external to the body or internal. External exposure comes from walking on contaminated soil or coming into contact with contaminated materials at nuclear accident sites. Internal exposure can come from breathing particles in the air that contain Cs-137, such as dust originating from contaminated soil, or ingesting contaminated water or foods. Because Cs-137 is not concentrated in a particular tissue, the ionizing radiation that it releases can expose all tissues and organs of the body.

How have researchers learned about cancer risks from nuclear power plant accidents?

Much of what is known about cancer caused by radiation exposures from nuclear power plant accidents comes from research on the April 1986 nuclear power plant disaster at Chernobyl, in what is now Ukraine. The radioactive isotopes released during the Chernobyl accident included I-131, Cs-137, and Sr-90.

Approximately 600 workers at the power plant during the emergency received very high doses of radiation and suffered from radiation sickness. All of those who received more than 6 grays (Gy) of radiation became very sick right away and subsequently died. Those who received less than 4 Gy had a better chance of survival. (A Gy is a measure of the amount of radiation absorbed by a person's body.)

Hundreds of thousands of people who worked as part of the cleanup crews in the years after the accident were exposed to lower external doses of ionizing radiation, ranging from approximately 0.14 Gy in 1986 to 0.04 Gy in 1989. In this group of people, there was an increased risk of leukemia.

Approximately 6.5 million residents of the contaminated areas surrounding Chernobyl received much lower amounts of radiation. From 1986 through 2005, these people received an accumulated average dose of 0.0092 Gy from external and internal sources of radiation. Children and adolescents exposed to I-131 showed an increased risk of developing thyroid cancer.

How long after exposure to I-131 is the risk of thyroid cancer increased?

Although the time it takes for the radiation to decrease by half (the half-life) of I-131 is only 8 days, the damage it causes can increase the risk of thyroid cancer for many years after the initial exposure.

A study led by National Cancer Institute (NCI) researchers followed more than 12,500 people who were younger than age 18 at the time they were exposed to high doses of I-131 (0.65 Gy on average) from the Chernobyl accident. A total of 65 new cases of thyroid cancer were found in this population between 1998 and 2007. Roughly half of these new cases were attributed to I-131 exposure. The researchers found that the higher a person's dose of I-131, the more likely they were to get thyroid cancer (with each Gy of exposure associated with a doubling of risk). They also found that this risk remained high for at least 20 years.

What should cancer patients do if they live in an area that may be contaminated due to a nuclear power plant accident?

Cancer patients who are being treated with systemic chemotherapy or radiation therapy should be evacuated from the area where a nuclear power plant accident has occurred so their medical treatment can continue without interruption. Patients should always keep a record of the treatments they have had in the past and that they may be currently receiving, including the names of any drugs and their doses. These records may be important in the aftermath not only of a nuclear power plant accident but also of other large-scale events that may disrupt medical services, when medical records may be lost.

Local or national authorities may also advise certain people (newborns, infants, children, adolescents, and women who are pregnant) in areas with high I-131 contamination to take potassium iodide (KI) to prevent the accumulation of I-131 in their thyroid. KI should not pose a danger to someone who previously received radiation therapy or chemotherapy. Patients who are actively being treated for cancer and who are advised to take KI should consult with their doctor before taking the medication, so their doctor can evaluate their treatment plan and their health status, including their nutritional status, to determine the safety of KI treatment for them.

Chapter 16

Radon and Cancer

What is radon?

Radon is a radioactive gas released from the normal decay of the elements uranium, thorium, and radium in rocks and soil. It is an invisible, odorless, tasteless gas that seeps up through the ground and diffuses into the air. In a few areas, depending on local geology, radon dissolves into ground water and can be released into the air when the water is used. Radon gas usually exists at very low levels outdoors. However, in areas without adequate ventilation, such as underground mines, radon can accumulate to levels that substantially increase the risk of lung cancer.

How is the general population exposed to radon?

Radon is present in nearly all air. Everyone breathes in radon every day, usually at very low levels. However, people who inhale high levels of radon are at an increased risk of developing lung cancer.

Radon can enter homes through cracks in floors, walls, or foundations, and collect indoors. It can also be released from building materials, or from water obtained from wells that contain radon. Radon levels can be higher in homes that are well insulated, tightly sealed, and/or built on soil rich in the elements uranium, thorium, and radium. Basement and first floors typically have the highest radon levels because of their closeness to the ground.

Text in this chapter is excerpted from "Radon and Cancer," National Cancer Institute at the National Institutes of Health (NIH), December 6, 2011.

How does radon cause cancer?

Radon decays quickly, giving off tiny radioactive particles. When inhaled, these radioactive particles can damage the cells that line the lung. Long-term exposure to radon can lead to lung cancer, the only cancer proven to be associated with inhaling radon. There has been a suggestion of increased risk of leukemia associated with radon exposure in adults and children; however, the evidence is not conclusive.

How many people develop lung cancer because of exposure to radon?

Cigarette smoking is the most common cause of lung cancer. Radon represents a far smaller risk for this disease, but it is the second leading cause of lung cancer in the United States. Scientists estimate that 15,000 to 22,000 lung cancer deaths in the United States each year are related to radon.

Exposure to the combination of radon gas and cigarette smoke creates a greater risk of lung cancer than exposure to either factor alone. The majority of radon-related cancer deaths occur among smokers. However, it is estimated that more than 10 percent of radon-related cancer deaths occur among nonsmokers.

How did scientists discover that radon plays a role in the development of lung cancer?

Radon was identified as a health problem when scientists noted that underground uranium miners who were exposed to it died of lung cancer at high rates. The results of miner studies have been confirmed by experimental animal studies, which show higher rates of lung tumors among rodents exposed to high radon levels.

What have scientists learned about the relationship between radon and lung cancer?

Scientists agree that radon causes lung cancer in humans. Recent research has focused on specifying the effect of residential radon on lung cancer risk. In these studies, scientists measure radon levels in the homes of people who have lung cancer and compare them to the levels of radon in the homes of people who have not developed lung cancer.

Researchers have combined and analyzed data from all radon studies conducted in Canada and the United States. By combining the data from these studies, scientists were able to analyze data from thousands of people. The results of this analysis demonstrated a slightly increased risk of lung cancer for individuals with elevated exposure to household radon. This increased risk was consistent with the estimated level of risk based on studies of underground miners.

Techniques to measure a person's exposure to radon over time have become more precise, thanks to a number of studies carried out in the 1990s and early 2000s.

How can people know if they have an elevated level of radon in their homes?

Testing is the only way to know if a person's home has elevated radon levels. Indoor radon levels are affected by the soil composition under and around the house, and the ease with which radon enters the house. Homes that are next door to each other can have different indoor radon levels, making a neighbor's test result a poor predictor of radon risk. In addition, rain or snow, barometric pressure, and other influences can cause radon levels to vary from month to month or day to day, which is why both short- and long-term tests are available.

Short-term detectors measure radon levels for 2 days to 90 days, depending on the device. Long-term tests determine the average concentration for more than 90 days. Because radon levels can vary from day to day and month to month, a long-term test is a better indicator of the average radon level. Both tests are relatively easy to use and inexpensive. A state or local radon official can explain the differences between testing devices and recommend the most appropriate test for a person's needs and conditions.

The U.S. Environmental Protection Agency (EPA) recommends taking action to reduce radon in homes that have a radon level at or above 4 picocuries per liter (pCi/L) of air. About 1 in 15 U.S. homes is estimated to have radon levels at or above this EPA action level. Scientists estimate that lung cancer deaths could be reduced by 2 to 4 percent, or about 5,000 deaths, by lowering radon levels in homes exceeding the EPA's action level.

The EPA has more information about residential radon exposure and what people can do about it in the Consumer's Guide to Radon Reduction.

Chapter 17

Cancer Prevention Overview

What Is Prevention?

Cancer prevention is action taken to lower the chance of getting cancer. In 2014, about 1.6 million people will be diagnosed with cancer in the United States. In addition to the physical problems and emotional distress caused by cancer, the high costs of care are also a burden to patients, their families, and to the public. By preventing cancer, the number of new cases of cancer is lowered. Hopefully, this will reduce the burden of cancer and lower the number of deaths caused by cancer.

Cancer is not a single disease but a group of related diseases. Many things in our genes, our lifestyle, and the environment around us may increase or decrease our risk of getting cancer.

Scientists are studying many different ways to help prevent cancer, including the following:

- Ways to avoid or control things known to cause cancer.

- Changes in diet and lifestyle.

- Finding precancerous conditions early. Precancerous conditions are conditions that may become cancer.

- Chemoprevention (medicines to treat a precancerous condition or to keep cancer from starting).

Text in this chapter is excerpted from "Cancer Prevention Overview," National Cancer Institute at the National Institutes of Health (NIH), April 17, 2014.

Carcinogenesis

Carcinogenesis is the process in which normal cells turn into cancer cells.

Carcinogenesis is the series of steps that take place as a normal cell becomes a cancer cell. Cells are the smallest units of the body and they make up the body's tissues. Each cell contains genes that guide the way the body grows, develops, and repairs itself. There are many genes that control whether a cell lives or dies, divides (multiplies), or takes on special functions, such as becoming a nerve cell or a muscle cell.

Changes (mutations) in genes occur during carcinogenesis.

Changes (mutations) in genes can cause normal controls in cells to break down. When this happens, cells do not die when they should and new cells are produced when the body does not need them. The buildup of extra cells may cause a mass (tumor) to form.

Tumors can be benign or malignant (cancerous). Malignant tumor cells invade nearby tissues and spread to other parts of the body. Benign tumor cells do not invade nearby tissues or spread.

Interventions That Are Known To Lower Cancer Risk

An intervention is a treatment or action taken to prevent or treat disease, or improve health in other ways. Many studies are being done to find ways to keep cancer from starting or recurring (coming back).

Chemoprevention is being studied in patients who have a high risk of developing cancer.

Chemoprevention is the use of substances to lower the risk of cancer, or keep it from recurring. The substances may be natural or made in the laboratory. Some chemo preventive agents are tested in people who are at high risk for a certain type of cancer. The risk may be because of a precancerous condition, family history, or lifestyle factors.

Some chemoprevention studies have shown good results. For example, selective estrogen receptor modulators (SERMS) such as tamoxifen or raloxifene have been shown to reduce the risk of breast cancer in women at high risk. Finasteride and dutasteride have been shown to reduce the risk of prostate cancer.

New ways to prevent cancer are being studied in clinical trials.

Chemoprevention agents that are being studied in clinical trials include COX-2 inhibitors. They are being studied for the prevention of colorectal and breast cancer. Aspirin is being studied for the prevention of colorectal cancer. Clinical trials are taking place in many parts of the country.

Interventions That Are Not Known To Lower Cancer Risk

Vitamin and dietary supplements have not been shown to prevent cancer.

An intervention is a treatment or action taken to prevent or treat disease, or improve health in other ways.

There is not enough proof that taking multivitamin and mineral supplements or single vitamins or minerals can prevent cancer. The following vitamins and mineral supplements have been studied, but have not been shown to lower the risk of cancer:

- Vitamin B6.

- Vitamin B12.

- Vitamin E.

- Vitamin C.

- Beta carotene.

- Folic acid.

- Selenium.

- Vitamin D.

The Selenium and Vitamin E Cancer Prevention Trial (SELECT) found that vitamin E taken alone increased the risk of prostate cancer. The risk continued even after the men stopped taking vitamin E. Taking selenium with vitamin E or taking selenium alone did not increase the risk of prostate cancer.

Vitamin D has also been studied to see if it has anticancer effects. Skin exposed to sunshine can make vitamin D. Vitamin D can also be consumed in the diet and in dietary supplements. Taking vitamin D in doses from 400–1100 IU / day has not been shown to lower the risk of cancer.

The Vitamin D and OmegA-3 TriaL (VITAL) is under way to study whether taking vitamin D (2000 IU/ day) and omega-3 fatty acids from marine (oily fish) sources lowers the risk of cancer.

The Physicians' Health Study found that men who have had cancer in the past and take a multivitamin daily may have a slightly lower risk of having a second cancer.

Chapter 18

Diet Factors

Chapter Contents

Section 18.1

Guide to Healthy Eating and Cooking Methods

This section includes excerpts from "Down Home Healthy Cooking,"
National Cancer Institute at the National Institutes of Health (NIH);
and text from "Cruciferous Vegetables and Cancer Prevention,"
National Cancer Institute at the National Institutes of Health (NIH),
June 7, 2012.

Table 18.1. The Right Food

Instead of This:	Use This:
Ham hocks and fat back	Turkey thighs
Pork bacon	Turkey bacon, lean ham, Canadian bacon
Lard, butter, or other hard fats	Small amount of vegetable oil
Pork sausage	Ground turkey breast
Ground beef and pork	Smoked turkey neck
Neck bone	Skinless chicken thighs
Regular bouillons and broths	Low sodium bouillon and broths
Cream	Evaporated skim milk
Regular cheese	Low fat or lite cheese
High fat cut of beef*	Top round, eye of round, round steak, rump roast, sirloin tip, chuck arm, pot roast, short loin, extra lean ground beef
High fat cut of pork*	Tenderloin, sirloin roast or chop, center cut loin chops
High fat cut of lamb*	Foreshank, leg roast, leg chop, loin chop

* Sometimes less tender cuts of meat like round or rump need marinating. To add flavor and tenderize, use an oil-free marinade. Place meat and marinade in a plastic bag and marinate for 1 to 2 hours in the refrigerator. Throw away the marinade. Don't use it for basing while cooking the meat.

Healthy cooking techniques

- Steam your vegetables whenever you can. Use garlic, onions, and herbs for flavor. Use very small amounts of butter, cheese, and sauces.

- Use more herbs and spices to flavor greens and other dishes. Cut down on the salt. Try adding Spanish onion and black pepper to black-eyed peas.

- Always use low-fat (1% or 2%) or skim milk for cooking instead of whole milk or cream.

- Put away that deep fat fryer. Try boiling, roasting, baking, grilling, braising, or stir-frying with a little oil instead.

What are cruciferous vegetables?

Cruciferous vegetables are part of the Brassica genus of plants. They include the following vegetables, among others:

- Arugula
- Bok choy
- Broccoli
- Brussels sprouts
- Cabbage
- Cauliflower
- Collard greens
- Horseradish
- Kale
- Radishes
- Rutabaga
- Turnips
- Watercress
- Wasabi

Why are cancer researchers studying cruciferous vegetables?

Cruciferous vegetables are rich in nutrients, including several carotenoids (beta-carotene, lutein, zeaxanthin); vitamins C, E, and K; folate; and minerals. They also are a good fiber source.

In addition, cruciferous vegetables contain a group of substances known as glucosinolates, which are sulfur-containing chemicals. These chemicals are responsible for the pungent aroma and bitter flavor of cruciferous vegetables.

During food preparation, chewing, and digestion, the glucosinolates in cruciferous vegetables are broken down to form biologically active compounds such as indoles, nitriles, thiocyanates, and isothiocyanates. Indole-3-carbinol (an indole) and sulforaphane (an isothiocyanate) have been most frequently examined for their anticancer effects.

Indoles and isothiocyanates have been found to inhibit the development of cancer in several organs in rats and mice, including the bladder, breast, colon, liver, lung, and stomach. Studies in animals and experiments with cells grown in the laboratory have identified several potential ways in which these compounds may help prevent cancer:

- They help protect cells from DNA damage.

- They help inactivate carcinogens.

- They have antiviral and antibacterial effects.

- They have anti-inflammatory effects.

- They induce cell death (apoptosis).

- They inhibit tumor blood vessel formation (angiogenesis) and tumor cell migration (needed for metastasis).

Studies in humans, however, have shown mixed results.

Is there evidence that cruciferous vegetables can help reduce cancer risk in people?

Researchers have investigated possible associations between intake of cruciferous vegetables and the risk of cancer. The evidence has been reviewed by various experts. Key studies regarding four common forms of cancer are described briefly below.

- Prostate cancer: Cohort studies in the Netherlands, United States, and Europe have examined a wide range of daily cruciferous vegetable intakes and found little or no association with prostate cancer risk. However, some case-control studies have found that people who ate greater amounts of cruciferous vegetables had a lower risk of prostate cancer.

- Colorectal cancer: Cohort studies in the United States and the Netherlands have generally found no association between cruciferous vegetable intake and colorectal cancer risk. The exception is one study in the Netherlands—the Netherlands Cohort Study on Diet and Cancer—in which women (but not men) who had a high intake of cruciferous vegetables had a reduced risk of colon (but not rectal) cancer.

- Lung cancer: Cohort studies in Europe, the Netherlands, and the United States have had varying results. Most studies have reported little association, but one U.S. analysis—using data from the Nurses' Health Study and the Health Professionals' Follow-up Study—showed that women who ate more than 5 servings of cruciferous vegetables per week had a lower risk of lung cancer.

- Breast cancer: One case-control study found that women who ate greater amounts of cruciferous vegetables had a lower risk of breast cancer. A meta-analysis of studies conducted in the United States, Canada, Sweden, and the Netherlands found no association between cruciferous vegetable intake and breast cancer risk. An additional cohort study of women in the United States similarly showed only a weak association with breast cancer risk.

A few studies have shown that the bioactive components of cruciferous vegetables can have beneficial effects on biomarkers of cancer-related processes in people. For example, one study found that indole-3-carbinol was more effective than placebo in reducing the growth of abnormal cells on the surface of the cervix.

In addition, several case-control studies have shown that specific forms of the gene that encodes glutathione S-transferase, which is the enzyme that metabolizes and helps eliminate isothiocyanates from the body, may influence the association between cruciferous vegetable intake and human lung and colorectal cancer risk.

Are cruciferous vegetables part of a healthy diet?

The federal government's Dietary Guidelines for Americans 2010 recommend consuming a variety of vegetables each day. Different vegetables are rich in different nutrients.

Vegetables are categorized into five subgroups: dark-green, red and orange, beans and peas (legumes), starchy, and other vegetables. Cruciferous vegetables fall into the "dark-green vegetables" category and the "other vegetables" category. More information about vegetables and diet, including how much of these foods should be eaten daily or weekly, is available from the U.S. Department of Agriculture website Choose My Plate.

Higher consumption of vegetables in general may protect against some diseases, including some types of cancer. However, when researchers try to distinguish cruciferous vegetables from other foods in the diet, it can be challenging to get clear results because study participants may have trouble remembering precisely what they ate. Also, people who eat cruciferous vegetables may be more likely than people who don't to have other healthy behaviors that reduce disease risk. It is also possible that some people, because of their genetic background, metabolize dietary isothiocyanates differently. However, research has not yet revealed a specific group of people who, because of their genetics, benefit more than other people from eating cruciferous vegetables.

Section 18.2

Antioxidants and Cancer Prevention

Text in this section is excerpted from "Antioxidants and Cancer Prevention," National Cancer Institute at the National Institutes of Health (NIH), January 16, 2014.

What are free radicals, and do they play a role in cancer development?

Free radicals are highly reactive chemicals that have the potential to harm cells. They are created when an atom or a molecule (a chemical that has two or more atoms) either gains or loses an electron (a small negatively charged particle found in atoms). Free radicals are formed naturally in the body and play an important role in many normal cellular processes. At high concentrations, however, free radicals can be hazardous to the body and damage all major components of cells, including DNA, proteins, and cell membranes. The damage to cells caused by free radicals, especially the damage to DNA, may play a role in the development of cancer and other health conditions.

Abnormally high concentrations of free radicals in the body can be caused by exposure to ionizing radiation and other environmental toxins. When ionizing radiation hits an atom or a molecule in a cell, an electron may be lost, leading to the formation of a free radical. The production of abnormally high levels of free radicals is the mechanism by which ionizing radiation kills cells. Moreover, some environmental toxins, such as cigarette smoke, some metals, and high-oxygen atmospheres, may contain large amounts of free radicals or stimulate the body's cells to produce more free radicals.

Free radicals that contain the element oxygen are the most common type of free radicals produced in living tissue. Another name for them is "reactive oxygen species," or "ROS".

What are antioxidants?

Antioxidants are chemicals that interact with and neutralize free radicals, thus preventing them from causing damage. Antioxidants are also known as "free radical scavengers."

The body makes some of the antioxidants it uses to neutralize free radicals. These antioxidants are called endogenous antioxidants. However, the body relies on external (exogenous) sources, primarily the diet, to obtain the rest of the antioxidants it needs. These exogenous antioxidants are commonly called dietary antioxidants. Fruits, vegetables, and grains are rich sources of dietary antioxidants. Some dietary antioxidants are also available as dietary supplements.

Examples of dietary antioxidants include beta-carotene, lycopene, and vitamins A, C, and E (alpha-tocopherol). The mineral element selenium is often thought to be a dietary antioxidant, but the antioxidant effects of selenium are most likely due to the antioxidant activity of proteins that have this element as an essential component (i.e., selenium-containing proteins), and not to selenium itself.

Can antioxidant supplements help prevent cancer?

In laboratory and animal studies, the presence of increased levels of exogenous antioxidants has been shown to prevent the types of free radical damage that have been associated with cancer development. Therefore, researchers have investigated whether taking dietary antioxidant supplements can help lower the risk of developing or dying from cancer in humans.

Many observational studies, including case-control studies and cohort studies, have been conducted to investigate whether the use of dietary antioxidant supplements is associated with reduced risks of cancer in humans. Overall, these studies have yielded mixed results.

Because observational studies cannot adequately control for biases that might influence study outcomes, the results of any individual observational study must be viewed with caution.

Randomized controlled clinical trials, however, lack most of the biases that limit the reliability of observational studies. Therefore, randomized trials are considered to provide the strongest and most reliable evidence of the benefit and/or harm of a health-related intervention. To date, nine randomized controlled trials of dietary antioxidant supplements for cancer prevention have been conducted worldwide. Many of the trials were sponsored by the National Cancer Institute. The results of these nine trials are summarized below:

- **Linxian General Population Nutrition Intervention Trial:** This trial was the first large-scale randomized trial to investigate the effects of antioxidant supplements on cancer risk. In the trial, healthy Chinese men and women at increased risk of developing esophageal cancer and gastric cancer were randomly assigned to take a combination of 15 milligrams (mg) beta-carotene, 30 mg alpha-tocopherol, and 50 micrograms (μg) selenium daily for 5 years or to take no antioxidant supplements. The initial results of the trial showed that people who took antioxidant supplements had a lower risk of death from gastric cancer but not from esophageal cancer. However, their risks of developing gastric cancer and/or esophageal cancer were not affected by antioxidant supplementation.

  In 2009, 15-year results from this trial were reported (10 years after antioxidant supplementation ended). In the updated results, a reduced risk of death from gastric cancer was no longer found for those who took antioxidant supplements compared with those who did not.

- **Alpha-Tocopherol/Beta-Carotene Cancer Prevention Study (ATBC):** This trial investigated whether the use of alpha-tocopherol and/or beta-carotene supplements for 5 to 8 years could help reduce the incidence of lung and other cancers in middle-aged male smokers in Finland. Initial results of the trial, reported in 1994, showed an increase in the incidence of lung cancer among the participants who took beta-carotene supplements (20 mg per day); in contrast, alpha-tocopherol supplementation (50 mg per day) had no effect on lung cancer incidence. Later results showed no effect of beta-carotene or alpha-tocopherol supplementation on the incidence of urothelial (bladder, ureter, or renal pelvis), pancreatic, colorectal, renal cell (kidney), or upper aerodigestive tract (oral/pharyngeal, esophageal, or laryngeal) cancers.

- **Carotene and Retinol Efficacy Trial (CARET):** This U.S. trial examined the effects of daily supplementation with beta-carotene and retinol (vitamin A) on the incidence of lung cancer, other cancers, and death among people who were at high risk of lung cancer because of a history of smoking or exposure to asbestos. The trial began in 1983 and ended in late 1995, 2 years earlier than originally planned. Results reported in 1996 showed that daily supplementation with both 15 mg beta-carotene and 25,000 International Units (IU) retinol was associated with increased lung cancer and increased death from all causes (all-cause mortality). A 2004 report showed that these adverse effects persisted up to 6 years after supplementation ended, although the elevated risks of lung cancer and all-cause mortality were no longer statistically significant. Additional results, reported in 2009, showed that beta-carotene and retinol supplementation had no effect on the incidence of prostate cancer.

- **Physicians' Health Study I (PHS I):** This trial examined the effects of long-term beta-carotene supplementation on cancer incidence, cancer mortality, and all-cause mortality among U.S. male physicians. The results of the study, reported in 1996, showed that beta-carotene supplementation (50 mg every other day for 12 years) had no effect on any of these outcomes in smokers or nonsmokers.

- **Women's Health Study (WHS):** This trial investigated the effects of beta-carotene supplementation (50 mg every other day), vitamin E supplementation (600 IU every other day), and aspirin (100 mg every other day) on the incidence of cancer and cardiovascular disease in U.S. women ages 45 and older. The results, reported in 1999, showed no benefit or harm associated with 2 years of beta-carotene supplementation. In 2005, similar results were reported for vitamin E supplementation.

- **Supplementation en Vitamines et Minéraux Antioxydants (SU.VI.MAX) Study:** This trial investigated the effects of daily supplementation with a combination of antioxidants and minerals on the incidence of cancer and cardiovascular disease in French men and women. The initial results of the study, reported

127

in 2004, showed that daily supplementation with vitamin C (120 mg), vitamin E (30 mg), beta-carotene (6 mg), and the minerals selenium (100 μg) and zinc (20 mg) for a median of 7.5 years had no effect on the incidence of cancer or cardiovascular disease or on all-cause mortality. However, when the data for men and women were analyzed separately, antioxidant and mineral supplementation was associated with lower total cancer incidence and all-cause mortality among men but not among women, and with an increase in skin cancer incidence, including melanoma, among women but not among men. The beneficial effects of the supplements for men disappeared within 5 years of ending supplementation, as did the increased risk of skin cancer among women.

- **Heart Outcomes Prevention Evaluation–The Ongoing Outcomes (HOPE–TOO) Study:** This international trial examined the effects of alpha-tocopherol supplementation on cancer incidence, death from cancer, and the incidence of major cardiovascular events (heart attack, stroke, or death from heart disease) in people diagnosed with cardiovascular disease or diabetes. The results, reported in 2005, showed no effect of daily supplementation with alpha-tocopherol (400 IU) for a median of 7 years on any of the outcomes.

- **Selenium and Vitamin E Cancer Prevention Trial (SELECT):** This U.S. trial investigated whether daily supplementation with selenium (200 μg), vitamin E (400 IU), or both would reduce the incidence of prostate cancer in men ages 50 and older. The study began in 2001 and was stopped in 2008, approximately 5 years earlier than originally planned. Results reported in late 2008 showed that the use of these supplements for a median duration of 5.5 years did not reduce the incidence of prostate or other cancers. Updated findings from the study, reported in 2011, showed that, after an average of 7 years (5.5 years on supplements and 1.5 years off supplements), there were 17 percent more cases of prostate cancer among men taking vitamin E alone than among men taking a placebo. No increase in prostate risk was observed for men assigned to take selenium alone or vitamin E plus selenium compared with men assigned to take a placebo.

- **Physicians' Health Study II (PHS II):** This trial examined whether supplementation with vitamin E, vitamin C, or both would reduce the incidence of cancer in male U.S. physicians ages

50 years and older. The results, reported in 2009, showed that the use of these supplements (400 IU vitamin E every other day, 500 mg vitamin C every day, or a combination of the two) for a median of 7.6 years did not reduce the incidence of prostate cancer or other cancers, including lymphoma, leukemia, melanoma, and cancers of the lung, bladder, pancreas, and colon and rectum.

Overall, these nine randomized controlled clinical trials did not provide evidence that dietary antioxidant supplements are beneficial in primary cancer prevention. In addition, a systematic review of the available evidence regarding the use of vitamin and mineral supplements for the prevention of chronic diseases, including cancer, conducted for the United States Preventive Services Task Force (USPSTF) likewise found no clear evidence of benefit in preventing cancer.

It is possible, however, that the lack of benefit in clinical studies can be explained by differences in the effects of the tested antioxidants when they are consumed as purified chemicals as opposed to when they are consumed in foods, which contain complex mixtures of antioxidants, vitamins, and minerals. Therefore, acquiring a more complete understanding of the antioxidant content of individual foods, how the various antioxidants and other substances in foods interact with one another, and factors that influence the uptake and distribution of food-derived antioxidants in the body are active areas of ongoing cancer prevention research.

Should people already diagnosed with cancer take antioxidant supplements?

Several randomized controlled trials, some including only small numbers of patients, have investigated whether taking antioxidant supplements during cancer treatment alters the effectiveness or reduces the toxicity of specific therapies. Although these trials had mixed results, some found that people who took antioxidant supplements during cancer therapy had worse outcomes, especially if they were smokers.

Additional large randomized controlled trials are needed to provide clear scientific evidence about the potential benefits or harms of taking antioxidant supplements during cancer treatment. Until more is known about the effects of antioxidant supplements in cancer patients, these supplements should be used with caution. Cancer patients should inform their doctors about their use of any dietary supplement.

129

Chapter 19

Cancer Screening

What Is Cancer Screening?

Cancer screening is looking for cancer before a person has any symptoms.

Screening tests can help find cancer at an early stage, before symptoms appear. When abnormal tissue or cancer is found early, it may be easier to treat or cure. By the time symptoms appear, the cancer may have grown and spread. This can make the cancer harder to treat or cure.

It is important to remember that when your 38doctor suggests a screening test, it does not always mean he or she thinks you have cancer. Screening tests are done when you have no cancer symptoms.

There are different kinds of screening tests.

Screening tests include the following:

- Physical exam and history: An exam of the body to check general signs of health, including checking for signs of disease, such as lumps or anything else that seems unusual. A history of the patient's health habits and past illnesses and treatments will also be taken.

- Laboratory tests: Medical procedures that test samples of tissue, blood, urine, or other substances in the body.

Text in this chapter is excerpted from "Cancer Screening Overview," National Cancer Institute at the National Institutes of Health (NIH), July 2, 2014.

- Imaging procedures: Procedures that make pictures of areas inside the body.

- Genetic tests: Tests that look for certain gene mutations (changes) that are linked to some types of cancer.

Screening tests have risks.

Not all screening tests are helpful and most have risks. It is important to know the risks of the test and whether it has been proven to decrease the chance of dying from cancer.

Some screening tests can cause serious problems.

Some screening procedures can cause bleeding or other problems. For example, colon cancer screening with sigmoidoscopy or colonoscopy can cause tears in the lining of the colon.

False-positive test results are possible.

Screening test results may appear to be abnormal even though there is no cancer. A false-positive test result (one that shows there is cancer when there really isn't) can cause anxiety and is usually followed by more tests and procedures, which also have risks.

False-negative test results are possible.

Screening test results may appear to be normal even though there is cancer. A person who receives a false-negative test result (one that shows there is no cancer when there really is) may delay seeking medical care even if there are symptoms.

Finding the cancer may not improve the person's health or help the person live longer.

Some cancers never cause symptoms or become life-threatening, but if found by a screening test, the cancer may be treated. There is no way to know if treating the cancer would help the person live longer than if no treatment were given. In both teenagers and adults, there is an increased risk of suicide in the first year after being diagnosed with cancer. Also, treatments for cancer have side effects.

For some cancers, finding and treating the cancer early does not improve the chance of a cure or help the person live longer.

What Are the Goals of Screening Tests?

Screening tests have many goals.

A screening test that works the way it should and is helpful does the following:

- Finds cancer before symptoms appear.

- Screens for a cancer that is easier to treat and cure when found early.

- Has few false-negative test results and false-positive test results.

- Decreases the chance of dying from cancer.

Screening tests are not meant to diagnose cancer.

Screening tests usually do not diagnose cancer. If a screening test result is abnormal, more tests may be done to check for cancer. For example, a screening mammogram may find a lump in the breast. A lump may be cancer or something else. More tests need to be done to find out if the lump is cancer. These are called diagnostic tests. Diagnostic tests may include a biopsy, in which cells or tissues are removed so a pathologist can check them under a microscope for signs of cancer.

Who Needs to Be Screened?

Certain screening tests may be suggested only for people who have a high risk for certain cancers.

Anything that increases the chance of cancer is called a cancer risk factor. Having a risk factor does not mean that you will get cancer; not having risk factors doesn't mean that you will not get cancer.

Some screening tests are used only for people who have known risk factors for certain types of cancer. People known to have a higher risk of cancer than others include those who:

- Have had cancer in the past; or

- Have two or more first-degree relatives (a parent, brother, or sister) who have had cancer; or

- Have certain gene mutations (changes) that have been linked to cancer.

People who have a high risk of cancer may need to be screened more often or at an earlier age than other people.

Cancer screening research includes finding out who has an increased risk of cancer.

Scientists are trying to better understand who is likely to get certain types of cancer. They study the things we do and the things around us to see if they cause cancer. This information helps doctors figure out who should be screened for cancer, which screening tests should be used, and how often the tests should be done.

Since 1973, the Surveillance, Epidemiology, and End Results (SEER) Program of the National Cancer Institute has been collecting information on people with cancer from different parts of the United States. Information from SEER, research studies, and other sources is used to study who is at risk.

How Is Cancer Risk Measured?

Cancer risk is measured in different ways. The findings from surveys and studies about cancer risk are studied and the results are explained in different ways. Some of the ways risk is explained include absolute risk, relative risk, and odds ratios.

Absolute risk

This is the risk a person has of developing a disease, in a given population (for example, the entire U.S. population) over a certain period of time. Researchers estimate the absolute risk by studying a large number of people that are part of a certain population (for example, women in a given age group). Researchers count the number of people in the group who get a certain disease over a certain period of time. For example, a group of 100,000 women between the ages of 20 and 29 are observed for one year, and 4 of them get breast cancer during that time. This means that the one-year absolute risk of breast cancer for a woman in this age group is 4 in 100,000, or 4 chances in 100,000.

Relative risk

This is often used in research studies to find out whether a trait or a factor can be linked to the risk of a disease. Researchers compare two groups of people who are a lot alike. However, the people in one of the groups must have the trait or factor being studied (they have been "exposed"). The people in the other group do not have it (they have not been exposed). To figure out relative risk, the percentage of people in the exposed group who have the disease is divided by the percentage of people in the unexposed group who have the disease.

Relative risks can be:

- Larger than 1: The trait or factor is linked to an increase in risk.

- Equal to 1: The trait or factor is not linked to risk.

- Less than 1: The trait or factor is linked to a decrease in risk.

Relative risks are also called risk ratios.

Odds ratio

In some types of studies, researchers don't have enough information to figure out relative risks. They use something called an odds ratio instead. An odds ratio can be an estimate of relative risk.

One type of study that uses an odds ratio instead of relative risk is called a case-control study. In a case-control study, two groups of people are compared. However, the individuals in each group are chosen based on whether or not they have a certain disease. Researchers look at the odds that the people in each group were exposed to something (a trait or factor) that might have caused the disease. Odds describes the number of times the trait or factor was present or happened, divided by the number of times it wasn't present or didn't happen. To get an odds ratio, the odds for one group are divided by the odds for the other group.

Odds ratios can be:

- Larger than 1: The trait or factor is linked to an increase in risk.

- Equal to 1: The trait or factor is not linked to risk.

- Less than 1: The trait or factor is linked to a decrease in risk.

Looking at traits and exposures in people with and without cancer can help find possible risk factors. Knowing who is at an increased risk for certain types of cancer can help doctors decide when and how often they should be screened.

Does Screening Help People Live Longer?

Finding some cancers at an early stage (before symptoms appear) may help decrease the chance of dying from those cancers.

For many cancers, the chance of recovery depends on the stage (the amount or spread of cancer in the body) of the cancer when it was diagnosed. Cancers that are diagnosed at earlier stages are often easier to treat or cure.

Studies of cancer screening compare the death rate of people screened for a certain cancer with the death rate from that cancer in people who were not screened. Some screening tests have been shown to be helpful both in finding cancers early and in decreasing the chance of dying from those cancers. Other tests are used because they have been shown to find a certain type of cancer in some people before symptoms appear, but they have not been proven to decrease the risk of dying from that cancer. If a cancer is fast-growing and spreads quickly, finding it early may not help the person survive the cancer.

Screening studies are done to see whether deaths from cancer decrease when people are screened.

When collecting information on how long cancer patients live, some studies define survival as living 5 years after the diagnosis. This is often used to measure how well cancer treatments work. However, to see if screening tests are useful, studies usually look at whether deaths from the cancer decrease in people who were screened. Over time, signs that a cancer screening test is working include:

- An increase in the number of early-stage cancers found.

- A decrease in the number of late-stage cancers found.

- A decrease in the number of deaths from the cancer.

The number of deaths from cancer is lower today than it was in the past. It is not always clear if this is because screening tests found the cancers earlier or because cancer treatments have gotten better, or both. The Surveillance, Epidemiology, and End Results (SEER) Program of the National Cancer Institute collects and reports information on survival times of people with cancer in the United States. This information is studied to see if finding cancer early affects how long these people live.

Certain factors may cause survival times to look like they are getting better when they are not.

These factors include lead-time bias and overdiagnosis.

- **Lead-time bias**
  Survival time for cancer patients is usually measured from the day the cancer is diagnosed until the day they die. Patients are often diagnosed after they have signs and symptoms of cancer. If a screening test leads to a diagnosis before a patient has any symptoms, the patient's survival time is increased because the date of diagnosis is earlier. This increase in survival time makes it seem as though screened patients are living longer when that may not be happening. This is called lead-time bias. It could be that the only reason

the survival time appears to be longer is that the date of diagnosis is earlier for the screened patients. But the screened patients may die at the same time they would have without the screening test.

- **Overdiagnosis**
Sometimes, screening tests find cancers that don't matter because they would have gone away on their own or never caused any symptoms. These cancers would never have been found if not for the screening test. Finding these cancers is called overdiagnosis. Overdiagnosis can make it seem like more people are surviving cancer longer, but in reality, these are people who would not have died from cancer anyway.

How Do Screening Tests Become Standard Tests?

Results from research studies help doctors decide when a screening test works well enough to be used as a standard test.

Evidence about how safe, accurate, and useful cancer screening tests are comes from clinical trials (research studies with people) and other kinds of research studies. When enough evidence has been collected to show that a screening test is safe, accurate, and useful, it becomes a standard test. Examples of cancer screening tests that were once under study but are now standard tests include:

- Colonoscopy for colorectal cancer.
- Mammograms for breast cancer.
- Pap tests (Pap smears) for cervical cancer.

Different types of research studies are done to study cancer screening.

Cancer screening trials study new ways of finding cancer in people before they have symptoms. Screening trials also study screening tests that may find cancer earlier or are more accurate than existing tests, or that may be easier, safer, or cheaper to use. Screening trials are designed to find the possible benefits and possible harms of cancer screening tests. Different clinical trial designs are used to study cancer screening tests.

The strongest evidence about screening comes from research done in clinical trials. However, clinical trials cannot always be used to study questions about screening. Findings from other types of studies can give useful information about how safe, useful, and accurate cancer screening tests are.

The following types of studies are used to get information about cancer screening tests:

Randomized controlled trials

Randomized controlled trials give the highest level of evidence about how safe, accurate, and useful cancer screening tests are. In these trials, volunteers are assigned randomly (by chance) to one of two or more groups. The people in one group (the control group) may be given a standard screening test (if one exists) or no screening test. The people in the other group(s) are given the new screening test(s). Test results for the groups are then compared to see if the new screening test works better than the standard test, and to see if there are any harmful side effects.

Using chance to assign people to groups means that the groups will probably be very much alike and that the trial results won't be affected by human choices or something else.

Nonrandomized controlled trials

In nonrandomized clinical trials, volunteers are not assigned randomly (by chance) to different groups. They choose which group they want to be in or the study leaders assign them. Evidence from this type of research is not as strong as evidence from randomized controlled trials.

Cohort studies

A cohort study follows a large number of people over time. The people are divided into groups, called cohorts, based on whether or not they have had a certain treatment or been exposed to certain things. In cohort studies, the information is collected and studied after certain outcomes (such as cancer or death) have occurred. For example, a cohort study might follow a group of women who have regular Pap tests, and divide them into those who test positive for the human papillomavirus (HPV) and those who test negative for HPV. The cohort study would show how the cervical cancer rates are different for the two groups over time.

Case-control studies

Case-control studies are like cohort studies but are done in a shorter time. They do not include many years of follow-up. Instead of looking forward in time, they look backward. In case-control studies, information is collected from cases (people who already have a certain disease) and compared with information collected from controls (people who do not have the disease). For example, a group of patients with melanoma and a group without melanoma might be asked about how they check their skin for abnormal growths and how often they check it. Based on the different answers from the two groups, the study may show that checking your skin is a useful screening test to decrease the number of melanoma cases and deaths from melanoma.

Evidence from case-control studies is not as strong as evidence from clinical trials or cohort studies.

Ecologic studies

Ecologic studies report information collected on entire groups of people, such as people in one city or county. Information is reported about the whole group, not about any single person in the group. These studies may give some evidence about whether a screening test is useful.

The evidence from ecologic studies is not as strong as evidence from clinical trials or other types of research studies.

Expert opinions

Expert opinions can be based on the experiences of doctors or reports of expert committees or panels. Expert opinions do not give strong evidence about the usefulness of screening tests.

Part Three

Cancer Types

Chapter 20

Neurological Cancers

Section 20.1

Adult Brain Tumors

Text in this section is excerpted from "Adult Brain Tumors
Treatment," National Cancer Institute at the National Institutes of
Health (NIH), February 13, 2015.

General Information About Adult Brain Tumors

*An adult brain tumor is a disease in which abnormal cells
form in the tissues of the brain.*

There are many types of brain and spinal cord tumors. The tumors
are formed by the abnormal growth of cells and may begin in different
parts of the brain or spinal cord. Together, the brain and spinal cord
make up the central nervous system (CNS).

The tumors may be either benign (not cancer) or malignant (cancer):

- Benign brain and spinal cord tumors grow and press on nearby
  areas of the brain. They rarely spread into other tissues and may
  recur (come back).
- Malignant brain and spinal cord tumors are likely to grow
  quickly and spread into other brain tissue.

When a tumor grows into or presses on an area of the brain, it
may stop that part of the brain from working the way it should. Both
benign and malignant brain tumors cause signs and symptoms and
need treatment.

Brain and spinal cord tumors can occur in both adults and children.
However, treatment for children may be different than treatment for
adults.

*A brain tumor that starts in another part of the body and
spreads to the brain is called a metastatic tumor.*

Tumors that start in the brain are called primary brain tumors.
Primary brain tumors may spread to other parts of the brain or to the
spine. They rarely spread to other parts of the body.

Often, tumors found in the brain have started somewhere else in the body and spread to one or more parts of the brain. These are called metastatic brain tumors (or brain metastases). Metastatic brain tumors are more common than primary brain tumors.

About half of metastatic brain tumors are from lung cancer. Other types of cancer that commonly spread to the brain are melanoma and cancer of the breast, colon, kidney, nasopharynx, and unknown primary site. Leukemia, lymphoma, breast cancer, and gastrointestinal cancer may spread to the leptomeninges (the two innermost membranes covering the brain and spinal cord). This is called leptomeningeal carcinomatosis.

There are different types of brain and spinal cord tumors.

Brain and spinal cord tumors are named based on the type of cell they formed in and where the tumor first formed in the CNS. The grade of a tumor may be used to tell the difference between slow-growing and fast-growing types of the tumor. The World Health Organization (WHO) tumor grades are based on how abnormal the cancer cells look under a microscope and how quickly the tumor is likely to grow and spread.

WHO Tumor Grading System

- Grade I (low-grade)—The tumor cells look more like normal cells under a microscope and grow and spread more slowly than grade II, III, and IV tumor cells. They rarely spread into nearby tissues. Grade I brain tumors may be cured if they are completely removed by surgery.

- Grade II—The tumor cells grow and spread more slowly than grade III and IV tumor cells. They may spread into nearby tissue and may recur (come back). Some tumors may become a higher-grade tumor.

- Grade III—The tumor cells look very different from normal cells under a microscope and grow more quickly than grade I and II tumor cells. They are likely to spread into nearby tissue.

- Grade IV (high-grade)—The tumor cells do not look like normal cells under a microscope and grow and spread very quickly. There may be areas of dead cells in the tumor. Grade IV tumors usually cannot be cured.

145

The following types of tumors can form in the brain or spinal cord:

Astrocytic Tumors

An astrocytic tumor begins in star-shaped brain cells called astrocytes, which help keep nerve cells healthy. An astrocyte is a type of glial cell. Glial cells sometimes form tumors called gliomas. Astrocytic tumors include the following:

- **Brain stem glioma (usually high grade)**: A brain stem glioma forms in the brain stem, which is the part of the brain connected to the spinal cord. It is often a high-grade tumor, which spreads widely through the brain stem and is hard to cure. Brain stem gliomas are rare in adults.

- **Pineal astrocytic tumor (any grade)**: A pineal astrocytic tumor forms in tissue around the pineal gland and may be any grade. The pineal gland is a tiny organ in the brain that makes melatonin, a hormone that helps control the sleeping and waking cycle.

- **Pilocytic astrocytoma (grade I)**: A pilocytic astrocytoma grows slowly in the brain or spinal cord. It may be in the form of a cyst and rarely spreads into nearby tissues. Pilocytic astrocytomas can often be cured.

- **Diffuse astrocytoma (grade II)**: A diffuse astrocytoma grows slowly, but often spreads into nearby tissues. The tumor cells look something like normal cells. In some cases, a diffuse astrocytoma can be cured. It is also called a low-grade diffuse astrocytoma.

- **Anaplastic astrocytoma (grade III)**: An anaplastic astrocytoma grows quickly and spreads into nearby tissues. The tumor cells look different from normal cells. This type of tumor usually cannot be cured. An anaplastic astrocytoma is also called a malignant astrocytoma or high-grade astrocytoma.

- **Glioblastoma (grade IV)**: A glioblastoma grows and spreads very quickly. The tumor cells look very different from normal cells. This type of tumor usually cannot be cured. It is also called glioblastoma multiforme.

Oligodendroglial Tumors

An oligodendroglial tumor begins in brain cells called oligodendrocytes, which help keep nerve cells healthy. An oligodendrocyte is a type of glial cell. Oligodendrocytes sometimes form tumors called oligodendrogliomas. Grades of oligodendroglial tumors include the following:

- **Oligodendroglioma (grade II):** An oligodendroglioma grows slowly, but often spreads into nearby tissues. The tumor cells look something like normal cells. In some cases, an oligodendroglioma can be cured.

- **Anaplastic oligodendroglioma (grade III):** An anaplastic oligodendroglioma grows quickly and spreads into nearby tissues. The tumor cells look different from normal cells. This type of tumor usually cannot be cured.

Mixed Gliomas

A mixed glioma is a brain tumor that has two types of tumor cells in it—oligodendrocytes and astrocytes. This type of mixed tumor is called an oligoastrocytoma.

- **Oligoastrocytoma (grade II):** An oligoastrocytoma is a slow-growing tumor. The tumor cells look something like normal cells. In some cases, an oligoastrocytoma can be cured.

- **Anaplastic oligoastrocytoma (grade III):** An anaplastic oligoastrocytoma grows quickly and spreads into nearby tissues. The tumor cells look different from normal cells. This type of tumor has a worse prognosis than oligoastrocytoma (grade II).

Ependymal Tumors

An ependymal tumor usually begins in cells that line the fluid -filled spaces in the brain and around the spinal cord. An ependymal tumor may also be called an ependymoma. Grades of ependymomas include the following:

- **Ependymoma (grade I or II):** A grade I or II ependymoma grows slowly and has cells that look something like normal cells. There are two types of grade I ependymoma—myxopapillary ependymoma and subependymoma. A grade II ependymoma grows in a ventricle (fluid-filled space in the brain) and its connecting paths or in the spinal cord. In some cases, a grade I or II ependymoma can be cured.

- **Anaplastic ependymoma (grade III):** An anaplastic ependymoma grows quickly and spreads into nearby tissues. The tumor cells look different from normal cells. This type of tumor usually has a worse prognosis than a grade I or II ependymoma.

Medulloblastomas

A medulloblastoma is a type of embryonal tumor. Medulloblastomas are most common in children or young adults.

Pineal Parenchymal Tumors

A pineal parenchymal tumor forms in parenchymal cells or pineocytes, which are the cells that make up most of the pineal gland. These tumors are different from pineal astrocytic tumors. Grades of pineal parenchymal tumors include the following:

- **Pineocytoma (grade II):** A pineocytoma is a slow-growing pineal tumor.

- **Pineoblastoma (grade IV):** A pineoblastoma is a rare tumor that is very likely to spread.

Meningeal Tumors

A meningeal tumor, also called a meningioma, forms in the meninges (thin layers of tissue that cover the brain and spinal cord). It can form from different types of brain or spinal cord cells. Meningiomas are most common in adults. Types of meningeal tumors include the following:

- **Meningioma (grade I):** A grade I meningioma is the most common type of meningeal tumor. A grade I meningioma is a slow-growing tumor. It forms most often in the dura mater. A grade I meningioma can be cured if it is completely removed by surgery.

- **Meningioma (grade II and III):** This is a rare meningeal tumor. It grows quickly and is likely to spread within the brain and spinal cord. The prognosis is worse than a grade I meningioma because the tumor usually cannot be completely removed by surgery.

A hemangiopericytoma is not a meningeal tumor but is treated like a grade II or III meningioma. A hemangiopericytoma usually forms in the dura mater. The prognosis is worse than a grade I meningioma because the tumor usually cannot be completely removed by surgery.

Germ Cell Tumors

A germ cell tumor forms in germ cells, which are the cells that develop into sperm in men or ova (eggs) in women. There are different types of germ cell tumors. These include germinomas, teratomas, embryonal yolk sac carcinomas, and choriocarcinomas. Germ cell tumors can be either benign or malignant.

Craniopharyngioma (Grade I)

A craniopharyngioma is a rare tumor that usually forms just above the pituitary gland (a pea-sized organ at the bottom of the brain that controls other glands). Craniopharyngiomas can form from different types of brain or spinal cord cells. They begin in the center of the brain, just above the back of the nose.

Recurrent Brain Tumors

A recurrent brain tumor is a tumor that has recurred (come back) after it has been treated. Brain tumors often recur, sometimes many years after the first tumor. The tumor may recur at the same place in the brain or in other parts of the central nervous system.

Having certain genetic syndromes may affect the risk of a brain tumor.

Anything that increases your chance of getting a disease is called a risk factor. Having a risk factor does not mean that you will get cancer; not having risk factors doesn't mean that you will not get cancer. Talk with your doctor if you think you may be at risk. There are few known risk factors for brain tumors. The following conditions may increase the risk of certain types of brain tumors:

- Being exposed to vinyl chloride may increase the risk of glioma.

- Infection with the Epstein-Barr virus, having AIDS (acquired immunodeficiency syndrome), or receiving an organ transplant may increase the risk of primary CNS lymphoma.

- Having certain genetic syndromes may increase the risk brain tumors:

  - Neurofibromatosis type 1 (NF1) or 2 (NF2).

  - von Hippel-Lindau disease.

- Tuberous sclerosis.

- Li-Fraumeni syndrome.

- Turcot syndrome type 1 or 2.

- Nevoid basal cell carcinoma syndrome.

The cause of most adult brain and spinal cord tumors is unknown.

The signs and symptoms of adult brain and spinal cord tumors are not the same in every person.

Signs and symptoms depend on the following:

- Where the tumor forms in the brain.

- What the affected part of the brain controls.

- The size of the tumor.

Signs and symptoms may be caused by brain tumors or by other conditions, including cancer that has spread to the brain. Check with your doctor if you have any of the following:

Brain Tumors

- Morning headache or headache that goes away after vomiting.

- Frequent nausea and vomiting.

- Loss of appetite.

- Vision, hearing, and speech problems.

- Loss of balance and trouble walking.

- Weakness.

- Unusual sleepiness or change in activity level.

- Changes in personality, mood, ability to focus, or behavior.

- Seizures.

Spinal Cord Tumors

- Back pain or pain that spreads from the back towards the arms or legs.

- A change in bowel habits or trouble urinating.
- Weakness in the legs.
- Trouble walking.

Tests that examine the brain and spinal cord are used to diagnose adult brain and spinal cord tumors.

The following tests and procedures may be used:

- **Physical exam and history:** An exam of the body to check general signs of health, including checking for signs of disease, such as lumps or anything else that seems unusual. A history of the patient's health habits and past illnesses and treatments will also be taken.

- **Neurological exam:** A series of questions and tests to check the brain, spinal cord, and nerve function. The exam checks a person's mental status, coordination, and ability to walk normally, and how well the muscles, senses, and reflexes work. This may also be called a neuro exam or a neurologic exam.

- **Visual field exam:** An exam to check a person's field of vision (the total area in which objects can be seen). This test measures both central vision (how much a person can see when looking straight ahead) and peripheral vision (how much a person can see in all other directions while staring straight ahead). Any loss of vision may be a sign of a tumor that has damaged or pressed on the parts of the brain that affect eyesight.

- **Tumor marker test:** A procedure in which a sample of blood, urine, or tissue is checked to measure the amounts of certain substances made by organs, tissues, or tumor cells in the body. Certain substances are linked to specific types of cancer when found in increased levels in the body. These are called tumor markers. This test may be done to diagnose a germ cell tumor.

- **Gene testing:** A laboratory test in which a sample of blood or tissue is tested for changes in a chromosome that has been linked with a certain type of brain tumor. This test may be done to diagnose an inherited syndrome.

- **CT scan (CAT scan):** A procedure that makes a series of detailed pictures of areas inside the body, taken from different angles. The pictures are made by a computer linked to an x-ray

machine. A dye may be injected into a vein or swallowed to help the organs or tissues show up more clearly. This procedure is also called computed tomography, computerized tomography, or computerized axial tomography.

- **MRI (magnetic resonance imaging) with gadolinium:** A procedure that uses a magnet, radio waves, and a computer to make a series of detailed pictures of the brain and spinal cord. A substance called gadolinium is injected into a vein. The gadolinium collects around the cancer cells so they show up brighter in the picture. This procedure is also called nuclear magnetic resonance imaging (NMRI). Sometimes a procedure called magnetic resonance spectroscopy (MRS) is done during the MRI scan. An MRS is used to diagnose tumors, based on their chemical make-up. MRI is often used to diagnose tumors in the spinal cord.

- **SPECT scan (single photon emission computed tomography scan):** A procedure that uses a special camera linked to a computer to make a 3-dimensional (3-D) picture of the brain. A small amount of a radioactive substance is injected into a vein or inhaled through the nose. As the substance travels through the blood, the camera rotates around the head and takes pictures of the brain. Blood flow and metabolism are higher than normal in areas where cancer cells are growing. These areas will show up brighter in the picture. This procedure may be done just before or after a CT scan. SPECT is used to tell the difference between a primary tumor and a tumor that has spread to the brain from somewhere else in the body.

- **PET scan (positron emission tomography scan):** A procedure to find malignant tumor cells in the body. A small amount of radioactive glucose (sugar) is injected into a vein. The PET scanner rotates around the body and makes a picture of where glucose is being used in the brain. Malignant tumor cells show up brighter in the picture because they are more active and take up more glucose than normal cells do. PET is used to tell the difference between a primary tumor and a tumor that has spread to the brain from somewhere else in the body.

- **Angiogram:** A procedure to look at blood vessels and the flow of blood in the brain. A contrast dye is injected into the blood vessel. As the contrast dye moves through the blood vessel, x-rays are taken to see if the vessel is blocked.

A biopsy is also used to diagnose a brain tumor.

If imaging tests show there may be a brain tumor, a biopsy is usually done. One of the following types of biopsies may be used:

- **Stereotactic biopsy:** When imaging tests show there may be a tumor deep in the brain in a hard to reach place, a stereotactic brain biopsy may be done. This kind of biopsy uses a computer and a 3-dimensional scanning device to find the tumor and guide the needle used to remove the tissue. A small incision is made in the scalp and a small hole is drilled through the skull. A biopsy needle is inserted through the hole to remove cells or tissues so they can be viewed under a microscope by a pathologist to check for signs of cancer.

- **Open biopsy:** When imaging tests show that there may be a tumor that can be removed by surgery, an open biopsy may be done. A part of the skull is removed in an operation called a craniotomy. A sample of brain tissue is removed and viewed under a microscope by a pathologist. If cancer cells are found, some or all of the tumor may be removed during the same surgery. Tests are done before surgery to find the areas around the tumor that are important for normal brain function. There are also ways to test brain function during surgery. The doctor will use the results of these tests to remove as much of the tumor as possible with the least damage to normal tissue in the brain.

The pathologist checks the biopsy sample to find out the type and grade of brain tumor. The grade of the tumor is based on how the tumor cells look under a microscope and how quickly the tumor is likely to grow and spread.

The following tests may be done on the tumor tissue that is removed:

- **Immunohistochemistry:** A test that uses antibodies to check for certain antigens in a sample of tissue. The antibody is usually linked to a radioactive substance or a dye that causes the tissue to light up under a microscope. This type of test may be used to tell the difference between different types of cancer.

- **Light and electron microscopy:** A laboratory test in which cells in a sample of tissue are viewed under regular and high-powered microscopes to look for certain changes in the cells.

- **Cytogenetic analysis:** A laboratory test in which cells in a sample of tissue are viewed under a microscope to look for certain changes in the chromosomes.

Sometimes a biopsy or surgery cannot be done.

For some tumors, a biopsy or surgery cannot be done safely because of where the tumor formed in the brain or spinal cord. These tumors are diagnosed and treated based on the results of imaging tests and other procedures.

Sometimes the results of imaging tests and other procedures show that the tumor is very likely to be benign and a biopsy is not done.

Certain factors affect prognosis (chance of recovery) and treatment options.

The prognosis (chance of recovery) and treatment options for primary brain and spinal cord tumors depend on the following:

- The type and grade of the tumor.
- Where the tumor is in the brain or spinal cord.
- Whether the tumor can be removed by surgery.
- Whether cancer cells remain after surgery.
- Whether there are certain changes in the chromosomes.
- Whether the cancer has just been diagnosed or has recurred (come back).
- The patient's general health.

The prognosis and treatment options for metastatic brain and spinal cord tumors depend on the following:

- Whether there are more than two tumors in the brain or spinal cord.
- Where the tumor is in the brain or spinal cord.
- How well the tumor responds to treatment.
- Whether the primary tumor continues to grow or spread.

Stages of Adult Brain Tumors

There is no standard staging system for adult brain and spinal cord tumors.

The extent or spread of cancer is usually described as stages. There is no standard staging system for brain and spinal cord tumors. Brain tumors that begin in the brain may spread to other parts of the brain and spinal cord, but they rarely spread to other parts of the body. Treatment of brain and spinal cord tumors is based on the following:

- The type of cell in which the tumor began.
- Where the tumor formed in the brain or spinal cord.
- The amount of cancer left after surgery.
- The grade of the tumor.

Treatment of brain tumors that have spread to the brain from other parts of the body is based on the number of tumors in the brain.

Treatment Option Overview

There are different types of treatment for patients with adult brain and spinal cord tumors.

Different types of treatment are available for patients with adult brain and spinal cord tumors. Some treatments are standard (the currently used treatment), and some are being tested in clinical trials. A treatment clinical trial is a research study meant to help improve current treatments or obtain information on new treatments for patients with cancer. When clinical trials show that a new treatment is better than the standard treatment, the new treatment may become the standard treatment. Patients may want to think about taking part in a clinical trial. Some clinical trials are open only to patients who have not started treatment.

Five types of standard treatment are used:

Watchful waiting

Watchful waiting is closely monitoring a patient's condition without giving any treatment until signs or symptoms appear or change.

Surgery

Surgery may be used to diagnose and treat adult brain and spinal cord tumors.

Even if the doctor removes all the cancer that can be seen at the time of the surgery, some patients may be given chemotherapy or radiation therapy after surgery to kill any cancer cells that are left. Treatment given after the surgery, to lower the risk that the cancer will come back, is called adjuvant therapy.

Radiation therapy

Radiation therapy is a cancer treatment that uses high-energy x-rays or other types of radiation to kill cancer cells or keep them from growing. There are two types of radiation therapy. External radiation therapy uses a machine outside the body to send radiation toward the cancer. Internal radiation therapy uses a radioactive substance sealed in needles, seeds, wires, or catheters that are placed directly into or near the cancer. The way the radiation therapy is given depends on the type of tumor and where it is in the brain or spinal cord.

The following ways of giving radiation therapy to the tumor cause less damage to the healthy tissue that is around the tumor:

- 3-dimensional conformal radiation therapy: A procedure that uses a computer to create a 3-dimensional (3-D) picture of the brain or spinal cord tumor. This allows doctors to give the highest possible dose of radiation to the tumor, with as little damage to normal tissue as possible. This type of radiation therapy is also called 3-dimensional radiation therapy and 3D-CRT.

- Intensity-modulated radiation therapy (IMRT): A type of 3-D radiation therapy that uses a computer to make pictures of the size and shape of the brain or spinal cord tumor. Thin beams of radiation of different intensities (strengths) are aimed at the tumor from many angles. This type of radiation therapy causes less damage to healthy tissue near the tumor.

- Stereotactic radiosurgery: A type of radiation therapy that uses a head frame attached to the skull to aim a single large dose of radiation directly to a brain tumor. This causes less damage to nearby healthy tissue. Stereotactic radiosurgery is also called stereotaxic radiosurgery, radiosurgery, and radiation surgery. This procedure does not involve surgery.

Chemotherapy

Chemotherapy is a cancer treatment that uses drugs to stop the growth of cancer cells, either by killing the cells or by stopping them from dividing. When chemotherapy is taken by mouth or injected into a vein or muscle, the drugs enter the bloodstream and can reach cancer cells throughout the body (systemic chemotherapy). When chemotherapy is placed directly into the cerebrospinal fluid, an organ, or a body cavity such as the abdomen, the drugs mainly affect cancer cells in those areas (regional chemotherapy). Combination chemotherapy is treatment using more than one anticancer drug. To treat brain tumors, a wafer that dissolves may be used to deliver an anticancer drug directly to the brain tumor site after the tumor has been removed by surgery. The way the chemotherapy is given depends on the type of tumor and where it is in the brain.

Anticancer drugs given by mouth or vein to treat brain and spinal cord tumors cannot cross the blood-brain barrier and enter the fluid that surrounds the brain and spinal cord. Instead, an anticancer drug is injected into the fluid-filled space to kill cancer cells there. This is called intrathecal chemotherapy.

Targeted therapy

Targeted therapy is a type of treatment that uses drugs or other substances to identify and attack specific cancer cells without harming normal cells.

Monoclonal antibody therapy is a type of targeted therapy that uses antibodies made in the laboratory from a single type of immune system cell. These antibodies can identify substances on cancer cells or normal substances that may help cancer cells grow. The antibodies attach to the substances and kill the cancer cells, block their growth, or keep them from spreading. Monoclonal antibodies are given by infusion. They may be used alone or to carry drugs, toxins, or radioactive material directly to cancer cells.

Bevacizumab is a monoclonal antibody that binds to a protein called vascular endothelial growth factor (VEGF) and may prevent the growth of new blood vessels that tumors need to grow. Bevacizumab is used in the treatment of recurrent glioblastoma.

157

Other types of targeted therapies are being studied for adult brain tumors, including tyrosine kinase inhibitors.

New types of treatment are being tested in clinical trials.

Proton beam radiation therapy

Proton beam radiation therapy is a type of high-energy, external radiation therapy that uses streams of protons (small, positively-charged pieces of matter) to make radiation. This type of radiation kills tumor cells with little damage to nearby tissues. It is used to treat cancers of the head, neck, and spine and organs such as the brain, eye, lung, and prostate. Proton beam radiation is different from x-ray radiation.

Biologic therapy

Biologic therapy is a treatment that uses the patient's immune system to fight cancer. Substances made by the body or made in a laboratory are used to boost, direct, or restore the body's natural defenses against cancer. This type of cancer treatment is also called biotherapy or immunotherapy.

Biologic therapy is being studied for the treatment of some types of brain tumors. Treatments may include the following:

- Dendritic cell vaccine therapy.
- Gene therapy.

Supportive care is given to lessen the problems caused by the disease or its treatment.

This therapy controls problems or side effects caused by the disease or its treatment and improves quality of life. For brain tumors, supportive care includes drugs to control seizures and fluid buildup or swelling in the brain.

Patients may want to think about taking part in a clinical trial.

For some patients, taking part in a clinical trial may be the best treatment choice. Clinical trials are part of the cancer research process. Clinical trials are done to find out if new cancer treatments are safe and effective or better than the standard treatment.

Many of today's standard treatments for cancer are based on earlier clinical trials. Patients who take part in a clinical trial may receive the standard treatment or be among the first to receive a new treatment.

Patients who take part in clinical trials also help improve the way cancer will be treated in the future. Even when clinical trials do not lead to effective new treatments, they often answer important questions and help move research forward.

Patients can enter clinical trials before, during, or after starting their cancer treatment.

Some clinical trials only include patients who have not yet received treatment. Other trials test treatments for patients whose cancer has not gotten better. There are also clinical trials that test new ways to stop cancer from recurring (coming back) or reduce the side effects of cancer treatment.

Follow-up tests may be needed.

Some of the tests that were done to diagnose the cancer or to find out the stage of the cancer may be repeated. Some tests will be repeated in order to see how well the treatment is working. Decisions about whether to continue, change, or stop treatment may be based on the results of these tests.

Some of the tests will continue to be done from time to time after treatment has ended. The results of these tests can show if your condition has changed or if the cancer has recurred (come back). These tests are sometimes called follow-up tests or check-ups.

The following tests and procedures may be used to check whether a brain tumor has come back after treatment:

- **SPECT scan (single photon emission computed tomography scan):** A procedure that uses a special camera linked to a computer to make a 3-dimensional (3-D) picture of the brain. A small amount of a radioactive substance is injected into a vein or inhaled through the nose. As the substance travels through the blood, the camera rotates around the head and takes pictures of the brain. Blood flow and metabolism are higher than normal in areas where cancer cells are growing. These areas will show up brighter in the picture. This procedure may be done just before or after a CT scan.

159

- **PET scan (positron emission tomography scan):** A proce-dure to find malignant tumor cells in the body. A small amount of radioactive glucose (sugar) is injected into a vein. The PET scanner rotates around the body and makes a picture of where glucose is being used in the brain. Malignant tumor cells show up brighter in the picture because they are more active and take up more glucose than normal cells do.

Section 20.2

Childhood Brain and Spinal Cord Tumors

Text in this section is excerpted from "Childhood Brain and Spinal Cord Tumors Treatment Overview," National Cancer Institute at the National Institutes of Health (NIH), May 13, 2015.

General Information About Childhood Brain and Spinal Cord Tumors

A childhood brain or spinal cord tumor is a disease in which abnormal cells form in the tissues of the brain or spinal cord.

There are many types of childhood brain and spinal cord tumors. The tumors are formed by the abnormal growth of cells and may begin in different areas of the brain or spinal cord.

The tumors may be benign (not cancer) or malignant (cancer). Benign brain tumors grow and press on nearby areas of the brain. They rarely spread into other tissues. Malignant brain tumors are likely to grow quickly and spread into other brain tissue. When a tumor grows into or presses on an area of the brain, it may stop that part of the brain from working the way it should. Both benign and malignant brain tumors can cause signs or symptoms and need treatment.

Brain and spinal cord tumors are a common type of childhood cancer.

Although cancer is rare in children, brain and spinal cord tumors are the third most common type of childhood cancer, after leukemia and lymphoma. Brain tumors can occur in both children and adults. Treatment for children is usually different than treatment for adults. **The cause of most childhood brain and spinal cord tumors is unknown.**

The signs and symptoms of childhood brain and spinal cord tumors are not the same in every child.

Signs and symptoms depend on the following:

- Where the tumor forms in the brain or spinal cord.
- The size of the tumor.
- How fast the tumor grows.
- The child's age and development.

Signs and symptoms may be caused by childhood brain and spinal cord tumors or by other conditions, including cancer that has spread to the brain. Check with your child's doctor if your child has any of the following:

Brain Tumor Signs and Symptoms

- Morning headache or headache that goes away after vomiting.
- Frequent nausea and vomiting.
- Vision, hearing, and speech problems.
- Loss of balance and trouble walking.
- Unusual sleepiness or change in activity level.
- Unusual changes in personality or behavior.
- Seizures.
- Increase in the head size (in infants).

Spinal Cord Tumor Signs and Symptoms

- Back pain or pain that spreads from the back towards the arms or legs.
- A change in bowel habits or trouble urinating.
- Weakness in the legs.
- Trouble walking.

In addition to these signs and symptoms of brain and spinal cord tumors, some children are unable to reach certain growth and development milestones such as sitting up, walking, and talking in sentences.

Tests that examine the brain and spinal cord are used to detect (find) childhood brain and spinal cord tumors.

The following tests and procedures may be used:

- **Physical exam and history:** An exam of the body to check general signs of health, including checking for signs of disease, such as lumps or anything else that seems unusual. A history of the patient's health habits and past illnesses and treatments will also be taken.

- **Neurological exam:** A series of questions and tests to check the brain, spinal cord, and nerve function. The exam checks a person's mental status, coordination, and ability to walk normally, and how well the muscles, senses, and reflexes work. This may also be called a neuro exam or a neurologic exam.

- **MRI (magnetic resonance imaging) with gadolinium:** A procedure that uses a magnet, radio waves, and a computer to make a series of detailed pictures of the brain and spinal cord. A substance called gadolinium is injected into a vein. The gadolinium collects around the cancer cells so they show up brighter in the picture. This procedure is also called nuclear magnetic resonance imaging (NMRI).

- **Serum tumor marker test:** A procedure in which a sample of blood is examined to measure the amounts of certain substances released into the blood by organs, tissues, or tumor cells in the body. Certain substances are linked to specific types of cancer when found in increased levels in the blood. These are called tumor markers.

Most childhood brain tumors are diagnosed and removed in surgery.

If doctors think there might be a brain tumor, a biopsy may be done to remove a sample of tissue. For tumors in the brain, the biopsy is done by removing part of the skull and using a needle to remove a sample of tissue. A pathologist views the tissue under a microscope to look for cancer cells. If cancer cells are found, the doctor may remove as much tumor as safely possible during the same surgery. The pathologist checks the cancer cells to find out the type and grade of brain tumor. The grade of the tumor is based on how abnormal the cancer cells look under a microscope and how quickly the tumor is likely to grow and spread.

The following test may be done on the sample of tissue that is removed:

- **Immunohistochemistry:** A test that uses antibodies to check for certain antigens in a sample of tissue. The antibody is usually linked to a radioactive substance or a dye that causes the tissue to light up under a microscope. This type of test may be used to tell the difference between different types of cancer.

Some childhood brain and spinal cord tumors are diagnosed by imaging tests.

Sometimes a biopsy or surgery cannot be done safely because of where the tumor formed in the brain or spinal cord. These tumors are diagnosed based on the results of imaging tests and other procedures.

Certain factors affect prognosis (chance of recovery).

The prognosis (chance of recovery) depends on the following:

- Whether there are any cancer cells left after surgery.
- The type of tumor.
- Where the tumor is in the body.
- The child's age.
- Whether the tumor has just been diagnosed or has recurred (come back).

Staging Childhood Brain and Spinal Cord Tumors

In childhood brain and spinal cord tumors, there is no standard staging system. Instead, the plan for cancer treatment depends on several factors:

Staging is the process used to find how much cancer there is and if cancer has spread within the brain, spinal cord, or to other parts of the body. It is important to know the stage in order to plan cancer treatment.

In childhood brain and spinal cord tumors, there is no standard staging system. Instead, the plan for cancer treatment depends on several factors:

- The type of tumor and where the tumor formed in the brain.

- Whether the tumor is newly diagnosed or recurrent. A newly diagnosed brain or spinal cord tumor is one that has never been treated. A recurrent childhood brain or spinal cord tumor is one that has recurred (come back) after it has been treated. Childhood brain and spinal cord tumors may come back in the same place or in another part of the brain, or spinal cord. Sometimes they come back in another part of the body. The tumor may come back many years after first being treated. Tests and procedures, including biopsy, that were done to diagnose and stage the tumor may be done to find out if the tumor has recurred.

- The grade of the tumor. The grade of the tumor is based on how abnormal the cancer cells look under a microscope and how quickly the tumor is likely to grow and spread. It is important to know the grade of the tumor and if there were any cancer cells remaining after surgery in order to plan treatment. The grade of the tumor is not used to plan treatment for all types of brain and spinal cord tumors.

- The tumor risk group. Risk groups are either average risk and poor risk or low, intermediate, and high risk. The risk groups are based on the amount of tumor remaining after surgery, the spread of cancer cells within the brain and spinal cord or to other parts of the body, where the tumor has formed, and the age of the child. The risk group is not used to plan treatment for all types of brain and spinal cord tumors.

The information from tests and procedures done to detect (find) childhood brain and spinal cord tumors is used to determine the tumor risk group.

After the tumor is removed in surgery, some of the tests used to detect childhood brain and spinal cord tumors are repeated to help determine the tumor risk group (see the General Information section). This is to find out how much tumor remains after surgery.

Other tests and procedures may be done to find out if cancer has spread:

- **Lumbar puncture:** A procedure used to collect cerebrospinal fluid from the spinal column. This is done by placing a needle into the spinal column. Lumbar puncture is usually not used to stage childhood spinal cord tumors. This procedure is also called an LP or spinal tap.

- **Bone scan:** A procedure to check if there are rapidly dividing cells, such as cancer cells, in the bone. A very small amount of radioactive material is injected into a vein and travels through the bloodstream. The radioactive material collects in the bones and is detected by a scanner.

- **Bone marrow aspiration and biopsy:** The removal of bone marrow, blood, and a small piece of bone by inserting a hollow needle into the hipbone or breastbone. A pathologist views the bone marrow, blood, and bone under a microscope to look for signs of cancer.

Childhood brain and spinal cord tumors may recur (come back) after treatment.

A recurrent childhood brain or spinal cord tumor is one that has recurred (come back) after it has been treated. Childhood brain and spinal cord tumors may come back in the same place or in another part of the brain. Sometimes they come back in another part of the body. The tumor may come back many years after first being treated. Diagnostic and staging tests and procedures, including biopsy, may be done to make sure that the tumor has recurred.

Treatment Option Overview

There are different types of treatment for children with brain and spinal cord tumors.

Different types of treatment are available for children with brain and spinal cord tumors. Some treatments are standard (the currently used treatment), and some are being tested in clinical trials. A treatment clinical trial is a research study meant to help improve current treatments or obtain information on new treatments for patients with cancer. When clinical trials show that a new treatment is better than the standard treatment, the new treatment may become the standard treatment.

165

Because cancer in children is rare, taking part in a clinical trial should be considered. Clinical trials are taking place in many parts of the country. Some clinical trials are open only to patients who have not started treatment.

Children with brain or spinal cord tumors should have their treatment planned by a team of health care providers who are experts in treating childhood brain and spinal cord tumors.

Treatment will be overseen by a pediatric oncologist, a doctor who specializes in treating children with cancer. The pediatric oncologist works with other health care providers who are experts in treating children with brain tumors and who specialize in certain areas of medicine. These may include the following specialists:

- Pediatrician.
- Neurosurgeon.
- Neurologist.
- Neuro-oncologist.
- Neuropathologist.
- Neuroradiologist.
- Radiation oncologist.
- Endocrinologist.
- Psychologist.
- Ophthalmologist.
- Rehabilitation specialist.
- Social worker.
- Nurse specialist.

Childhood brain and spinal cord tumors may cause signs or symptoms that begin before the cancer is diagnosed and continue for months or years.

Childhood brain and spinal cord tumors may cause signs or symptoms that continue for months or years. Signs or symptoms caused by the tumor may begin before diagnosis. Signs or symptoms caused by treatment may begin during or right after treatment.

Some cancer treatments cause side effects months or years after treatment has ended.

These are called late effects. Late effects of cancer treatment may include the following:

- Physical problems.

- Changes in mood, feelings, thinking, learning, or memory.

- Second cancers (new types of cancer).

Some late effects may be treated or controlled. It is important to talk with your child's doctors about the effects cancer treatment can have on your child.

Three types of standard treatment are used:

Surgery

Surgery may be used to diagnose and treat childhood brain and spinal cord tumors.

Radiation therapy

Radiation therapy is a cancer treatment that uses high-energy x-rays or other types of radiation to kill cancer cells or keep them from growing. There are two types of radiation therapy. External radiation therapy uses a machine outside the body to send radiation toward the cancer. Internal radiation therapy uses a radioactive substance sealed in needles, seeds, wires, or catheters that are placed directly into or near the cancer. The way the radiation therapy is given depends on the type and stage of the cancer being treated.

Chemotherapy

Chemotherapy is a cancer treatment that uses drugs to stop the growth of cancer cells, either by killing the cells or by stopping them from dividing. When chemotherapy is taken by mouth or injected into a vein or muscle, the drugs enter the bloodstream and can reach cancer cells throughout the body (systemic chemotherapy). When chemotherapy is placed directly in the cerebrospinal fluid, an organ, or a body cavity such as the abdomen, the drugs mainly affect cancer cells in those areas (regional chemotherapy). The way the chemotherapy is given depends on the type and stage of the cancer being treated.

Anticancer drugs given by mouth or vein to treat brain and spinal cord tumors cannot cross the blood-brain barrier and enter the fluid that surrounds the brain and spinal cord. Instead, an anticancer drug is injected into the fluid-filled space to kill cancer cells there. This is called intrathecal chemotherapy.

New types of treatment are being tested in clinical trials.

High-dose chemotherapy with stem cell transplant

High-dose chemotherapy with stem cell transplant is a way of giving high doses of chemotherapy and replacing blood-forming cells destroyed by the cancer treatment. Stem cells (immature blood cells) are removed from the blood or bone marrow of the patient or a donor and are frozen and stored. After the chemotherapy is completed, the stored stem cells are thawed and given back to the patient through an infusion. These reinfused stem cells grow into (and restore) the body's blood cells.

Section 20.3

Neuroblastoma

Text in this section is excerpted from "Neuroblastoma Treatment," National Cancer Institute at the National Institutes of Health (NIH), May 21, 2015.

General Information About Neuroblastoma

Neuroblastoma is a disease in which malignant (cancer) cells form in nerve tissue of the adrenal gland, neck, chest, or spinal cord.

Neuroblastoma often begins in the nerve tissue of the adrenal glands. There are two adrenal glands, one on top of each kidney in the back of the upper abdomen. The adrenal glands make important hormones that help control heart rate, blood pressure, blood sugar, and the way the body reacts to stress. Neuroblastoma may also begin in the abdomen, in the chest, in nerve tissue near the spine in the neck, or in the spinal cord.

Neuroblastoma most often begins during early childhood, usually in children younger than 5 years of age. It is found when the tumor begins to grow and cause signs or symptoms. Sometimes it forms before birth and is found during a fetal ultrasound.

By the time neuroblastoma is diagnosed, the cancer has usually metastasized (spread). Neuroblastoma spreads most often to the lymph nodes, bones, bone marrow, liver, and in infants, skin.

Neuroblastoma is sometimes caused by a gene mutation (change) passed from the parent to the child.

The gene mutation that increases the risk of neuroblastoma is sometimes inherited (passed from the parent to the child). In patients with this gene mutation, neuroblastoma usually occurs at a younger age and more than one tumor may form in the adrenal medulla.

Signs and symptoms of neuroblastoma include bone pain and a lump in the abdomen, neck, or chest.

The most common signs and symptoms of neuroblastoma are caused by the tumor pressing on nearby tissues as it grows or by cancer spreading to the bone. These and other signs and symptoms may be caused by neuroblastoma or by other conditions.

Check with your child's doctor if your child has any of the following:

- Lump in the abdomen, neck, or chest.
- Bulging eyes.
- Dark circles around the eyes ("black eyes").
- Bone pain.
- Swollen stomach and trouble breathing (in infants).
- Painless, bluish lumps under the skin (in infants).
- Weakness or paralysis (loss of ability to move a body part).

Less common signs and symptoms of neuroblastoma include the following:

- Fever.

- Shortness of breath.

- Feeling tired.

- Easy bruising or bleeding.

- Petechiae (flat, pinpoint spots under the skin caused by bleeding).

- High blood pressure.

- Severe watery diarrhea.

- Jerky muscle movements.

- Uncontrolled eye movement.

Tests that examine many different body tissues and fluids are used to detect (find) and diagnose neuroblastoma.

The following tests and procedures may be used:

- **Physical exam and history:** An exam of the body to check general signs of health, including checking for signs of disease, such as lumps or anything else that seems unusual. A history of the patient's health habits and past illnesses and treatments will also be taken.

- **Neurological exam:** A series of questions and tests to check the brain, spinal cord, and nerve function. The exam checks a person's mental status, coordination, and ability to walk normally, and how well the muscles, senses, and reflexes work. This may also be called a neuro exam or a neurologic exam.

- **Urine catecholamine studies:** A procedure in which a urine sample is checked to measure the amount of certain substances, vanillylmandelic acid (VMA) and homovanillic acid (HVA), that are made when catecholamines break down and are released into the urine. A higher than normal amount of VMA or HVA can be a sign of neuroblastoma.

- **Blood chemistry studies:** A procedure in which a blood sample is checked to measure the amounts of certain substances released into the blood by organs and tissues in the body.

An unusual (higher or lower than normal) amount of a substance can be a sign of disease.

- **Hormone test:** A procedure in which a blood sample is checked to measure the amount of hormones released into the blood by the adrenal medulla. A higher than normal amount of the hormones dopamine and norepinephrine may be a sign of neuroblastoma.

- **mIBG (metaiodobenzylguanidine) scan:** A procedure used to find neuroendocrine tumors, such as neuroblastoma and pheochromocytoma. A very small amount of a substance called radioactive mIBG is injected into a vein and travels through the bloodstream. Neuroendocrine tumor cells take up the radioactive mIBG and are detected by a scanner. Scans may be taken over 1-3 days. An iodine solution may be given before or during the test to keep the thyroid gland from absorbing too much of the mIBG. This test is also used to find out how well the tumor is responding to treatment. mIBG is used in high doses to treat neuroblastoma.

- **Bone marrow aspiration and biopsy:** The removal of bone marrow, blood, and a small piece of bone by inserting a hollow needle into the hipbone or breastbone. A pathologist views the bone marrow, blood, and bone under a microscope to look for signs of cancer.

- **X-ray:** An x-ray is a type of energy beam that can go through the body and onto film, making a picture of areas inside the body.

- **CT scan (CAT scan):** A procedure that makes a series of detailed pictures of areas inside the body, taken from different angles. The pictures are made by a computer linked to an x-ray machine. A dye may be injected into a vein or swallowed to help the organs or tissues show up more clearly. This procedure is also called computed tomography, computerized tomography, or computerized axial tomography.

- **MRI (magnetic resonance imaging) with gadolinium:** A procedure that uses a magnet, radio waves, and a computer to make a series of detailed pictures of areas inside the body. A substance called gadolinium is injected into a vein. The gadolinium collects around the cancer cells so they show up brighter in the picture. This procedure is also called nuclear magnetic resonance imaging (NMRI).

- **Ultrasound exam:** A procedure in which high-energy sound waves (ultrasound) are bounced off internal tissues or organs and make echoes. The echoes form a picture of body tissues called a sonogram. The picture can be printed to be looked at later.

A biopsy is done to diagnose neuroblastoma.

Cells and tissues are removed during a biopsy so they can be viewed under a microscope by a pathologist to check for signs of cancer. The way the biopsy is done depends on where the tumor is in the body. Sometimes the whole tumor is removed at the same time the biopsy is done.

The following tests may be done on the tissue that is removed:

- **Cytogenetic analysis:** A laboratory test in which cells in a sample of tissue are viewed under a microscope to look for certain changes in the chromosomes.

- **Light and electron microscopy:** A laboratory test in which cells in a sample of tissue are viewed under regular and high-powered microscopes to look for certain changes in the cells.

- **Immunohistochemistry:** A test that uses antibodies to check for certain antigens in a sample of tissue. The antibody is usually linked to a radioactive substance or a dye that causes the tissue to light up under a microscope. This type of test may be used to tell the difference between different types of cancer.

- **MYC-N amplification study:** A laboratory study in which tumor or bone marrow cells are checked for the level of *MYC-N*. *MYC-N* is important for cell growth. A higher level of *MYC-N* (more than 10 copies of the gene) is called *MYC-N* amplification. Neuroblastoma with *MYC-N* amplification is more likely to spread in the body and less likely to respond to treatment.

Children who are 6 months old or younger may not need a biopsy or surgery to remove the tumor because the tumor may disappear without treatment.

Certain factors affect prognosis (chance of recovery) and treatment options.

The prognosis (chance of recovery) and treatment options depend on the following:

- Age of the child at diagnosis.
- Stage of the cancer.

- Tumor histology (the shape, function, and structure of the tumor cells).

- Whether there is cancer in the lymph nodes on the same side of the body as the cancer or whether there is cancer in the lymph nodes on the opposite side of the body.

- How the tumor responds to treatment.

- Whether there are certain changes in the chromosomes.

- How much time passed between diagnosis and when the cancer recurred (for recurrent cancer).

Prognosis and treatment options for neuroblastoma are also affected by tumor biology, which includes:

- The patterns of the tumor cells.

- How different the tumor cells are from normal cells.

- How fast the tumor cells are growing.

- Whether the tumor shows *MYC-N* amplification.

The tumor biology is said to be favorable or unfavorable, depending on these factors. A favorable tumor biology means there is a better chance of recovery.

In some children who are 6 months old and younger, neuroblastoma may disappear without treatment. The child is closely watched for signs or symptoms of neuroblastoma. If signs or symptoms occur, treatment may be needed.

Stages of Neuroblastoma

After neuroblastoma has been diagnosed, tests are done to find out if cancer has spread from where it started to other parts of the body.

The process used to find out the extent or spread of cancer is called staging. The information gathered from the staging process helps determine the stage of the disease. For neuroblastoma, stage is one of the factors used to plan treatment. The results of tests and procedures used to diagnose neuroblastoma may also be used for staging.

The following tests and procedures also may be used to determine the stage:

- **Lumbar puncture:** A procedure used to collect cerebrospinal fluid from the spinal column. This is done by placing a needle into the spinal column. This procedure is also called an LP or spinal tap.

- **Lymph node biopsy:** The removal of all or part of a lymph node. A pathologist views the tissue under a microscope to look for cancer cells. One of the following types of biopsies may be done:

    - **Excisional biopsy:** The removal of an entire lymph node.

    - **Incisional biopsy:** The removal of part of a lymph node.

    - **Core biopsy:** The removal of tissue from a lymph node using a wide needle.

    - **Fine-needle aspiration (FNA) biopsy:** The removal of tissue or fluid from a lymph node using a thin needle.

- **X-rays of the chest, bones, and abdomen:** An x-ray is a type of energy beam that can go through the body and onto film, making a picture of areas inside the body.

- **Bone scan:** A procedure to check if there are rapidly dividing cells, such as cancer cells, in the bone. A very small amount of radioactive material is injected into a vein and travels through the bloodstream. The radioactive material collects in the bones with cancer and is detected by a scanner.

There are three ways that cancer spreads in the body.

Cancer can spread through tissue, the lymph system, and the blood:

- Tissue. The cancer spreads from where it began by growing into nearby areas.

- Lymph system. The cancer spreads from where it began by getting into the lymph system. The cancer travels through the lymph vessels to other parts of the body.

- Blood. The cancer spreads from where it began by getting into the blood. The cancer travels through the blood vessels to other parts of the body.

Cancer may spread from where it began to other parts of the body.

When cancer spreads to another part of the body, it is called metastasis. Cancer cells break away from where they began (the primary tumor) and travel through the lymph system or blood.

- Lymph system. The cancer gets into the lymph system, travels through the lymph vessels, and forms a tumor (metastatic tumor) in another part of the body.

- Blood. The cancer gets into the blood, travels through the blood vessels, and forms a tumor (metastatic tumor) in another part of the body.

The metastatic tumor is the same type of cancer as the primary tumor. For example, if neuroblastoma spreads to the liver, the cancer cells in the liver are actually neuroblastoma cells. The disease is metastatic neuroblastoma, not liver cancer.

The following stages are used for neuroblastoma:

Stage 1

In stage 1, the tumor is in only one area and all of the tumor that can be seen is completely removed during surgery.

Stage 2

Stage 2 is divided into stages 2A and 2B.

- Stage 2A: The tumor is in only one area and all of the tumor that can be seen cannot be completely removed during surgery.

- Stage 2B: The tumor is in only one area and all of the tumor that can be seen may be completely removed during surgery. Cancer cells are found in the lymph nodes near the tumor.

Stage 3

In stage 3, one of the following is true:

- the tumor cannot be completely removed during surgery and has spread from one side of the body to the other side and may also have spread to nearby lymph nodes; or

- the tumor is in only one area, on one side of the body, but has spread to lymph nodes on the other side of the body; or

- the tumor is in the middle of the body and has spread to tissues or lymph nodes on both sides of the body, and the tumor cannot be removed by surgery.

Stage 4

Stage 4 is divided into stages 4 and 4S.

- In stage 4, the tumor has spread to distant lymph nodes or other parts of the body.

- In stage 4S:

  - the child is younger than 12 months; and

  - the cancer has spread to the skin, liver, and/or bone marrow; and

  - the tumor is in only one area and all of the tumor that can be seen may be completely removed during surgery; and/or

  - cancer cells may be found in the lymph nodes near the tumor.

Treatment of neuroblastoma is based on risk groups.

For many types of cancer, stages are used to plan treatment. For neuroblastoma, treatment depends on risk groups. The stage of neuroblastoma is one factor used to determine risk group. Other factors are the age of the child, tumor histology, and tumor biology.

There are three risk groups: low risk, intermediate risk, and high risk.

- Low-risk and intermediate-risk neuroblastoma have a good chance of being cured.

- High-risk neuroblastoma may be hard to cure.

Treatment Option Overview

There are different types of treatment for patients with neuroblastoma.

Different types of treatment are available for patients with neuroblastoma. Some treatments are standard (the currently used treatment),

176

and some are being tested in clinical trials. A treatment clinical trial is a research study meant to help improve current treatments or obtain information on new treatments for patients with cancer. When clinical trials show that a new treatment is better than the standard treatment, the new treatment may become the standard treatment.

Because cancer in children is rare, taking part in a clinical trial should be considered. Some clinical trials are open only to patients who have not started treatment.

Children with neuroblastoma should have their treatment planned by a team of doctors with expertise in treating childhood cancer, especially neuroblastoma.

Treatment will be overseen by a pediatric oncologist, a doctor who specializes in treating children with cancer. The pediatric oncologist works with other pediatric health care providers who are experts in treating children with neuroblastoma and who specialize in certain areas of medicine. These may include the following specialists:

- Pediatric surgeon.
- Radiation oncologist.
- Endocrinologist.
- Neurologist.
- Neuropathologist.
- Neuroradiologist.
- Pediatrician.
- Pediatric nurse specialist.
- Social worker.
- Child life professional.
- Rehabilitation specialist.
- Psychologist.

Children who are treated for neuroblastoma may have an increased risk of second cancers.

Some cancer treatments cause side effects that continue or appear years after cancer treatment has ended. These are called late effects. Late effects of cancer treatment may include:

- Physical problems.

- Changes in mood, feelings, thinking, learning, or memory.

- Second cancers (new types of cancer).

Some late effects may be treated or controlled. It is important that parents of children who are treated for neuroblastoma talk with their doctors about the possible late effects caused by some treatments.

Five types of standard treatment are used:

Observation

Observation is closely monitoring a patient's condition without giving any treatment until signs or symptoms appear or change.

Surgery

Surgery is used to treat neuroblastoma unless it has spread to other parts of the body. Depending on where the tumor is, as much of the tumor as is safely possible will be removed. If the tumor cannot be removed, a biopsy may be done instead.

Radiation therapy

Radiation therapy is a cancer treatment that uses high-energy x-rays or other types of radiation to kill cancer cells or keep them from growing. There are two types of radiation therapy. External radiation therapy uses a machine outside the body to send radiation toward the cancer. Internal radiation therapy uses a radioactive substance sealed in needles, seeds, wires, or catheters that are placed directly into or near the cancer.

The way the radiation therapy is given depends on the type and stage of the cancer being treated. External radiation therapy is used to treat neuroblastoma.

High-risk neuroblastoma that comes back after initial treatment is sometimes treated with mIBG (radioactive iodine therapy). Radioactive iodine is given through an intravenous (IV) line and enters the bloodstream which carries radiation directly to tumor cells. Radioactive iodine collects in neuroblastoma cells and kills them with the radiation that is given off.

Chemotherapy

Chemotherapy is a cancer treatment that uses drugs to stop the growth of cancer cells, either by killing the cells or by stopping them from dividing. When chemotherapy is taken by mouth or injected into a vein or muscle, the drugs enter the bloodstream and can reach cancer cells throughout the body (systemic chemotherapy). When chemotherapy is placed directly into the cerebrospinal fluid, an organ, or a body cavity such as the abdomen, the drugs mainly affect cancer cells in those areas (regional chemotherapy). The way the chemotherapy is given depends on the type and stage of the cancer being treated.

The use of two or more anticancer drugs is called combination chemotherapy.

High-dose chemotherapy and radiation therapy with stem cell rescue

High-dose chemotherapy and radiation therapy with stem cell rescue is a way of giving high doses of chemotherapy and radiation therapy and replacing blood-forming cells destroyed by cancer treatment for high-risk neuroblastoma. Stem cells (immature blood cells) are removed from the blood or bone marrow of the patient and are frozen and stored. After chemotherapy and radiation therapy are completed, the stored stem cells are thawed and given back to the patient through an infusion. These reinfused stem cells grow into (and restore) the body's blood cells.

Maintenance therapy is given after high-dose chemotherapy and radiation therapy with stem cell rescue to kill any cancer cells that may regrow and cause the disease to come back. Maintenance therapy is given for 6 months and includes the following treatments:

- Isotretinoin: A vitamin-like drug that slows the cancer's ability to make more cancer cells and changes how these cells look and act. This drug is taken by mouth.

- Anti-GD2 antibody ch14.18: A type of monoclonal antibody therapy that uses an antibody (ch14.18) made in the laboratory from a single type of immune system cell. ch14.18 identifies and attaches to a substance, called GD2, on the surface of neuro-blastoma cells. Once the ch14.18 attaches to the GD2, a signal is sent to the immune system that a foreign substance has been found and needs to be killed. Then the body's immune system kills the neuroblastoma cell. This drug is given by infusion.

- Granulocyte-macrophage colony-stimulating factor (GM-CSF): A cytokine that helps make more immune system cells, especially granulocytes and macrophages (white blood cells), which can attack and kill cancer cells.

179

- Interleukin-2 (IL-2): A type of biologic therapy that boosts the growth and activity of many immune cells, especially lymphocytes (a type of white blood cell). Lymphocytes can attack and kill cancer cells.

New types of treatment are being tested in clinical trials.

Targeted therapy

Targeted therapy is a type of treatment that uses drugs or other substances to identify and attack specific cancer cells without harming normal cells. Tyrosine kinase inhibitor (TKI) therapy is one type of targeted therapy being studied in the treatment of neuroblastoma.

TKI therapy blocks signals needed for tumors to grow. TKIs block the enzyme, tyrosine kinase, that causes stem cells to become more white blood cells (granulocytes or blasts) than the body needs. Crizotinib is one of the TKIs being studied to treat neuroblastoma that has come back after treatment. TKIs may be used in combination with other anticancer drugs as adjuvant therapy (treatment given after the initial treatment, to lower the risk that the cancer will come back).

Vaccine therapy

Vaccine therapy is a type of biologic therapy. Biologic therapy is a treatment that uses the patient's immune system to fight cancer. Substances made by the body or made in a laboratory are used to boost, direct, or restore the body's natural defenses against cancer. This type of cancer treatment is also called biotherapy or immunotherapy.

Other drug therapy

Lenalidomide is a type of angiogenesis inhibitor. It prevents the growth of new blood vessels that are needed by a tumor to grow.

Section 20.4

Pituitary Tumors

Text in this section is excerpted from "Pituitary Tumors Treatment (PDQ®)," National Cancer Institute at the National Institutes of Health (NIH), March 11, 2015.

General Information About Pituitary Tumors

A pituitary tumor is a growth of abnormal cells in the tissues of the pituitary gland.

Pituitary tumors form in the pituitary gland, a pea-sized organ in the center of the brain, just above the back of the nose. The pituitary gland is sometimes called the "master endocrine gland" because it makes hormones that affect the way many parts of the body work. It also controls hormones made by many other glands in the body.

Pituitary tumors are divided into three groups:

- Benign pituitary adenomas: Tumors that are not cancer. These tumors grow very slowly and do not spread from the pituitary gland to other parts of the body.

- Invasive pituitary adenomas: Benign tumors that may spread to bones of the skull or the sinus cavity below the pituitary gland.

- Pituitary carcinomas: Tumors that are malignant (cancer). These pituitary tumors spread into other areas of the central nervous system (brain and spinal cord) or outside of the central nervous system. Very few pituitary tumors are malignant.

Pituitary tumors may be either non-functioning or functioning.

- Non-functioning pituitary tumors do not make extra amounts of hormones.

- Functioning pituitary tumors make more than the normal amount of one or more hormones. Most pituitary tumors are functioning tumors. The extra hormones made by pituitary tumors may cause certain signs or symptoms of disease.

The pituitary gland hormones control many other glands in the body.

Hormones made by the pituitary gland include:

- Prolactin: A hormone that causes a woman's breasts to make milk during and after pregnancy.

- Adrenocorticotropic hormone (ACTH): A hormone that causes the adrenal glands to make a hormone called cortisol. Cortisol helps control the use of sugar, protein, and fats in the body and helps the body deal with stress.

- Growth hormone: A hormone that helps control body growth and the use of sugar and fat in the body. Growth hormone is also called somatotropin.

- Thyroid-stimulating hormone: A hormone that causes the thyroid gland to make other hormones that control growth, body temperature, and heart rate. Thyroid-stimulating hormone is also called thyrotropin.

- Luteinizing hormone (LH) and follicle-stimulating hormone (FSH): Hormones that control the menstrual cycle in women and the making of sperm in men.

Having certain genetic conditions increases the risk of developing a pituitary tumor.

Anything that increases your risk of getting a disease is called a risk factor. Having a risk factor does not mean that you will get cancer; not having risk factors doesn't mean that you will not get cancer. Talk with your doctor if you think you may be at risk. Risk factors for pituitary tumors include having the following hereditary diseases:

- Multiple endocrine neoplasia type 1 (MEN1) syndrome.

- Carney complex.

- Isolated familial acromegaly.

Signs of a pituitary tumor include problems with vision and certain physical changes.

Signs and symptoms can be caused by the growth of the tumor and/ or by hormones the tumor makes or by other conditions. Some tumors may not cause signs or symptoms. Check with your doctor if you have any of these problems.

Signs and symptoms of a non-functioning pituitary tumor

Sometimes, a pituitary tumor may press on or damage parts of the pituitary gland, causing it to stop making one or more hormones. Too little of a certain hormone will affect the work of the gland or organ that the hormone controls. The following signs and symptoms may occur:

- Headache.
- Some loss of vision.
- Loss of body hair.
- In women, less frequent or no menstrual periods or no milk from the breasts.
- In men, loss of facial hair, growth of breast tissue, and impotence.
- In women and men, lower sex drive.
- In children, slowed growth and sexual development.
- Most of the tumors that make LH and FSH do not make enough extra hormone to cause signs and symptoms. These tumors are considered to be non-functioning tumors.

Signs and symptoms of a functioning pituitary tumor

When a functioning pituitary tumor makes extra hormones, the signs and symptoms will depend on the type of hormone being made.

Too much prolactin may cause:

- Headache.
- Some loss of vision.
- Less frequent or no menstrual periods or menstrual periods with a very light flow.
- Trouble becoming pregnant or an inability to become pregnant.
- Impotence in men.
- Lower sex drive.

- Flow of breast milk in a woman who is not pregnant or breast-feeding.

Too much ACTH may cause:

- Headache.
- Some loss of vision.
- Weight gain in the face, neck, and trunk of the body, and thin arms and legs.
- A lump of fat on the back of the neck.
- Thin skin that may have purple or pink stretch marks on the chest or abdomen.
- Easy bruising.
- Growth of fine hair on the face, upper back, or arms.
- Bones that break easily.
- Anxiety, irritability, and depression.

Too much growth hormone may cause:

- Headache.
- Some loss of vision.
- In adults, acromegaly (growth of the bones in the face, hands, and feet). In children, the whole body may grow much taller and larger than normal.
- Tingling or numbness in the hands and fingers.
- Snoring or pauses in breathing during sleep.
- Joint pain.
- Sweating more than usual.
- Dysmorphophobia (extreme dislike of or concern about one or more parts of the body).

Too much thyroid-stimulating hormone may cause:

- Irregular heartbeat.
- Shakiness.
- Weight loss.

- Trouble sleeping.
- Frequent bowel movements.
- Sweating.

Other general signs and symptoms of pituitary tumors:

- Nausea and vomiting.
- Confusion.
- Dizziness.
- Seizures.
- Runny or "drippy" nose (cerebrospinal fluid that surrounds the brain and spinal cord leaks into the nose).

Imaging studies and tests that examine the blood and urine are used to detect (find) and diagnose a pituitary tumor.

The following tests and procedures may be used:

- **Physical exam and history:** An exam of the body to check general signs of health, including checking for signs of disease, such as lumps or anything else that seems unusual. A history of the patient's health habits and past illnesses and treatments will also be taken.

- **Eye exam:** An exam to check vision and the general health of the eyes.

- **Visual field exam:** An exam to check a person's field of vision (the total area in which objects can be seen). This test measures both central vision (how much a person can see when looking straight ahead) and peripheral vision (how much a person can see in all other directions while staring straight ahead). The eyes are tested one at a time. The eye not being tested is covered.

- **Neurological exam:** A series of questions and tests to check the brain, spinal cord, and nerve function. The exam checks a person's mental status, coordination, and ability to walk normally, and how well the muscles, senses, and reflexes work. This may also be called a neuro exam or a neurologic exam.

- **MRI (magnetic resonance imaging) with gadolinium:** A procedure that uses a magnet, radio waves, and a computer to make a series of detailed pictures of areas inside the brain and spinal cord. A substance called gadolinium is injected into a vein. The gadolinium collects around the cancer cells so they show up brighter in the picture. This procedure is also called nuclear magnetic resonance imaging (NMRI).

- **Blood chemistry study:** A procedure in which a blood sample is checked to measure the amounts of certain substances, such as glucose (sugar), released into the blood by organs and tissues in the body. An unusual (higher or lower than normal) amount of a substance can be a sign of disease in the organ or tissue that makes it.

- **Blood tests:** Tests to measure the levels of testosterone or estrogen in the blood. A higher or lower than normal amount of these hormones may be a sign of pituitary tumor.

- **Twenty-four-hour urine test:** A test in which urine is collected for 24 hours to measure the amounts of certain substances. An unusual (higher or lower than normal) amount of a substance can be a sign of disease in the organ or tissue that makes it. A higher than normal amount of the hormone cortisol may be a sign of a pituitary tumor and Cushing syndrome.

- **High-dose dexamethasone suppression test:** A test in which one or more high doses of dexamethasone are given. The level of cortisol is checked from a sample of blood or from urine that is collected for three days.

- **Low-dose dexamethasone suppression test:** A test in which one or more small doses of dexamethasone are given. The level of cortisol is checked from a sample of blood or from urine that is collected for three days.

- **Venous sampling for pituitary tumors:** A procedure in which a sample of blood is taken from veins coming from the pituitary gland. The sample is checked to measure the amount of ACTH released into the blood by the gland. Venous sampling may be done if blood tests show there is a tumor making ACTH, but the pituitary gland looks normal in the imaging tests.

- **Biopsy:** The removal of cells or tissues so they can be viewed under a microscope by a pathologist to check for signs of cancer.

The following tests may be done on the sample of tissue that is removed:

- **Immunohistochemistry:** A test that uses antibodies to check for certain antigens in a sample of tissue. The antibody is usually linked to a radioactive substance or a dye that causes the tissue to light up under a microscope. This type of test may be used to tell the difference between different types of cancer.

- **Immunocytochemistry:** A test that uses antibodies to check for certain antigens in a sample of cells. The antibody is usually linked to a radioactive substance or a dye that causes the cells to light up under a microscope. This type of test may be used to tell the difference between different types of cancer.

- **Light and electron microscopy:** A laboratory test in which cells in a sample of tissue are viewed under regular and high-powered microscopes to look for certain changes in the cells.

Certain factors affect prognosis (chance of recovery) and treatment options.

The prognosis (chance of recovery) depends on the type of tumor and whether the tumor has spread into other areas of the central nervous system (brain and spinal cord) or outside of the central nervous system to other parts of the body.

Treatment options depend on the following:

- The type and size of the tumor.
- Whether the tumor is making hormones.
- Whether the tumor is causing problems with vision or other signs or symptoms.
- Whether the tumor has spread into the brain around the pituitary gland or to other parts of the body.
- Whether the tumor has just been diagnosed or has recurred (come back).

Chapter 21

Head and Neck Cancer

Chapter Contents

Section 21.1

Laryngeal Cancer

Text in this section is excerpted from "Laryngeal Cancer Treatment,"
National Cancer Institute at the National Institutes of Health (NIH),
May 19, 2015.

General Information About Hypopharyngeal Cancer

**Laryngeal cancer is a disease in which malignant (cancer)
cells form in the tissues of the larynx.**

The larynx is a part of the throat, between the base of the tongue
and the trachea. The larynx contains the vocal cords, which vibrate
and make sound when air is directed against them. The sound echoes
through the pharynx, mouth, and nose to make a person's voice.

There are three main parts of the larynx:

- Supraglottis: The upper part of the larynx above the vocal cords,
  including the epiglottis.

- Glottis: The middle part of the larynx where the vocal cords are
  located.

- Subglottis: The lower part of the larynx between the vocal cords
  and the trachea (windpipe).

Most laryngeal cancers form in squamous cells, the thin, flat cells
lining the inside of the larynx.
Laryngeal cancer is a type of head and neck cancer.

**Use of tobacco products and drinking too much alcohol can
affect the risk of laryngeal cancer.**

Anything that increases your risk of getting a disease is called a
risk factor. Having a risk factor does not mean that you will get cancer;
not having risk factors doesn't mean that you will not get cancer. Talk
with your doctor if you think you may be at risk.

190

Signs and symptoms of laryngeal cancer include a sore throat and ear pain.

These and other signs and symptoms may be caused by laryngeal cancer or by other conditions. Check with your doctor if you have any of the following:

- A sore throat or cough that does not go away.
- Trouble or pain when swallowing.
- Ear pain.
- A lump in the neck or throat.
- A change or hoarseness in the voice.

Tests that examine the throat and neck are used to help detect (find), diagnose, and stage laryngeal cancer.

The following tests and procedures may be used:

- **Physical exam of the throat and neck:** An exam to check the throat and neck for abnormal areas. The doctor will feel the inside of the mouth with a gloved finger and examine the mouth and throat with a small long-handled mirror and light. This will include checking the insides of the cheeks and lips; the gums; the back, roof, and floor of the mouth; the top, bottom, and sides of the tongue; and the throat. The neck will be felt for swollen lymph nodes. A history of the patient's health habits and past illnesses and medical treatments will also be taken.
- **Biopsy:**
  - Laryngoscopy
  - Endoscopy
- **CT scan (CAT scan) MRI (magnetic resonance imaging)**
- **PET scan (positron emission tomography scan) Bone scan**
- **Barium swallow**

Certain factors affect prognosis (chance of recovery) and treatment options.

Prognosis (chance of recovery) depends on the following:

- The stage of the disease.

191

- The location and size of the tumor.
- The grade of the tumor.
- The patient's age, gender, and general health, including whether the patient is anemic.

Treatment options depend on the following:

- The stage of the disease.
- The location and size of the tumor.
- Keeping the patient's ability to talk, eat, and breathe as normal as possible.
- Whether the cancer has come back (recurred).

Smoking tobacco and drinking alcohol decrease the effectiveness of treatment for laryngeal cancer. Patients with laryngeal cancer who continue to smoke and drink are less likely to be cured and more likely to develop a second tumor. After treatment for laryngeal cancer, frequent and careful follow-up is important.

Stages of Laryngeal Cancer

After laryngeal cancer has been diagnosed, tests are done to find out if cancer cells have spread within the larynx or to other parts of the body.

The process used to find out if cancer has spread within the larynx or to other parts of the body is called staging. The information gathered from the staging process determines the stage of the disease. It is important to know the stage of the disease in order to plan treatment. The results of some of the tests used to diagnose laryngeal cancer are often also used to stage the disease.

There are three ways that cancer spreads in the body.

Cancer can spread through tissue, the lymph system, and the blood:

- Tissue. The cancer spreads from where it began by growing into nearby areas.
- Lymph system. The cancer spreads from where it began by getting into the lymph system. The cancer travels through the lymph vessels to other parts of the body.

- Blood. The cancer spreads from where it began by getting into the blood. The cancer travels through the blood vessels to other parts of the body.

Cancer may spread from where it began to other parts of the body.

When cancer spreads to another part of the body, it is called metastasis. Cancer cells break away from where they began (the primary tumor) and travel through the lymph system or blood.

- Lymph system. The cancer gets into the lymph system, travels through the lymph vessels, and forms a tumor (metastatic tumor) in another part of the body.

- Blood. The cancer gets into the blood, travels through the blood vessels, and forms a tumor (metastatic tumor) in another part of the body.

The metastatic tumor is the same type of cancer as the primary tumor. For example, if laryngeal cancer spreads to the lung, the cancer cells in the lung are actually laryngeal cancer cells. The disease is metastatic laryngeal cancer, not lung cancer.

The following stages are used for laryngeal cancer:

Stage 0 (Carcinoma in Situ)

In stage 0, abnormal cells are found in the lining of the larynx. These abnormal cells may become cancer and spread into nearby normal tissue. Stage 0 is also called carcinoma in situ.

Stage I

In stage I, cancer has formed. Stage I laryngeal cancer depends on where cancer began in the larynx:

- Supraglottis: Cancer is in one area of the supraglottis only and the vocal cords can move normally.

- Glottis: Cancer is in one or both vocal cords and the vocal cords can move normally.

- Subglottis: Cancer is in the subglottis only.

Stage II

In stage II, cancer is in the larynx only. Stage II laryngeal cancer depends on where cancer began in the larynx:

- Supraglottis: Cancer is in more than one area of the supraglottis or surrounding tissues.

- Glottis: Cancer has spread to the supraglottis and/or the subglottis and/or the vocal cords cannot move normally.

- Subglottis: Cancer has spread to one or both vocal cords, which may not move normally.

Stage III

Stage III laryngeal cancer depends on whether cancer has spread from the supraglottis, glottis, or subglottis.

In stage III cancer of the supraglottis:

- cancer is in the larynx only and the vocal cords cannot move, and/or cancer is in tissues next to the larynx. Cancer may have spread to one lymph node on the same side of the neck as the original tumor and the lymph node is 3 centimeters or smaller; or

- cancer is in one area of the supraglottis and in one lymph node on the same side of the neck as the original tumor; the lymph node is 3 centimeters or smaller and the vocal cords can move normally; or

- cancer is in more than one area of the supraglottis or surrounding tissues and in one lymph node on the same side of the neck as the original tumor; the lymph node is 3 centimeters or smaller.

In stage III cancer of the glottis:

- cancer is in the larynx only and the vocal cords cannot move, and/or cancer is in tissues next to the larynx; cancer may have spread to one lymph node on the same side of the neck as the original tumor and the lymph node is 3 centimeters or smaller; or

- cancer is in one or both vocal cords and in one lymph node on the same side of the neck as the original tumor; the lymph node is 3 centimeters or smaller and the vocal cords can move normally; or

- cancer has spread to the supraglottis and/or the subglottis and/or the vocal cords cannot move normally. Cancer has also spread to one lymph node on the same side of the neck as the original tumor and the lymph node is 3 centimeters or smaller.

In stage III cancer of the subglottis:

- cancer is in the larynx and the vocal cords cannot move; cancer may have spread to one lymph node on the same side of the neck as the original tumor and the lymph node is 3 centimeters or smaller; or

- cancer is in the subglottis and in one lymph node on the same side of the neck as the original tumor; the lymph node is 3 centimeters or smaller; or

- cancer has spread to one or both vocal cords, which may not move normally. Cancer has also spread to one lymph node on the same side of the neck as the original tumor and the lymph node is 3 centimeters or smaller.

Stage IV

Stage IV is divided into stage IVA, stage IVB, and stage IVC. Each substage is the same for cancer in the supraglottis, glottis, or subglottis.

- In stage IVA:

  - cancer has spread through the thyroid cartilage and/or has spread to tissues beyond the larynx such as the neck, trachea, thyroid, or esophagus. Cancer may have spread to one lymph node on the same side of the neck as the original tumor and the lymph node is 3 centimeters or smaller; or

  - cancer has spread to one lymph node on the same side of the neck as the original tumor and the lymph node is larger than 3 centimeters but not larger than 6 centimeters, or has spread to more than one lymph node anywhere in the neck with none larger than 6 centimeters. Cancer may have spread to tissues beyond the larynx, such as the neck, trachea, thyroid, or esophagus. The vocal cords may not move normally.

- In stage IVB:

  - cancer has spread to the space in front of the spinal column, surrounds the carotid artery, or has spread to parts of the chest. Cancer may have spread to one or more lymph nodes anywhere in the neck and the lymph nodes may be any size; or

  - cancer has spread to a lymph node that is larger than 6 centimeters and may have spread as far as the space in front of the spinal column, around the carotid artery, or to parts of the chest. The vocal cords may not move normally.

- In stage IVC, cancer has spread to other parts of the body, such as the lungs, liver, or bone.

Treatment Option Overview

There are different types of treatment for patients with laryngeal cancer.

Different types of treatment are available for patients with laryngeal cancer. Some treatments are standard (the currently used treatment), and some are being tested in clinical trials. A treatment clinical trial is a research study meant to help improve current treatments or obtain information on new treatments for patients with cancer. When clinical trials show that a new treatment is better than the standard treatment, the new treatment may become the standard treatment. Patients may want to think about taking part in a clinical trial. Some clinical trials are open only to patients who have not started treatment.

Three types of standard treatment are used:

Radiation therapy

Radiation therapy is a cancer treatment that uses high-energy x-rays or other types of radiation to kill cancer cells. There are two types of radiation therapy. External radiation therapy uses a machine outside the body to send radiation toward the cancer. Internal radiation therapy uses a radioactive substance sealed in needles, seeds, wires, or catheters that are placed directly into or near the cancer. The way the radiation therapy is given depends on the type and stage of the cancer being treated.

Radiation therapy may work better in patients who have stopped smoking before beginning treatment. External radiation therapy to the thyroid or the pituitary gland may change the way the thyroid gland works. The doctor may test the thyroid gland before and after therapy to make sure it is working properly.

Hyperfractionated radiation therapy and new types of radiation therapy are being studied in the treatment of laryngeal cancer.

Surgery

Surgery (removing the cancer in an operation) is a common treatment for all stages of laryngeal cancer. The following surgical procedures may be used:

- Cordectomy: Surgery to remove the vocal cords only.

- Supraglottic laryngectomy: Surgery to remove the supraglottis only.

- Hemilaryngectomy: Surgery to remove half of the larynx (voice box). A hemilaryngectomy saves the voice.

- Partial laryngectomy: Surgery to remove part of the larynx (voice box). A partial laryngectomy helps keep the patient's ability to talk.

- Total laryngectomy: Surgery to remove the whole larynx. During this operation, a hole is made in the front of the neck to allow the patient to breathe. This is called a tracheostomy.

- Thyroidectomy: The removal of all or part of the thyroid gland.

- Laser surgery: A surgical procedure that uses a laser beam (a narrow beam of intense light) as a knife to make bloodless cuts in tissue or to remove a surface lesion such as a tumor.

Even if the doctor removes all the cancer that can be seen at the time of the surgery, some patients may be given chemotherapy or radiation therapy after surgery to kill any cancer cells that are left. Treatment given after the surgery, to lower the risk that the cancer will come back, is called adjuvant therapy.

Chemotherapy

Chemotherapy is a cancer treatment that uses drugs to stop the growth of cancer cells, either by killing the cells or by stopping the cells from dividing. When chemotherapy is taken by mouth or injected into a vein or muscle, the drugs enter the bloodstream and can reach cancer cells throughout the body (systemic chemotherapy). When chemotherapy is placed directly into the cerebrospinal fluid, an organ, or a body cavity such as the abdomen, the drugs mainly affect cancer cells in those areas (regional chemotherapy). The way the chemotherapy is given depends on the type and stage of the cancer being treated.

New types of treatment are being tested in clinical trials.

Chemoprevention

Chemoprevention is the use of drugs, vitamins, or other substances to reduce the risk of developing cancer or to reduce the risk cancer will recur (come back). The drug isotretinoin is being studied to prevent the development of a second cancer in patients who have had cancer of the head or neck.

Radiosensitizers

Radiosensitizers are drugs that make tumor cells more sensitive to radiation therapy. Combining radiation therapy with radiosensitizers may kill more tumor cells.

Patients may want to think about taking part in a clinical trial.

For some patients, taking part in a clinical trial may be the best treatment choice. Clinical trials are part of the cancer research process. Clinical trials are done to find out if new cancer treatments are safe and effective or better than the standard treatment.

Many of today's standard treatments for cancer are based on earlier clinical trials. Patients who take part in a clinical trial may receive the standard treatment or be among the first to receive a new treatment.

Patients who take part in clinical trials also help improve the way cancer will be treated in the future. Even when clinical trials do not lead to effective new treatments, they often answer important questions and help move research forward.

Patients can enter clinical trials before, during, or after starting their cancer treatment.

Some clinical trials only include patients who have not yet received treatment. Other trials test treatments for patients whose cancer has

not gotten better. There are also clinical trials that test new ways to stop cancer from recurring (coming back) or reduce the side effects of cancer treatment.

Clinical trials are taking place in many parts of the country.

Follow-up tests may be needed.

Some of the tests that were done to diagnose the cancer or to find out the stage of the cancer may be repeated. Some tests will be repeated in order to see how well the treatment is working. Decisions about whether to continue, change, or stop treatment may be based on the results of these tests.

Some of the tests will continue to be done from time to time after treatment has ended. The results of these tests can show if your condition has changed or if the cancer has recurred (come back). These tests are sometimes called follow-up tests or check-ups.

Section 21.2

Lip and Oral Cavity Cancer

Text in this section is excerpted from "Lip and Oral Cavity Cancer Treatment," National Cancer Institute at the National Institutes of Health (NIH), May 19, 2015.

General information about lip and oral cavity cancer

Lip and oral cavity cancer is a disease in which malignant (cancer) cells form in the lips or mouth.

The oral cavity includes the following:

- The front two thirds of the tongue.

- The gingiva (gums).

- The buccal mucosa (the lining of the inside of the cheeks).

- The floor (bottom) of the mouth under the tongue.

199

- The hard palate (the roof of the mouth).

- The retromolar trigone (the small area behind the wisdom teeth).

Most lip and oral cavity cancers start in squamous cells, the thin, flat cells that line the lips and oral cavity. These are called squamous cell carcinomas. Cancer cells may spread into deeper tissue as the cancer grows. Squamous cell carcinoma usually develops in areas of leukoplakia (white patches of cells that do not rub off).

Lip and oral cavity cancer is a type of head and neck cancer.

Tobacco and alcohol use can affect the risk of lip and oral cavity cancer.

Anything that increases your risk of getting a disease is called a risk factor. Having a risk factor does not mean that you will get cancer; not having risk factors doesn't mean that you will not get cancer. Talk with your doctor if you think you may be at risk. Risk factors for lip and oral cavity cancer include the following:

- Using tobacco products.

- Heavy alcohol use.

- Being exposed to natural sunlight or artificial sunlight (such as from tanning beds) over long periods of time.

- Being male.

Signs of lip and oral cavity cancer include a sore or lump on the lips or in the mouth.

These and other signs and symptoms may be caused by lip and oral cavity cancer or by other conditions. Check with your doctor if you have any of the following:

- A sore on the lip or in the mouth that does not heal.

- A lump or thickening on the lips or gums or in the mouth.

- A white or red patch on the gums, tongue, or lining of the mouth.

- Bleeding, pain, or numbness in the lip or mouth.

- Change in voice.

- Loose teeth or dentures that no longer fit well.

- Trouble chewing or swallowing or moving the tongue or jaw.

- Swelling of jaw.

- Sore throat or feeling that something is caught in the throat.

Lip and oral cavity cancer may not have any symptoms and is sometimes found during a regular dental exam.

Tests that examine the mouth and throat are used to detect (find), diagnose, and stage lip and oral cavity cancer.

The following tests and procedures may be used:

- **Physical exam of the lips and oral cavity:** An exam to check the lips and oral cavity for abnormal areas. The medical doctor or dentist will feel the entire inside of the mouth with a gloved finger and examine the oral cavity with a small long-handled mirror and lights. This will include checking the insides of the cheeks and lips; the gums; the roof and floor of the mouth; and the top, bottom, and sides of the tongue. The neck will be felt for swollen lymph nodes. A history of the patient's health habits and past illnesses and medical and dental treatments will also be taken.

- **Endoscopy**

- **Biopsy**

- **Exfoliative cytology:** A procedure to collect cells from the lip or oral cavity. A piece of cotton, a brush, or a small wooden stick is used to gently scrape cells from the lips, tongue, mouth, or throat. The cells are viewed under a microscope to find out if they are abnormal.

- **MRI (magnetic resonance imaging)**

- **CT scan (CAT scan) Barium swallow**

- **PET scan (positron emission tomography scan)**

- **Bone scan**

Certain factors affect prognosis (chance of recovery) and treatment options.

Prognosis (chance of recovery) depends on the following:

- The stage of the cancer.

- Where the tumor is in the lip or oral cavity.

- Whether the cancer has spread to blood vessels.

201

For patients who smoke, the chance of recovery is better if they stop smoking before beginning radiation therapy.

Treatment options depend on the following:

- The stage of the cancer.
- The size of the tumor and where it is in the lip or oral cavity.
- Whether the patient's appearance and ability to talk and eat can stay the same.
- The patient's age and general health.

Patients who have had lip and oral cavity cancer have an increased risk of developing a second cancer in the head or neck. Frequent and careful follow-up is important. Clinical trials are studying the use of retinoid drugs to reduce the risk of a second head and neck cancer.

Stages of Lip and Oral Cavity Cancer

After lip and oral cavity cancer has been diagnosed, tests are done to find out if cancer cells have spread within the lip and oral cavity or to other parts of the body.

The process used to find out if cancer has spread within the lip and oral cavity or to other parts of the body is called staging. The information gathered from the staging process determines the stage of the disease. It is important to know the stage in order to plan treatment. The results of the tests used to diagnose lip and oral cavity cancer are also used to stage the disease.

There are three ways that cancer spreads in the body.

Cancer can spread through tissue, the lymph system, and the blood:

Tissue. The cancer spreads from where it began by growing into nearby areas.

Lymph system. The cancer spreads from where it began by getting into the lymph system. The cancer travels through the lymph vessels to other parts of the body.

Blood. The cancer spreads from where it began by getting into the blood. The cancer travels through the blood vessels to other parts of the body.

Cancer may spread from where it began to other parts of the body.

When cancer spreads to another part of the body, it is called metastasis. Cancer cells break away from where they began (the primary tumor) and travel through the lymph system or blood.

- Lymph system. The cancer gets into the lymph system, travels through the lymph vessels, and forms a tumor (metastatic tumor) in another part of the body.

- Blood. The cancer gets into the blood, travels through the blood vessels, and forms a tumor (metastatic tumor) in another part of the body.

The metastatic tumor is the same type of cancer as the primary tumor. For example, if lip cancer spreads to the lung, the cancer cells in the lung are actually lip cancer cells. The disease is metastatic lip cancer, not lung cancer.

The following stages are used for lip and oral cavity cancer:

Stage 0 (Carcinoma in Situ)

In stage 0, abnormal cells are found in the lining of the lips and oral cavity. These abnormal cells may become cancer and spread into nearby normal tissue. Stage 0 is also called carcinoma in situ.

Stage I

In stage I, cancer has formed and the tumor is 2 centimeters or smaller. Cancer has not spread to the lymph nodes.

Stage II

In stage II, the tumor is larger than 2 centimeters but not larger than 4 centimeters, and cancer has not spread to the lymph nodes.

Stage III

In stage III, the tumor:

- may be any size and has spread to one lymph node that is 3 centimeters or smaller, on the same side of the neck as the tumor; or

- is larger than 4 centimeters.

Stage IV

Stage IV is divided into stages IVA, IVB, and IVC.

- In stage IVA, the tumor:
- has spread through tissue in the lip or oral cavity into nearby tissue and/or bone (jaw, tongue, floor of mouth, maxillary sinus, or skin on the chin or nose); cancer may have spread to one lymph node that is 3 centimeters or smaller, on the same side of the neck as the tumor; or
- is any size or has spread through tissue in the lip or oral cavity into nearby tissue and/or bone (jaw, tongue, floor of mouth, maxillary sinus, or skin on the chin or nose), and cancer has spread:
  - to one lymph node on the same side of the neck as the tumor and the lymph node is larger than 3 centimeters but not larger than 6 centimeters; or
  - to more than one lymph node on the same side of the neck as the tumor and the lymph nodes are not larger than 6 centimeters; or
  - to lymph nodes on the opposite side of the neck as the tumor or on both sides of the neck, and the lymph nodes are not larger than 6 centimeters.
- In stage IVB, the tumor:
  - may be any size and has spread to one or more lymph nodes that are larger than 6 centimeters; or
  - has spread further into the muscles or bones in the oral cavity, or to the base of the skull and/or the carotid artery. Cancer may have spread to one or more lymph nodes anywhere in the neck.
- In stage IVC, the tumor has spread beyond the lip or oral cavity to distant parts of the body, such as the lungs. The tumor may be any size and may have spread to the lymph nodes.

Treatment Option Overview

There are different types of treatment for patients with lip and oral cavity cancer.

Different types of treatment are available for patients with lip and oral cavity cancer. Some treatments are standard (the currently used treatment), and some are being tested in clinical trials. A treatment clinical trial is a research study meant to help improve current treatments or obtain information on new treatments for patients with cancer. When clinical trials show that a new treatment is better than the standard treatment, the new treatment may become the standard treatment. Patients may want to think about taking part in a clinical trial. Some clinical trials are open only to patients who have not started treatment.

Patients with lip and oral cavity cancer should have their treatment planned by a team of doctors who are expert in treating head and neck cancer.

Treatment will be overseen by a medical oncologist, a doctor who specializes in treating people with cancer. Because the lips and oral cavity are important for breathing, eating, and talking, patients may need special help adjusting to the side effects of the cancer and its treatment. The medical oncologist may refer the patient to other health professionals with special training in the treatment of patients with head and neck cancer. These include the following:

- Head and neck surgeon.
- Radiation oncologist.
- Dentist.
- Speech therapist.
- Dietitian.
- Psychologist.
- Rehabilitation specialist.
- Plastic surgeon.

Two types of standard treatment are used:

Surgery

Surgery (removing the cancer in an operation) is a common treatment for all stages of lip and oral cavity cancer. Surgery may include the following:

- Wide local excision: Removal of the cancer and some of the healthy tissue around it. If cancer has spread into bone, surgery may include removal of the involved bone tissue.

- Neck dissection: Removal of lymph nodes and other tissues in the neck. This is done when cancer may have spread from the lip and oral cavity.

- Plastic surgery: An operation that restores or improves the appearance of parts of the body. Dental implants, a skin graft, or other plastic surgery may be needed to repair parts of the mouth, throat, or neck after removal of large tumors.

Even if the doctor removes all the cancer that can be seen at the time of the surgery, some patients may be given chemotherapy or radiation therapy after surgery to kill any cancer cells that are left. Treatment given after the surgery, to lower the risk that the cancer will come back, is called adjuvant therapy.

Radiation therapy

Radiation therapy is a cancer treatment that uses high-energy x-rays or other types of radiation to kill cancer cells. There are two types of radiation therapy. External radiation therapy uses a machine outside the body to send radiation toward the cancer. Internal radiation therapy uses a radioactive substance sealed in needles, seeds, wires, or catheters that are placed directly into or near the cancer. The way the radiation therapy is given depends on the type and stage of the cancer being treated.

For patients who smoke, radiation therapy works better when smoking is stopped before beginning treatment. It is also important for patients to have a dental exam before radiation therapy begins, so that existing problems can be treated.

New types of treatment are being tested in clinical trials.

Chemotherapy

Chemotherapy is a cancer treatment that uses drugs to stop the growth of cancer cells, either by killing the cells or by stopping the cells from dividing. When chemotherapy is taken by mouth or injected into a vein or muscle, the drugs enter the bloodstream and can reach cancer cells throughout the body (systemic chemotherapy). When chemotherapy is placed directly into the cerebrospinal fluid, an organ, or a body cavity such as the abdomen, the drugs mainly affect cancer cells in those areas (regional chemotherapy). The way the chemotherapy is given depends on the type and stage of the cancer being treated.

Hyperfractionated radiation therapy

Hyperfractionated radiation therapy is radiation treatment in which the total dose of radiation is divided into small doses and the treatments are given more than once a day.

Hyperthermia therapy

Hyperthermia therapy is a treatment in which body tissue is heated above normal temperature to damage and kill cancer cells or to make cancer cells more sensitive to the effects of radiation and certain anti-cancer drugs.

Patients may want to think about taking part in a clinical trial.

For some patients, taking part in a clinical trial may be the best treatment choice. Clinical trials are part of the cancer research process. Clinical trials are done to find out if new cancer treatments are safe and effective or better than the standard treatment.

Many of today's standard treatments for cancer are based on earlier clinical trials. Patients who take part in a clinical trial may receive the standard treatment or be among the first to receive a new treatment.

Patients who take part in clinical trials also help improve the way cancer will be treated in the future. Even when clinical trials do not lead to effective new treatments, they often answer important questions and help move research forward.

Patients can enter clinical trials before, during, or after starting their cancer treatment.

Some clinical trials only include patients who have not yet received treatment. Other trials test treatments for patients whose cancer has not gotten better. There are also clinical trials that test new ways to stop cancer from recurring (coming back) or reduce the side effects of cancer treatment.

Clinical trials are taking place in many parts of the country.

Follow-up tests may be needed.

Some of the tests that were done to diagnose the cancer or to find out the stage of the cancer may be repeated. Some tests will be repeated in order to see how well the treatment is working. Decisions about whether to continue, change, or stop treatment may be based on the results of these tests.

Some of the tests will continue to be done from time to time after treatment has ended. The results of these tests can show if your condition has changed or if the cancer has recurred (come back). These tests are sometimes called follow-up tests or check-ups.

Section 21.3

Metastatic Squamous Neck Cancer with Occult Primary

Text in this section is excerpted from "Metastatic Squamous Neck Cancer with Occult Primary Treatment," National Cancer Institute at the National Institutes of Health (NIH), July 3, 2014.

General Information About Metastatic Squamous Neck Cancer with Occult Primary

Metastatic squamous neck cancer with occult primary is a disease in which squamous cell cancer spreads to lymph nodes in the neck and it is not known where the cancer first formed in the body.

Squamous cells are thin, flat cells found in tissues that form the surface of the skin and the lining of body cavities such as the mouth, hollow organs such as the uterus and blood vessels, and the lining of the respiratory (breathing) and digestive tracts. Some organs with squamous cells are the esophagus, lungs, kidneys, and uterus. Cancer can begin in squamous cells anywhere in the body and metastasize (spread) through the blood or lymph system to other parts of the body.

When squamous cell cancer spreads to lymph nodes in the neck or around the collarbone, it is called metastatic squamous neck cancer. The doctor will try to find the primary tumor (the cancer that first formed in the body), because treatment for metastatic cancer is the same as treatment for the primary tumor. For example, when lung cancer spreads to the neck, the cancer cells in the neck are lung cancer cells and they are treated the same as the cancer in the lung. Sometimes doctors cannot find where in the body the cancer first began to grow. When tests cannot find a primary tumor, it is called an occult (hidden) primary tumor. In many cases, the primary tumor is never found.

Signs and symptoms of metastatic squamous neck cancer with occult primary include a lump or pain in the neck or throat.

Check with your doctor if you have a lump or pain in your neck or throat that doesn't go away. These and other signs and symptoms may be caused by metastatic squamous neck cancer with occult primary. Other conditions may cause the same signs and symptoms.

Tests that examine the tissues of the neck, respiratory tract, and upper part of the digestive tract are used to detect (find) and diagnose metastatic squamous neck cancer and the primary tumor.

Tests will include checking for a primary tumor in the organs and tissues of the respiratory tract (part of the trachea), the upper part of the digestive tract (including the lips, mouth, tongue, nose, throat, vocal cords, and part of the esophagus), and the genitourinary system.

The following procedures may be used:

- **Physical exam and history:** An exam of the body, especially the head and neck, to check general signs of health. This includes checking for signs of disease, such as lumps or anything else that seems unusual. A history of the patient's health habits and past illnesses and treatments will also be taken.

- **Biopsy:** The removal of cells or tissues so they can be viewed under a microscope by a pathologist or tested in the laboratory to check for signs of cancer.

Three types of biopsy may be done:

    - **Fine-needle aspiration (FNA) biopsy:** The removal of tissue or fluid using a thin needle.

209

- **Core needle biopsy:** The removal of tissue using a wide needle.

- **Excisional biopsy:** The removal of an entire lump of tissue.

The following procedures are used to remove samples of cells or tissue:

- **Tonsillectomy: Surgery to remove both tonsils.**

- **Endoscopy**

One or more of the following laboratory tests may be done to study the tissue samples:

- **Immunohistochemistry**

- **Light and electron microscopy**

- **Epstein-Barr virus (EBV) and human papillomavirus (HPV) test**

- **MRI (magnetic resonance imaging)**

- **CT scan (CAT scan)**

- **PET scan (positron emission tomography scan)**

A diagnosis of occult primary tumor is made if the primary tumor is not found during testing or treatment.

Certain factors affect prognosis (chance of recovery) and treatment options.

The prognosis (chance of recovery) and treatment options depend on the following:

- The number and size of lymph nodes that have cancer in them.

- Whether the cancer has responded to treatment or has recurred (come back).

- How different from normal the cancer cells look under a microscope.

- The patient's age and general health.

Treatment options also depend on the following:

- Which part of the neck the cancer is in.

- Whether certain tumor markers are found.

Stages of Metastatic Squamous Neck Cancer with Occult Primary

After metastatic squamous neck cancer with occult primary has been diagnosed, tests are done to find out if cancer cells have spread to other parts of the body.

The process used to find out if cancer has spread to other parts of the body is called staging. The results from tests and procedures used to detect and diagnose the primary tumor are also used to find out if cancer has spread to other parts of the body.

There is no standard staging system for metastatic squamous neck cancer with occult primary. The tumors are described as untreated or recurrent. Untreated metastatic squamous neck cancer with occult primary is cancer that is newly diagnosed and has not been treated, except to relieve signs and symptoms caused by the cancer.

There are three ways that cancer spreads in the body.

Cancer can spread through tissue, the lymph system, and the blood:

- Tissue. The cancer spreads from where it began by growing into nearby areas.

- Lymph system. The cancer spreads from where it began by getting into the lymph system. The cancer travels through the lymph vessels to other parts of the body.

- Blood. The cancer spreads from where it began by getting into the blood. The cancer travels through the blood vessels to other parts of the body.

Treatment option overview

There are different types of treatment for patients with metastatic squamous neck cancer with occult primary.

Different types of treatment are available for patients with metastatic squamous neck cancer with occult primary. Some treatments are standard (the currently used treatment), and some are being tested in clinical trials. A treatment clinical trial is a research study meant to help improve current treatments or obtain information on new treatments for patients with cancer. When clinical trials show that a new treatment is better than the standard treatment, the new treatment may become the standard treatment. Patients may want to think about taking part in a clinical trial. Some clinical trials are open only to patients who have not started treatment.

Two types of standard treatment are used:

Surgery

Surgery may include neck dissection. There are different types of neck dissection, based on the amount of tissue that is removed.

- Radical neck dissection: Surgery to remove tissues in one or both sides of the neck between the jawbone and the collarbone, including the following:

  - All lymph nodes.

  - The jugular vein.

  - Muscles and nerves that are used for face, neck, and shoulder movement, speech, and swallowing.

  The patient may need physical therapy of the throat, neck, shoulder, and/or arm after radical neck dissection. Radical neck dissection may be used when cancer has spread widely in the neck.

- Modified radical neck dissection: Surgery to remove all the lymph nodes in one or both sides of the neck without removing the neck muscles. The nerves and/or the jugular vein may be removed.

- Partial neck dissection: Surgery to remove some of the lymph nodes in the neck. This is also called selective neck dissection.

Even if the doctor removes all the cancer that can be seen at the time of surgery, some patients may be given radiation therapy after surgery to kill any cancer cells that are left. Treatment given after surgery, to lower the risk that the cancer will come back, is called adjuvant therapy.

Radiation therapy

Radiation therapy is a cancer treatment that uses high-energy x-rays or other types of radiation to kill cancer cells or keep them from growing. There are two types of radiation therapy. External radiation therapy uses a machine outside the body to send radiation toward the cancer. Internal radiation therapy uses a radioactive substance sealed in needles, seeds, wires, or catheters that are placed directly into or near the cancer.

Intensity-modulated radiation therapy (IMRT) is a type of 3-dimensional (3-D) radiation therapy that uses a computer to make pictures of the size and shape of the tumor. Thin beams of radiation of different intensities (strengths) are aimed at the tumor from many angles. This type of radiation therapy is less likely to cause dry mouth, trouble swallowing, and damage to the skin.

Radiation therapy to the neck may change the way the thyroid gland works. The gland will be tested before treatment and at regular checkups after treatment.

New types of treatment are being tested in clinical trials.

Chemotherapy
Hyperfractionated radiation therapy

Patients may want to think about taking part in a clinical trial.

For some patients, taking part in a clinical trial may be the best treatment choice. Clinical trials are part of the cancer research process. Clinical trials are done to find out if new cancer treatments are safe and effective or better than the standard treatment.

Many of today's standard treatments for cancer are based on earlier clinical trials. Patients who take part in a clinical trial may receive the standard treatment or be among the first to receive a new treatment.

Patients who take part in clinical trials also help improve the way cancer will be treated in the future. Even when clinical trials do not lead to effective new treatments, they often answer important questions and help move research forward.

Patients can enter clinical trials before, during, or after starting their cancer treatment.

Some clinical trials only include patients who have not yet received treatment. Other trials test treatments for patients whose cancer has not gotten better. There are also clinical trials that test new ways to stop cancer from recurring (coming back) or reduce the side effects of cancer treatment.

213

Clinical trials are taking place in many parts of the country.

Follow-up tests may be needed.

Some of the tests that were done to diagnose the cancer or to find out the stage of the cancer may be repeated. Some tests will be repeated in order to see how well the treatment is working. Decisions about whether to continue, change, or stop treatment may be based on the results of these tests.

Some of the tests will continue to be done from time to time after treatment has ended. The results of these tests can show if your condition has changed or if the cancer has recurred (come back). These tests are sometimes called follow-up tests or check-ups.

Section 21.4

Thyroid Cancer

Text in this section is excerpted from "Thyroid Cancer Treatment," National Cancer Institute at the National Institutes of Health (NIH), April 2, 2015.

General Information About Thyroid Cancer

Thyroid cancer is a disease in which malignant (cancer) cells form in the tissues of the thyroid gland.

The thyroid is a gland at the base of the throat near the trachea (windpipe). It is shaped like a butterfly, with a right lobe and a left lobe. The isthmus, a thin piece of tissue, connects the two lobes. A healthy thyroid is a little larger than a quarter. It usually cannot be felt through the skin.

The thyroid uses iodine, a mineral found in some foods and in iodized salt, to help make several hormones. Thyroid hormones do the following:

- Control heart rate, body temperature, and how quickly food is changed into energy (metabolism).

214

- Control the amount of calcium in the blood.

There are four main types of thyroid cancer:

- Papillary thyroid cancer: The most common type of thyroid cancer.

- Follicular thyroid cancer. Hürthle cell carcinoma is a form of follicular thyroid cancer and is treated the same way.

- Medullary thyroid cancer.

- Anaplastic thyroid cancer.

Age, gender, and exposure to radiation can affect the risk of thyroid cancer.

Anything that increases your risk of getting a disease is called a risk factor. Having a risk factor does not mean that you will get cancer; not having risk factors doesn't mean that you will not get cancer. Talk with your doctor if you think you may be at risk. Risk factors for thyroid cancer include the following:

- Being between 25 and 65 years old.

- Being female.

- Being exposed to radiation to the head and neck as a child or being exposed to radiation from an atomic bomb. The cancer may occur as soon as 5 years after exposure.

- Having a history of goiter (enlarged thyroid).

- Having a family history of thyroid disease or thyroid cancer.

- Having certain genetic conditions such as familial medullary thyroid cancer (FMTC), multiple endocrine neoplasia type 2A syndrome, and multiple endocrine neoplasia type 2B syndrome.

- Being Asian.

Medullary thyroid cancer is sometimes caused by a change in a gene that is passed from parent to child.

The genes in cells carry hereditary information from parent to child. A certain change in a gene that is passed from parent to child (inherited) may cause medullary thyroid cancer. A test has been developed that can find the changed gene before medullary thyroid cancer appears. The patient is tested first to see if he or she has the changed gene. If the patient has it, other family members may also be tested. Family members, including young children, who have the changed gene can decrease the chance of developing medullary thyroid cancer by having a thyroidectomy (surgery to remove the thyroid).

Signs of thyroid cancer include a swelling or lump in the neck.

Thyroid cancer may not cause early signs or symptoms. It is sometimes found during a routine physical exam. Signs or symptoms may occur as the tumor gets bigger. Other conditions may cause the same signs or symptoms. Check with your doctor if you have any of the following:

- A lump in the neck.
- Trouble breathing.
- Trouble swallowing.
- Hoarseness.

Tests that examine the thyroid, neck, and blood are used to detect (find) and diagnose thyroid cancer.

The following tests and procedures may be used:

- **Physical exam and history:** An exam of the body to check general signs of health, including checking for signs of disease, such as lumps or swelling in the neck, voice box, and lymph nodes, and anything else that seems unusual. A history of the patient's health habits and past illnesses and treatments will also be taken.

- **Laryngoscopy:** A procedure in which the doctor checks the larynx (voice box) with a mirror or with a laryngoscope. A laryngoscope is a thin, tube-like instrument with a light and a lens for viewing. A thyroid tumor may press on vocal cords. The laryngoscopy is done to see if the vocal cords are moving normally.

- **Blood hormone studies:** A procedure in which a blood sample is checked to measure the amounts of certain hormones released into the blood by organs and tissues in the body. An unusual (higher or lower than normal) amount of a substance can be a sign of disease in the organ or tissue that makes it. The blood may be checked for abnormal levels of thyroid-stimulating hormone (TSH). TSH is made by the pituitary gland in the brain. It stimulates the release of thyroid hormone and controls how fast follicular thyroid cells grow. The blood may also be checked for high levels of the hormone calcitonin and antithyroid antibodies.

- **Blood chemistry studies:** A procedure in which a blood sample is checked to measure the amounts of certain substances, such as calcium, released into the blood by organs and tissues in the body. An unusual (higher or lower than normal) amount of a substance can be a sign of disease in the organ or tissue that makes it.

- **Ultrasound exam:** A procedure in which high-energy sound waves (ultrasound) are bounced off internal tissues or organs and make echoes. The echoes form a picture of body tissues called a sonogram. The picture can be printed to be looked at later. This procedure can show the size of a thyroid tumor and whether it is solid or a fluid-filled cyst. Ultrasound may be used to guide a fine-needle aspiration biopsy.

- **CT scan (CAT scan):** A procedure that makes a series of detailed pictures of areas inside the body, taken from different angles. The pictures are made by a computer linked to an x-ray machine. A dye may be injected into a vein or swallowed to help the organs or tissues show up more clearly. This procedure is also called computed tomography, computerized tomography, or computerized axial tomography.

- **Fine-needle aspiration biopsy of the thyroid:** The removal of thyroid tissue using a thin needle. The needle is inserted through the skin into the thyroid. Several tissue samples are removed from different parts of the thyroid. A pathologist views the tissue samples under a microscope to look for cancer cells. Because the type of thyroid cancer can be hard to diagnose, patients should ask to have biopsy samples checked by a pathologist who has experience diagnosing thyroid cancer.

- **Surgical biopsy:** The removal of the thyroid nodule or one lobe of the thyroid during surgery so the cells and tissues can be viewed under a microscope by a pathologist to check for signs of cancer. Because the type of thyroid cancer can be hard to diagnose, patients should ask to have biopsy samples checked by a pathologist who has experience diagnosing thyroid cancer.

Certain factors affect prognosis (chance of recovery) and treatment options.

The prognosis (chance of recovery) and treatment options depend on the following:

- The age of the patient.
- The type of thyroid cancer.
- The stage of the cancer.
- The patient's general health.
- Whether the patient has multiple endocrine neoplasia type 2B (MEN 2B).
- Whether the cancer has just been diagnosed or has recurred (come back).

Stages of Thyroid Cancer

After thyroid cancer has been diagnosed, tests are done to find out if cancer cells have spread within the thyroid or to other parts of the body.

The process used to find out if cancer has spread within the thyroid or to other parts of the body is called staging. The information gathered from the staging process determines the stage of the disease. It is important to know the stage in order to plan treatment. The following tests and procedures may be used in the staging process:

- **CT scan (CAT scan) Ultrasound exam**
- **Chest x-ray**
- **Sentinel lymph node biopsy**

There are three ways that cancer spreads in the body.

Cancer can spread through tissue, the lymph system, and the blood:

- Tissue. The cancer spreads from where it began by growing into nearby areas.
- Lymph system. The cancer spreads from where it began by getting into the lymph system. The cancer travels through the lymph vessels to other parts of the body.

- Blood. The cancer spreads from where it began by getting into the blood. The cancer travels through the blood vessels to other parts of the body.

Cancer may spread from where it began to other parts of the body.

When cancer spreads to another part of the body, it is called metastasis. Cancer cells break away from where they began (the primary tumor) and travel through the lymph system or blood.

- Lymph system. The cancer gets into the lymph system, travels through the lymph vessels, and forms a tumor (metastatic tumor) in another part of the body.
- Blood. The cancer gets into the blood, travels through the blood vessels, and forms a tumor (metastatic tumor) in another part of the body.

The metastatic tumor is the same type of cancer as the primary tumor. For example, if thyroid cancer spreads to the lung, the cancer cells in the lung are actually thyroid cancer cells. The disease is metastatic thyroid cancer, not lung cancer.

The following stages are used for papillary and follicular thyroid cancer in patients younger than 45 years:

Stage I

In stage I papillary and follicular thyroid cancer, the tumor is any size, may be in the thyroid, or may have spread to nearby tissues and lymph nodes. Cancer has not spread to other parts of the body.

Stage II

In stage II papillary and follicular thyroid cancer, the tumor is any size and cancer has spread from the thyroid to other parts of the body, such as the lungs or bone, and may have spread to lymph nodes.

The following stages are used for papillary and follicular thyroid cancer in patients 45 years and older:

Stage I

In stage I papillary and follicular thyroid cancer, cancer is found only in the thyroid and the tumor is 2 centimeters or smaller.

Stage II

In stage II papillary and follicular thyroid cancer, cancer is only in the thyroid and the tumor is larger than 2 centimeters but not larger than 4 centimeters.

Stage III

In stage III papillary and follicular thyroid cancer, either of the following is found:

- the tumor is larger than 4 centimeters and only in the thyroid or the tumor is any size and cancer has spread to tissues just outside the thyroid, but not to lymph nodes; or

- the tumor is any size and cancer may have spread to tissues just outside the thyroid and has spread to lymph nodes near the trachea or the larynx (voice box).

Stage IV

Stage IV papillary and follicular thyroid cancer is divided into stages IVA, IVB, and IVC.

- In stage IVA, either of the following is found:
  - the tumor is any size and cancer has spread outside the thyroid to tissues under the skin, the trachea, the esophagus, the larynx (voice box), and/or the recurrent laryngeal nerve (a nerve with two branches that go to the larynx); cancer may have spread to nearby lymph nodes; or
  - the tumor is any size and cancer may have spread to tissues just outside the thyroid. Cancer has spread to lymph nodes on one or both sides of the neck or between the lungs.

- In stage IVB, cancer has spread to tissue in front of the spinal column or has surrounded the carotid artery or the blood vessels in the area between the lungs; cancer may have spread to lymph nodes.

- In stage IVC, the tumor is any size and cancer has spread to other parts of the body, such as the lungs and bones, and may have spread to lymph nodes.

The following stages are used for medullary thyroid cancer:

Stage 0

Stage 0 medullary thyroid cancer is found only with a special screening test. No tumor can be found in the thyroid.

Stage I

Stage I medullary thyroid cancer is found only in the thyroid and is 2 centimeters or smaller.

Stage II

In stage II medullary thyroid cancer, either of the following is found:

- the tumor is larger than 2 centimeters and only in the thyroid; or

- the tumor is any size and has spread to tissues just outside the thyroid, but not to lymph nodes.

Stage III

In stage III medullary thyroid cancer, the tumor is any size, has spread to lymph nodes near the trachea and the larynx (voice box), and may have spread to tissues just outside the thyroid.

Stage IV

Stage IV medullary thyroid cancer is divided into stages IVA, IVB, and IVC.

- In stage IVA, either of the following is found:

  - the tumor is any size and cancer has spread outside the thyroid to tissues under the skin, the trachea, the esophagus, the larynx (voice box), and/or the recurrent laryngeal nerve (a nerve with 2 branches that go to the larynx); cancer may have spread to lymph nodes near the trachea or the larynx; or

  - the tumor is any size and cancer may have spread to tissues just outside the thyroid. Cancer has spread to lymph nodes on one or both sides of the neck or between the lungs.

- In stage IVB, cancer has spread to tissue in front of the spinal column or has surrounded the carotid artery or the blood vessels in the area between the lungs. Cancer may have spread to lymph nodes.

- In stage IVC, the tumor is any size and cancer has spread to other parts of the body, such as the lungs and bones, and may have spread to lymph nodes.

Anaplastic thyroid cancer is considered stage IV thyroid cancer.

Anaplastic thyroid cancer grows quickly and has usually spread within the neck when it is found. Stage IV anaplastic thyroid cancer is divided into stages IVA, IVB, and IVC.

- In stage IVA, cancer is found in the thyroid and may have spread to lymph nodes.

- In stage IVB, cancer has spread to tissue just outside the thyroid and may have spread to lymph nodes.

- In stage IVC, cancer has spread to other parts of the body, such as the lungs and bones, and may have spread to lymph nodes.

Treatment Option Overview

There are different types of treatment for patients with thyroid cancer.

Different types of treatment are available for patients with thyroid cancer. Some treatments are standard (the currently used treatment), and some are being tested in clinical trials. A treatment clinical trial is a research study meant to help improve current treatments or obtain information on new treatments for patients with cancer. When clinical trials show that a new treatment is better than the standard treatment, the new treatment may become the standard treatment. Patients may want to think about taking part in a clinical trial. Some clinical trials are open only to patients who have not started treatment.

Five types of standard treatment are used:

Surgery

Surgery is the most common treatment of thyroid cancer. One of the following procedures may be used:

- Lobectomy: Removal of the lobe in which thyroid cancer is found. Biopsies of lymph nodes in the area may be done to see if they contain cancer.

- Near-total thyroidectomy: Removal of all but a very small part of the thyroid.

- Total thyroidectomy: Removal of the whole thyroid.

- Lymphadenectomy: Removal of lymph nodes in the neck that contain cancer.

Radiation therapy, including radioactive iodine therapy

Radiation therapy is a cancer treatment that uses high-energy x-rays or other types of radiation to kill cancer cells or keep them from growing. There are two types of radiation therapy. External radiation therapy uses a machine outside the body to send radiation toward the cancer. Internal radiation therapy uses a radioactive substance sealed in needles, seeds, wires, or catheters that are placed directly into or near the cancer. The way the radiation therapy is given depends on the type and stage of the cancer being treated.

Radiation therapy may be given after surgery to kill any thyroid cancer cells that were not removed. Follicular and papillary thyroid cancers are sometimes treated with radioactive iodine (RAI) therapy. RAI is taken by mouth and collects in any remaining thyroid tissue, including thyroid cancer cells that have spread to other places in the body. Since only thyroid tissue takes up iodine, the RAI destroys thyroid tissue and thyroid cancer cells without harming other tissue. Before a full treatment dose of RAI is given, a small test-dose is given to see if the tumor takes up the iodine.

Chemotherapy

Chemotherapy is a cancer treatment that uses drugs to stop the growth of cancer cells, either by killing the cells or by stopping them from dividing. When chemotherapy is taken by mouth or injected into a vein or muscle, the drugs enter the bloodstream and can reach cancer cells throughout the body (systemic chemotherapy). When chemotherapy is placed directly into the cerebrospinal fluid, an organ, or a body cavity such as the abdomen, the drugs mainly affect cancer cells in those areas (regional chemotherapy).

Thyroid hormone therapy

Hormone therapy is a cancer treatment that removes hormones or blocks their action and stops cancer cells from growing. Hormones are substances made by glands in the body and circulated in the bloodstream. In the treatment of thyroid cancer, drugs may be given to prevent the body from making thyroid-stimulating hormone (TSH), a hormone that can increase the chance that thyroid cancer will grow or recur.

Also, because thyroid cancer treatment kills thyroid cells, the thyroid is not able to make enough thyroid hormone. Patients are given thyroid hormone replacement pills.

Targeted therapy

Targeted therapy is a type of treatment that uses drugs or other substances to identify and attack specific cancer cells without harming normal cells. Tyrosine kinase inhibitor therapy is a type of targeted therapy that blocks signals needed for tumors to grow.

Vandetanib and sorafenib are tyrosine kinase inhibitors that are used to treat certain types of thyroid cancer.

Patients may want to think about taking part in a clinical trial.

For some patients, taking part in a clinical trial may be the best treatment choice. Clinical trials are part of the cancer research process. Clinical trials are done to find out if new cancer treatments are safe and effective or better than the standard treatment.

Many of today's standard treatments for cancer are based on earlier clinical trials. Patients who take part in a clinical trial may receive the standard treatment or be among the first to receive a new treatment.

Patients who take part in clinical trials also help improve the way cancer will be treated in the future. Even when clinical trials do not lead to effective new treatments, they often answer important questions and help move research forward.

Patients can enter clinical trials before, during, or after starting their cancer treatment.

Some clinical trials only include patients who have not yet received treatment. Other trials test treatments for patients whose cancer has not gotten better. There are also clinical trials that test new ways to stop cancer from recurring (coming back) or reduce the side effects of cancer treatment.

Clinical trials are taking place in many parts of the country.

Follow-up tests may be needed.

Some of the tests that were done to diagnose the cancer or to find out the stage of the cancer may be repeated. Some tests will be repeated in order to see how well the treatment is working. Decisions about whether to continue, change, or stop treatment may be based on the results of these tests.

Some of the tests will continue to be done from time to time after treatment has ended. The results of these tests can show if your condition has changed or if the cancer has recurred (come back). These tests are sometimes called follow-up tests or check-ups.

Chapter 22

Respiratory / Thoracic Cancer

Chapter Contents

Section 22.1

Non-Small Cell Lung Cancer

Text in this section is excerpted from "Non-Small Cell Lung Cancer Treatment," National Cancer Institute at the National Institutes of Health (NIH), May 12, 2015.

General Information About Non-Small Cell Lung Cancer

Non-small cell lung cancer is a disease in which malignant (cancer) cells form in the tissues of the lung.

The lungs are a pair of cone-shaped breathing organs in the chest. The lungs bring oxygen into the body as you breathe in. They release carbon dioxide, a waste product of the body's cells, as you breathe out. Each lung has sections called lobes. The left lung has two lobes. The right lung is slightly larger and has three lobes. Two tubes called bronchi lead from the trachea (windpipe) to the right and left lungs. The bronchi are sometimes also involved in lung cancer. Tiny air sacs called alveoli and small tubes called bronchioles make up the inside of the lungs.

A thin membrane called the pleura covers the outside of each lung and lines the inside wall of the chest cavity. This creates a sac called the pleural cavity. The pleural cavity normally contains a small amount of fluid that helps the lungs move smoothly in the chest when you breathe.

There are two main types of lung cancer: non-small cell lung cancer and small cell lung cancer.

There are several types of non-small cell lung cancer.

Each type of non-small cell lung cancer has different kinds of cancer cells. The cancer cells of each type grow and spread in different ways. The types of non-small cell lung cancer are named for the kinds of cells found in the cancer and how the cells look under a microscope:

- Squamous cell carcinoma: Cancer that begins in squamous cells, which are thin, flat cells that look like fish scales. This is also called epidermoid carcinoma.

- Large cell carcinoma: Cancer that may begin in several types of large cells.

- Adenocarcinoma: Cancer that begins in the cells that line the alveoli and make substances such as mucus.

Other less common types of non-small cell lung cancer are: pleomorphic, carcinoid tumor, salivary gland carcinoma, and unclassified carcinoma.

Smoking increases the risk of non-small cell lung cancer.

Smoking cigarettes, pipes, or cigars is the most common cause of lung cancer. The earlier in life a person starts smoking, the more often a person smokes, and the more years a person smokes, the greater the risk of lung cancer. If a person has stopped smoking, the risk becomes lower as the years pass.

Anything that increases your chance of getting a disease is called a risk factor. Having a risk factor does not mean that you will get cancer; not having risk factors doesn't mean that you will not get cancer. Talk with your doctor if you think you may be at risk.

Risk factors for lung cancer include the following:

- Smoking cigarettes, pipes, or cigars, now or in the past.

- Being exposed to secondhand smoke.

- Having a family history of lung cancer.

- Being treated with radiation therapy to the breast or chest.

- Being exposed to asbestos, chromium, nickel, arsenic, soot, or tar in the workplace.

- Being exposed to radon in the home or workplace.

- Living where there is air pollution.

- Being infected with the human immunodeficiency virus (HIV).

- Using beta carotene supplements and being a heavy smoker.

When smoking is combined with other risk factors, the risk of lung cancer is increased.

Signs of non-small cell lung cancer include a cough that doesn't go away and shortness of breath.

Sometimes lung cancer does not cause any signs or symptoms. It may be found during a chest x-ray done for another condition. Signs and symptoms may be caused by lung cancer or by other conditions. Check with your doctor if you have any of the following:

- Chest discomfort or pain.
- A cough that doesn't go away or gets worse over time.
- Trouble breathing.
- Wheezing.
- Blood in sputum (mucus coughed up from the lungs).
- Hoarseness.
- Loss of appetite.
- Weight loss for no known reason.
- Feeling very tired.
- Trouble swallowing.
- Swelling in the face and/or veins in the neck.

Tests that examine the lungs are used to detect (find), diagnose, and stage non-small cell lung cancer.

Tests and procedures to detect, diagnose, and stage non-small cell lung cancer are often done at the same time. Some of the following tests and procedures may be used:

- **Physical exam and history:** An exam of the body to check general signs of health, including checking for signs of disease, such as lumps or anything else that seems unusual. A history of the patient's health habits, including smoking, and past jobs, illnesses, and treatments will also be taken.

- **Laboratory tests:** Medical procedures that test samples of tissue, blood, urine, or other substances in the body. These tests help to diagnose disease, plan and check treatment, or monitor the disease over time.

- **Chest x-ray:** An x-ray of the organs and bones inside the chest. An x-ray is a type of energy beam that can go through the body and onto film, making a picture of areas inside the body.

- **X-ray of the chest.** X-rays are used to take pictures of organs and bones of the chest. X-rays pass through the patient onto film.

- **CT scan (CAT scan):** A procedure that makes a series of detailed pictures of areas inside the body, such as the chest, taken from different angles. The pictures are made by a computer linked to an x-ray machine. A dye may be injected into a vein or swallowed to help the organs or tissues show up more clearly. This procedure is also called computed tomography, computerized tomography, or computerized axial tomography.

- **Sputum cytology:** A procedure in which a pathologist views a sample of sputum (mucus coughed up from the lungs) under a microscope, to check for cancer cells.

- **Fine-needle aspiration (FNA) biopsy of the lung:** The removal of tissue or fluid from the lung using a thin needle. A CT scan, ultrasound, or other imaging procedure is used to locate the abnormal tissue or fluid in the lung. A small incision may be made in the skin where the biopsy needle is inserted into the abnormal tissue or fluid. A sample is removed with the needle and sent to the laboratory. A pathologist then views the sample under a microscope to look for cancer cells. A chest x-ray is done after the procedure to make sure no air is leaking from the lung into the chest.

- **Bronchoscopy:** A procedure to look inside the trachea and large airways in the lung for abnormal areas. A bronchoscope is inserted through the nose or mouth into the trachea and lungs. A bronchoscope is a thin, tube-like instrument with a light and a lens for viewing. It may also have a tool to remove tissue samples, which are checked under a microscope for signs of cancer.

- **Bronchoscopy.** A bronchoscope is inserted through the mouth, trachea, and major bronchi into the lung, to look for abnormal areas. A bronchoscope is a thin, tube-like instrument with a light and a lens for viewing. It may also have a cutting tool. Tissue samples may be taken to be checked under a microscope for signs of disease.

- **Thoracoscopy:** A surgical procedure to look at the organs inside the chest to check for abnormal areas. An incision (cut) is made between two ribs, and a thoracoscope is inserted into the chest. A thoracoscope is a thin, tube-like instrument with a light and a lens for viewing. It may also have a tool to remove tissue or lymph node samples, which are checked under a microscope for signs of cancer. In some cases, this procedure is used to remove part of the esophagus or lung. If certain tissues, organs, or lymph nodes can't be reached, a thoracotomy may be done. In this procedure, a larger incision is made between the ribs and the chest is opened.

- **Thoracentesis:** The removal of fluid from the space between the lining of the chest and the lung, using a needle. A pathologist views the fluid under a microscope to look for cancer cells.

- **Light and electron microscopy**: A laboratory test in which cells in a sample of tissue are viewed under regular and high-powered microscopes to look for certain changes in the cells.

- **Immunohistochemistry:** A test that uses antibodies to check for certain antigens in a sample of tissue. The antibody is usually linked to a radioactive substance or a dye that causes the tissue to light up under a microscope. This type of test may be used to tell the difference between different types of cancer.

Certain factors affect prognosis (chance of recovery) and treatment options.

The prognosis (chance of recovery) and treatment options depend on the following:

- The stage of the cancer (the size of the tumor and whether it is in the lung only or has spread to other places in the body).

- The type of lung cancer.

- Whether the cancer has mutations (changes) in certain genes, such as the epidermal growth factor receptor (EGFR) gene or the anaplastic lymphoma kinase (ALK) gene.

- Whether there are signs and symptoms such as coughing or trouble breathing.

- The patient's general health.

For most patients with non-small cell lung cancer, current treatments do not cure the cancer.

If lung cancer is found, taking part in one of the many clinical trials being done to improve treatment should be considered. Clinical trials are taking place in most parts of the country for patients with all stages of non-small cell lung cancer.

Stages of Non-Small Cell Lung Cancer

After lung cancer has been diagnosed, tests are done to find out if cancer cells have spread within the lungs or to other parts of the body.

The process used to find out if cancer has spread within the lungs or to other parts of the body is called staging. The information gathered from the staging process determines the stage of the disease. It is important to know the stage in order to plan treatment. Some of the tests used to diagnose non-small cell lung cancer are also used to stage the disease. Other tests and procedures that may be used in the staging process include the following:

- **MRI (magnetic resonance imaging):** A procedure that uses a magnet, radio waves, and a computer to make a series of detailed pictures of areas inside the body, such as the brain. This procedure is also called nuclear magnetic resonance imaging (NMRI).

- **CT scan (CAT scan):** A procedure that makes a series of detailed pictures of areas inside the body, such as the brain and abdomen, taken from different angles. The pictures are made by a computer linked to an x-ray machine. A dye may be injected into a vein or swallowed to help the organs or tissues show up more clearly. This procedure is also called computed tomography, computerized tomography, or computerized axial tomography.

- **PET scan (positron emission tomography scan):** A procedure to find malignant tumor cells in the body. A small amount of radioactive glucose (sugar) is injected into a vein. The PET scanner rotates around the body and makes a picture of where glucose is being used in the body. Malignant tumor cells show up brighter in the picture because they are more active and take up more glucose than normal cells do.

- **Radionuclide bone scan:** A procedure to check if there are rapidly dividing cells, such as cancer cells, in the bone. A very small amount of radioactive material is injected into a vein and travels through the bloodstream. The radioactive material collects in the bones and is detected by a scanner.

233

- **Pulmonary function test (PFT):** A test to see how well the lungs are working. It measures how much air the lungs can hold and how quickly air moves into and out of the lungs. It also measures how much oxygen is used and how much carbon dioxide is given off during breathing. This is also called lung function test.

- **Endoscopic ultrasound (EUS):** A procedure in which an endoscope is inserted into the body. An endoscope is a thin, tube-like instrument with a light and a lens for viewing. A probe at the end of the endoscope is used to bounce high-energy sound waves (ultrasound) off internal tissues or organs and make echoes. The echoes form a picture of body tissues called a sonogram. This procedure is also called endosonography. EUS may be used to guide fine needle aspiration (FNA) biopsy of the lung, lymph nodes, or other areas.

- **Mediastinoscopy:** A surgical procedure to look at the organs, tissues, and lymph nodes between the lungs for abnormal areas. An incision (cut) is made at the top of the breastbone and a mediastinoscope is inserted into the chest. A mediastinoscope is a thin, tube-like instrument with a light and a lens for viewing. It may also have a tool to remove tissue or lymph node samples, which are checked under a microscope for signs of cancer.

- **Anterior mediastinotomy:** A surgical procedure to look at the organs and tissues between the lungs and between the breastbone and heart for abnormal areas. An incision (cut) is made next to the breastbone and a mediastinoscope is inserted into the chest. A mediastinoscope is a thin, tube-like instrument with a light and a lens for viewing. It may also have a tool to remove tissue or lymph node samples, which are checked under a microscope for signs of cancer. This is also called the Chamberlain procedure.

- **Lymph node biopsy:** The removal of all or part of a lymph node. A pathologist views the tissue under a microscope to look for cancer cells.

- **Bone marrow aspiration and biopsy:** The removal of bone marrow, blood, and a small piece of bone by inserting a hollow needle into the hipbone or breastbone. A pathologist views the bone marrow, blood, and bone under a microscope to look for signs of cancer.

There are three ways that cancer spreads in the body.

Cancer can spread through tissue, the lymph system, and the blood:

- Tissue. The cancer spreads from where it began by growing into nearby areas.

- Lymph system. The cancer spreads from where it began by getting into the lymph system. The cancer travels through the lymph vessels to other parts of the body.

- Blood. The cancer spreads from where it began by getting into the blood. The cancer travels through the blood vessels to other parts of the body.

Cancer may spread from where it began to other parts of the body.

When cancer spreads to another part of the body, it is called metastasis. Cancer cells break away from where they began (the primary tumor) and travel through the lymph system or blood.

- Lymph system. The cancer gets into the lymph system, travels through the lymph vessels, and forms a tumor (metastatic tumor) in another part of the body.

- Blood. The cancer gets into the blood, travels through the blood vessels, and forms a tumor (metastatic tumor) in another part of the body.

The metastatic tumor is the same type of cancer as the primary tumor. For example, if non-small cell lung cancer spreads to the brain, the cancer cells in the brain are actually lung cancer cells. The disease is metastatic lung cancer, not brain cancer.

The following stages are used for non-small cell lung cancer:

Occult (hidden) stage

In the occult (hidden) stage, cancer cannot be seen by imaging or bronchoscopy. Cancer cells are found in sputum (mucus coughed up from the lungs) or bronchial washing (a sample of cells taken from inside the airways that lead to the lung). Cancer may have spread to other parts of the body.

235

Stage 0 (carcinoma in situ)

In stage 0, abnormal cells are found in the lining of the airways. These abnormal cells may become cancer and spread into nearby normal tissue. Stage 0 is also called carcinoma in situ.

Stage I

In stage I, cancer has formed. Stage I is divided into stages IA and IB:

- Stage IA: The tumor is in the lung only and is 3 centimeters or smaller.

- Stage IB: Cancer has not spread to the lymph nodes and one or more of the following is true:

  - The tumor is larger than 3 centimeters but not larger than 5 centimeters.

  - Cancer has spread to the main bronchus and is at least 2 centimeters below where the trachea joins the bronchus.

  - Cancer has spread to the innermost layer of the membrane that covers the lung.

  - Part of the lung has collapsed or developed pneumonitis (inflammation of the lung) in the area where the trachea joins the bronchus.

Stage II

Stage II is divided into stages IIA and IIB. Stage IIA and IIB are each divided into two sections depending on the size of the tumor, where the tumor is found, and whether there is cancer in the lymph nodes.

Stage IIA:

(1) Cancer has spread to lymph nodes on the same side of the chest as the tumor. The lymph nodes with cancer are within the lung or near the bronchus. Also, one or more of the following is true:

- The tumor is not larger than 5 centimeters.

- Cancer has spread to the main bronchus and is at least 2 centimeters below where the trachea joins the bronchus.

- Cancer has spread to the innermost layer of the membrane that covers the lung.

- Part of the lung has collapsed or developed pneumonitis (inflammation of the lung) in the area where the trachea joins the bronchus.

or

(2) Cancer has not spread to lymph nodes and one or more of the following is true:

- The tumor is larger than 5 centimeters but not larger than 7 centimeters.

- Cancer has spread to the main bronchus and is at least 2 centimeters below where the trachea joins the bronchus.

- Cancer has spread to the innermost layer of the membrane that covers the lung.

- Part of the lung has collapsed or developed pneumonitis (inflammation of the lung) in the area where the trachea joins the bronchus.

Stage IIB:

(1) Cancer has spread to nearby lymph nodes on the same side of the chest as the tumor. The lymph nodes with cancer are within the lung or near the bronchus. Also, one or more of the following is true:

- The tumor is larger than 5 centimeters but not larger than 7 centimeters.

- Cancer has spread to the main bronchus and is at least 2 centimeters below where the trachea joins the bronchus.

- Cancer has spread to the innermost layer of the membrane that covers the lung.

- Part of the lung has collapsed or developed pneumonitis (inflammation of the lung) in the area where the trachea joins the bronchus.

or

(2) Cancer has not spread to lymph nodes and one or more of the following is true:

- The tumor is larger than 7 centimeters.

237

- Cancer has spread to the main bronchus (and is less than 2 centimeters below where the trachea joins the bronchus), the chest wall, the diaphragm, or the nerve that controls the diaphragm.
- Cancer has spread to the membrane around the heart or lining the chest wall.
- The whole lung has collapsed or developed pneumonitis (inflammation of the lung).
- There are one or more separate tumors in the same lobe of the lung.

Stage IIIA

Stage IIIA is divided into three sections depending on the size of the tumor, where the tumor is found, and which lymph nodes have cancer (if any).

(1) Cancer has spread to lymph nodes on the same side of the chest as the tumor. The lymph nodes with cancer are near the sternum (chest bone) or where the bronchus enters the lung. Also:

- The tumor may be any size.
- Part of the lung (where the trachea joins the bronchus) or the whole lung may have collapsed or developed pneumonitis (inflammation of the lung).
- There may be one or more separate tumors in the same lobe of the lung.

Cancer may have spread to any of the following:

- Main bronchus, but not the area where the trachea joins the bronchus.
- Chest wall.
- Diaphragm and the nerve that controls it.
- Membrane around the lung or lining the chest wall.
- Membrane around the heart.

or

(2) Cancer has spread to lymph nodes on the same side of the chest as the tumor. The lymph nodes with cancer are within the lung or near the bronchus. Also:

- The tumor may be any size.
- The whole lung may have collapsed or developed pneumonitis (inflammation of the lung).

- There may be one or more separate tumors in any of the lobes of the lung with cancer.

Cancer may have spread to any of the following:

- Main bronchus, but not the area where the trachea joins the bronchus.
- Chest wall.
- Diaphragm and the nerve that controls it.
- Membrane around the lung or lining the chest wall.
- Heart or the membrane around it.
- Major blood vessels that lead to or from the heart.
- Trachea.
- Esophagus.
- Nerve that controls the larynx (voice box).
- Sternum (chest bone) or backbone.
- Carina (where the trachea joins the bronchi).
  or

(3) Cancer has not spread to the lymph nodes and the tumor may be any size. Cancer has spread to any of the following:

- Heart.
- Major blood vessels that lead to or from the heart.
- Trachea.
- Esophagus.
- Nerve that controls the larynx (voice box).
- Sternum (chest bone) or backbone.
- Carina (where the trachea joins the bronchi).

Stage IIIB

Stage IIIB is divided into two sections depending on the size of the tumor, where the tumor is found, and which lymph nodes have cancer.

(1) Cancer has spread to lymph nodes above the collarbone or to lymph nodes on the opposite side of the chest as the tumor. Also:

- The tumor may be any size.
- Part of the lung (where the trachea joins the bronchus) or the whole lung may have collapsed or developed pneumonitis (inflammation of the lung).
- There may be one or more separate tumors in any of the lobes of the lung with cancer.

Cancer may have spread to any of the following:

- Main bronchus.
- Chest wall.
- Diaphragm and the nerve that controls it.
- Membrane around the lung or lining the chest wall.
- Heart or the membrane around it.
- Major blood vessels that lead to or from the heart.
- Trachea.
- Esophagus.
- Nerve that controls the larynx (voice box).
- Sternum (chest bone) or backbone.
- Carina (where the trachea joins the bronchi).
  or

(2) Cancer has spread to lymph nodes on the same side of the chest as the tumor. The lymph nodes with cancer are near the sternum (chest bone) or where the bronchus enters the lung. Also:

- The tumor may be any size.
- There may be separate tumors in different lobes of the same lung.

Cancer has spread to any of the following:

- Heart.
- Major blood vessels that lead to or from the heart.
- Trachea.

- Esophagus.

- Nerve that controls the larynx (voice box).

- Sternum (chest bone) or backbone.

- Carina (where the trachea joins the bronchi).

Stage IV

In stage IV, the tumor may be any size and cancer may have spread to lymph nodes. One or more of the following is true:

- There are one or more tumors in both lungs.

- Cancer is found in fluid around the lungs or the heart.

- Cancer has spread to other parts of the body, such as the brain, liver, adrenal glands, kidneys, or bone.

Treatment Option Overview

There are different types of treatment for patients with non-small cell lung cancer.

- Different types of treatments are available for patients with non-small cell lung cancer. Some treatments are standard (the currently used treatment), and some are being tested in clinical trials. A treatment clinical trial is a research study meant to help improve current treatments or obtain information on new treatments for patients with cancer. When clinical trials show that a new treatment is better than the standard treatment, the new treatment may become the standard treatment. Patients may want to think about taking part in a clinical trial. Some clinical trials are open only to patients who have not started treatment.

Nine types of standard treatment are used:

Surgery

Four types of surgery are used to treat lung cancer:

- Wedge resection: Surgery to remove a tumor and some of the normal tissue around it. When a slightly larger amount of tissue is taken, it is called a segmental resection.

241

- Lobectomy: Surgery to remove a whole lobe (section) of the lung.

- Pneumonectomy. The whole lung is removed.

- Sleeve resection: Surgery to remove part of the bronchus.

- Even if the doctor removes all the cancer that can be seen at the time of the surgery, some patients may be given chemotherapy or radiation therapy after surgery to kill any cancer cells that are left. Treatment given after the surgery, to lower the risk that the cancer will come back, is called adjuvant therapy.

Radiation therapy

- Radiation therapy is a cancer treatment that uses high-energy x-rays or other types of radiation to kill cancer cells or keep them from growing. There are two types of radiation therapy. External radiation therapy uses a machine outside the body to send radiation toward the cancer. Internal radiation therapy uses a radioactive substance sealed in needles, seeds, wires, or catheters that are placed directly into or near the cancer.

- Radiosurgery is a method of delivering radiation directly to the tumor with little damage to healthy tissue. It does not involve surgery and may be used to treat certain tumors in patients who cannot have surgery.

- The way the radiation therapy is given depends on the type and stage of the cancer being treated. It also depends on where the cancer is found. For tumors in the airways, radiation is given directly to the tumor through an endoscope.

Chemotherapy

- Chemotherapy is a cancer treatment that uses drugs to stop the growth of cancer cells, either by killing the cells or by stopping them from dividing. When chemotherapy is taken by mouth or injected into a vein or muscle, the drugs enter the bloodstream and can reach cancer cells throughout the body (systemic chemotherapy). When chemotherapy is placed directly into the cerebrospinal fluid, an organ, or a body cavity such as the abdomen, the drugs mainly affect cancer cells in those areas (regional chemotherapy). The way the chemotherapy is given depends on the type and stage of the cancer being treated.

Targeted therapy

- Targeted therapy is a type of treatment that uses drugs or other substances to attack specific cancer cells. Targeted therapies usually cause less harm to normal cells than chemotherapy or radiation therapy do. Monoclonal antibodies and small-molecule tyrosine kinase inhibitors are the two main types of targeted therapy being used in the treatment of non-small cell lung cancer.

- Monoclonal antibody therapy is a cancer treatment that uses antibodies made in the laboratory from a single type of immune system cell. These antibodies can identify substances on cancer cells or normal substances in the blood or tissues that may help cancer cells grow. The antibodies attach to the substances and kill the cancer cells, block their growth, or keep them from spreading. Monoclonal antibodies are given by infusion. They may be used alone or to carry drugs, toxins, or radioactive material directly to cancer cells.

- Monoclonal antibodies used to treat non-small cell lung cancer include bevacizumab and cetuximab. Bevacizumab binds to vascular endothelial growth factor (VEGF) in the blood and tissues and may prevent the growth of new blood vessels that tumors need to grow. Cetuximab is a monoclonal antibody that acts as a tyrosine kinase inhibitor. It binds to epidermal growth factor receptor (EGFR), which is a tyrosine kinase protein, on the surface of cancer cells and works to stop the cells from growing and dividing.

- Small-molecule tyrosine kinase inhibitors are targeted therapy drugs that work inside cancer cells and block signals needed for tumors to grow. Small-molecule tyrosine kinase inhibitors may be used with other anticancer drugs as adjuvant therapy.

- Small-molecule tyrosine kinase inhibitors used to treat non-small cell lung cancer include erlotinib and gefitinib. They are types of epidermal growth factor receptor (EGFR) tyrosine kinase inhibitors.

- Crizotinib is another type of small-molecule tyrosine kinase inhibitor that is used to treat non-small cell lung cancer. It is used to treat non-small cell lung cancer that has certain mutations (changes) in the anaplastic lymphoma kinase (ALK) gene. The protein made by the ALK gene has tyrosine kinase activity.

243

Laser therapy

- Laser therapy is a cancer treatment that uses a laser beam (a narrow beam of intense light) to kill cancer cells.

Photodynamic therapy (PDT)

- Photodynamic therapy (PDT) is a cancer treatment that uses a drug and a certain type of laser light to kill cancer cells. A drug that is not active until it is exposed to light is injected into a vein. The drug collects more in cancer cells than in normal cells. Fiberoptic tubes are then used to carry the laser light to the cancer cells, where the drug becomes active and kills the cells. Photodynamic therapy causes little damage to healthy tissue. It is used mainly to treat tumors on or just under the skin or in the lining of internal organs. When the tumor is in the airways, PDT is given directly to the tumor through an endoscope.

Cryosurgery

- Cryosurgery is a treatment that uses an instrument to freeze and destroy abnormal tissue, such as carcinoma in situ. This type of treatment is also called cryotherapy. For tumors in the airways, cryosurgery is done through an endoscope.

Electrocautery

- Electrocautery is a treatment that uses a probe or needle heated by an electric current to destroy abnormal tissue. For tumors in the airways, electrocautery is done through an endoscope.

Watchful waiting

- Watchful waiting is closely monitoring a patient's condition without giving any treatment until signs or symptoms appear or change. This may be done in certain rare cases of non-small cell lung cancer.

New types of treatment are being tested in clinical trials.

Chemoprevention

- Chemoprevention is the use of drugs, vitamins, or other substances to reduce the risk of cancer or to reduce the risk cancer will recur (come back).

New combinations

- New combinations of treatments are being studied in clinical trials.

Patients may want to think about taking part in a clinical trial.

- For some patients, taking part in a clinical trial may be the best treatment choice. Clinical trials are part of the cancer research process. Clinical trials are done to find out if new cancer treatments are safe and effective or better than the standard treatment.

- Many of today's standard treatments for cancer are based on earlier clinical trials. Patients who take part in a clinical trial may receive the standard treatment or be among the first to receive a new treatment.

- Patients who take part in clinical trials also help improve the way cancer will be treated in the future. Even when clinical trials do not lead to effective new treatments, they often answer important questions and help move research forward.

Patients can enter clinical trials before, during, or after starting their cancer treatment.

- Some clinical trials only include patients who have not yet received treatment. Other trials test treatments for patients whose cancer has not gotten better. There are also clinical trials that test new ways to stop cancer from recurring (coming back) or reduce the side effects of cancer treatment.

- Clinical trials are taking place in many parts of the country.

Follow-up tests may be needed.

- Some of the tests that were done to diagnose the cancer or to find out the stage of the cancer may be repeated. Some tests will be repeated in order to see how well the treatment is working. Decisions about whether to continue, change, or stop treatment may be based on the results of these tests.

- Some of the tests will continue to be done from time to time after treatment has ended. The results of these tests can show if your condition has changed or if the cancer has recurred (come back). These tests are sometimes called follow-up tests or check-ups.

Section 22.2

Small Cell Lung Cancer

Text in this section is excerpted from "Small Cell Lung Cancer Treatment," National Cancer Institute at the National Institutes of Health (NIH), May 12, 2015.

General Information About Small Cell Lung Cancer

Small cell lung cancer is a disease in which malignant (cancer) cells form in the tissues of the lung.

The lungs are a pair of cone-shaped breathing organs that are found in the chest. The lungs bring oxygen into the body when you breathe in and take out carbon dioxide when you breathe out. Each lung has sections called lobes. The left lung has two lobes. The right lung, which is slightly larger, has three. A thin membrane called the pleura surrounds the lungs. Two tubes called bronchi lead from the trachea (windpipe) to the right and left lungs. The bronchi are sometimes also affected by lung cancer. Small tubes called bronchioles and tiny air sacs called alveoli make up the inside of the lungs.

There are two types of lung cancer: small cell lung cancer and non-small cell lung cancer.

There are two main types of small cell lung cancer.

These two types include many different types of cells. The cancer cells of each type grow and spread in different ways. The types of small cell lung cancer are named for the kinds of cells found in the cancer and how the cells look when viewed under a microscope:

- Small cell carcinoma (oat cell cancer).

- Combined small cell carcinoma.

Smoking increases the risk of small cell lung cancer.

Smoking cigarettes, pipes, or cigars is the most common cause of lung cancer. The earlier in life a person starts smoking, the more often a person smokes, and the more years a person smokes, the greater the risk of lung cancer. If a person has stopped smoking, the risk becomes lower as the years pass.

Anything that increases your chance of getting a disease is called a risk factor. Having a risk factor does not mean that you will get cancer; not having risk factors doesn't mean that you will not get cancer. Talk to your doctor if you think you may be at risk.

Risk factors for small cell lung cancer include:

- Smoking cigarettes, pipes, or cigars now or in the past.
- Being exposed to secondhand smoke.
- Having a family history of lung cancer.
- Being treated with radiation therapy to the breast or chest.
- Being exposed to asbestos, chromium, nickel, arsenic, soot, or tar in the workplace.
- Being exposed to radon in the home or workplace.
- Living where there is air pollution.
- Being infected with the human immunodeficiency virus (HIV).
- Using beta carotene supplements and being a heavy smoker.

When smoking is combined with other risk factors, the risk of lung cancer is increased.

Signs and symptoms of small cell lung cancer include coughing, shortness of breath, and chest pain.

These and other signs and symptoms may be caused by small cell lung cancer or by other conditions. Check with your doctor if you have any of the following:

- Chest discomfort or pain.
- A cough that doesn't go away or gets worse over time.
- Trouble breathing.
- Wheezing.
- Blood in sputum (mucus coughed up from the lungs).
- Hoarseness.

- Trouble swallowing.
- Loss of appetite.
- Weight loss for no known reason.
- Feeling very tired.
- Swelling in the face and/or veins in the neck.

Tests and procedures that examine the lungs are used to detect (find), diagnose, and stage small cell lung cancer.

The following tests and procedures may be used:

- **Physical exam and history:** An exam of the body to check general signs of health, including checking for signs of disease, such as lumps or anything else that seems unusual. A history of the patient's health habits, including smoking, and past jobs, illnesses, and treatments will also be taken.

- **Laboratory tests:** Medical procedures that test samples of tissue, blood, urine, or other substances in the body. These tests help to diagnose disease, plan and check treatment, or monitor the disease over time.

- **Chest x-ray:** An x-ray of the organs and bones inside the chest. An x-ray is a type of energy beam that can go through the body and onto film, making a picture of areas inside the body.

- **CT scan (CAT scan) of the brain, chest, and abdomen:** A procedure that makes a series of detailed pictures of areas inside the body, taken from different angles. The pictures are made by a computer linked to an x-ray machine. A dye may be injected into a vein or swallowed to help the organs or tissues show up more clearly. This procedure is also called computed tomography, computerized tomography, or computerized axial tomography.

- **Sputum cytology:** A microscope is used to check for cancer cells in the sputum (mucus coughed up from the lungs).

- **Biopsy:** The removal of cells or tissues so they can be viewed under a microscope by a pathologist to check for signs of cancer. The different ways a biopsy can be done include the following:

- **Fine-needle aspiration (FNA) biopsy of the lung:** The removal of tissue or fluid from the lung, using a thin needle. A

CT scan, ultrasound, or other imaging procedure is used to find the abnormal tissue or fluid in the lung. A small incision may be made in the skin where the biopsy needle is inserted into the abnormal tissue or fluid. A sample is removed with the needle and sent to the laboratory. A pathologist then views the sample under a microscope to look for cancer cells. A chest x-ray is done after the procedure to make sure no air is leaking from the lung into the chest.

- **Thoracoscopy:** A surgical procedure to look at the organs inside the chest to check for abnormal areas. An incision (cut) is made between two ribs, and a thoracoscope is inserted into the chest. A thoracoscope is a thin, tube-like instrument with a light and a lens for viewing. It may also have a tool to remove tissue or lymph node samples, which are checked under a microscope for signs of cancer. In some cases, this procedure is used to remove part of the esophagus or lung. If certain tissues, organs, or lymph nodes can't be reached, a thoracotomy may be done. In this procedure, a larger incision is made between the ribs and the chest is opened.

- **Thoracentesis:** The removal of fluid from the space between the lining of the chest and the lung, using a needle. A pathologist views the fluid under a microscope to look for cancer cells.

- **Mediastinoscopy:** A surgical procedure to look at the organs, tissues, and lymph nodes between the lungs for abnormal areas. An incision (cut) is made at the top of the breastbone and a mediastinoscope is inserted into the chest. A mediastinoscope is a thin, tube-like instrument with a light and a lens for viewing. It may also have a tool to remove tissue or lymph node samples, which are checked under a microscope for signs of cancer.

- **Light and electron microscopy:** A laboratory test in which cells in a sample of tissue are viewed under regular and high-powered microscopes to look for certain changes in the cells.

- **Immunohistochemistry:** A test that uses antibodies to check for certain antigens in a sample of tissue. The antibody is usually linked to a radioactive substance or a dye that causes the tissue to light up under a microscope. This type of test may be used to tell the difference between different types of cancer.

Certain factors affect prognosis (chance of recovery) and treatment options.

The prognosis (chance of recovery) and treatment options depend on the following:

- The stage of the cancer (whether it is in the chest cavity only or has spread to other places in the body).

- The patient's age, gender, and general health.

For certain patients, prognosis also depends on whether the patient is treated with both chemotherapy and radiation.

For most patients with small cell lung cancer, current treatments do not cure the cancer.

If lung cancer is found, patients should think about taking part in one of the many clinical trials being done to improve treatment. Clinical trials are taking place in most parts of the country for patients with all stages of small cell lung cancer.

Stages of Small Cell Lung Cancer

After small cell lung cancer has been diagnosed, tests are done to find out if cancer cells have spread within the chest or to other parts of the body.

The process used to find out if cancer has spread within the chest or to other parts of the body is called staging. The information gathered from the staging process determines the stage of the disease. It is important to know the stage in order to plan treatment. Some of the tests used to diagnose small cell lung cancer are also used to stage the disease.

Other tests and procedures that may be used in the staging process include the following:

- **MRI (magnetic resonance imaging) of the brain:** A procedure that uses a magnet, radio waves, and a computer to make a series of detailed pictures of areas inside the body. This procedure is also called nuclear magnetic resonance imaging (NMRI).

- **CT scan (CAT scan):** A procedure that makes a series of detailed pictures of areas inside the body, such as the brain, chest or upper abdomen, taken from different angles. The pictures are made by a computer linked to an x-ray machine. A dye may be injected into a vein or swallowed to help the organs or tissues show up more clearly. This procedure is also called computed tomography, computerized tomography, or computerized axial tomography.

- **PET scan (positron emission tomography scan):** A procedure to find malignant tumor cells in the body. A small amount of radioactive glucose (sugar) is injected into a vein. The PET scanner rotates around the body and makes a picture of where glucose is being used in the body. Malignant tumor cells show up brighter in the picture because they are more active and take up more glucose than normal cells do. A PET scan and CT scan may be done at the same time. This is called a PET-CT.

- **Bone scan:** A procedure to check if there are rapidly dividing cells, such as cancer cells, in the bone. A very small amount of radioactive material is injected into a vein and travels through the bloodstream. The radioactive material collects in the bones and is detected by a scanner.

There are three ways that cancer spreads in the body.

Cancer can spread through tissue, the lymph system, and the blood:

- Tissue. The cancer spreads from where it began by growing into nearby areas.

- Lymph system. The cancer spreads from where it began by getting into the lymph system. The cancer travels through the lymph vessels to other parts of the body.

- Blood. The cancer spreads from where it began by getting into the blood. The cancer travels through the blood vessels to other parts of the body.

Cancer may spread from where it began to other parts of the body.

When cancer spreads to another part of the body, it is called metastasis. Cancer cells break away from where they began (the primary tumor) and travel through the lymph system or blood.

- Lymph system. The cancer gets into the lymph system, travels through the lymph vessels, and forms a tumor (metastatic tumor) in another part of the body.

251

- Blood. The cancer gets into the blood, travels through the blood vessels, and forms a tumor (metastatic tumor) in another part of the body.

The metastatic tumor is the same type of cancer as the primary tumor. For example, if small cell lung cancer spreads to the brain, the cancer cells in the brain are actually lung cancer cells. The disease is metastatic small cell lung cancer, not brain cancer.

The following stages are used for small cell lung cancer:

Limited-Stage Small Cell Lung Cancer

In limited-stage, cancer is in the lung where it started and may have spread to the area between the lungs or to the lymph nodes above the collarbone.

Extensive-Stage Small Cell Lung Cancer

In extensive-stage, cancer has spread beyond the lung or the area between the lungs or the lymph nodes above the collarbone to other places in the body.

Recurrent Small Cell Lung Cancer

Recurrent small cell lung cancer is cancer that has recurred (come back) after it has been treated. The cancer may come back in the chest, central nervous system, or in other parts of the body.

Treatment Option Overview

There are different types of treatment for patients with small cell lung cancer.

Different types of treatment are available for patients with small cell lung cancer. Some treatments are standard (the currently used treatment), and some are being tested in clinical trials. A treatment clinical trial is a research study meant to help improve current treatments or obtain information on new treatments for patients with cancer. When clinical trials show that a new treatment is better than the standard treatment, the new treatment may become the standard treatment. Patients may want to think about taking part in a clinical trial. Some clinical trials are open only to patients who have not started treatment.

Five types of standard treatment are used:

Surgery

Surgery may be used if the cancer is found in one lung and in nearby lymph nodes only. Because this type of lung cancer is usually found in both lungs, surgery alone is not often used. During surgery, the doctor will also remove lymph nodes to find out if they have cancer in them. Sometimes, surgery may be used to remove a sample of lung tissue to find out the exact type of lung cancer.

Even if the doctor removes all the cancer that can be seen at the time of the operation, some patients may be given chemotherapy or radiation therapy after surgery to kill any cancer cells that are left. Treatment given after the surgery, to lower the risk that the cancer will come back, is called adjuvant therapy.

Chemotherapy

Chemotherapy is a cancer treatment that uses drugs to stop the growth of cancer cells, either by killing the cells or by stopping them from dividing. When chemotherapy is taken by mouth or injected into a vein or muscle, the drugs enter the bloodstream and can reach cancer cells throughout the body (systemic chemotherapy). When chemotherapy is placed directly into the cerebrospinal fluid, an organ, or a body cavity such as the abdomen, the drugs mainly affect cancer cells in those areas (regional chemotherapy). The way the chemotherapy is given depends on the type and stage of the cancer being treated.

Radiation therapy

Radiation therapy is a cancer treatment that uses high-energy x-rays or other types of radiation to kill cancer cells or keep them from growing. There are two types of radiation therapy. External radiation therapy uses a machine outside the body to send radiation toward the cancer. Internal radiation therapy uses a radioactive substance sealed in needles, seeds, wires, or catheters that are placed directly into or near the cancer. Prophylactic cranial irradiation (radiation therapy to the brain to reduce the risk that cancer will spread to the brain) may also be given. The way the radiation therapy is given depends on the type and stage of the cancer being treated.

Laser therapy

Laser therapy is a cancer treatment that uses a laser beam (a narrow beam of intense light) to kill cancer cells.

Endoscopic stent placement

An endoscope is a thin, tube-like instrument used to look at tissues inside the body. An endoscope has a light and a lens for viewing and may be used to place a stent in a body structure to keep the structure open. An endoscopic stent can be used to open an airway blocked by abnormal tissue.

Patients may want to think about taking part in a clinical trial.

For some patients, taking part in a clinical trial may be the best treatment choice. Clinical trials are part of the cancer research process. Clinical trials are done to find out if new cancer treatments are safe and effective or better than the standard treatment.

Many of today's standard treatments for cancer are based on earlier clinical trials. Patients who take part in a clinical trial may receive the standard treatment or be among the first to receive a new treatment.

Patients who take part in clinical trials also help improve the way cancer will be treated in the future. Even when clinical trials do not lead to effective new treatments, they often answer important questions and help move research forward.

Patients can enter clinical trials before, during, or after starting their cancer treatment.

Some clinical trials only include patients who have not yet received treatment. Other trials test treatments for patients whose cancer has not gotten better. There are also clinical trials that test new ways to stop cancer from recurring (coming back) or reduce the side effects of cancer treatment.

Clinical trials are taking place in many parts of the country.

Follow-up tests may be needed.

Some of the tests that were done to diagnose the cancer or to find out the stage of the cancer may be repeated. Some tests will be repeated in order to see how well the treatment is working. Decisions about whether to continue, change, or stop treatment may be based on the results of these tests.

Some of the tests will continue to be done from time to time after treatment has ended. The results of these tests can show if your condition has changed or if the cancer has recurred (come back). These tests are sometimes called follow-up tests or check-ups.

Section 22.3

Malignant Mesothelioma

Text in this section is excerpted from "Malignant Mesothelioma Treatment," National Cancer Institute at the National Institutes of Health (NIH), April 2, 2015.

General Information About Malignant Mesothelioma

Malignant mesothelioma is a disease in which malignant (cancer) cells form in the lining of the chest or abdomen.

Malignant mesothelioma is a disease in which malignant (cancer) cells are found in the pleura (the thin layer of tissue that lines the chest cavity and covers the lungs) or the peritoneum (the thin layer of tissue that lines the abdomen and covers most of the organs in the abdomen). Malignant mesothelioma may also form in the heart or testicles, but this is rare.

Being exposed to asbestos can affect the risk of malignant mesothelioma.

Anything that increases your chance of getting a disease is called a risk factor. Having a risk factor does not mean that you will get cancer; not having risk factors doesn't mean that you will not get cancer. Talk to your doctor if you think you may be at risk.

Most people with malignant mesothelioma have worked or lived in places where they inhaled or swallowed asbestos. After being exposed to asbestos, it usually takes a long time for malignant mesothelioma to form. Living with a person who works near asbestos is also a risk factor for malignant mesothelioma.

Signs and symptoms of malignant mesothelioma include shortness of breath and pain under the rib cage.

Sometimes the cancer causes fluid to collect in the chest or in the abdomen. Signs and symptoms may be caused by the fluid, malignant mesothelioma, or other conditions. Check with your doctor if you have any of the following:

- Trouble breathing.
- Cough.
- Pain under the rib cage.
- Pain or swelling in the abdomen.
- Lumps in the abdomen.
- Constipation.
- Problems with blood clots (clots form when they shouldn't).
- Weight loss for no known reason.
- Feeling very tired.

Tests that examine the inside of the chest and abdomen are used to detect (find) and diagnose malignant mesothelioma.

Sometimes it is hard to tell the difference between malignant mesothelioma in the chest and lung cancer.

The following tests and procedures may be used to diagnose malignant mesothelioma in the chest or peritoneum:

- **Physical exam and history:** An exam of the body to check general signs of health, including checking for signs of disease, such as lumps or anything else that seems unusual. A history of the patient's health habits, exposure to asbestos, and past illnesses and treatments will also be taken.

- **Chest x-ray:** An x-ray of the organs and bones inside the chest. An x-ray is a type of energy beam that can go through the body and onto film, making a picture of areas inside the body.

- **CT scan (CAT scan):** A procedure that makes a series of detailed pictures of the chest and abdomen, taken from different angles. The pictures are made by a computer linked to an x-ray machine. A dye may be injected into a vein or swallowed to help the organs or tissues show up more clearly. This procedure is also called computed tomography, computerized tomography, or computerized axial tomography.

- **Biopsy:** The removal of cells or tissues from the pleura or peritoneum so they can be viewed under a microscope by a pathologist to check for signs of cancer.

Procedures used to collect the cells or tissues include the following:

- **Fine-needle (FNA)** aspiration biopsy of the lung: The removal of tissue or fluid using a thin needle. An imaging procedure is used to locate the abnormal tissue or fluid in the lung. A small incision may be made in the skin where the biopsy needle is inserted into the abnormal tissue or fluid, and a sample is removed.

- **Thoracoscopy:** An incision (cut) is made between two ribs and a thoracoscope (a thin, tube-like instrument with a light and a lens for viewing) is inserted into the chest.

- **Thoracotomy:** An incision (cut) is made between two ribs to check inside the chest for signs of disease.

- **Peritoneoscopy:** An incision (cut) is made in the abdominal wall and a peritoneoscope (a thin, tube-like instrument with a light and a lens for viewing) is inserted into the abdomen.

- **Laparotomy:** An incision (cut) is made in the wall of the abdomen to check the inside of the abdomen for signs of disease.

- **Open biopsy:** A procedure in which an incision (cut) is made through the skin to expose and remove tissues to check for signs of disease.

The following tests may be done on the cells and tissue samples that are taken:

- **Cytologic exam:** An exam of cells under a microscope to check for anything abnormal. For mesothelioma, fluid is taken from the chest or from the abdomen. A pathologist checks the fluid for signs of cancer.

- **Immunohistochemistry:** A test that uses antibodies to check for certain antigens in a sample of tissue. The antibody is usually linked to a radioactive substance or a dye that causes the tissue to light up under a microscope. This type of test may be used to tell the difference between different types of cancer.

- **Electron microscopy:** A laboratory test in which cells in a sample of tissue are viewed under a high-powered microscope to look for certain changes in the cells. An electron microscope shows tiny details better than other types of microscopes.

Certain factors affect prognosis (chance of recovery) and treatment options.

The prognosis (chance of recovery) and treatment options depend on the following:

- The stage of the cancer.
- The size of the tumor.
- Whether the tumor can be removed completely by surgery.
- The amount of fluid in the chest or abdomen.
- The patient's age.
- The patient's activity level.
- The patient's general health, including lung and heart health.
- The type of mesothelioma cells and how they look under a microscope.
- The number of white blood cells and how much hemoglobin is in the blood.
- Whether the patient is male or female.
- Whether the cancer has just been diagnosed or has recurred (come back).

Stages Of Malignant Mesothelioma

After malignant mesothelioma has been diagnosed, tests are done to find out if cancer cells have spread to other parts of the body.

The process used to find out if cancer has spread outside the pleura or peritoneum is called staging. The information gathered from the staging process determines the stage of the disease. It is important to know whether the cancer has spread in order to plan treatment.

The following tests and procedures may be used in the staging process:

- **CT scan (CAT scan):** A procedure that makes a series of detailed pictures of the chest and abdomen, taken from different angles. The pictures are made by a computer linked to an x-ray machine. A dye may be injected into a vein or swallowed to help the organs or tissues show up more clearly. This procedure is also called computed tomography, computerized tomography, or computerized axial tomography.

- **PET scan (positron emission tomography scan):** A procedure to find malignant tumor cells in the body. A small amount of radioactive glucose (sugar) is injected into a vein. The PET scanner rotates around the body and makes a picture of where glucose is being used in the body. Malignant tumor cells show up brighter in the picture because they are more active and take up more glucose than normal cells do.

- **Endoscopic ultrasound (EUS):** A procedure in which an endoscope is inserted into the body. An endoscope is a thin, tube-like instrument with a light and a lens for viewing. A probe at the end of the endoscope is used to bounce high-energy sound waves (ultrasound) off internal tissues or organs and make echoes. The echoes form a picture of body tissues called a sonogram. This procedure is also called endosonography. EUS may be used to guide fine-needle aspiration (FNA) biopsy of the lung, lymph nodes, or other areas.

- **Pulmonary function test (PFT):** A test to see how well the lungs are working. It measures how much air the lungs can hold and how quickly air moves into and out of the lungs. It also measures how much oxygen is used and how much carbon dioxide is given off during breathing. This is also called lung function test.

There are three ways that cancer spreads in the body.

Cancer can spread through tissue, the lymph system, and the blood:

- Tissue. The cancer spreads from where it began by growing into nearby areas.

- Lymph system. The cancer spreads from where it began by getting into the lymph system. The cancer travels through the lymph vessels to other parts of the body.

- Blood. The cancer spreads from where it began by getting into the blood. The cancer travels through the blood vessels to other parts of the body.

Cancer may spread from where it began to other parts of the body.

When cancer spreads to another part of the body, it is called metastasis. Cancer cells break away from where they began (the primary tumor) and travel through the lymph system or blood.

- Lymph system. The cancer gets into the lymph system, travels through the lymph vessels, and forms a tumor (metastatic tumor) in another part of the body.

- Blood. The cancer gets into the blood, travels through the blood vessels, and forms a tumor (metastatic tumor) in another part of the body.

The metastatic tumor is the same type of cancer as the primary tumor. For example, if malignant mesothelioma spreads to the brain, the cancer cells in the brain are actually malignant mesothelioma cells. The disease is metastatic malignant mesothelioma, not brain cancer.

The following stages are used for malignant mesothelioma:

Stage I (Localized)

Stage I is divided into stages IA and IB:

- In stage IA, cancer is found in one side of the chest in the lining of the chest wall and may also be found in the lining of the chest cavity between the lungs and/or the lining that covers the diaphragm. Cancer has not spread to the lining that covers the lung.

- In stage IB, cancer is found in one side of the chest in the lining of the chest wall and the lining that covers the lung. Cancer may also be found in the lining of the chest cavity between the lungs and/or the lining that covers the diaphragm.

Stage II (Advanced)

In stage II, cancer is found in one side of the chest in the lining of the chest wall, the lining of the chest cavity between the lungs, the lining that covers the diaphragm, and the lining that covers the lung. Also, cancer has spread into one or both of the following:

- Lung tissue.
- Diaphragm.

Stage III (Advanced)

In stage III, either of the following is true:

Cancer is found in one side of the chest in the lining of the chest wall. Cancer may have spread to:

- the lining of the chest cavity between the lungs;
- the lining that covers the diaphragm;
- the lining that covers the lung;
- the lung tissue;
- the diaphragm.

Cancer has spread to lymph nodes where the lung joins the bronchus, along the trachea and esophagus, between the lung and diaphragm, or below the trachea.
or
Cancer is found in one side of the chest in the lining of the chest wall, the lining of the chest cavity between the lungs, the lining that covers the diaphragm, and the lining that covers the lung. Cancer has spread into one or more of the following:

- Tissue between the ribs and the lining of the chest wall.
- Fat in the area between the lungs.
- Soft tissues of the chest wall.
- Sac around the heart.

Cancer may have spread to lymph nodes where the lung joins the bronchus, along the trachea and esophagus, between the lung and diaphragm, or below the trachea.

Stage IV (Advanced)

In stage IV, cancer cannot be removed by surgery and is found in one or both sides of the body. Cancer may have spread to lymph nodes anywhere in the chest or above the collarbone. Cancer has spread in one or more of the following ways:

- Through the diaphragm into the peritoneum (the thin layer of tissue that lines the abdomen and covers most of the organs in the abdomen).

- To the tissue lining the chest on the opposite side of the body as the tumor.

- To the chest wall and may be found in the rib.

- Into the organs in the center of the chest cavity.

- Into the spine.

- Into the sac around the heart or into the heart muscle.

- To distant parts of the body such as the brain, spine, thyroid, or prostate.

Treatment Options for Malignant Mesothelioma

There are different types of treatment for patients with malignant mesothelioma.

Different types of treatments are available for patients with malignant mesothelioma. Some treatments are standard (the currently used treatment), and some are being tested in clinical trials. A treatment clinical trial is a research study meant to help improve current treatments or obtain information on new treatments for patients with cancer. When clinical trials show that a new treatment is better than the standard treatment, the new treatment may become the standard treatment. Patients may want to think about taking part in a clinical trial. Some clinical trials are open only to patients who have not started treatment.

Three types of standard treatment are used:

Surgery

The following surgical treatments may be used for malignant mesothelioma in the chest:

- Wide local excision: Surgery to remove the cancer and some of the healthy tissue around it.

- Pleurectomy and decortication: Surgery to remove part of the covering of the lungs and lining of the chest and part of the outside surface of the lungs.

- Extrapleural pneumonectomy: Surgery to remove one whole lung and part of the lining of the chest, the diaphragm, and the lining of the sac around the heart.

- Pleurodesis: A surgical procedure that uses chemicals or drugs to make a scar in the space between the layers of the pleura. Fluid is first drained from the space using a catheter or chest tube and the chemical or drug is put into the space. The scarring stops the build-up of fluid in the pleural cavity.

Even if the doctor removes all the cancer that can be seen at the time of the surgery, some patients may be given chemotherapy or radiation therapy after surgery to kill any cancer cells that are left. Treatment given after surgery, to lower the risk that the cancer will come back, is called adjuvant therapy.

Radiation therapy

Radiation therapy is a cancer treatment that uses high-energy x-rays or other types of radiation to kill cancer cells or keep them from growing. There are two types of radiation therapy. External radiation therapy uses a machine outside the body to send radiation toward the cancer. Internal radiation therapy uses a radioactive substance sealed in needles, seeds, wires, or catheters that are placed directly into or near the cancer.

The way the radiation therapy is given depends on the type and stage of the cancer being treated.

Chemotherapy

Chemotherapy is a cancer treatment that uses drugs to stop the growth of cancer cells, either by killing the cells or by stopping them from dividing. When chemotherapy is taken by mouth or injected into a vein or muscle, the drugs enter the bloodstream and can reach cancer cells throughout the body (systemic chemotherapy). When chemotherapy is placed directly into the cerebrospinal fluid, an organ, or a body cavity such as the chest or peritoneum, the drugs mainly affect cancer cells in those areas (regional chemotherapy). Combination chemotherapy is the use of more than one anticancer drug.

263

Hyperthermic intraperitoneal chemotherapy is used in the treatment of mesothelioma that has spread to the peritoneum (tissue that lines the abdomen and covers most of the organs in the abdomen). After the surgeon removes all the cancer that can be seen, a solution containing anticancer drugs is heated and pumped into and out of the abdomen to kill cancer cells that remain. Heating the anticancer drugs may kill more cancer cells.

The way the chemotherapy is given depends on the type and stage of the cancer being treated.

New types of treatment are being tested in clinical trials.

Biologic therapy

Biologic therapy is a treatment that uses the patient's immune system to fight cancer. Substances made by the body or made in a laboratory are used to boost, direct, or restore the body's natural defenses against cancer. This type of cancer treatment is also called biotherapy or immunotherapy.

Patients may want to think about taking part in a clinical trial.

For some patients, taking part in a clinical trial may be the best treatment choice. Clinical trials are part of the cancer research process. Clinical trials are done to find out if new cancer treatments are safe and effective or better than the standard treatment.

Many of today's standard treatments for cancer are based on earlier clinical trials. Patients who take part in a clinical trial may receive the standard treatment or be among the first to receive a new treatment.

Patients who take part in clinical trials also help improve the way cancer will be treated in the future. Even when clinical trials do not lead to effective new treatments, they often answer important questions and help move research forward.

Patients can enter clinical trials before, during, or after starting their cancer treatment.

Some clinical trials only include patients who have not yet received treatment. Other trials test treatments for patients whose cancer has not gotten better. There are also clinical trials that test new ways to stop cancer from recurring (coming back) or reduce the side effects of cancer treatment.

Clinical trials are taking place in many parts of the country.

Follow-up tests may be needed.

Some of the tests that were done to diagnose the cancer or to find out the stage of the cancer may be repeated. Some tests will be repeated in order to see how well the treatment is working. Decisions about whether to continue, change, or stop treatment may be based on the results of these tests.

Some of the tests will continue to be done from time to time after treatment has ended. The results of these tests can show if your condition has changed or if the cancer has recurred (come back). These tests are sometimes called follow-up tests or check-ups.

Section 22.4

Thymoma and Thymic Carcinoma

Text in this section is excerpted from "Thymoma and Thymic Carcinoma Treatment," National Cancer Institute at the National Institutes of Health (NIH), April 2, 2015.

General Information About Thymoma and Thymic Carcinoma

Thymoma and thymic carcinoma are diseases in which malignant (cancer) cells form on the outside surface of the thymus.

The thymus, a small organ that lies in the upper chest under the breastbone, is part of the lymph system. It makes white blood cells, called lymphocytes, that protect the body against infections.

There are different types of tumors of the thymus. Thymomas and thymic carcinomas are rare tumors of the cells that are on the outside surface of the thymus. The tumor cells in a thymoma look similar to the normal cells of the thymus, grow slowly, and rarely spread beyond the thymus. On the other hand, the tumor cells in a thymic carcinoma look very different from the normal cells of the thymus, grow more quickly, and have usually spread to other parts of the body when the cancer is found. Thymic carcinoma is more difficult to treat than thymoma.

Thymoma is linked with myasthenia gravis and other autoimmune diseases.

People with thymoma often have autoimmune diseases as well. These diseases cause the immune system to attack healthy tissue and organs. They include:

- Myasthenia gravis.
- Acquired pure red cell aplasia.
- Hypogammaglobulinemia.
- Polymyositis.
- Lupus erythematosus.
- Rheumatoid arthritis.
- Thyroiditis.
- Sjögren syndrome.

Signs and symptoms of thymoma and thymic carcinoma include a cough and chest pain.

Thymoma and thymic carcinoma may not cause early signs or symptoms. The cancer may be found during a routine chest x-ray. Signs and symptoms may be caused by thymoma, thymic carcinoma, or other conditions. Check with your doctor if you have any of the following:

- A cough that doesn't go away.
- Chest pain.
- Trouble breathing.

Tests that examine the thymus are used to detect (find) thymoma or thymic carcinoma.

The following tests and procedures may be used:

- **Physical exam and history:** An exam of the body to check general signs of health, including checking for signs of disease, such as lumps or anything else that seems unusual. A history of the patient's health habits and past illnesses and treatments will also be taken.

- **Chest x-ray:** An x-ray of the organs and bones inside the chest. An x-ray is a type of energy beam that can go through the body and onto film, making a picture of areas inside the body.

- **CT scan (CAT scan):** A procedure that makes a series of detailed pictures of areas inside the body, such as the chest, taken from different angles. The pictures are made by a computer linked to an x-ray machine. A dye may be injected into a vein or swallowed to help the organs or tissues show up more clearly. This procedure is also called computed tomography, computerized tomography, or computerized axial tomography.

- **MRI (magnetic resonance imaging):** A procedure that uses a magnet, radio waves, and a computer to make a series of detailed pictures of areas inside the body, such as the chest. This procedure is also called nuclear magnetic resonance imaging (NMRI).

- **PET scan (positron emission tomography scan):** A procedure to find malignant tumor cells in the body. A small amount of radioactive glucose (sugar) is injected into a vein. The PET scanner rotates around the body and makes a picture of where glucose is being used in the body. Malignant tumor cells show up brighter in the picture because they are more active and take up more glucose than normal cells do.

Thymoma and thymic carcinoma are usually diagnosed, staged, and treated during surgery.

A biopsy of the tumor is done to diagnose the disease. The biopsy may be done before or during surgery (a mediastinoscopy or mediastinotomy), using a thin needle to remove a sample of cells. This is called a fine-needle aspiration (FNA) biopsy. Sometimes a wide needle is used to remove a sample of cells and this is called a core biopsy. A pathologist will view the sample under a microscope to check for cancer. If thymoma or thymic carcinoma is diagnosed, the pathologist will determine the type of cancer cell in the tumor. There may be more than one type of cancer cell in a thymoma. The surgeon will decide if all or part of the tumor can be removed by surgery. In some cases, lymph nodes and other tissues may be removed as well.

Certain factors affect prognosis (chance of recovery) and treatment options.

The prognosis (chance of recovery) and treatment options depend on the following:

- The stage of the cancer.
- The type of cancer cell.
- Whether the tumor can be removed completely by surgery.
- The patient's general health.
- Whether the cancer has just been diagnosed or has recurred (come back).

Stages of Thymoma and Thymic Carcinoma

Tests done to detect thymoma or thymic carcinoma are also used to stage the disease.

Staging is the process used to find out if cancer has spread from the thymus to other parts of the body. The findings made during surgery and the results of tests and procedures are used to determine the stage of the disease. It is important to know the stage in order to plan treatment.

There are three ways that cancer spreads in the body.

Cancer can spread through tissue, the lymph system, and the blood:

- Tissue. The cancer spreads from where it began by growing into nearby areas.
- Lymph system. The cancer spreads from where it began by getting into the lymph system. The cancer travels through the lymph vessels to other parts of the body.
- Blood. The cancer spreads from where it began by getting into the blood. The cancer travels through the blood vessels to other parts of the body.

Cancer may spread from where it began to other parts of the body.

When cancer spreads to another part of the body, it is called metastasis. Cancer cells break away from where they began (the primary tumor) and travel through the lymph system or blood.

- Lymph system. The cancer gets into the lymph system, travels through the lymph vessels, and forms a tumor (metastatic tumor) in another part of the body.

- Blood. The cancer gets into the blood, travels through the blood vessels, and forms a tumor (metastatic tumor) in another part of the body.

The metastatic tumor is the same type of cancer as the primary tumor. For example, if thymic carcinoma spreads to the bone, the cancer cells in the bone are actually thymic carcinoma cells. The disease is metastatic thymic carcinoma, not bone cancer.

The following stages are used for thymoma:

Stage I

In stage I, cancer is found only within the thymus. All cancer cells are inside the capsule (sac) that surrounds the thymus.

Stage II

In stage II, cancer has spread through the capsule and into the fat around the thymus or into the lining of the chest cavity.

Stage III

In stage III, cancer has spread to nearby organs in the chest, including the lung, the sac around the heart, or large blood vessels that carry blood to the heart.

Stage IV

Stage IV is divided into stage IVA and stage IVB, depending on where the cancer has spread.

- In stage IVA, cancer has spread widely around the lungs and heart.

- In stage IVB, cancer has spread to the blood or lymph system.

Thymic carcinomas have usually spread to other parts of the body when diagnosed.

The staging system used for thymomas is sometimes used for thymic carcinomas.

Treatment Option Overview

There are different types of treatment for patients with thymoma and thymic carcinoma.

Different types of treatments are available for patients with thymoma and thymic carcinoma. Some treatments are standard (the currently used treatment), and some are being tested in clinical trials. A treatment clinical trial is a research study meant to help improve current treatments or obtain information on new treatments for patients with cancer. When clinical trials show that a new treatment is better than the standard treatment, the new treatment may become the standard treatment. Patients may want to think about taking part in a clinical trial. Some clinical trials are open only to patients who have not started treatment.

Four types of standard treatment are used:

Surgery

Surgery to remove the tumor is the most common treatment of thymoma.

Even if the doctor removes all the cancer that can be seen at the time of the surgery, some patients may be given radiation therapy after surgery to kill any cancer cells that are left. Treatment given after the surgery, to lower the risk that the cancer will come back, is called adjuvant therapy.

Radiation therapy

Radiation therapy is a cancer treatment that uses high-energy x-rays or other types of radiation to kill cancer cells or keep them from growing. There are two types of radiation therapy. External radiation therapy uses a machine outside the body to send radiation toward the cancer. Internal radiation therapy uses a radioactive substance sealed in needles, seeds, wires, or catheters that are placed directly into or near the cancer. The way the radiation therapy is given depends on the type and stage of the cancer being treated.

Chemotherapy

Chemotherapy is a cancer treatment that uses drugs to stop the growth of cancer cells, either by killing the cells or by stopping them from dividing. When chemotherapy is taken by mouth or injected into a vein or muscle, the drugs enter the bloodstream and can reach cancer cells throughout the body (systemic chemotherapy). When chemotherapy is placed directly into the cerebrospinal fluid, an organ, or a body cavity such as the abdomen, the drugs mainly affect cancer cells in those areas (regional chemotherapy). The way the chemotherapy is given depends on the type and stage of the cancer being treated.

Chemotherapy may be used to shrink the tumor before surgery or radiation therapy. This is called neoadjuvant chemotherapy.

Hormone therapy

Hormone therapy is a cancer treatment that removes hormones or blocks their action and stops cancer cells from growing. Hormones are substances produced by glands in the body and circulated in the bloodstream. Some hormones can cause certain cancers to grow. If tests show that the cancer cells have places where hormones can attach (receptors), drugs, surgery, or radiation therapy is used to reduce the production of hormones or block them from working.

Hormone therapy with drugs called corticosteroids may be used to treat thymoma or thymic carcinoma.

Patients may want to think about taking part in a clinical trial.

For some patients, taking part in a clinical trial may be the best treatment choice. Clinical trials are part of the cancer research process. Clinical trials are done to find out if new cancer treatments are safe and effective or better than the standard treatment.

Many of today's standard treatments for cancer are based on earlier clinical trials. Patients who take part in a clinical trial may receive the standard treatment or be among the first to receive a new treatment.

Patients who take part in clinical trials also help improve the way cancer will be treated in the future. Even when clinical trials do not lead to effective new treatments, they often answer important questions and help move research forward.

Patients can enter clinical trials before, during, or after starting their cancer treatment.

Some clinical trials only include patients who have not yet received treatment. Other trials test treatments for patients whose cancer has

not gotten better. There are also clinical trials that test new ways to stop cancer from recurring (coming back) or reduce the side effects of cancer treatment.

Clinical trials are taking place in many parts of the country.

Follow-up tests may be needed.

Some of the tests that were done to diagnose the cancer or to find out the stage of the cancer may be repeated. Some tests will be repeated in order to see how well the treatment is working. Decisions about whether to continue, change, or stop treatment may be based on the results of these tests.

Some of the tests will continue to be done from time to time after treatment has ended. The results of these tests can show if your condition has changed or if the cancer has recurred (come back). These tests are sometimes called follow-up tests or check-ups.

Section 22.5

Breast Cancer

Text in this section is excerpted from "Breast Cancer Treatment,"
National Cancer Institute at the National Institutes of Health (NIH),
April 3, 2015.

Female

General Information About Breast Cancer

Breast cancer is a disease in which malignant (cancer) cells form in the tissues of the breast.

The breast is made up of lobes and ducts. Each breast has 15 to 20 sections called lobe. Each lobe has many smaller sections called lobules. Lobules end in dozens of tiny bulbs that can make milk. The lobes, lobules, and bulbs are linked by thin tubes called ducts.

Each breast also has blood vessels and lymph vessels. The lymph vessels carry an almost colorless fluid called lymph. Lymph vessels carry lymph between lymph nodes. Lymph nodes are small bean-shaped structures that are found throughout the body. They filter substances in lymph and help fight infection and disease. Clusters of lymph nodes are found near the breast in the axilla (under the arm), above the collarbone, and in the chest.

The most common type of breast cancer is ductal carcinoma, which begins in the cells of the ducts. Cancer that begins in the lobes or lobules is called lobular carcinoma and is more often found in both breasts than are other types of breast cancer. Inflammatory breast cancer is an uncommon type of breast cancer in which the breast is warm, red, and swollen.

Having a family history of breast cancer and other factors increase the risk of breast cancer.

Anything that increases your chance of getting a disease is called a risk factor. Having a risk factor does not mean that you will get cancer; not having risk factors doesn't mean that you will not get cancer. Talk with your doctor if you think you may be at risk.

Older age is the main risk factor for most cancers. The chance of getting cancer increases as you get older. Other risk factors for breast cancer include:

- A family history of breast cancer in a first-degree relative (mother, daughter, or sister).
- Inherited changes in the *BRCA1* and *BRCA2* genes or in other genes that increase the risk of breast cancer.
- Drinking alcoholic beverages.
- Breast tissue that is dense on a mammogram.
- Exposure of breast tissue to estrogen made by the body:
    - Menstruating at an early age.
    - Older age at first birth or never having given birth.
    - Starting menopause at a later age.
- Taking hormones such as estrogen combined with progestin for symptoms of menopause.
- Taking oral contraceptives ("the pill").
- Obesity.
- A personal history of invasive breast cancer, ductal carcinoma in situ (DCIS), or lobular carcinoma in situ (LCIS).

- A personal history of benign (noncancer) breast disease.
- Being white.
- Treatment with radiation therapy to the breast/chest.

Breast cancer is sometimes caused by inherited gene mutations (changes).

The genes in cells carry the hereditary information that is received from a person's parents. Hereditary breast cancer makes up about 5% to 10% of all breast cancer. Some mutated genes related to breast cancer are more common in certain ethnic groups.

Women who have certain gene mutations, such as a *BRCA1* or *BRCA2* mutation, have an increased risk of breast cancer. These women also have an increased risk of ovarian cancer, and may have an increased risk of other cancers. Men who have a mutated gene related to breast cancer also have an increased risk of breast cancer.

There are tests that can detect (find) mutated genes. These genetic tests are sometimes done for members of families with a high risk of cancer.

Decreasing the length of time a woman's breast tissue is exposed to estrogen decreases the risk of breast cancer.

Anything that decreases your chance of getting a disease is called a protective factor.

Protective factors for breast cancer include the following:

- Taking any of the following:
  - Estrogen-only hormone therapy after a hysterectomy.
  - Selective estrogen receptor modulators (SERMs).
  - Aromatase inhibitors.
- Less exposure of breast tissue to estrogen made by the body:
  - Early pregnancy.
  - Breastfeeding.
  - Late menstruation.
  - Early menopause.
- Getting enough exercise.

- Having any of the following procedures:
- Risk-reducing mastectomy.
- Risk-reducing oophorectomy.
- Ovarian ablation.

Signs of breast cancer include a lump or change in the breast.

These and other signs may be caused by breast cancer or by other conditions. Check with your doctor if you have any of the following:

- A lump or thickening in or near the breast or in the underarm area.
- A change in the size or shape of the breast.
- A dimple or puckering in the skin of the breast.
- A nipple turned inward into the breast.
- Fluid, other than breast milk, from the nipple, especially if it's bloody.
- Scaly, red, or swollen skin on the breast, nipple, or areola (the dark area of skin that is around the nipple).
- Dimples in the breast that look like the skin of an orange, called peau d'orange.

Tests that examine the breasts are used to detect (find) and diagnose breast cancer.

Check with your doctor if you notice any changes in your breasts. The following tests and procedures may be used:

- **Physical exam and history**: An exam of the body to check general signs of health, including checking for signs of disease, such as lumps or anything else that seems unusual. A history of the patient's health habits and past illnesses and treatments will also be taken.
- **Clinical breast exam (CBE):** An exam of the breast by a doctor or other health professional. The doctor will carefully feel the breasts and under the arms for lumps or anything else that seems unusual.

- **Mammogram:** An x-ray of the breast.

- **MRI (magnetic resonance imaging):** A procedure that uses a magnet, radio waves, and a computer to make a series of detailed pictures of both breasts. This procedure is also called nuclear magnetic resonance imaging (NMRI).

- **Blood chemistry studies:** A procedure in which a blood sample is checked to measure the amounts of certain substances released into the blood by organs and tissues in the body. An unusual (higher or lower than normal) amount of a substance can be a sign of disease.

- **Biopsy:** The removal of cells or tissues so they can be viewed under a microscope by a pathologist to check for signs of cancer. If a lump in the breast is found, the doctor may need to remove a small piece of the lump.

  There are four types of biopsy used to check for breast cancer:

  - **Excisional biopsy:** The removal of an entire lump of tissue.

  - **Incisional biopsy:** The removal of part of a lump or a sample of tissue.

  - **Core biopsy:** The removal of tissue using a wide needle.

  - **Fine-needle aspiration (FNA) biopsy:** The removal of tissue or fluid, using a thin needle.

If cancer is found, tests are done to study the cancer cells.

Decisions about the best treatment are based on the results of these tests. The tests give information about:

- how quickly the cancer may grow.

- how likely it is that the cancer will spread through the body.

- how well certain treatments might work.

- how likely the cancer is to recur (come back).

Tests include the following:

- **Estrogen and progesterone receptor test:** A test to measure the amount of estrogen and progesterone (hormones) receptors in cancer tissue. If there are more estrogen and

276

progesterone receptors than normal, the cancer is called estrogen and/or progesterone receptor positive. This type of breast cancer may grow more quickly. The test results show whether treatment to block estrogen and progesterone may stop the cancer from growing.

- **Human epidermal growth factor type 2 receptor (HER2/neu) test:** A laboratory test to measure how many HER2/neu genes there are and how much HER2/neu protein is made in a sample of tissue. If there are more HER2/neu genes or higher levels of HER2/neu protein than normal, the cancer is called HER2/neu positive. This type of breast cancer may grow more quickly and is more likely to spread to other parts of the body. The cancer may be treated with drugs that target the HER2/neu protein, such as trastuzumab and pertuzumab.

- **Multigene tests:** Tests in which samples of tissue are studied to look at the activity of many genes at the same time. These tests may help predict whether cancer will spread to other parts of the body or recur (come back).

  - **Oncotype DX:** This test helps predict whether stage I or stage II breast cancer that is estrogen receptor positive and node-negative will spread to other parts of the body. If the risk of the cancer spreading is high, chemotherapy may be given to lower the risk.

  - **MammaPrint:** This test helps predict whether stage I or stage II breast cancer that is node-negative will spread to other parts of the body. If the risk of the cancer spreading is high, chemotherapy may be given to lower the risk.

Based on these tests, breast cancer is described as:

- Hormone-receptor positive (estrogen and/or progesterone receptor positive) or hormone-receptor negative (estrogen and/or progesterone receptor negative).

- HER2/neu positive or HER2/neu negative.

- Triple negative (estrogen receptor, progesterone receptor, and HER2/neu negative).

This information helps the doctor decide which treatments will work best for your cancer.

277

Certain factors affect prognosis (chance of recovery) and treatment options.

The prognosis (chance of recovery) and treatment options depend on the following:

- The stage of the cancer (the size of the tumor and whether it is in the breast only or has spread to lymph nodes or other places in the body).

- The type of breast cancer.

- Estrogen receptor and progesterone receptor levels in the tumor tissue.

- Human epidermal growth factor type 2 receptor (HER2/neu) levels in the tumor tissue.

- Whether the tumor tissue is triple-negative (cells that do not have estrogen receptors, progesterone receptors, or high levels of HER2/neu).

- How fast the tumor is growing.

- How likely the tumor is to recur (come back).

- A woman's age, general health, and menopausal status (whether a woman is still having menstrual periods).

- Whether the cancer has just been diagnosed or has recurred (come back).

Stages of Breast Cancer

After breast cancer has been diagnosed, tests are done to find out if cancer cells have spread within the breast or to other parts of the body.

The process used to find out whether the cancer has spread within the breast or to other parts of the body is called staging. The information gathered from the staging process determines the stage of the disease. It is important to know the stage in order to plan treatment. The following tests and procedures may be used in the staging process:

- **Sentinel lymph node biopsy:** The removal of the sentinel lymph node during surgery. The sentinel lymph node is the first lymph node to receive lymphatic drainage from a tumor. It is the first lymph node the cancer is likely to spread to from the tumor.

A radioactive substance and/or blue dye is injected near the tumor. The substance or dye flows through the lymph ducts to the lymph nodes. The first lymph node to receive the substance or dye is removed. A pathologist views the tissue under a microscope to look for cancer cells. If cancer cells are not found, it may not be necessary to remove more lymph nodes.

- **Chest x-ray:** An x-ray of the organs and bones inside the chest. An x-ray is a type of energy beam that can go through the body and onto film, making a picture of areas inside the body.

- **CT scan (CAT scan):** A procedure that makes a series of detailed pictures of areas inside the body, taken from different angles. The pictures are made by a computer linked to an x-ray machine. A dye may be injected into a vein or swallowed to help the organs or tissues show up more clearly. This procedure is also called computed tomography, computerized tomography, or computerized axial tomography.

- **Bone scan:** A procedure to check if there are rapidly dividing cells, such as cancer cells, in the bone. A very small amount of radioactive material is injected into a vein and travels through the bloodstream. The radioactive material collects in the bones and is detected by a scanner.

- **PET scan (positron emission tomography scan):** A procedure to find malignant tumor cells in the body. A small amount of radioactive glucose (sugar) is injected into a vein. The PET scanner rotates around the body and makes a picture of where glucose is being used in the body. Malignant tumor cells show up brighter in the picture because they are more active and take up more glucose than normal cells do.

There are three ways that cancer spreads in the body.

Cancer can spread through tissue, the lymph system, and the blood:

- Tissue. The cancer spreads from where it began by growing into nearby areas.

- Lymph system. The cancer spreads from where it began by getting into the lymph system. The cancer travels through the lymph vessels to other parts of the body.

- Blood. The cancer spreads from where it began by getting into the blood. The cancer travels through the blood vessels to other parts of the body.

Cancer may spread from where it began to other parts of the body.

When cancer spreads to another part of the body, it is called metastasis. Cancer cells break away from where they began (the primary tumor) and travel through the lymph system or blood.

- Lymph system. The cancer gets into the lymph system, travels through the lymph vessels, and forms a tumor (metastatic tumor) in another part of the body.

- Blood. The cancer gets into the blood, travels through the blood vessels, and forms a tumor (metastatic tumor) in another part of the body.

The metastatic tumor is the same type of cancer as the primary tumor. For example, if breast cancer spreads to the bone, the cancer cells in the bone are actually breast cancer cells. The disease is metastatic breast cancer, not bone cancer.

The following stages are used for breast cancer:

This section describes the stages of breast cancer. The breast cancer stage is based on the results of testing that is done on the tumor and lymph nodes removed during surgery and other tests.

Stage 0 (carcinoma in situ)

There are 3 types of breast carcinoma in situ:

Ductal carcinoma in situ (DCIS) is a noninvasive condition in which abnormal cells are found in the lining of a breast duct. The abnormal cells have not spread outside the duct to other tissues in the breast. In some cases, DCIS may become invasive cancer and spread to other tissues. At this time, there is no way to know which lesions could become invasive.

Lobular carcinoma in situ (LCIS) is a condition in which abnormal cells are found in the lobules of the breast. This condition seldom becomes invasive cancer.

Paget disease of the nipple is a condition in which abnormal cells are found in the nipple only.

Stage I

Stage I breast cancer. In stage IA, the tumor is 2 centimeters or smaller and has not spread outside the breast. In stage IB, no tumor is found in the breast or the tumor is 2 centimeters or smaller. Small clusters of cancer cells (larger than 0.2 millimeter but not larger than 2 millimeters) are found in the lymph nodes.

In stage I, cancer has formed. Stage I is divided into stages IA and IB.

- In stage IA, the tumor is 2 centimeters or smaller. Cancer has not spread outside the breast.

- In stage IB, small clusters of breast cancer cells (larger than 0.2 millimeter but not larger than 2 millimeters) are found in the lymph nodes and either:

    - no tumor is found in the breast; or

    - the tumor is 2 centimeters or smaller.

Stage II

Stage II is divided into stages IIA and IIB.

- In stage IIA:

    - no tumor is found in the breast or the tumor is 2 centimeters or smaller. Cancer (larger than 2 millimeters) is found in 1 to 3 axillary lymph nodes or in the lymph nodes near the breastbone (found during a sentinel lymph node biopsy); or

    - the tumor is larger than 2 centimeters but not larger than 5 centimeters. Cancer has not spread to the lymph nodes.

- In stage IIB, the tumor is:

    - larger than 2 centimeters but not larger than 5 centimeters. Small clusters of breast cancer cells (larger than 0.2 millimeter but not larger than 2 millimeters) are found in the lymph nodes; or

    - larger than 2 centimeters but not larger than 5 centimeters. Cancer has spread to 1 to 3 axillary lymph nodes or to the lymph nodes near the breastbone (found during a sentinel lymph node biopsy); or

    - larger than 5 centimeters. Cancer has not spread to the lymph nodes.

Stage IIIA

In stage IIIA:

- no tumor is found in the breast or the tumor may be any size. Cancer is found in 4 to 9 axillary lymph nodes or in the lymph

281

nodes near the breastbone (found during imaging tests or a physical exam); or

- the tumor is larger than 5 centimeters. Small clusters of breast cancer cells (larger than 0.2 millimeter but not larger than 2 millimeters) are found in the lymph nodes; or

- the tumor is larger than 5 centimeters. Cancer has spread to 1 to 3 axillary lymph nodes or to the lymph nodes near the breastbone (found during a sentinel lymph node biopsy).

Stage IIIB

In stage IIIB, the tumor may be any size and cancer has spread to the chest wall and/or to the skin of the breast and caused swelling or an ulcer. Also, cancer may have spread to:

- up to 9 axillary lymph nodes; or

- the lymph nodes near the breastbone.

Cancer that has spread to the skin of the breast may also be inflammatory breast cancer.

Stage IIIC

In stage IIIC, no tumor is found in the breast or the tumor may be any size. Cancer may have spread to the skin of the breast and caused swelling or an ulcer and/or has spread to the chest wall. Also, cancer has spread to:

- 10 or more axillary lymph nodes; or

- lymph nodes above or below the collarbone; or

- axillary lymph nodes and lymph nodes near the breastbone.

Cancer that has spread to the skin of the breast may also be inflammatory breast cancer.

For treatment, stage IIIC breast cancer is divided into operable and inoperable stage IIIC.

Stage IV

In stage IV, cancer has spread to other organs of the body, most often the bones, lungs, liver, or brain.

Treatment Option Overview

There are different types of treatment for patients with breast cancer.

Different types of treatment are available for patients with breast cancer. Some treatments are standard (the currently used treatment), and some are being tested in clinical trials. A treatment clinical trial is a research study meant to help improve current treatments or obtain information on new treatments for patients with cancer. When clinical trials show that a new treatment is better than the standard treatment, the new treatment may become the standard treatment. Patients may want to think about taking part in a clinical trial. Some clinical trials are open only to patients who have not started treatment.

Six types of standard treatment are used:

Surgery

Most patients with breast cancer have surgery to remove the cancer from the breast. Some of the lymph nodes under the arm are usually taken out and looked at under a microscope to see if they contain cancer cells.

Breast-conserving surgery, an operation to remove the cancer but not the breast itself, includes the following:

- Lumpectomy: Surgery to remove a tumor (lump) and a small amount of normal tissue around it.

- Partial mastectomy: Surgery to remove the part of the breast that has cancer and some normal tissue around it. The lining over the chest muscles below the cancer may also be removed. This procedure is also called a segmental mastectomy.

Patients who are treated with breast-conserving surgery may also have some of the lymph nodes under the arm removed for biopsy. This procedure is called lymph node dissection. It may be done at the same time as the breast-conserving surgery or after. Lymph node dissection is done through a separate incision.

Other types of surgery include the following:

- Total mastectomy: Surgery to remove the whole breast that has cancer. This procedure is also called a simple mastectomy. Some of the lymph nodes under the arm may be removed for biopsy

283

at the same time as the breast surgery or after. This is done through a separate incision.

- Modified radical mastectomy: Surgery to remove the whole breast that has cancer, many of the lymph nodes under the arm, the lining over the chest muscles, and sometimes, part of the chest wall muscles.

Chemotherapy may be given before surgery to remove the tumor. When given before surgery, chemotherapy will shrink the tumor and reduce the amount of tissue that needs to be removed during surgery. Treatment given before surgery is called neoadjuvant therapy.

Even if the doctor removes all the cancer that can be seen at the time of the surgery, some patients may be given radiation therapy, chemotherapy, or hormone therapy after surgery to kill any cancer cells that are left. Treatment given after the surgery, to lower the risk that the cancer will come back, is called adjuvant therapy.

If a patient is going to have a mastectomy, breast reconstruction (surgery to rebuild a breast's shape after a mastectomy) may be considered. Breast reconstruction may be done at the time of the mastectomy or at a future time. The reconstructed breast may be made with the patient's own (nonbreast) tissue or by using implants filled with saline or silicone gel.

Sentinel lymph node biopsy followed by surgery

Sentinel lymph node biopsy is the removal of the sentinel lymph node during surgery. The sentinel lymph node is the first lymph node to receive lymphatic drainage from a tumor. It is the first lymph node the cancer is likely to spread to from the tumor. A radioactive substance and/or blue dye is injected near the tumor. The substance or dye flows through the lymph ducts to the lymph nodes. The first lymph node to receive the substance or dye is removed. A pathologist views the tissue under a microscope to look for cancer cells. If cancer cells are not found, it may not be necessary to remove more lymph nodes. After the sentinel lymph node biopsy, the surgeon removes the tumor (breast-conserving surgery or mastectomy).

Radiation therapy

Radiation therapy is a cancer treatment that uses high-energy x-rays or other types of radiation to kill cancer cells or keep them from growing. There are two types of radiation therapy. External radiation therapy uses a machine outside the body to send radiation toward the cancer. Internal radiation therapy uses a radioactive substance sealed in needles, seeds, wires, or catheters that are placed directly into or near the cancer. The way the radiation therapy is given depends on the type and stage of the cancer being treated.

Chemotherapy

Chemotherapy is a cancer treatment that uses drugs to stop the growth of cancer cells, either by killing the cells or by stopping them from dividing. When chemotherapy is taken by mouth or injected into a vein or muscle, the drugs enter the bloodstream and can reach cancer cells throughout the body (systemic chemotherapy). When chemotherapy is placed directly into the cerebrospinal fluid, an organ, or a body cavity such as the abdomen, the drugs mainly affect cancer cells in those areas (regional chemotherapy). The way the chemotherapy is given depends on the type and stage of the cancer being treated.

Hormone therapy

Hormone therapy is a cancer treatment that removes hormones or blocks their action and stops cancer cells from growing. Hormones are substances made by glands in the body and circulated in the bloodstream. Some hormones can cause certain cancers to grow. If tests show that the cancer cells have places where hormones can attach (receptors), drugs, surgery, or radiation therapy is used to reduce the production of hormones or block them from working. The hormone estrogen, which makes some breast cancers grow, is made mainly by the ovaries. Treatment to stop the ovaries from making estrogen is called ovarian ablation.

Hormone therapy with tamoxifen is often given to patients with early stages of breast cancer and those with metastatic breast cancer (cancer that has spread to other parts of the body). Hormone therapy with tamoxifen or estrogens can act on cells all over the body and may increase the chance of developing endometrial cancer. Women taking tamoxifen should have a pelvic exam every year to look for any signs of cancer. Any vaginal bleeding, other than menstrual bleeding, should be reported to a doctor as soon as possible.

Hormone therapy with an aromatase inhibitor is given to some postmenopausal women who have hormone-dependent breast cancer. Hormone-dependent breast cancer needs the hormone estrogen to grow. Aromatase inhibitors decrease the body's estrogen by blocking an enzyme called aromatase from turning androgen into estrogen.

For the treatment of early stage breast cancer, certain aromatase inhibitors may be used as adjuvant therapy instead of tamoxifen or after 2 or more years of tamoxifen. For the treatment of metastatic breast cancer, aromatase inhibitors are being tested in clinical trials to compare them to hormone therapy with tamoxifen.

Targeted therapy

Targeted therapy is a type of treatment that uses drugs or other substances to identify and attack specific cancer cells without harming normal cells. Monoclonal antibodies and tyrosine kinase inhibitors are two types of targeted therapies used in the treatment of breast cancer. PARP inhibitors are a type of targeted therapy being studied for the treatment of triple-negative breast cancer.

Monoclonal antibody therapy is a cancer treatment that uses antibodies made in the laboratory, from a single type of immune system cell. These antibodies can identify substances on cancer cells or normal substances that may help cancer cells grow. The antibodies attach to the substances and kill the cancer cells, block their growth, or keep them from spreading. Monoclonal antibodies are given by infusion. They may be used alone or to carry drugs, toxins, or radioactive material directly to cancer cells. Monoclonal antibodies may be used in combination with chemotherapy as adjuvant therapy.

Trastuzumab is a monoclonal antibody that blocks the effects of the growth factor protein HER2, which sends growth signals to breast cancer cells. About one-fourth of patients with breast cancer have tumors that may be treated with trastuzumab combined with chemotherapy.

Pertuzumab is a monoclonal antibody that may be combined with trastuzumab and chemotherapy to treat breast cancer. It may be used to treat certain patients with HER2-positive breast cancer that has metastasized (spread to other parts of the body). It may also be used as neoadjuvant therapy in certain patients with early-stage HER2-positive breast cancer.

Ado-trastuzumab emtansine is a monoclonal antibody linked to an anticancer drug. This is called an antibody-drug conjugate. It is used to treat HER2-positive breast cancer that has spread to other parts of the body or recurred (come back).

Tyrosine kinase inhibitors are targeted therapy drugs that block signals needed for tumors to grow. Tyrosine kinase inhibitors may be used with other anticancer drugs as adjuvant therapy.

Lapatinib is a tyrosine kinase inhibitor that blocks the effects of the HER2 protein and other proteins inside tumor cells. It may be used with other drugs to treat patients with HER2-positive breast cancer that has progressed after treatment with trastuzumab.

PARP inhibitors are a type of targeted therapy that block DNA repair and may cause cancer cells to die. PARP inhibitor therapy is being studied for the treatment of triple-negative breast cancer.

New types of treatment are being tested in clinical trials.

High-dose chemotherapy with stem cell transplant

High-dose chemotherapy with stem cell transplant is a way of giving high doses of chemotherapy and replacing blood -forming cells destroyed by the cancer treatment. Stem cells (immature blood cells) are removed from the blood or bone marrow of the patient or a donor and are frozen and stored. After the chemotherapy is completed, the stored stem cells are thawed and given back to the patient through an infusion. These reinfused stem cells grow into (and restore) the body's blood cells.

Studies have shown that high-dose chemotherapy followed by stem cell transplant does not work better than standard chemotherapy in the treatment of breast cancer. Doctors have decided that, for now, high-dose chemotherapy should be tested only in clinical trials. Before taking part in such a trial, women should talk with their doctors about the serious side effects, including death, that may be caused by high-dose chemotherapy.

Patients may want to think about taking part in a clinical trial.

For some patients, taking part in a clinical trial may be the best treatment choice. Clinical trials are part of the cancer research process. Clinical trials are done to find out if new cancer treatments are safe and effective or better than the standard treatment.

Many of today's standard treatments for cancer are based on earlier clinical trials. Patients who take part in a clinical trial may receive the standard treatment or be among the first to receive a new treatment.

Patients who take part in clinical trials also help improve the way cancer will be treated in the future. Even when clinical trials do not lead to effective new treatments, they often answer important questions and help move research forward.

Patients can enter clinical trials before, during, or after starting their cancer treatment.

Some clinical trials only include patients who have not yet received treatment. Other trials test treatments for patients whose cancer has not gotten better. There are also clinical trials that test new ways to stop cancer from recurring (coming back) or reduce the side effects of cancer treatment.

Clinical trials are taking place in many parts of the country.

Follow-up tests may be needed.

Some of the tests that were done to diagnose the cancer or to find out the stage of the cancer may be repeated. Some tests will be repeated in order to see how well the treatment is working. Decisions about whether to continue, change, or stop treatment may be based on the results of these tests.

Some of the tests will continue to be done from time to time after treatment has ended. The results of these tests can show if your condition has changed or if the cancer has recurred (come back). These tests are sometimes called follow-up tests or check-ups.

Male

General Information about Male Breast Cancer

Male breast cancer is a disease in which malignant (cancer) cells form in the tissues of the breast.

Breast cancer may occur in men. Men at any age may develop breast cancer, but it is usually detected (found) in men between 60 and 70 years of age. Male breast cancer makes up less than 1% of all cases of breast cancer.

The following types of breast cancer are found in men:

- Infiltrating ductal carcinoma: Cancer that has spread beyond the cells lining ducts in the breast. Most men with breast cancer have this type of cancer.

- Ductal carcinoma in situ: Abnormal cells that are found in the lining of a duct; also called intraductal carcinoma.

- Inflammatory breast cancer: A type of cancer in which the breast looks red and swollen and feels warm.

- Paget disease of the nipple: A tumor that has grown from ducts beneath the nipple onto the surface of the nipple.

Lobular carcinoma in situ (abnormal cells found in one of the lobes or sections of the breast), which sometimes occurs in women, has not been seen in men.

Radiation exposure, high levels of estrogen, and a family history of breast cancer can increase a man's risk of breast cancer.

Anything that increases your risk of getting a disease is called a risk factor. Having a risk factor does not mean that you will get cancer; not having risk factors doesn't mean that you will not get cancer. Talk with your doctor if you think you may be at risk. Risk factors for breast cancer in men may include the following:

- Being exposed to radiation.

- Having a disease linked to high levels of estrogen in the body, such as cirrhosis (liver disease) or Klinefelter syndrome (a genetic disorder.)

- Having several female relatives who have had breast cancer, especially relatives who have an alteration of the BRCA2 gene.

Male breast cancer is sometimes caused by inherited gene mutations (changes).

The genes in cells carry the hereditary information that is received from a person's parents. Hereditary breast cancer makes up about 5% to 10% of all breast cancer. Some mutated genes related to breast cancer are more common in certain ethnic groups. Men who have a mutated gene related to breast cancer have an increased risk of this disease.

Men with breast cancer usually have lumps that can be felt.

Lumps and other signs may be caused by male breast cancer or by other conditions. Check with your doctor if you notice a change in your breasts.

Tests that examine the breasts are used to detect (find) and diagnose breast cancer in men.

The following tests and procedures may be used:

- **Physical exam and history:** An exam of the body to check general signs of health, including checking for signs of disease, such as lumps or anything else that seems unusual. A history of the patient's health habits and past illnesses and treatments will also be taken.

- **Clinical breast exam (CBE):** An exam of the breast by a doctor or other health professional. The doctor will carefully feel the breasts and under the arms for lumps or anything else that seems unusual.

- **Ultrasound exam:** A procedure in which high-energy sound waves (ultrasound) are bounced off internal tissues or organs and make echoes. The echoes form a picture of body tissues called a sonogram. The picture can be printed to be looked at later.

- **MRI (magnetic resonance imaging):** A procedure that uses a magnet, radio waves, and a computer to make a series of detailed pictures of areas inside the body. This procedure is also called nuclear magnetic resonance imaging (NMRI).

- **Blood chemistry studies:** A procedure in which a blood sample is checked to measure the amounts of certain substances released into the blood by organs and tissues in the body. An unusual (higher or lower than normal) amount of a substance can be a sign of disease in the organ or tissue that makes it.

- **Biopsy:** The removal of cells or tissues so they can be viewed under a microscope by a pathologist to check for signs of cancer. The following are different types of biopsies:
  - Fine-needle aspiration (FNA) biopsy: The removal of tissue or fluid using a thin needle.
  - Core biopsy: The removal of tissue using a wide needle.
  - Excisional biopsy: The removal of an entire lump of tissue.

If cancer is found, tests are done to study the cancer cells.

Decisions about the best treatment are based on the results of these tests. The tests give information about:

- How quickly the cancer may grow.

- How likely it is that the cancer will spread through the body.

- How well certain treatments might work.

- How likely the cancer is to recur (come back).

Tests include the following:

- **Estrogen and progesterone receptor test:** A test to measure the amount of estrogen and progesterone (hormones) receptors in cancer tissue. If cancer is found in the breast, tissue from the tumor is checked in the laboratory to find out whether estrogen and progesterone could affect the way cancer grows. The test results show whether hormone therapy may stop the cancer from growing.

- **HER2 test:** A test to measure the amount of HER2 in cancer tissue. HER2 is a growth factor protein that sends growth signals to cells. When cancer forms, the cells may make too much of the protein, causing more cancer cells to grow. If cancer is found in the breast, tissue from the tumor is checked in the laboratory to find out if there is too much HER2 in the cells. The test results show whether monoclonal antibody therapy may stop the cancer from growing.

Survival for men with breast cancer is similar to survival for women with breast cancer.

Survival for men with breast cancer is similar to that for women with breast cancer when their stage at diagnosis is the same. Breast cancer in men, however, is often diagnosed at a later stage. Cancer found at a later stage may be less likely to be cured.

Certain factors affect prognosis (chance of recovery) and treatment options.

The prognosis (chance of recovery) and treatment options depend on the following:

- The stage of the cancer (whether it is in the breast only or has spread to other places in the body).

- The type of breast cancer.

- Estrogen-receptor and progesterone-receptor levels in the tumor tissue.

- Whether the cancer is also found in the other breast.

- The patient's age and general health.

Stages of Male Breast Cancer

After breast cancer has been diagnosed, tests are done to find out if cancer cells have spread within the breast or to other parts of the body.

After breast cancer has been diagnosed, tests are done to find out if cancer cells have spread within the breast or to other parts of the body. This process is called staging. The information gathered from the staging process determines the stage of the disease. It is important to know the stage in order to plan treatment. Breast cancer in men is staged the same as it is in women. The spread of cancer from the breast to lymph nodes and other parts of the body appears to be similar in men and women.

The following tests and procedures may be used in the staging process:

- **Sentinel lymph node biopsy:** The removal of the sentinel lymph node during surgery. The sentinel lymph node is the first lymph node to receive lymphatic drainage from a tumor. It is the first lymph node the cancer is likely to spread to from the tumor. A radioactive substance and/or blue dye is injected near the tumor. The substance or dye flows through the lymph ducts to the lymph nodes. The first lymph node to receive the substance or dye is removed. A pathologist views the tissue under a microscope to look for cancer cells. If cancer cells are not found, it may not be necessary to remove more lymph nodes.

- **Chest x-ray:** An x-ray of the organs and bones inside the chest. An x-ray is a type of energy beam that can go through the body and onto film, making a picture of areas inside the body.

- **CT scan (CAT scan):** A procedure that makes a series of detailed pictures of areas inside the body, taken from different angles. The pictures are made by a computer linked to an x-ray machine. A dye may be injected into a vein or swallowed to help the organs or tissues show up more clearly. This procedure is also called computed tomography, computerized tomography, or computerized axial tomography.

- **Bone scan:** A procedure to check if there are rapidly dividing cells, such as cancer cells, in the bone. A very small amount of radioactive material is injected into a vein and travels through the bloodstream. The radioactive material collects in the bones and is detected by a scanner.

- **PET scan (positron emission tomography scan):** A procedure to find malignant tumor cells in the body. A small amount of radioactive glucose (sugar) is injected into a vein. The PET scanner rotates around the body and makes a picture of where glucose is being used in the body. Malignant tumor cells show up brighter in the picture because they are more active and take up more glucose than normal cells do.

There are three ways that cancer spreads in the body.

Cancer can spread through tissue, the lymph system, and the blood:

- Tissue. The cancer spreads from where it began by growing into nearby areas.

- Lymph system. The cancer spreads from where it began by getting into the lymph system. The cancer travels through the lymph vessels to other parts of the body.

- Blood. The cancer spreads from where it began by getting into the blood. The cancer travels through the blood vessels to other parts of the body.

Cancer may spread from where it began to other parts of the body.

When cancer spreads to another part of the body, it is called metastasis. Cancer cells break away from where they began (the primary tumor) and travel through the lymph system or blood.

- Lymph system. The cancer gets into the lymph system, travels through the lymph vessels, and forms a tumor (metastatic tumor) in another part of the body.

- Blood. The cancer gets into the blood, travels through the blood vessels, and forms a tumor (metastatic tumor) in another part of the body.

The metastatic tumor is the same type of cancer as the primary tumor. For example, if breast cancer spreads to the bone, the cancer cells in the bone are actually breast cancer cells. The disease is metastatic breast cancer, not bone cancer.

293

The following stages are used for male breast cancer:

This section describes the stages of breast cancer. The breast cancer stage is based on the results of testing that is done on the tumor and lymph nodes removed during surgery and other tests.

Stage 0 (carcinoma in situ)

There are 3 types of breast carcinoma in situ:

- Ductal carcinoma in situ (DCIS) is a noninvasive condition in which abnormal cells are found in the lining of a breast duct. The abnormal cells have not spread outside the duct to other tissues in the breast. In some cases, DCIS may become invasive cancer and spread to other tissues. At this time, there is no way to know which lesions could become invasive.

- Paget disease of the nipple is a condition in which abnormal cells are found in the nipple only.

- Lobular carcinoma in situ (LCIS) is a condition in which abnormal cells are found in the lobules of the breast. This condition has not been seen in men.

Stage I

In stage I, cancer has formed. Stage I is divided into stages IA and IB.

- In stage IA, the tumor is 2 centimeters or smaller. Cancer has not spread outside the breast.

- In stage IB, small clusters of breast cancer cells (larger than 0.2 millimeter but not larger than 2 millimeters) are found in the lymph nodes and either:

  - no tumor is found in the breast; or

  - the tumor is 2 centimeters or smaller.

Stage II

Stage II is divided into stages IIA and IIB.

- In stage IIA

  - no tumor is found in the breast or the tumor is 2 centimeters or smaller. Cancer (larger than 2 millimeters) is found in 1

to 3 axillary lymph nodes or in the lymph nodes near the
breastbone (found during a sentinel lymph node biopsy); or

- the tumor is larger than 2 centimeters but not larger than 5
centimeters. Cancer has not spread to the lymph nodes.

- In stage IIB, the tumor is:
  - larger than 2 centimeters but not larger than 5 centimeters.
  Small clusters of breast cancer cells (larger than 0.2 millimeter but not larger than 2 millimeters) are found in the lymph
  nodes; or
  - larger than 2 centimeters but not larger than 5 centimeters.
  Cancer has spread to 1 to 3 axillary lymph nodes or to the
  lymph nodes near the breastbone (found during a sentinel
  lymph node biopsy); or
  - larger than 5 centimeters. Cancer has not spread to the
  lymph nodes.

Stage IIIA

In stage IIIA:

- no tumor is found in the breast or the tumor may be any size.
Cancer is found in 4 to 9 axillary lymph nodes or in the lymph
nodes near the breastbone (found during imaging tests or a
physical exam); or
- the tumor is larger than 5 centimeters. Small clusters of breast
cancer cells (larger than 0.2 millimeter but not larger than 2
millimeters) are found in the lymph nodes; or
- the tumor is larger than 5 centimeters. Cancer has spread to 1
to 3 axillary lymph nodes or to the lymph nodes near the breastbone (found during a sentinel lymph node biopsy).

Stage IIIB

In stage IIIB, the tumor may be any size and cancer has spread to
the chest wall and/or to the skin of the breast and caused swelling or
an ulcer. Also, cancer may have spread to:

- up to 9 axillary lymph nodes; or
- the lymph nodes near the breastbone.

Cancer that has spread to the skin of the breast may also be inflammatory breast cancer.

295

Stage IIIC

In stage IIIC, no tumor is found in the breast or the tumor may be any size. Cancer may have spread to the skin of the breast and caused swelling or an ulcer and/or has spread to the chest wall. Also, cancer has spread to:

- 10 or more axillary lymph nodes; or
- lymph nodes above or below the collarbone; or
- axillary lymph nodes and lymph nodes near the breastbone.

Cancer that has spread to the skin of the breast may also be inflammatory breast cancer.

For treatment, stage IIIC breast cancer is divided into operable and inoperable stage IIIC.

Stage IV

In stage IV, cancer has spread to other organs of the body, most often the bones, lungs, liver, or brain.

Inflammatory Male Breast Cancer

In inflammatory breast cancer, cancer has spread to the skin of the breast and the breast looks red and swollen and feels warm. The redness and warmth occur because the cancer cells block the lymph vessels in the skin. The skin of the breast may also show the dimpled appearance called peau d'orange (like the skin of an orange). There may not be any lumps in the breast that can be felt. Inflammatory breast cancer may be stage IIIB, stage IIIC, or stage IV.

Treatment Option Overview

There are different types of treatment for men with breast cancer.

Different types of treatment are available for men with breast cancer. Some treatments are standard (the currently used treatment), and some are being tested in clinical trials. A treatment clinical trial is a research study meant to help improve current treatments or obtain information on new treatments for patients with cancer. When clinical trials show that a new treatment is better than the standard treatment, the new treatment may become the standard treatment.

For some patients, taking part in a clinical trial may be the best treatment choice. Many of today's standard treatments for cancer are based on earlier clinical trials. Patients who take part in a clinical trial may receive the standard treatment or be among the first to receive a new treatment.

Patients who take part in clinical trials also help improve the way cancer will be treated in the future. Even when clinical trials do not lead to effective new treatments, they often answer important questions and help move research forward.

Some clinical trials only include patients who have not yet received treatment. Other trials test treatments for patients whose cancer has not gotten better. There are also clinical trials that test new ways to stop cancer from recurring (coming back) or reduce the side effects of cancer treatment.

Five types of standard treatment are used to treat men with breast cancer:

Surgery

Surgery for men with breast cancer is usually a modified radical mastectomy (removal of the breast, many of the lymph nodes under the arm, the lining over the chest muscles, and sometimes part of the chest wall muscles).

Breast-conserving surgery, an operation to remove the cancer but not the breast itself, is also used for some men with breast cancer. A lumpectomy is done to remove the tumor (lump) and a small amount of normal tissue around it. Radiation therapy is given after surgery to kill any cancer cells that are left.

Chemotherapy

Chemotherapy is a cancer treatment that uses drugs to stop the growth of cancer cells, either by killing the cells or by stopping them from dividing. When chemotherapy is taken by mouth or injected into a vein or muscle, the drugs enter the bloodstream and can reach cancer cells throughout the body (systemic chemotherapy). When chemotherapy is placed directly into the cerebrospinal fluid, an organ, or a body cavity such as the abdomen, the drugs mainly affect cancer cells in those areas (regional chemotherapy). The way the chemotherapy is given depends on the type and stage of the cancer being treated.

Hormone therapy

Hormone therapy is a cancer treatment that removes hormones or blocks their action and stops cancer cells from growing. Hormones are substances made by glands in the body and circulated in the bloodstream. Some hormones can cause certain cancers to grow. If tests show that the cancer cells have places where hormones can attach (receptors), drugs, surgery, or radiation therapy is used to reduce the production of hormones or block them from working.

Radiation therapy

Radiation therapy is a cancer treatment that uses high-energy x-rays or other types of radiation to kill cancer cells or keep them from growing. There are two types of radiation therapy. External radiation therapy uses a machine outside the body to send radiation toward the cancer. Internal radiation therapy uses a radioactive substance sealed in needles, seeds, wires, or catheters that are placed directly into or near the cancer. The way the radiation therapy is given depends on the type and stage of the cancer being treated.

Targeted therapy

Targeted therapy is a type of treatment that uses drugs or other substances to identify and attack specific cancer cells without harming normal cells. Monoclonal antibody therapy is a type of targeted therapy used to treat men with breast cancer.

Monoclonal antibody therapy uses antibodies made in the laboratory from a single type of immune system cell. These antibodies can identify substances on cancer cells or normal substances that may help cancer cells grow. The antibodies attach to the substances and kill the cancer cells, block their growth, or keep them from spreading. Monoclonal antibodies are given by infusion. They may be used alone or to carry drugs, toxins, or radioactive material directly to cancer cells. Monoclonal antibodies are also used with chemotherapy as adjuvant therapy (treatment given after surgery to lower the risk that the cancer will come back).

Trastuzumab is a monoclonal antibody that blocks the effects of the growth factor protein HER2.

Chapter 23

Gastrointestinal / Digestive Cancer

Chapter Contents

Section 23.1

Gastrointestinal Carcinoid Tumor

Text in this section is excerpted from "Gastrointestinal Carcinoid Tumors Treatment," National Cancer Institute at the National Institutes of Health (NIH), April 2, 2015.

General Information About Gastrointestinal Carcinoid Tumors

A gastrointestinal carcinoid tumor is cancer that forms in the lining of the gastrointestinal tract.

The gastrointestinal (GI) tract is part of the body's digestive system. It helps to digest food, takes nutrients (vitamins, minerals, carbohydrates, fats, proteins, and water) from food to be used by the body and helps pass waste material out of the body.

The GI tract is made up of these and other organs:

- Stomach.
- Small intestine (duodenum, jejunum, and ileum).
- Colon.
- Rectum.

Gastrointestinal carcinoid tumors form from a certain type of neuroendocrine cell (a type of cell that is like a nerve cell and a hormone -making cell). These cells are scattered throughout the chest and abdomen but most are found in the GI tract. Neuroendocrine cells make hormones that help control digestive juices and the muscles used in moving food through the stomach and intestines. A GI carcinoid tumor may also make hormones and release them into the body.

GI carcinoid tumors are rare and most grow very slowly. Most of them occur in the small intestine, rectum, and appendix. Sometimes more than one tumor will form.

Health history can affect the risk of gastrointestinal carcinoid tumors.

Anything that increases a person's chance of developing a disease is called a risk factor. Having a risk factor does not mean that you will get cancer; not having risk factors doesn't mean that you will not get cancer. Talk to your doctor if you think you may be at risk.

Risk factors for GI carcinoid tumors include the following:

- Having a family history of multiple endocrine neoplasia type 1 (MEN1) syndrome or neurofibromatosis type 1 (NF1) syndrome.

- Having certain conditions that affect the stomach's ability to make stomach acid, such as atrophic gastritis, pernicious anemia, or Zollinger-Ellison syndrome.

Some gastrointestinal carcinoid tumors have no signs or symptoms in the early stages.

Signs and symptoms may be caused by the growth of the tumor and/or the hormones the tumor makes. Some tumors, especially tumors of the stomach or appendix, may not cause signs or symptoms. Carcinoid tumors are often found during tests or treatments for other conditions.

Carcinoid tumors in the small intestine (duodenum, jejunum, and ileum), colon, and rectum sometimes cause signs or symptoms as they grow or because of the hormones they make. Other conditions may cause the same signs or symptoms. Check with your doctor if you have any of the following:

Duodenum
Signs and symptoms of GI carcinoid tumors in the duodenum (first part of the small intestine, that connects to the stomach) may include the following:

- Abdominal pain.
- Constipation.
- Diarrhea.
- Change in stool color.
- Nausea.
- Vomiting.

301

- Jaundice (yellowing of the skin and whites of the eyes).
- Heartburn.

Jejunum and ileum

Signs and symptoms of GI carcinoid tumors in the jejunum (middle part of the small intestine) and ileum (last part of the small intestine, that connects to the colon) may include the following:

- Abdominal pain.
- Weight loss for no known reason.
- Feeling very tired.
- Feeling bloated
- Diarrhea.
- Nausea.
- Vomiting.

Colon

Signs and symptoms of GI carcinoid tumors in the colon may include the following:

- Abdominal pain.
- Weight loss for no known reason.

Rectum

Signs and symptoms of GI carcinoid tumors in the rectum may include the following:

- Blood in the stool.
- Pain in the rectum.
- Constipation.

Carcinoid syndrome may occur if the tumor spreads to the liver or other parts of the body.

The hormones made by gastrointestinal carcinoid tumors are usually destroyed by liver enzymes in the blood. If the tumor has spread to the liver and the liver enzymes cannot destroy the extra hormones made by the tumor, high amounts of these hormones may remain in the body and cause carcinoid syndrome. This can also happen if tumor cells enter the blood.

Signs and symptoms of carcinoid syndrome include the following:

- Redness or a feeling of warmth in the face and neck.
- Abdominal pain.
- Feeling bloated.
- Diarrhea.
- Wheezing or other trouble breathing.
- Fast heartbeat.

These signs and symptoms may be caused by gastrointestinal carcinoid tumors or by other conditions. Talk to your doctor if you have any of these signs or symptoms.

Imaging studies and tests that examine the blood and urine are used to detect (find) and diagnose gastrointestinal carcinoid tumors.

The following tests and procedures may be used:

- **Physical exam and history:** An exam of the body to check general signs of health, including checking for signs of disease, such as lumps or anything else that seems unusual. A history of the patient's health habits and past illnesses and treatments will also be taken.

- **Blood chemistry studies:** A procedure in which a blood sample is checked to measure the amounts of certain substances, such as hormones, released into the blood by organs and tissues in the body. An unusual (higher or lower than normal) amount of a substance can be a sign of disease in the organ or tissue that produces it. The blood sample is checked to see if it contains a hormone produced by carcinoid tumors. This test is used to help diagnose carcinoid syndrome.

- **Tumor marker test:** A procedure in which a sample of blood, urine, or tissue is checked to measure the amounts of certain substances, such as chromogranin A, made by organs, tissues, or tumor cells in the body. Chromogranin A is a tumor marker. It has been linked to neuroendocrine tumors when found in increased levels in the body.

- **Twenty-four-hour urine test:** A test in which urine is collected for 24 hours to measure the amounts of certain substances, such as 5-HIAA or serotonin (hormone). An unusual (higher or lower than normal) amount of a substance can be a sign of disease in the organ or tissue that makes it. This test is used to help diagnose carcinoid syndrome.

- **MIBG scan:** A procedure used to find neuroendocrine tumors, such as carcinoid tumors. A very small amount of radioactive material called MIBG (metaiodobenzylguanidine) is injected into a vein and travels through the bloodstream. Carcinoid tumors take up the radioactive material and are detected by a device that measures radiation.

- **CT scan (CAT scan):** A procedure that makes a series of detailed pictures of areas inside the body, taken from different angles. The pictures are made by a computer linked to an x-ray machine. A dye may be injected into a vein or swallowed to help the organs or tissues show up more clearly. This procedure is also called computed tomography, computerized tomography, or computerized axial tomography.

- **MRI (magnetic resonance imaging):** A procedure that uses a magnet, radio waves, and a computer to make a series of detailed pictures of areas inside the body. This procedure is also called nuclear magnetic resonance imaging

- **PET scan (positron emission tomography scan):** A procedure to find malignant tumor cells in the body. A small amount of radioactive glucose (sugar) is injected into a vein. The PET scanner rotates around the body and makes a picture of where glucose is being used in the body. Malignant tumor cells show up brighter in the picture because they are more active and take up more glucose than normal cells.

- **Endoscopic ultrasound (EUS):** A procedure in which an endoscope is inserted into the body, usually through the mouth or rectum. An endoscope is a thin, tube-like instrument with a light and a lens for viewing. A probe at the end of the endoscope is used to bounce high-energy sound waves (ultrasound) off internal tissues or organs, such as the stomach, small intestine, colon, or rectum, and make echoes. The echoes form a picture of body tissues called a sonogram. This procedure is also called endosonography.

- **Upper endoscopy:** A procedure to look at organs and tissues inside the body to check for abnormal areas. An endoscope is inserted through the mouth and passed through the esophagus into the stomach. Sometimes the endoscope also is passed from the stomach into the small intestine. An endoscope is a thin, tube-like instrument with a light and a lens for viewing. It may also have a tool to remove tissue or lymph node samples, which are checked under a microscope for signs of disease.

- **Colonoscopy:** A procedure to look inside the rectum and colon for polyps, abnormal areas, or cancer. A colonoscope is inserted through the rectum into the colon. A colonoscope is a thin, tube-like instrument with a light and a lens for viewing. It may also have a tool to remove polyps or tissue samples, which are checked under a microscope for signs of cancer.

- **Capsule endoscopy:** A procedure used to see all of the small intestine. The patient swallows a capsule that contains a tiny camera. As the capsule moves through the gastrointestinal tract, the camera takes pictures and sends them to a receiver worn on the outside of the body.

- **Biopsy:** The removal of cells or tissues so they can be viewed under a microscope to check for signs of cancer. Tissue samples may be taken during endoscopy and colonoscopy.

Certain factors affect prognosis (chance of recovery) and treatment options.

The prognosis (chance of recovery) and treatment options depend on the following:

- Where the tumor is in the gastrointestinal tract.
- The size of the tumor.
- Whether the cancer has spread from the stomach and intestines to other parts of the body, such as the liver or lymph nodes.
- Whether the patient has carcinoid syndrome or has carcinoid heart syndrome.
- Whether the cancer can be completely removed by surgery.
- Whether the cancer is newly diagnosed or has recurred.

305

Stages of Gastrointestinal Carcinoid Tumors

After a gastrointestinal carcinoid tumor has been diagnosed, tests are done to find out if cancer cells have spread within the stomach and intestines or to other parts of the body.

Staging is the process used to find out how far the cancer has spread. The information gathered from the staging process determines the stage of the disease. The results of tests and procedures used to diagnose gastrointestinal (GI) carcinoid tumors may also be used for staging. A bone scan may be done to check if there are rapidly dividing cells, such as cancer cells, in the bone. A very small amount of radioactive material is injected into a veinand travels through the bloodstream. The radioactive material collects in the bones and is detected by a scanner.

There are three ways that cancer spreads in the body.

Cancer can spread through tissue, the lymph system, and the blood:

- Tissue. The cancer spreads from where it began by growing into nearby areas.
- Lymph system. The cancer spreads from where it began by getting into the lymph system. The cancer travels through the lymph vessels to other parts of the body.
- Blood. The cancer spreads from where it began by getting into the blood. The cancer travels through the blood vessels to other parts of the body.

Cancer may spread from where it began to other parts of the body.

When cancer spreads to another part of the body, it is called metastasis. Cancer cells break away from where they began (the primary tumor) and travel through the lymph system or blood.

- Lymph system. The cancer gets into the lymph system, travels through the lymph vessels, and forms a tumor (metastatic tumor) in another part of the body.
- Blood. The cancer gets into the blood, travels through the blood vessels, and forms a tumor (metastatic tumor) in another part of the body.

The metastatic tumor is the same type of tumor as the primary tumor. For example, if a gastrointestinal (GI) carcinoid tumor spreads to the liver, the tumor cells in the liver are actually GI carcinoid tumor cells. The disease is metastatic GI carcinoid tumor, not liver cancer.

The plan for cancer treatment depends on where the carcinoid tumor is found and whether it can be removed by surgery.

For many cancers it is important to know the stage of the cancer in order to plan treatment. However, the treatment of gastrointestinal carcinoid tumors is not based on the stage of the cancer. Treatment depends mainly on whether the tumor can be removed by surgery and if the tumor has spread.

Treatment is based on whether the tumor:

- Can be completely removed by surgery.

- Has spread to other parts of the body.

- Has come back after treatment. The tumor may come back in the stomach or intestines or in other parts of the body.

- Has not gotten better with treatment.

Treatment Option Overview

There are different types of treatment for patients with gastrointestinal carcinoid tumors.

Different types of treatment are available for patients with gastrointestinal carcinoid tumor. Some treatments are standard (the currently used treatment), and some are being tested in clinical trials. A treatment clinical trial is a research study meant to help improve current treatments or obtain information on new treatments for patients with cancer. When clinical trials show that a new treatment is better than the standard treatment, the new treatment may become the standard treatment. Patients may want to think about taking part in a clinical trial. Some clinical trials are open only to patients who have not started treatment.

Four types of standard treatment are used:

Surgery

Treatment of GI carcinoid tumors usually includes surgery. One of the following surgical procedures may be used:

- Endoscopic resection: Surgery to remove a small tumor that is on the inside lining of the GI tract. An endoscope is inserted through the mouth and passed through the esophagus to the stomach and sometimes, the duodenum. An endoscope is a thin, tube-like instrument with a light, a lens for viewing, and a tool for removing tumor tissue.

- Local excision: Surgery to remove the tumor and a small amount of normal tissue around it.

- Resection: Surgery to remove part or all of the organ that contains cancer. Nearby lymph nodes may also be removed.

- Cryosurgery: A treatment that uses an instrument to freeze and destroy carcinoid tumor tissue. This type of treatment is also called cryotherapy. The doctor may use ultrasound to guide the instrument.

- Radiofrequency ablation: The use of a special probe with tiny electrodes that release high-energy radio waves (similar to microwaves) that kill cancer cells. The probe may be inserted through the skin or through an incision (cut) in the abdomen.

- Liver transplant: Surgery to remove the whole liver and replace it with a healthy donated liver.

- Hepatic artery embolization: A procedure to embolize (block) the hepatic artery, which is the main blood vessel that brings blood into the liver. Blocking the flow of blood to the liver helps kill cancer cells growing there.

Radiation therapy

Radiation therapy is a cancer treatment that uses high-energy x-rays or other types of radiation to kill cancer cells. There are two types of radiation therapy. External radiation therapy uses a machine outside the body to send radiation toward the cancer. Internal radiation therapy uses a radioactive substance sealed in needles, seeds, wires, or catheters that are placed directly into or near the cancer. The way the radiation therapy is given depends on the type and stage of the cancer being treated.

Radiopharmaceutical therapy is a type of radiation therapy. Radiation is given to the tumor using a drug that has a radioactive substance, such as iodine I 131, attached to it. The radioactive substance kills the tumor cells.

Chemotherapy

Chemotherapy is a cancer treatment that uses drugs to stop the growth of cancer cells, either by killing the cells or by stopping the cells from dividing. When chemotherapy is taken by mouth or injected into a vein or muscle, the drugs enter the bloodstream and can reach cancer cells throughout the body (systemic chemotherapy). When chemotherapy is placed directly into the cerebrospinal fluid, an organ, or a body cavity such as the abdomen, the drugs mainly affect cancer cells in those areas (regional chemotherapy).

Chemoembolization of the hepatic artery is a type of regional chemotherapy that may be used to treat a gastrointestinal carcinoid tumor that has spread to the liver. The anticancer drug is injected into the hepatic artery through a catheter (thin tube). The drug is mixed with a substance that embolizes (blocks) the artery, and cuts off blood flow to the tumor. Most of the anticancer drug is trapped near the tumor and only a small amount of the drug reaches other parts of the body. The blockage may be temporary or permanent, depending on the substance used to block the artery. The tumor is prevented from getting the oxygen and nutrients it needs to grow. The liver continues to receive blood from the hepatic portal vein, which carries blood from the stomach and intestine.

The way the chemotherapy is given depends on the type and stage of the cancer being treated.

Hormone therapy

Hormone therapy with a somatostatin analogue is a treatment that stops extra hormones from being made. GI carcinoid tumors are treated with octreotide or lanreotide which are injected under the skin or into the muscle. Octreotide and lanreotide may also have a small effect on stopping tumor growth.

Treatment for carcinoid syndrome may also be needed.

Treatment of carcinoid syndrome may include the following:

* Hormone therapy with a somatostatin analogue stops extra hormones from being made. Carcinoid syndrome is treated

with octreotide or lanreotide to lessen flushing and diarrhea. Octreotide and lanreotide may also help slow tumor growth.

- Interferon therapy stimulates the body's immune system to work better and lessens flushing and diarrhea. Interferon may also help slow tumor growth.

- Taking medicine for diarrhea.

- Taking medicine for skin rashes.

- Taking medicine to breathe easier.

- Taking medicine before having anesthesia for a medical procedure.

Other ways to help treat carcinoid syndrome include avoiding things that cause flushing or difficulty breathing such as alcohol, nuts, certain cheeses and foods with capsaicin, such as chili peppers. Avoiding stressful situations and certain types of physical activity can also help treat carcinoid syndrome.

For some patients with carcinoid heart syndrome, a heart valve replacement may be done.

New types of treatment are being tested in clinical trials.

Targeted therapy

Targeted therapy is a type of treatment that uses drugs or other substances to identify and attack specific cancer cells without harming normal cells. Several types of targeted therapy are being studied in the treatment of GI carcinoid tumors.

Patients may want to think about taking part in a clinical trial.

For some patients, taking part in a clinical trial may be the best treatment choice. Clinical trials are part of the cancer research process. Clinical trials are done to find out if new cancer treatments are safe and effective or better than the standard treatment.

Many of today's standard treatments for cancer are based on earlier clinical trials. Patients who take part in a clinical trial may receive the standard treatment or be among the first to receive a new treatment.

Patients who take part in clinical trials also help improve the way cancer will be treated in the future. Even when clinical trials do not lead to effective new treatments, they often answer important questions and help move research forward.

Patients can enter clinical trials before, during, or after starting their cancer treatment.

Some clinical trials only include patients who have not yet received treatment. Other trials test treatments for patients whose cancer has not gotten better. There are also clinical trials that test new ways to stop cancer from recurring (coming back) or reduce the side effects of cancer treatment.

Clinical trials are taking place in many parts of the country.

Follow-up tests may be needed.

Some of the tests that were done to diagnose the cancer or to find out the stage of the cancer may be repeated. Some tests will be repeated in order to see how well the treatment is working. Decisions about whether to continue, change, or stop treatment may be based on the results of these tests.

Some of the tests will continue to be done from time to time after treatment has ended. The results of these tests can show if your condition has changed or if the cancer has recurred (come back). These tests are sometimes called follow-up tests or check-ups.

Section 23.2

Esophageal Cancer

Text in this section is excerpted from "Esophageal Cancer
Treatment," National Cancer Institute at the National Institutes of
Health (NIH), May 12, 2015.

General Information About Esophageal Cancer

**Esophageal cancer is a disease in which malignant (cancer)
cells form in the tissues of the esophagus.**

The esophagus is the hollow, muscular tube that moves food and
liquid from the throat to the stomach. The wall of the esophagus is
made up of several layers of tissue, including mucous membrane,
muscle, and connective tissue. Esophageal cancer starts at the inside
lining of the esophagus and spreads outward through the other layers
as it grows.

The two most common forms of esophageal cancer are named for
the type of cells that become malignant (cancerous):

- Squamous cell carcinoma: Cancer that forms in squamous cells,
  the thin, flat cells lining the esophagus. This cancer is most
  often found in the upper and middle part of the esophagus, but
  can occur anywhere along the esophagus. This is also called epidermoid carcinoma.

- Adenocarcinoma: Cancer that begins in glandular (secretory)
  cells. Glandular cells in the lining of the esophagus produce and
  release fluids such as mucus. Adenocarcinomas usually form in
  the lower part of the esophagus, near the stomach.

**Smoking, heavy alcohol use, and Barrett esophagus can
increase the risk of developing esophageal cancer.**

Anything that increases your risk of getting a disease is called a
risk factor. Having a risk factor does not mean that you will get cancer;

not having risk factors doesn't mean that you will not get cancer. Talk with your doctor if you think you may be at risk.

Risk factors include the following:

- Tobacco use.
- Heavy alcohol use.
- Barrett esophagus: A condition in which the cells lining the lower part of the esophagus have changed or been replaced with abnormal cells that could lead to cancer of the esophagus. Gastric reflux (the backing up of stomach contents into the lower section of the esophagus) may irritate the esophagus and, over time, cause Barrett esophagus.
- Older age.
- Being male.
- Being African-American.

Signs and symptoms of esophageal cancer are weight loss and painful or difficult swallowing.

These and other signs and symptoms may be caused by esophageal cancer or by other conditions. Check with your doctor if you have any of the following:

- Painful or difficult swallowing.
- Weight loss.
- Pain behind the breastbone.
- Hoarseness and cough.
- Indigestion and heartburn.

Tests that examine the esophagus are used to detect (find) and diagnose esophageal cancer.

The following tests and procedures may be used:

- **Physical exam and history:** An exam of the body to check general signs of health, including checking for signs of disease, such as lumps or anything else that seems unusual. A history of the patient's health habits and past illnesses and treatments will also be taken.

- **Chest x-ray:** An x-ray of the organs and bones inside the chest. An x-ray is a type of energy beam that can go through the body and onto film, making a picture of areas inside the body.

- **Barium swallow:** A series of x-rays of the esophagus and stomach. The patient drinks a liquid that contains barium (a silver-white metallic compound). The liquid coats the esophagus and stomach, and x-rays are taken. This procedure is also called an upper GI series.

- **Esophagoscopy:** A procedure to look inside the esophagus to check for abnormal areas. An esophagoscope is inserted through the mouth or nose and down the throat into the esophagus. An esophagoscope is a thin, tube-like instrument with a light and a lens for viewing. It may also have a tool to remove tissue samples, which are checked under a microscope for signs of cancer. When the esophagus and stomach are looked at, it is called an upper endoscopy.

- **Biopsy:** The removal of cells or tissues so they can be viewed under a microscope by a pathologist to check for signs of cancer. The biopsy is usually done during an esophagoscopy. Sometimes a biopsy shows changes in the esophagus that are not cancer but may lead to cancer.

Certain factors affect prognosis (chance of recovery) and treatment options.

The prognosis (chance of recovery) and treatment options depend on the following:

- The stage of the cancer (whether it affects part of the esophagus, involves the whole esophagus, or has spread to other places in the body).

- The size of the tumor.

- The patient's general health.

When esophageal cancer is found very early, there is a better chance of recovery. Esophageal cancer is often in an advanced stage when it is diagnosed. At later stages, esophageal cancer can be treated but rarely can be cured. Taking part in one of the clinical trials being done to improve treatment should be considered.

Stages of Esophageal Cancer

After esophageal cancer has been diagnosed, tests are done to find out if cancer cells have spread within the esophagus or to other parts of the body.

The process used to find out if cancer cells have spread within the esophagus or to other parts of the body is called staging. The information gathered from the staging process determines the stage of the disease. It is important to know the stage in order to plan treatment.

The following tests and procedures may be used in the staging process:

- **Bronchoscopy:** A procedure to look inside the trachea and large airways in the lung for abnormal areas. A bronchoscope is inserted through the nose or mouth into the trachea and lungs. A bronchoscope is a thin, tube-like instrument with a light and a lens for viewing. It may also have a tool to remove tissue samples, which are checked under a microscope for signs of cancer.

- **CT scan (CAT scan):** A procedure that makes a series of detailed pictures of areas inside the body, such as the chest, abdomen, and pelvis, taken from different angles. The pictures are made by a computer linked to an x-ray machine. A dye may be injected into a vein or swallowed to help the organs or tissues show up more clearly. This procedure is also called computed tomography, computerized tomography, or computerized axial tomography.

- **PET scan (positron emission tomography scan):** A procedure to find malignant tumor cells in the body. A small amount of radioactive glucose (sugar) is injected into a vein. The PET scanner rotates around the body and makes a picture of where glucose is being used in the body. Malignant tumor cells show up brighter in the picture because they are more active and take up more glucose than normal cells do. A PET scan and CT scan may be done at the same time. This is called a PET-CT.

- **MRI (magnetic resonance imaging):** A procedure that uses a magnet, radio waves, and a computer to make a series of detailed pictures of areas inside the body. This procedure is also called nuclear magnetic resonance imaging (NMRI).

- **Endoscopic ultrasound (EUS):** A procedure in which an endoscope is inserted into the body, usually through the mouth

315

or rectum. An endoscope is a thin, tube-like instrument with a light and a lens for viewing. A probe at the end of the endoscope is used to bounce high-energy sound waves (ultrasound) off internal tissues or organs and make echoes. The echoes form a picture of body tissues called a sonogram. This procedure is also called endosonography.

- **Thoracoscopy:** A surgical procedure to look at the organs inside the chest to check for abnormal areas. An incision (cut) is made between two ribs and a thoracoscope is inserted into the chest. A thoracoscope is a thin, tube-like instrument with a light and a lens for viewing. It may also have a tool to remove tissue or lymph node samples, which are checked under a microscope for signs of cancer. In some cases, this procedure may be used to remove part of the esophagus or lung.

- **Laparoscopy:** A surgical procedure to look at the organs inside the abdomen to check for signs of disease. Small incisions (cuts) are made in the wall of the abdomen and a laparoscope (a thin, lighted tube) is inserted into one of the incisions. Other instruments may be inserted through the same or other incisions to perform procedures such as removing organs or taking tissue samples to be checked under a microscope for signs of disease.

There are three ways that cancer spreads in the body.

Cancer can spread through tissue, the lymph system, and the blood:

- Tissue. The cancer spreads from where it began by growing into nearby areas.

- Lymph system. The cancer spreads from where it began by getting into the lymph system. The cancer travels through the lymph vessels to other parts of the body.

- Blood. The cancer spreads from where it began by getting into the blood. The cancer travels through the blood vessels to other parts of the body.

Cancer may spread from where it began to other parts of the body.

When cancer spreads to another part of the body, it is called metastasis. Cancer cells break away from where they began (the primary tumor) and travel through the lymph system or blood.

- Lymph system. The cancer gets into the lymph system, travels through the lymph vessels, and forms a tumor (metastatic tumor) in another part of the body.

- Blood. The cancer gets into the blood, travels through the blood vessels, and forms a tumor (metastatic tumor) in another part of the body.

The metastatic tumor is the same type of cancer as the primary tumor. For example, if esophageal cancer spreads to the lung, the cancer cells in the lung are actually esophageal cancer cells. The disease is metastatic esophageal cancer, not lung cancer.

The grade of the tumor is also used to describe the cancer and plan treatment.

The grade of the tumor describes how abnormal the cancer cells look under a microscope and how quickly the tumor is likely to grow and spread. Grades 1 to 3 are used to describe esophageal cancer:

- In grade 1, the cancer cells look more like normal cells under a microscope and grow and spread more slowly than grade 2 and 3 cancer cells.

- In grade 2, the cancer cells look more abnormal under a microscope and grow and spread more quickly than grade 1 cancer cells.

- In grade 3, the cancer cells look more abnormal under a microscope and grow and spread more quickly than grade 1 and 2 cancer cells.

The following stages are used for squamous cell carcinoma of the esophagus:

Stage 0 (High-grade Dysplasia)

In stage 0, abnormal cells are found in the mucosa or submucosa layer of the esophagus wall. These abnormal cells may become cancer and spread into nearby normal tissue. Stage 0 is also called high-grade dysplasia.

Stage I squamous cell carcinoma of the esophagus

Stage I is divided into Stage IA and Stage IB, depending on where the cancer is found.

317

- Stage IA: Cancer has formed in the mucosa or submucosa layer of the esophagus wall. The cancer cells are grade 1. Grade 1 cancer cells look more like normal cells under a microscope and grow and spread more slowly than grade 2 and 3 cancer cells.

- Stage IB: Cancer has formed:

  - in the mucosa or submucosa layer of the esophagus wall. The cancer cells are grade 2 and 3; or

  - in the mucosa or submucosa layer and spread into the muscle layer or the connective tissue layer of the esophagus wall. The cancer cells are grade 1. The tumor is in the lower esophagus or it is not known where the tumor is.

Grade 1 cancer cells look more like normal cells under a microscope and grow and spread more slowly than grade 2 and 3 cancer cells.

Stage II squamous cell carcinoma of the esophagus

Stage II is divided into Stage IIA and Stage IIB, depending on where the cancer has spread.

- Stage IIA: Cancer has spread:

  - into the muscle layer or the connective tissue layer of the esophagus wall. The cancer cells are grade 1. The tumor is in either the upper or middle esophagus; or

  - into the muscle layer or the connective tissue layer of the esophagus wall. The cancer cells are grade 2 and 3. The tumor is in the lower esophagus or it is not known where the tumor is.

Grade 1 cancer cells look more like normal cells under a microscope and grow and spread more slowly than grade 2 and 3 cancer cells.

- Stage IIB: Cancer:

  - has spread into the muscle layer or the connective tissue layer of the esophagus wall. The cancer cells are grade 2 and 3. Grade 2 and 3 cancer cells look more abnormal under a microscope and grow and spread more quickly than grade 1 cancer cells. The tumor is in either the upper or middle esophagus; or

  - is in the mucosa or submucosa layer and may have spread into the muscle layer of the esophagus wall. Cancer is found in 1 or 2 lymph nodes near the tumor.

Stage III squamous cell carcinoma of the esophagus

Stage III is divided into Stage IIIA, Stage IIIB, and Stage IIIC, depending on where the cancer has spread.

- Stage IIIA: Cancer:
  - is in the mucosa or submucosa layer and may have spread into the muscle layer of the esophagus wall. Cancer is found in 3 to 6 lymph nodes near the tumor; or
  - has spread into the connective tissue layer of the esophagus wall. Cancer is found in 1 or 2 lymph nodes near the tumor; or
  - has spread into the diaphragm, pleura (tissue that covers the lungs and lines the inner wall of the chest cavity), or sac around the heart. The cancer can be removed by surgery.
- Stage IIIB: Cancer has spread into the connective tissue layer of the esophagus wall. Cancer is found in 3 to 6 lymph nodes near the tumor.
- Stage IIIC: Cancer has spread:
  - into the diaphragm, pleura (tissue that covers the lungs and lines the inner wall of the chest cavity), or sac around the heart. The cancer can be removed by surgery. Cancer is found in 1 to 6 lymph nodes near the tumor; or
  - into other nearby organs such as the aorta, trachea, or spine, and the cancer cannot be removed by surgery; or
  - to 7 or more lymph nodes near the tumor.

Stage IV squamous cell carcinoma of the esophagus

In stage IV, cancer has spread to other parts of the body.

The following stages are used for adenocarcinoma of the esophagus:

Stage 0 (High-grade Dysplasia)

In stage 0, abnormal cells are found in the mucosa or submucosa layer of the esophagus wall. These abnormal cells may become cancer and spread into nearby normal tissue. Stage 0 is also called high-grade dysplasia.

319

Stage I adenocarcinoma of the esophagus

Stage I is divided into Stage IA and Stage IB, depending on where the cancer is found.

- Stage IA: Cancer has formed in the mucosa or submucosa layer of the esophagus wall. The cancer cells are grade 1 or 2. Grade 1 and 2 cancer cells look more like normal cells under a microscope and grow and spread more slowly than grade 3 cancer cells.

- Stage IB: Cancer has formed:

  - in the mucosa or submucosa layer of the esophagus wall. The cancer cells are grade 3; or

  - in the mucosa or submucosa layer and spread into the muscle layer of the esophagus wall. The cancer cells are grade 1 or 2.

Stage II adenocarcinoma of the esophagus

Stage II is divided into Stage IIA and Stage IIB, depending on where the cancer has spread.

- Stage IIA: Cancer has spread into the muscle layer of the esophagus wall. The cancer cells are grade 3. Grade 3 cancer cells look more abnormal under a microscope and grow and spread more quickly than grade 1 and 2 cancer cells.

- Stage IIB: Cancer:

  - has spread into the connective tissue layer of the esophagus wall; or

  - is in the mucosa or submucosa layer and may have spread into the muscle layer of the esophagus wall. Cancer is found in 1 or 2 lymph nodes near the tumor.

Stage III adenocarcinoma of the esophagus

Stage III is divided into Stage IIIA, Stage IIIB, and Stage IIIC, depending on where the cancer has spread.

- Stage IIIA: Cancer:

  - is in the mucosa or submucosa layer and may have spread into the muscle layer of the esophagus wall. Cancer is found in 3 to 6 lymph nodes near the tumor; or

- has spread into the connective tissue layer of the esophagus wall. Cancer is found in 1 or 2 lymph nodes near the tumor; or

- has spread into the diaphragm, pleura (tissue that covers the lungs and lines the inner wall of the chest cavity), or sac around the heart. The cancer can be removed by surgery.

- Stage IIIB: Cancer has spread into the connective tissue layer of the esophagus wall. Cancer is found in 3 to 6 lymph nodes near the tumor.

- Stage IIIC: Cancer has spread:

  - into the diaphragm, pleura (tissue that covers the lungs and lines the inner wall of the chest cavity), or sac around the heart. The cancer can be removed by surgery. Cancer is found in 1 to 6 lymph nodes near the tumor; or

  - into other nearby organs such as the aorta, trachea, or spine, and the cancer cannot be removed by surgery; or

  - to 7 or more lymph nodes near the tumor.

Stage IV adenocarcinoma of the esophagus

In stage IV, cancer has spread to other parts of the body.

Treatment Options Overview

There are different types of treatment for patients with esophageal cancer.

Different types of treatment are available for patients with esophageal cancer. Some treatments are standard (the currently used treatment), and some are being tested in clinical trials. A treatment clinical trial is a research study meant to help improve current treatments or obtain information on new treatments for patients with cancer. When clinical trials show that a new treatment is better than the standard treatment, the new treatment may become the standard treatment. Patients may want to think about taking part in a clinical trial. Some clinical trials are open only to patients who have not started treatment.

Patients have special nutritional needs during treatment for esophageal cancer.

Many people with esophageal cancer find it hard to eat because they have trouble swallowing. The esophagus may be narrowed by the tumor or as a side effect of treatment. Some patients may receive nutrients directly into a vein. Others may need a feeding tube (a flexible plastic tube that is passed through the nose or mouth into the stomach) until they are able to eat on their own.

Six types of standard treatment are used:

Surgery

Surgery is the most common treatment for cancer of the esophagus. Part of the esophagus may be removed in an operation called an esophagectomy.

The doctor will connect the remaining healthy part of the esophagus to the stomach so the patient can still swallow. A plastic tube or part of the intestine may be used to make the connection. Lymph nodes near the esophagus may also be removed and viewed under a microscope to see if they contain cancer. If the esophagus is partly blocked by the tumor, an expandable metal stent (tube) may be placed inside the esophagus to help keep it open.

Radiation therapy

Radiation therapy is a cancer treatment that uses high-energy x-rays or other types of radiation to kill cancer cells or keep them from growing. There are two types of radiation therapy. External radiation therapy uses a machine outside the body to send radiation toward the cancer. Internal radiation therapy uses a radioactive substance sealed in needles, seeds, wires, or catheters that are placed directly into or near the cancer. The way the radiation therapy is given depends on the type and stage of the cancer being treated.

A plastic tube may be inserted into the esophagus to keep it open during radiation therapy. This is called intraluminal intubation and dilation.

Chemotherapy

Chemotherapy is a cancer treatment that uses drugs to stop the growth of cancer cells, either by killing the cells or by stopping them from dividing. When chemotherapy is taken by mouth or injected into a vein or muscle, the drugs enter the bloodstream and can reach cancer cells throughout the body (systemic chemotherapy). When chemotherapy is placed directly into the cerebrospinal fluid, an organ, or a body cavity such as the abdomen, the drugs mainly affect cancer cells in those areas (regional chemotherapy). The way the chemotherapy is given depends on the type and stage of the cancer being treated.

Chemoradiation therapy

Chemoradiation therapy combines chemotherapy and radiation therapy to increase the effects of both.

Laser therapy

Laser therapy is a cancer treatment that uses a laser beam (a narrow beam of intense light) to kill cancer cells.

Electrocoagulation

Electrocoagulation is the use of an electric current to kill cancer cells.

Patients may want to think about taking part in a clinical trial.

For some patients, taking part in a clinical trial may be the best treatment choice. Clinical trials are part of the cancer research process. Clinical trials are done to find out if new cancer treatments are safe and effective or better than the standard treatment.

Many of today's standard treatments for cancer are based on earlier clinical trials. Patients who take part in a clinical trial may receive the standard treatment or be among the first to receive a new treatment.

Patients who take part in clinical trials also help improve the way cancer will be treated in the future. Even when clinical trials do not lead to effective new treatments, they often answer important questions and help move research forward.

Patients can enter clinical trials before, during, or after starting their cancer treatment.

Some clinical trials only include patients who have not yet received treatment. Other trials test treatments for patients whose cancer has not gotten better. There are also clinical trials that test new ways to stop cancer from recurring (coming back) or reduce the side effects of cancer treatment.

Clinical trials are taking place in many parts of the country.

Follow-up tests may be needed.

Some of the tests that were done to diagnose the cancer or to find out the stage of the cancer may be repeated. Some tests will be repeated in order to see how well the treatment is working. Decisions about whether to continue, change, or stop treatment may be based on the results of these tests.

Some of the tests will continue to be done from time to time after treatment has ended. The results of these tests can show if your child's condition has changed or if the cancer has recurred (come back). These tests are sometimes called follow-up tests or check-ups.

Treatment Options By Stage

Stage 0 (High-grade Dysplasia)

Treatment of stage 0 is usually surgery.

Stage I Esophageal Cancer

Treatment of stage I esophageal squamous cell carcinoma or adeno-carcinoma may include the following:

- Surgery.
- Chemoradiation therapy followed by surgery.
- Clinical trials.

For more specific results, refine the search by using other search features, such as the location of the trial, the type of treatment, or the name of the drug. Talk with your doctor about clinical trials that may be right for you.

Stage II Esophageal Cancer

Treatment of stage II esophageal squamous cell carcinoma or adeno-carcinoma may include the following:

- Chemoradiation therapy followed by surgery.
- Chemoradiation therapy alone.
- Surgery alone.

For more specific results, refine the search by using other search features, such as the location of the trial, the type of treatment, or the name of the drug. Talk with your doctor about clinical trials that may be right for you.

Stage III Esophageal Cancer

Treatment of stage III esophageal squamous cell carcinoma or adeno-carcinoma may include the following:

- Chemoradiation therapy followed by surgery.

- Chemoradiation therapy alone.

For more specific results, refine the search by using other search features, such as the location of the trial, the type of treatment, or the name of the drug. Talk with your doctor about clinical trials that may be right for you.

Stage IV Esophageal Cancer

Treatment of stage IV esophageal squamous cell carcinoma or adeno-carcinoma may include the following:

- An esophageal stent as palliative therapy to relieve symptoms and improve quality of life.

- External or internal radiation therapy as palliative therapy to relieve symptoms and improve quality of life.

- Laser surgery or electrocoagulation as palliative therapy to relieve symptoms and improve quality of life.

- Chemotherapy.

- Clinical trials of chemotherapy.

For more specific results, refine the search by using other search features, such as the location of the trial, the type of treatment, or the name of the drug. Talk with your doctor about clinical trials that may be right for you.

Section 23.3

Adult Primary Liver Cancer

Text in this section is excerpted from "Adult Primary Liver Cancer
Treatment," National Cancer Institute at the National Institutes of
Health (NIH), March 18, 2015.

General Information About Adult Primary Liver Cancer

*Adult primary liver cancer is a disease in which malignant
(cancer) cells form in the tissues of the liver.*

The liver is one of the largest organs in the body. It has four lobes and
fills the upper right side of the abdomen inside the rib cage. Three of
the many important functions of the liver are:

- To filter harmful substances from the blood so they can be
  passed from the body in stools and urine.

- To make bile to help digest fat that comes from food.

- To store glycogen (sugar), which the body uses for energy.

There are two types of adult primary liver cancer.

The two types of adult primary liver cancer are:

- Hepatocellular carcinoma.

- Cholangiocarcinoma (bile duct cancer).

The most common type of adult primary liver cancer is hepatocellular carcinoma. This type of liver cancer is the third leading cause of
cancer-related deaths worldwide.

*Having hepatitis or cirrhosis can affect the risk of adult
primary liver cancer.*

Anything that increases your chance of getting a disease is called a
risk factor. Having a risk factor does not mean that you will get cancer;

not having risk factors doesn't mean that you will not get cancer. Talk with your doctor if you think you may be at risk.

The following are risk factors for adult primary liver cancer:

- Having hepatitis B or hepatitis C. Having both hepatitis B and hepatitis C increases the risk even more.

- Having cirrhosis, which can be caused by:

  - hepatitis (especially hepatitis C); or

  - drinking large amounts of alcohol for many years or being an alcoholic.

- Having metabolic syndrome, a set of conditions that occur together, including extra fat around the abdomen, high blood sugar, high blood pressure, high levels of triglycerides and low levels of high-density lipoproteins in the blood.

- Having liver injury that is long-lasting, especially if it leads to cirrhosis.

- Having hemochromatosis, a condition in which the body takes up and stores more iron than it needs. The extra iron is stored in the liver, heart, and pancreas.

- Eating foods tainted with aflatoxin (poison from a fungus that can grow on foods, such as grains and nuts,that have not been stored properly).

Signs and symptoms of adult primary liver cancer include a lump or pain on the right side.

These and other signs and symptoms may be caused by adult primary liver cancer or by other conditions. Check with your doctor if you have any of the following:

- A hard lump on the right side just below the rib cage.

- Discomfort in the upper abdomen on the right side.

- A swollen abdomen.

- Pain near the right shoulder blade or in the back.

- Jaundice (yellowing of the skin and whites of the eyes).

- Easy bruising or bleeding.

- Unusual tiredness or weakness.

- Nausea and vomiting.

- Loss of appetite or feelings of fullness after eating a small meal.

- Weight loss for no known reason.

- Pale, chalky bowel movements and dark urine.

- Fever.

Tests that examine the liver and the blood are used to detect (find) and diagnose adult primary liver cancer.

The following tests and procedures may be used:

- **Physical exam and history:** An exam of the body to check general signs of health, including checking for signs of disease, such as lumps or anything else that seems unusual. A history of the patient's health habits and past illnesses and treatments will also be taken.

- **Serum tumor marker test:** A procedure in which a sample of blood is examined to measure the amounts of certain substances released into the blood by organs, tissues, or tumor cells in the body. Certain substances are linked to specific types of cancer when found in increased levels in the blood. These are called tumor markers. An increased level of alpha-fetoprotein (AFP) in the blood may be a sign of liver cancer. Other cancers and certain noncancerous conditions, including cirrhosis and hepatitis, may also increase AFP levels. Sometimes the AFP level is normal even when there is liver cancer.

- **Liver function tests:** A procedure in which a blood sample is checked to measure the amounts of certain substances released into the blood by the liver. A higher than normal amount of a substance can be a sign of liver cancer.

- **CT scan (CAT scan):** A procedure that makes a series of detailed pictures of areas inside the body, such as the abdomen, taken from different angles. The pictures are made by a computer linked to an x-ray machine. A dye may be injected into a vein or swallowed to help the organs or tissues show up more clearly. This procedure is also called computed tomography, computerized tomography, or computerized axial tomography. Images may be taken at three different times after the dye is injected, to get the best picture of abnormal areas in the liver. This is called triple-phase CT. A spiral or helical CT scan makes a series of very detailed pictures of areas inside the body using an x-ray machine that scans the body in a spiral path.

- **MRI (magnetic resonance imaging):** A procedure that uses a magnet, radio waves, and a computer to make a series of detailed pictures of areas inside the body, such as the liver. This procedure is also called nuclear magnetic resonance imaging (NMRI). To create detailed pictures of blood vessels in and near the liver, dye is injected into a vein. This procedure is called MRA (magnetic resonance angiography). Images may be taken at three different times after the dye is injected, to get the best picture of abnormal areas in the liver. This is called triple-phase MRI.

- **Ultrasound exam:** A procedure in which high-energy sound waves (ultrasound) are bounced off internal tissues or organs and make echoes. The echoes form a picture of body tissues called a sonogram. The picture can be printed to be looked at later.

- **Biopsy:** The removal of cells or tissues so they can be viewed under a microscope by a pathologist to check for signs of cancer. Procedures used to collect the sample of cells or tissues include the following:

  - **Fine-needle aspiration biopsy:** The removal of cells, tissue or fluid using a thin needle.

  - **Core needle biopsy:** The removal of cells or tissue using a slightly wider needle.

  - **Laparoscopy:** A surgical procedure to look at the organs inside the abdomen to check for signs of disease. Small incisions (cuts) are made in the wall of the abdomen and a laparoscope (a thin, lighted tube) is inserted into one of the incisions. Another instrument is inserted through the same or another incision to remove the tissue samples.

A biopsy is not always needed to diagnose adult primary liver cancer.

Certain factors affect prognosis (chance of recovery) and treatment options.

The prognosis (chance of recovery) and treatment options depend on the following:

- The stage of the cancer (the size of the tumor, whether it affects part or all of the liver, or has spread to other places in the body).

- How well the liver is working.

- The patient's general health, including whether there is cirrhosis of the liver.

Stages of Adult Primary Liver Cancer

After adult primary liver cancer has been diagnosed, tests are done to find out if cancer cells have spread within the liver or to other parts of the body.

The process used to find out if cancer has spread within the liver or to other parts of the body is called staging. The information gathered from the staging process determines the stage of the disease. It is important to know the stage in order to plan treatment.

The following tests and procedures may be used in the staging process:

- **CT scan (CAT scan):** A procedure that makes a series of detailed pictures of areas inside the body, such as the chest, abdomen, and pelvis, taken from different angles. The pictures are made by a computer linked to an x-ray machine. A dye may be injected into a vein or swallowed to help the organs or tissues show up more clearly. This procedure is also called computed tomography, computerized tomography, or computerized axial tomography.

- **MRI (magnetic resonance imaging):** A procedure that uses a magnet, radio waves, and a computer to make a series of detailed pictures of areas inside the body. This procedure is also called nuclear magnetic resonance imaging (NMRI).

- **PET scan (positron emission tomography scan):** A procedure to find malignant tumor cells in the body. A small amount of radioactive glucose (sugar) is injected into a vein. The PET scanner rotates around the body and makes a picture of where glucose is being used in the body. Malignant tumor cells show up brighter in the picture because they are more active and take up more glucose than normal cells do.

There are three ways that cancer spreads in the body.

Cancer can spread through tissue, the lymph system, and the blood:

- Tissue. The cancer spreads from where it began by growing into nearby areas.

- Lymph system. The cancer spreads from where it began by getting into the lymph system. The cancer travels through the lymph vessels to other parts of the body.

- Blood. The cancer spreads from where it began by getting into the blood. The cancer travels through the blood vessels to other parts of the body.

Cancer may spread from where it began to other parts of the body.

When cancer spreads to another part of the body, it is called metastasis. Cancer cells break away from where they began (the primary tumor) and travel through the lymph system or blood.

- Lymph system. The cancer gets into the lymph system, travels through the lymph vessels, and forms a tumor (metastatic tumor) in another part of the body.

- Blood. The cancer gets into the blood, travels through the blood vessels, and forms a tumor (metastatic tumor) in another part of the body.

The metastatic tumor is the same type of cancer as the primary tumor. For example, if primary liver cancer spreads to the lung, the cancer cells in the lung are actually liver cancer cells. The disease is metastatic liver cancer, not lung cancer.

The Barcelona Clinic Liver Cancer Staging System may be used to stage adult primary liver cancer.

There are several staging systems for liver cancer. The Barcelona Clinic Liver Cancer (BCLC) Staging System is widely used and is described below. This system is used to predict the patient's chance of recovery and to plan treatment, based on the following:

- Whether the cancer has spread within the liver or to other parts of the body.

- How well the liver is working.

- The general health and wellness of the patient.

- The symptoms caused by the cancer.

The BCLC staging system has five stages:

- Stage 0: Very early
- Stage A: Early
- Stage B: Intermediate
- Stage C: Advanced
- Stage D: End-stage

The following groups are used to plan treatment.

BCLC stages 0, A, and B

Treatment to cure the cancer is given for BCLC stages 0, A, and B.

BCLC stages C and D

Treatment to relieve the symptoms caused by liver cancer and improve the patient's quality of life is given for BCLC stages C and D. Treatments are not likely to cure the cancer.

Treatment Option Overview

There are different types of treatment for patients with adult primary liver cancer.

Different types of treatments are available for patients with adult primary liver cancer. Some treatments are standard (the currently used treatment), and some are being tested in clinical trials. A treatment clinical trial is a research study meant to help improve current treatments or obtain information on new treatments for patients with cancer. When clinical trials show that a new treatment is better than the standard treatment, the new treatment may become the standard treatment. Patients may want to think about taking part in a clinical trial. Some clinical trials are open only to patients who have not started treatment.

Patients with liver cancer are treated by a team of specialists who are experts in treating liver cancer.

The patient's treatment will be overseen by a medical oncologist, a doctor who specializes in treating people with cancer. The medical oncologist may refer the patient to other health professionals who have special training in treating patients with liver cancer. These may include the following specialists:

- Hepatologist (specialist in liver disease).
- Surgical oncologist.
- Transplant surgeon.
- Radiation oncologist.
- Interventional radiologist (a specialist who diagnoses and treats diseases using imaging and the smallest incisions possible).
- Pathologist.

Seven types of standard treatment are used:

Surveillance

Surveillance for lesions smaller than 1 centimeter found during screening. Follow-up every three months is common.

Surgery

A partial hepatectomy (surgery to remove the part of the liver where cancer is found) may be done. A wedge of tissue, an entire lobe, or a larger part of the liver, along with some of the healthy tissue around it is removed. The remaining liver tissue takes over the functions of the liver and may regrow.

Liver transplant

In a liver transplant, the entire liver is removed and replaced with a healthy donated liver. A liver transplant may be done when the disease is in the liver only and a donated liver can be found. If the patient has to wait for a donated liver, other treatment is given as needed.

Ablation therapy

Ablation therapy removes or destroys tissue. Different types of ablation therapy are used for liver cancer:

- Radiofrequency ablation: The use of special needles that are inserted directly through the skin or through an incision in the abdomen to reach the tumor. High-energy radio waves heat the needles and tumor which kills cancer cells.

- Microwave therapy: A type of treatment in which the tumor is exposed to high temperatures created by microwaves. This can damage and kill cancer cells or make them more sensitive to the effects of radiation and certain anticancer drugs.

- Percutaneous ethanol injection: A cancer treatment in which a small needle is used to inject ethanol (pure alcohol) directly into a tumor to kill cancer cells. Several treatments may be needed. Usually local anesthesia is used, but if the patient has many tumors in the liver, general anesthesia may be used.

- Cryoablation: A treatment that uses an instrument to freeze and destroy cancer cells. This type of treatment is also called cryotherapy and cryosurgery. The doctor may use ultrasound to guide the instrument.

- Electroporation therapy: A treatment that sends electrical pulses through an electrode placed in a tumor to kill cancer cells. Electroporation therapy is being studied in clinical trials.

Embolization therapy

Embolization therapy is the use of substances to block or decrease the flow of blood through the hepatic artery to the tumor. When the tumor does not get the oxygen and nutrients it needs, it will not continue to grow. Embolization therapy is used for patients who cannot have surgery to remove the tumor or ablation therapy and whose tumor has not spread outside the liver.

The liver receives blood from the hepatic portal vein and the hepatic artery. Blood that comes into the liver from the hepatic portal vein usually goes to the healthy liver tissue. Blood that comes from the hepatic artery usually goes to the tumor. When the hepatic artery is blocked during embolization therapy, the healthy liver tissue continues to receive blood from the hepatic portal vein.

There are two main types of embolization therapy:

- Transarterial embolization (TAE): A small incision (cut) is made in the inner thigh and a catheter (thin, flexible tube) is inserted and threaded up into the hepatic artery. Once the catheter is in place, a substance that blocks the hepatic artery and stops blood flow to the tumor is injected.

- Transarterial chemoembolization (TACE): This procedure is like TAE except an anticancer drug is also given. The procedure can be done by attaching the anticancer drug to small beads that are injected into the hepatic artery or by injecting the anticancer drug through the catheter into the hepatic artery and then injecting the substance to block the hepatic artery. Most of the anticancer drug is trapped near the tumor and only a small amount of the drug reaches other parts of the body. This type of treatment is also called chemoembolization.

Targeted therapy

Targeted therapy is a treatment that uses drugs or other substances to identify and attack specific cancer cells without harming normal cells. Adult liver cancer may be treated with a targeted therapy drug that stops cells from dividing and prevents the growth of new blood vessels that tumors need to grow.

Radiation therapy

Radiation therapy is a cancer treatment that uses high-energy x-rays or other types of radiation to kill cancer cells or keep them from growing. Radiation therapy is given in different ways:

- External radiation therapy uses a machine outside the body to send radiation toward the cancer.

- 3-D conformal radiation therapy uses a computer to create a 3-dimensional picture of the tumor. This allows doctors to give the highest possible dose of radiation to the tumor, while preventing damage to normal tissue as much as possible.

- Stereotactic body radiation therapy uses special equipment to position a patient and deliver radiation directly to the tumors. The total dose of radiation is divided into smaller doses given over several days. This type of radiation therapy helps prevent damage to normal tissue. This type of radiation therapy is being studied in clinical trials.

- Proton-beam radiation therapy is a type of high-energy radiation therapy that uses streams of protons (small, positively-charged particles of matter) to kill tumor cells. This type of radiation therapy is being studied in clinical trials.

Patients may want to think about taking part in a clinical trial.

For some patients, taking part in a clinical trial may be the best treatment choice. Clinical trials are part of the cancer research process.

Clinical trials are done to find out if new cancer treatments are safe and effective or better than the standard treatment.

Many of today's standard treatments for cancer are based on earlier clinical trials. Patients who take part in a clinical trial may receive the standard treatment or be among the first to receive a new treatment.

Patients who take part in clinical trials also help improve the way cancer will be treated in the future. Even when clinical trials do not lead to effective new treatments, they often answer important questions and help move research forward.

Patients can enter clinical trials before, during, or after starting their cancer treatment.

Some clinical trials only include patients who have not yet received treatment. Other trials test treatments for patients whose cancer has not gotten better. There are also clinical trials that test new ways to stop cancer from recurring (coming back) or reduce the side effects of cancer treatment.

Clinical trials are taking place in many parts of the country.

Follow-up tests may be needed.

Some of the tests that were done to diagnose the cancer or to find out the stage of the cancer may be repeated. Some tests will be repeated in order to see how well the treatment is working. Decisions about whether to continue, change, or stop treatment may be based on the results of these tests.

Some of the tests will continue to be done from time to time after treatment has ended. The results of these tests can show if your condition has changed or if the cancer has recurred (come back). These tests are sometimes called follow-up tests or check-ups.

Treatment of Adult Primary Liver Cancer

Stages 0, A, and B Adult Primary Liver Cancer

Treatment of stages 0, A, and B adult primary liver cancer may include the following:

- Surveillance for lesions smaller than 1 centimeter.

- Partial hepatectomy.

- Total hepatectomy and liver transplant.

- Ablation of the tumor using one of the following methods:
  - Radiofrequency ablation.
  - Microwave therapy.
  - Percutaneous ethanol injection.
  - Cryoablation.
- A clinical trial of electroporation therapy.

Stages C and D Adult Primary Liver Cancer

Treatment of stages C and D adult primary liver cancer may include the following:

- Embolization therapy using one of the following methods:
  - Transarterial embolization (TAE).
  - Transarterial chemoembolization (TACE).
- Targeted therapy.
- Radiation therapy.
  - A clinical trial of targeted therapy after chemoembolization or combined with chemotherapy.
  - A clinical trial of new targeted therapy drugs.
  - A clinical trial of targeted therapy with or without stereotactic body radiation therapy.
  - A clinical trial of stereotactic body radiation therapy or proton-beam radiation therapy.

Section 23.4

Extrahepatic Bile Duct Cancer

Text in this section is excerpted from "Extrahepatic Bile Duct Cancer
Treatment," National Cancer Institute at the National Institutes of
Health (NIH), October 13, 2013.

General Information About Extrahepatic Bile Duct Cancer

Extrahepatic bile duct cancer is a rare disease in which malignant (cancer) cells form in the ducts that are outside the liver.

The extrahepatic bile duct is made up of two parts:

- Common hepatic duct, which is also called the perihilar part of the extrahepatic duct.

- Common bile duct, which is also called the distal part of the extrahepatic duct.

The extrahepatic bile duct is part of a network of ducts (tubes) that connect the liver, gallbladder, and small intestine. This network begins in the liver where many small ducts collect bile (a fluid made by the liver to break down fats during digestion). The small ducts come together to form the right and left hepatic ducts, which lead out of the liver. The two ducts join outside the liver and form the common hepatic duct. Bile from the liver passes through the hepatic ducts, common hepatic duct and cystic duct and is stored in the gallbladder.

When food is being digested, bile stored in the gallbladder is released and passes through the cystic duct to the common bile duct and into the small intestine.

Having colitis or certain liver diseases can increase the risk of extrahepatic bile duct cancer.

Anything that increases your risk of getting a disease is called a risk factor. Having a risk factor does not mean that you will get cancer;

not having risk factors doesn't mean that you will not get cancer. Talk with your doctor if you think you may be at risk. Risk factors include having any of the following disorders:

- Primary sclerosing cholangitis.

- Chronic ulcerative colitis.

- Choledochal cysts.

- Infection with a Chinese liver fluke parasite.

Signs and symptoms of extrahepatic bile duct cancer include jaundice and pain.

These and other signs and symptoms may be caused by extrahepatic bile duct cancer or by other conditions. Check with your doctor if you have any of the following:

- Jaundice (yellowing of the skin or whites of the eyes).

- Pain in the abdomen.

- Fever.

- Itchy skin.

Tests that examine the bile duct and liver are used to detect (find) and diagnose extrahepatic bile duct cancer.

The following tests and procedures may be used:

- **Physical exam and history:** An exam of the body to check general signs of health, including checking for signs of disease, such as lumps or anything else that seems unusual. A history of the patient's health habits and past illnesses and treatments will also be taken.

- **Ultrasound exam:** A procedure in which high-energy sound waves (ultrasound) are bounced off internal tissues or organs and make echoes. The echoes form a picture of body tissues called a sonogram. The picture can be printed to be looked at later.

- **CT scan (CAT scan):** A procedure that makes a series of detailed pictures of areas inside the body, taken from different angles. The pictures are made by a computer linked to an x-ray machine. A dye may be injected into a vein or swallowed to help the organs or tissues show up more clearly. This procedure is also called computed tomography, computerized tomography, or computerized axial tomography. A spiral or helical CT scan makes detailed pictures of areas inside the body using an x-ray machine that scans the body in a spiral path.

- **MRI (magnetic resonance imaging)**: A procedure that uses a magnet, radio waves, and a computer to make a series of detailed pictures of areas inside the body. This procedure is also called nuclear magnetic resonance imaging (NMRI).

- **PET scan (positron emission tomography scan)**: A procedure to find malignant tumor cells in the body. A small amount of radioactive glucose (sugar) is injected into a vein. The PET scanner rotates around the body and makes a picture of where glucose is being used in the body. Malignant tumor cells show up brighter in the picture because they are more active and take up more glucose than normal cells do.

- **ERCP (endoscopic retrograde cholangiopancreatography)**: A procedure used to x-ray the ducts (tubes) that carry bile from the liver to the gallbladder and from the gallbladder to the small intestine. Sometimes bile duct cancer causes these ducts to narrow and block or slow the flow of bile, causing jaundice. An endoscope is passed through the mouth, esophagus, and stomach into the first part of the small intestine. An endoscope is a thin, tube-like instrument with a light and a lens for viewing. A catheter (a smaller tube) is then inserted through the endoscope into the pancreatic ducts. A dye is injected through the catheter into the ducts and an x-ray is taken. If the ducts are blocked by a tumor, a fine tube may be inserted into the duct to unblock it. This tube (or stent) may be left in place to keep the duct open. Tissue samples may also be taken and checked under a microscope for signs of cancer.

- **PTC (percutaneous transhepatic cholangiography)**: A procedure used to x-ray the liver and bile ducts. A thin needle is inserted through the skin below the ribs and into the liver. Dye is injected into the liver or bile ducts and an x-ray is taken. If a blockage is found, a thin, flexible tube called a stent is sometimes left in the liver to drain bile into the small intestine or a collection bag outside the body.

- **Biopsy**: The removal of cells or tissues so they can be viewed under a microscope to check for signs of cancer. The sample may be taken using a thin needle inserted into the duct during an x-ray or ultrasound. This is called a fine-needle aspiration (FNA) biopsy.

The biopsy is usually done during PTC or ERCP. Tissue, including part of a lymph node, may also be removed during surgery.

- **Liver function tests:** A procedure in which a blood sample is checked to measure the amounts of certain substances released into the blood by the liver. A higher than normal amount of a substance can be a sign of liver disease that may be caused by extrahepatic bile duct cancer.

- **Tumor marker test:** A procedure in which a sample of blood, urine, or tissue is checked to measure the amounts of certain substances made by organs, tissues, or tumor cells in the body. Certain substances are linked to specific types of cancer when found in increased levels in the body. These are called tumor markers. Carcinoembryonic antigen (CEA) and CA 19-9 are associated with extrahepatic bile duct cancer when found in increased levels in the body.

Certain factors affect prognosis (chance of recovery) and treatment options.

The prognosis (chance of recovery) and treatment options depend on the following:

- The stage of the cancer (whether it affects only the bile duct or has spread to other places in the body).
- Whether the tumor can be completely removed by surgery.
- Whether the tumor is in the upper or lower part of the duct.
- Whether the cancer has just been diagnosed or has recurred (come back).

Treatment options may also depend on the symptoms caused by the tumor. Extrahepatic bile duct cancer is usually found after it has spread and can rarely be removed completely by surgery. Palliative therapy may relieve symptoms and improve the patient's quality of life.

Stages of Extrahepatic Bile Duct Cancer

After extrahepatic bile duct cancer has been diagnosed, tests are done to find out if cancer cells have spread within the bile duct or to other parts of the body.

The process used to find out if cancer has spread within the extrahepatic bile duct or to other parts of the body is called staging. The information gathered from the staging process determines the stage of the disease. It is important to know the stage in order to plan treatment.

Extrahepatic bile duct cancer may be staged following a laparotomy. A surgical incision is made in the wall of the abdomen to check the inside of the abdomen for signs of disease and to remove tissue and fluid for examination under a microscope. The results of the diagnostic imaging tests, laparotomy, and biopsy are viewed together to determine the stage of the cancer. Sometimes, a laparoscopy will be done before the laparotomy to see if the cancer has spread. If the cancer has spread and cannot be removed by surgery, the surgeon may decide not to do a laparotomy.

There are three ways that cancer spreads in the body.

Cancer can spread through tissue, the lymph system, and the blood:

- Tissue. The cancer spreads from where it began by growing into nearby areas.

- Lymph system. The cancer spreads from where it began by getting into the lymph system. The cancer travels through the lymph vessels to other parts of the body.

- Blood. The cancer spreads from where it began by getting into the blood. The cancer travels through the blood vessels to other parts of the body.

Cancer may spread from where it began to other parts of the body.

When cancer spreads to another part of the body, it is called metastasis. Cancer cells break away from where they began (the primary tumor) and travel through the lymph system or blood.

- Lymph system. The cancer gets into the lymph system, travels through the lymph vessels, and forms a tumor (metastatic tumor) in another part of the body.

- Blood. The cancer gets into the blood, travels through the blood vessels, and forms a tumor (metastatic tumor) in another part of the body.

The metastatic tumor is the same type of cancer as the primary tumor. For example, if extrahepatic bile duct cancer spreads to the liver, the cancer cells in the liver are actually extrahepatic bile duct cancer cells. The disease is metastatic extrahepatic bile duct cancer, not liver cancer.

There are two staging systems for extrahepatic bile duct cancer.

Extrahepatic bile duct cancer has two staging systems. The staging system used depends on where in the extrahepatic bile duct the cancer first formed.

- *Perihilar* or proximal extrahepatic bile duct tumors (perihilar bile duct tumors) form in the area where the bile duct leaves the liver. This type of tumor is also called a Klatskin tumor.

- *Distal* extrahepatic bile duct tumors (distal bile duct tumors) form in the area where the bile duct empties into the small intestine.

The following stages are used for **perihilar extrahepatic bile duct cancer:**

Stage 0 (Carcinoma in Situ)

In stage 0, abnormal cells are found in the innermost layer of tissue lining the perihilar bile duct. These abnormal cells may become cancer and spread into nearby normal tissue. Stage 0 is also called carcinoma in situ.

Stage I

In stage I, cancer has formed in the innermost layer of the wall of the perihilar bile duct and has spread into the muscle and fibrous tissue of the wall.

Stage II

In stage II, cancer has spread through the wall of the perihilar bile duct to nearby fatty tissue or to the liver.

Stage III

Stage III is divided into stages IIIA and IIIB.

- Stage IIIA: The tumor has spread to one branch of the hepatic artery or of the portal vein.

- Stage IIIB: The tumor has spread to nearby lymph nodes. Cancer has also spread into the wall of the perihilar bile duct and may have spread through the wall to nearby fatty tissue, the liver, or to one branch of the hepatic artery or of the portal vein.

Stage IV

Stage IV is divided into stages IVA and IVB.

- Stage IVA: The tumor may have spread to nearby lymph nodes and has spread to one or more of the following:

  - the main part of the portal vein or both branches of the portal vein;

  - the hepatic artery;

  - the right and left hepatic ducts;

  - the right hepatic duct and the left branch of the hepatic artery or of the portal vein;

  - the left hepatic duct and the right branch of the hepatic artery or of the portal vein.

- Stage IVB: The tumor has spread to other parts of the body, such as the liver.

The following stages are used for **distal** extrahepatic bile duct cancer:

Stage 0 (Carcinoma in Situ)

In stage 0, abnormal cells are found in the innermost layer of tissue lining the distal bile duct. These abnormal cells may become cancer and spread into nearby normal tissue. Stage 0 is also called carcinoma in situ.

Stage I

In stage I, cancer has formed. Stage I is divided into stages IA and IB.

- Stage IA: Cancer is found in the distal bile duct only.

- Stage IB: Cancer has spread all the way through the wall of the distal bile duct.

Stage II

Stage II is divided into stages IIA and IIB.

- Stage IIA: Cancer has spread from the distal bile duct to the gallbladder, pancreas, small intestine, or other nearby organs.
- Stage IIB: Cancer has spread from the distal bile duct to nearby lymph nodes. Cancer may have spread through the wall of the distal bile duct or to the gallbladder, pancreas, small intestine, or other nearby organs.

Stage III

In stage III, cancer has spread to the large vessels that carry blood to the organs in the abdomen. Cancer may have spread to nearby lymph nodes.

Stage IV

In stage IV, cancer has spread to other parts of the body, such as the liver or lungs.

Extrahepatic bile duct cancer can also be grouped according to how the cancer may be treated. There are two treatment groups:

Localized (and resectable)

The cancer is in an area where it can be removed completely by surgery.

Unresectable, recurrent, or metastatic

Unresectable cancer cannot be removed completely by surgery. Most patients with extrahepatic bile duct cancer have unresectable cancer.

Recurrent cancer is cancer that has recurred (come back) after it has been treated. Extrahepatic bile duct cancer may come back in the bile duct or in other parts of the body.

Metastasis is the spread of cancer from the primary site (place where it started) to other places in the body. Metastatic extrahepatic bile duct cancer may have spread to nearby blood vessels, the liver, the common bile duct, nearby lymph nodes, other parts of the abdominal cavity, or to distant parts of the body.

Treatment Option Overview

There are different types of treatment for patients with extrahepatic bile duct cancer.

Different types of treatment are available for patients with extra-hepatic bile duct cancer. Some treatments are standard (the currently used treatment), and some are being tested in clinical trials. A treatment clinical trial is a research study meant to help improve current treatments or obtain information on new treatments for patients with cancer. When clinical trials show that a new treatment is better than the standard treatment, the new treatment may become the standard treatment. Patients may want to think about taking part in a clinical trial. Some clinical trials are open only to patients who have not started treatment.

Three types of standard treatment are used:

Surgery

The following types of surgery are used to treat extrahepatic bile duct cancer:

- Removal of the bile duct: If the tumor is small and only in the bile duct, the entire bile duct may be removed. A new duct is made by connecting the duct openings in the liver to the intestine. Lymph nodes are removed and viewed under a microscope to see if they contain cancer.

- Partial hepatectomy: Removal of the part of the liver where cancer is found. The part removed may be a wedge of tissue, an entire lobe, or a larger part of the liver, along with some normal tissue around it.

- Whipple procedure: A surgical procedure in which the head of the pancreas, the gallbladder, part of the stomach, part of the small intestine, and the bile duct are removed. Enough of the pancreas is left to make digestive juices and insulin.

- Surgical biliary bypass: If the tumor cannot be removed but is blocking the small intestine and causing bile to build up in the gallbladder, a biliary bypass may be done. During this operation, the gallbladder or bile duct will be cut and sewn to the small intestine to create a new pathway around the blocked area. This procedure helps to relieve jaundice caused by the build-up of bile.

- Stent placement: If the tumor is blocking the bile duct, a stent (a thin tube) may be placed in the duct to drain bile that has built up in the area. The stent may drain to the outside of the body or it may go around the blocked area and drain the bile into the small intestine. The doctor may place the stent during surgery or PTC, or with an endoscope.

Radiation therapy

Radiation therapy is a cancer treatment that uses high-energy x-rays or other types of radiation to kill cancer cells or keep them from growing. There are two types of radiation therapy. External radiation therapy uses a machine outside the body to send radiation toward the cancer. Internal radiation therapy uses a radioactive substance sealed in needles, seeds, wires, or catheters that are placed directly into or near the cancer. The way the radiation therapy is given depends on the type and stage of the cancer being treated.

Chemotherapy

Chemotherapy is a cancer treatment that uses drugs to stop the growth of cancer cells, either by killing the cells or by stopping them from dividing. When chemotherapy is taken by mouth or injected into a vein or muscle, the drugs enter the bloodstream and can reach cancer cells throughout the body (systemic chemotherapy). When chemotherapy is placed directly into the cerebrospinal fluid, an organ, or a body cavity such as the abdomen, the drugs mainly affect cancer cells in those areas (regional chemotherapy). The way the chemotherapy is given depends on the type and stage of the cancer being treated.

New types of treatment are being tested in clinical trials.

Radiation sensitizers

Clinical trials are studying ways to improve the effect of radiation therapy on tumor cells, including the following:

- Hyperthermia therapy: A treatment in which body tissue is exposed to high temperatures to damage and kill cancer cells or to make cancer cells more sensitive to the effects of radiation therapy and certain anticancer drugs.
- Radiosensitizers: Drugs that make tumor cells more sensitive to radiation therapy. Combining radiation therapy with radiosensitizers may kill more tumor cells.

Patients may want to think about taking part in a clinical trial.

For some patients, taking part in a clinical trial may be the best treatment choice. Clinical trials are part of the cancer research process. Clinical trials are done to find out if new cancer treatments are safe and effective or better than the standard treatment.

Many of today's standard treatments for cancer are based on earlier clinical trials. Patients who take part in a clinical trial may receive the standard treatment or be among the first to receive a new treatment.

Patients who take part in clinical trials also help improve the way cancer will be treated in the future. Even when clinical trials do not lead to effective new treatments, they often answer important questions and help move research forward.

Patients can enter clinical trials before, during, or after starting their cancer treatment.

Some clinical trials only include patients who have not yet received treatment. Other trials test treatments for patients whose cancer has not gotten better. There are also clinical trials that test new ways to stop cancer from recurring (coming back) or reduce the side effects of cancer treatment.

Clinical trials are taking place in many parts of the country.

Follow-up tests may be needed.

Some of the tests that were done to diagnose the cancer or to find out the stage of the cancer may be repeated. Some tests will be repeated in order to see how well the treatment is working. Decisions about whether to continue, change, or stop treatment may be based on the results of these tests.

Some of the tests will continue to be done from time to time after treatment has ended. The results of these tests can show if your condition has changed or if the cancer has recurred (come back). These tests are sometimes called follow-up tests or check-ups.

Section 23.5

Gallbladder Cancer

Text in this section is excerpted from "Gallbladder Cancer Treatment," National Cancer Institute at the National Institutes of Health (NIH), April 13, 2014.

General Information About Gallbladder Cancer

Gallbladder cancer is a disease in which malignant (cancer) cells form in the tissues of the gallbladder.

Gallbladder cancer is a rare disease in which malignant (cancer) cells are found in the tissues of the gallbladder. The gallbladder is a pear-shaped organ that lies just under the liver in the upper abdomen. The gallbladder stores bile, a fluid made by the liver to digest fat. When food is being broken down in the stomach and intestines, bile is released from the gallbladder through a tube called the common bile duct, which connects the gallbladder and liver to the first part of the small intestine.

The wall of the gallbladder has 3 main layers of tissue.

- Mucosal (inner) layer.
- Muscularis (middle, muscle) layer.
- Serosal (outer) layer.

Between these layers is supporting connective tissue. Primary gallbladder cancer starts in the inner layer and spreads through the outer layers as it grows.

Being female can increase the risk of developing gallbladder cancer.

Anything that increases your chance of getting a disease is called a risk factor. Having a risk factor does not mean that you will get cancer; not having risk factors doesn't mean that you will not get cancer. Talk with your doctor if you think you may be at risk.

Risk factors for gallbladder cancer include the following:

- Being female.
- Being Native American.

Signs and symptoms of gallbladder cancer include jaundice, fever, and pain.

These and other signs and symptoms may be caused by gallbladder cancer or by other conditions. Check with your doctor if you have any of the following:

- Jaundice (yellowing of the skin and whites of the eyes).
- Pain above the stomach.
- Fever.
- Nausea and vomiting.
- Bloating.
- Lumps in the abdomen.

Gallbladder cancer is difficult to detect (find) and diagnose early.

Gallbladder cancer is difficult to detect and diagnose for the following reasons:

- There are no signs or symptoms in the early stages of gallbladder cancer.
- The symptoms of gallbladder cancer, when present, are like the symptoms of many other illnesses.
- The gallbladder is hidden behind the liver.

Gallbladder cancer is sometimes found when the gallbladder is removed for other reasons. Patients with gallstones rarely develop gallbladder cancer.

Tests that examine the gallbladder and nearby organs are used to detect (find), diagnose, and stage gallbladder cancer.

Procedures that make pictures of the gallbladder and the area around it help diagnose gallbladder cancer and show how far the cancer has spread. The process used to find out if cancer cells have spread within and around the gallbladder is called staging.

In order to plan treatment, it is important to know if the gallbladder cancer can be removed by surgery. Tests and procedures to detect, diagnose, and stage gallbladder cancer are usually done at the same time.

The following tests and procedures may be used:

- **Physical exam and history:** An exam of the body to check general signs of health, including checking for signs of disease, such as lumps or anything else that seems unusual. A history of the patient's health habits and past illnesses and treatments will also be taken.

- **Liver function tests:** A procedure in which a blood sample is checked to measure the amounts of certain substances released into the blood by the liver. A higher than normal amount of a substance can be a sign of liver disease that may be caused by gallbladder cancer.

- **Carcinoembryonic antigen (CEA) assay:** A test that measures the level of CEA in the blood. CEA is released into the bloodstream from both cancer cells and normal cells. When found in higher than normal amounts, it can be a sign of gallbladder cancer or other conditions.

- **CA 19-9 assay:** A test that measures the level of CA 19-9 in the blood. CA 19-9 is released into the bloodstream from both cancer cells and normal cells. When found in higher than normal amounts, it can be a sign of gallbladder cancer or other conditions.

- **Blood chemistry studies:** A procedure in which a blood sample is checked to measure the amounts of certain substances released into the blood by organs and tissues in the body. An unusual (higher or lower than normal) amount of a substance can be a sign of disease in the organ or tissue that makes it.

- **CT scan (CAT scan):** A procedure that makes a series of detailed pictures of areas inside the body, such as the chest, abdomen, and pelvis, taken from different angles. The pictures are made by a computer linked to an x-ray machine. A dye may be injected into a vein or swallowed to help the organs or tissues show up more clearly. This procedure is also called computed tomography, computerized tomography, or computerized axial tomography.

- **Ultrasound exam:** A procedure in which high-energy sound waves (ultrasound) are bounced off internal tissues or organs and make echoes. The echoes form a picture of body tissues called a sonogram. An abdominal ultrasound is done to diagnose gallbladder cancer.

- **PTC (percutaneous transhepatic cholangiography):** A procedure used to x-ray the liver and bile ducts. A thin needle is inserted through the skin below the ribs and into the liver. Dye is injected into the liver or bile ducts and an x-ray is taken. If a blockage is found, a thin, flexible tube called a stent is sometimes left in the liver to drain bile into the small intestine or a collection bag outside the body.

- **Chest x-ray:** An x-ray of the organs and bones inside the chest. An x-ray is a type of energy beam that can go through the body and onto film, making a picture of areas inside the body.

- **ERCP (endoscopic retrograde cholangiopancreatography):** A procedure used to x-ray the ducts (tubes) that carry bile from the liver to the gallbladder and from the gallbladder to the small intestine. Sometimes gallbladder cancer causes these ducts to narrow and block or slow the flow of bile, causing jaundice. An endoscope (a thin, lighted tube) is passed through the mouth, esophagus, and stomach into the first part of the small intestine. A catheter (a smaller tube) is then inserted through the endoscope into the bile ducts. A dye is injected through the catheter into the ducts and an x-ray is taken. If the ducts are blocked by a tumor, a fine tube may be inserted into the duct to unblock it. This tube (or stent) may be left in place to keep the duct open. Tissue samples may also be taken.

- **Laparoscopy:** A surgical procedure to look at the organs inside the abdomen to check for signs of disease. Small incisions (cuts) are made in the wall of the abdomen and a laparoscope (a thin, lighted tube) is inserted into one of the incisions. Other instruments may be inserted through the same or other incisions to perform procedures such as removing organs or taking tissue samples for biopsy. The laparoscopy helps to find out if the cancer is within the gallbladder only or has spread to nearby tissues and if it can be removed by surgery.

- **Biopsy:** The removal of cells or tissues so they can be viewed under a microscope by a pathologist to check for signs of cancer. The biopsy may be done after surgery to remove the tumor. If the tumor clearly cannot be removed by surgery, the biopsy may be done using a fine needle to remove cells from the tumor.

Certain factors affect the prognosis (chance of recovery) and treatment options.

The prognosis (chance of recovery) and treatment options depend on the following:

- The stage of the cancer (whether the cancer has spread from the gallbladder to other places in the body).

- Whether the cancer can be completely removed by surgery.

- The type of gallbladder cancer (how the cancer cell looks under a microscope).

- Whether the cancer has just been diagnosed or has recurred (come back).

Treatment may also depend on the age and general health of the patient and whether the cancer is causing signs or symptoms.

Gallbladder cancer can be cured only if it is found before it has spread, when it can be removed by surgery. If the cancer has spread, palliative treatment can improve the patient's quality of life by controlling the symptoms and complications of this disease.

Taking part in one of the clinical trials being done to improve treatment should be considered.

Stages of Gallbladder Cancer

There are three ways that cancer spreads in the body.

Cancer can spread through tissue, the lymph system, and the blood:

- Tissue. The cancer spreads from where it began by growing into nearby areas.

- Lymph system. The cancer spreads from where it began by getting into the lymph system. The cancer travels through the lymph vessels to other parts of the body.

- Blood. The cancer spreads from where it began by getting into the blood. The cancer travels through the blood vessels to other parts of the body.

Cancer may spread from where it began to other parts of the body.

When cancer spreads to another part of the body, it is called metastasis. Cancer cells break away from where they began (the primary tumor) and travel through the lymph system or blood.

- Lymph system. The cancer gets into the lymph system, travels through the lymph vessels, and forms a tumor (metastatic tumor) in another part of the body.

- Blood. The cancer gets into the blood, travels through the blood vessels, and forms a tumor (metastatic tumor) in another part of the body.

The metastatic tumor is the same type of cancer as the primary tumor. For example, if gallbladder cancer spreads to the liver, the cancer cells in the liver are actually gallbladder cancer cells. The disease is metastatic gallbladder cancer, not liver cancer.

The following stages are used for gallbladder cancer:

Stage 0 (Carcinoma in Situ)

In stage 0, abnormal cells are found in the inner (mucosal) layer of the gallbladder. These abnormal cells may become cancer and spread into nearby normal tissue. Stage 0 is also called carcinoma in situ.

Stage I

In stage I, cancer has formed and has spread beyond the inner (mucosal) layer to a layer of tissue with blood vessels or to the muscle layer.

Stage II

In stage II, cancer has spread beyond the muscle layer to the connective tissue around the muscle.

Stage IIIA

In stage IIIA, cancer has spread through the thin layers of tissue that cover the gallbladder and/or to the liver and/or to one nearby organ (such as the stomach, small intestine, colon, pancreas, or bile ducts outside the liver).

Stage IIIB

In stage IIIB, cancer has spread to nearby lymph nodes and:

- beyond the inner layer of the gallbladder to a layer of tissue with blood vessels or to the muscle layer; or
- beyond the muscle layer to the connective tissue around the muscle; or
- through the thin layers of tissue that cover the gallbladder and/or to the liver and/or to one nearby organ (such as the stomach, small intestine, colon, pancreas, or bile ducts outside the liver).

Stage IVA

In stage IVA, cancer has spread to a main blood vessel of the liver or to 2 or more nearby organs or areas other than the liver. Cancer may have spread to nearby lymph nodes.

Stage IVB

In stage IVB, cancer has spread to either:

- lymph nodes along large arteries in the abdomen and/or near the lower part of the backbone; or
- to organs or areas far away from the gallbladder.

For gallbladder cancer, stages are also grouped according to how the cancer may be treated. There are two treatment groups:

Localized (Stage I)

Cancer is found in the wall of the gallbladder and can be completely removed by surgery.

Unresectable, recurrent, or metastatic (Stage II, Stage III, and Stage IV)

Unresectable cancer cannot be removed completely by surgery. Most patients with gallbladder cancer have unresectable cancer.

Recurrent cancer is cancer that has recurred (come back) after it has been treated. Gallbladder cancer may come back in the gallbladder or in other parts of the body.

Metastasis is the spread of cancer from the primary site (place where it started) to other places in the body. Metastatic gallbladder cancer may spread to surrounding tissues, organs, throughout the abdominal cavity, or to distant parts of the body.

Treatment Option Overview

There are different types of treatment for patients with gallbladder cancer.

Different types of treatments are available for patients with gallbladder cancer. Some treatments are standard (the currently used treatment), and some are being tested in clinical trials. A treatment clinical trial is a research study meant to help improve current treatments or obtain information on new treatments for patients with cancer. When clinical trials show that a new treatment is better than the standard treatment, the new treatment may become the standard treatment. Patients may want to think about taking part in a clinical trial. Some clinical trials are open only to patients who have not started treatment.

Three types of standard treatment are used:

Surgery

Gallbladder cancer may be treated with a cholecystectomy, surgery to remove the gallbladder and some of the tissues around it. Nearby lymph nodes may be removed. Alaparoscope is sometimes used to guide gallbladder surgery. The laparoscope is attached to a video camera and inserted through an incision (port) in the abdomen. Surgical instruments are inserted through other ports to perform the surgery. Because there is a risk that gallbladder cancer cells may spread to these ports, tissue surrounding the port sites may also be removed.

If the cancer has spread and cannot be removed, the following types of palliative surgery may relieve symptoms:

- Surgical biliary bypass: If the tumor is blocking the small intestine and bile is building up in the gallbladder, a biliary bypass may be done. During this operation, the gallbladder or bile duct will be cut and sewn to the small intestine to create a new pathway around the blocked area.

- Endoscopic stent placement: If the tumor is blocking the bile duct, surgery may be done to put in a stent (a thin, flexible tube) to drain bile that has built up in the area. The stent may be placed through a catheter that drains to the outside of the body or the stent may go around the blocked area and drain the bile into the small intestine.

- Percutaneous transhepatic biliary drainage: A procedure done to drain bile when there is a blockage and endoscopic stent placement is not possible. An x-ray of the liver and bile ducts is done to locate the blockage. Images made by ultrasound are used to guide placement of a stent, which is left in the liver to drain bile into the small intestine or a collection bag outside the body. This procedure may be done to relieve jaundice before surgery.

Radiation therapy

Radiation therapy is a cancer treatment that uses high-energy x-rays or other types of radiation to kill cancer cells. There are two types of radiation therapy. External radiation therapy uses a machine outside the body to send radiation toward the cancer. Internal radiation therapy uses a radioactive substance sealed in needles, seeds, wires, or catheters that are placed directly into or near the cancer. The way the radiation therapy is given depends on the type and stage of the cancer being treated.

Chemotherapy

Chemotherapy is a cancer treatment that uses drugs to stop the growth of cancer cells, either by killing the cells or by stopping the cells from dividing. When chemotherapy is taken by mouth or injected into a vein or muscle, the drugs enter the bloodstream and can reach cancer cells throughout the body (systemic chemotherapy). When chemotherapy is placed directly into the cerebrospinal fluid, an organ, or a body cavity such as the abdomen, the drugs mainly affect cancer cells in those areas (regional chemotherapy). The way the chemotherapy is given depends on the type and stage of the cancer being treated.

New types of treatment are being tested in clinical trials.

Radiation sensitizers

Clinical trials are studying ways to improve the effect of radiation therapy on tumor cells, including the following:

- Hyperthermia therapy: A treatment in which body tissue is exposed to high temperatures to damage and kill cancer cells or to make cancer cells more sensitive to the effects of radiation therapy and certain anticancer drugs.

- Radiosensitizers: Drugs that make tumor cells more sensitive to radiation therapy. Giving radiation therapy together with radio-sensitizers may kill more tumor cells.

Patients may want to think about taking part in a clinical trial.

For some patients, taking part in a clinical trial may be the best treatment choice. Clinical trials are part of the cancer research process. Clinical trials are done to find out if new cancer treatments are safe and effective or better than the standard treatment.

Many of today's standard treatments for cancer are based on earlier clinical trials. Patients who take part in a clinical trial may receive the standard treatment or be among the first to receive a new treatment.

Patients who take part in clinical trials also help improve the way cancer will be treated in the future. Even when clinical trials do not lead to effective new treatments, they often answer important questions and help move research forward.

Patients can enter clinical trials before, during, or after starting their cancer treatment.

Some clinical trials only include patients who have not yet received treatment. Other trials test treatments for patients whose cancer has not gotten better. There are also clinical trials that test new ways to stop cancer from recurring (coming back) or reduce the side effects of cancer treatment.

Clinical trials are taking place in many parts of the country.

Follow-up tests may be needed.

Some of the tests that were done to diagnose the cancer or to find out the stage of the cancer may be repeated. Some tests will be repeated in order to see how well the treatment is working. Decisions about whether to continue, change, or stop treatment may be based on the results of these tests.

Some of the tests will continue to be done from time to time after treatment has ended. The results of these tests can show if your condition has changed or if the cancer has recurred (come back). These tests are sometimes called follow-up tests or check-ups.

358

Section 23.6

Pancreatic Cancer

Text in this section is excerpted from "Pancreatic Cancer Treatment," National Cancer Institute at the National Institutes of Health (NIH), April 2, 2015.

General Information About Pancreatic Cancer

Pancreatic cancer is a disease in which malignant (cancer) cells form in the tissues of the pancreas.

The pancreas is a gland about 6 inches long that is shaped like a thin pear lying on its side. The wider end of the pancreas is called the head, the middle section is called the body, and the narrow end is called the tail. The pancreas lies between the stomach and the spine.

The pancreas has two main jobs in the body:

- To make juices that help digest (break down) food.

- To make hormones, such as insulin and glucagon, that help control blood sugar levels. Both of these hormones help the body use and store the energy it gets from food.

The digestive juices are made by exocrine pancreas cells and the hormones are made by endocrine pancreas cells. About 95% of pancreatic cancers begin in exocrine cells.

Smoking and health history can affect the risk of pancreatic cancer.

Anything that increases your risk of getting a disease is called a risk factor. Having a risk factor does not mean that you will get cancer; not having risk factors doesn't mean that you will not get cancer. Talk with your doctor if you think you may be at risk.

Risk factors for pancreatic cancer include the following:

- Smoking.
- Being very overweight.
- Having a personal history of diabetes or chronic pancreatitis.
- Having a family history of pancreatic cancer or pancreatitis.
- Having certain hereditary conditions, such as:
  - Multiple endocrine neoplasia type 1 (MEN1) syndrome.
  - Hereditary nonpolyposis colon cancer (HNPCC; Lynch syndrome).
  - von Hippel-Lindau syndrome.
  - Peutz-Jeghers syndrome.
  - Hereditary breast and ovarian cancer syndrome.
  - Familial atypical multiple mole melanoma (FAMMM) syndrome.

Signs and symptoms of pancreatic cancer include jaundice, pain, and weight loss.

Pancreatic cancer may not cause early signs or symptoms. Signs and symptoms may be caused by pancreatic cancer or by other conditions. Check with your doctor if you have any of the following:

- Jaundice (yellowing of the skin and whites of the eyes).
- Light-colored stools.
- Dark urine.
- Pain in the upper or middle abdomen and back.
- Weight loss for no known reason.
- Loss of appetite.
- Feeling very tired.
- Pancreatic cancer is difficult to detect (find) and diagnose early.

Pancreatic cancer is difficult to detect and diagnose for the following reasons:

- There aren't any noticeable signs or symptoms in the early stages of pancreatic cancer.

- The signs and symptoms of pancreatic cancer, when present, are like the signs and symptoms of many other illnesses.

- The pancreas is hidden behind other organs such as the stomach, small intestine, liver, gallbladder, spleen, and bile ducts.

Tests that examine the pancreas are used to detect (find), diagnose, and stage pancreatic cancer.

Pancreatic cancer is usually diagnosed with tests and procedures that make pictures of the pancreas and the area around it. The process used to find out if cancer cells have spread within and around the pancreas is called staging. Tests and procedures to detect, diagnose, and stage pancreatic cancer are usually done at the same time. In order to plan treatment, it is important to know the stage of the disease and whether or not the pancreatic cancer can be removed by surgery.

The following tests and procedures may be used:

- **Physical exam and history:** An exam of the body to check general signs of health, including checking for signs of disease, such as lumps or anything else that seems unusual. A history of the patient's health habits and past illnesses and treatments will also be taken.

- **Blood chemistry studies:** A procedure in which a blood sample is checked to measure the amounts of certain substances, such as bilirubin, released into the blood by organs and tissues in the body. An unusual (higher or lower than normal) amount of a substance can be a sign of disease in the organ or tissue that makes it.

- **Tumor marker test:** A procedure in which a sample of blood, urine, or tissue is checked to measure the amounts of certain substances, such as CA 19-9, and carcinoembryonic antigen (CEA), made by organs, tissues, or tumor cells in the body. Certain substances are linked to specific types of cancer when found in increased levels in the body. These are called tumor markers.

- **MRI (magnetic resonance imaging):** A procedure that uses a magnet, radio waves, and a computer to make a series of detailed pictures of areas inside the body. This procedure is also called nuclear magnetic resonance imaging (NMRI).

- **CT scan (CAT scan):** A procedure that makes a series of detailed pictures of areas inside the body, taken from different angles. The pictures are made by a computer linked to an x-ray machine. A dye may be injected into a vein or swallowed to help the organs or tissues show up more clearly. This procedure is also called computed tomography, computerized tomography, or computerized axial tomography. A spiral or helical CT scan makes a series of very detailed pictures of areas inside the body using an x-ray machine that scans the body in a spiral path.

- **PET scan (positron emission tomography scan):** A procedure to find malignant tumor cells in the body. A small amount of radioactive glucose (sugar) is injected into a vein. The PET scanner rotates around the body and makes a picture of where glucose is being used in the body. Malignant tumor cells show up brighter in the picture because they are more active and take up more glucose than normal cells do. A PET scan and CT scan may be done at the same time. This is called a PET-CT.

- **Abdominal ultrasound:** An ultrasound exam used to make pictures of the inside of the abdomen. The ultrasound transducer is pressed against the skin of the abdomen and directs high-energy sound waves (ultrasound) into the abdomen. The sound waves bounce off the internal tissues and organs and make echoes. The transducer receives the echoes and sends them to a computer, which uses the echoes to make pictures called sonograms. The picture can be printed to be looked at later.

- **Endoscopic ultrasound (EUS):** A procedure in which an endoscope is inserted into the body, usually through the mouth or rectum. An endoscope is a thin, tube-like instrument with a light and a lens for viewing. A probe at the end of the endoscope is used to bounce high-energy sound waves (ultrasound) off internal tissues or organs and make echoes. The echoes form a picture of body tissues called a sonogram. This procedure is also called endosonography.

- **Endoscopic retrograde cholangiopancreatography (ERCP):** A procedure used to x-ray the ducts (tubes) that carry bile from the liver to the gallbladder and from the gallbladder to the small intestine. Sometimes pancreatic cancer causes these ducts to narrow and block or slow the flow of bile, causing jaundice. An endoscope (a thin, lighted tube) is passed through the mouth, esophagus, and stomach into the first part of the small

362

intestine. A catheter (a smaller tube) is then inserted through the endoscope into the pancreatic ducts. A dye is injected through the catheter into the ducts and an x-ray is taken. If the ducts are blocked by a tumor, a fine tube may be inserted into the duct to unblock it. This tube (or stent) may be left in place to keep the duct open. Tissue samples may also be taken.

- **Percutaneous transhepatic cholangiography (PTC):** A procedure used to x-ray the liver and bile ducts. A thin needle is inserted through the skin below the ribs and into the liver. Dye is injected into the liver or bile ducts and an x-ray is taken. If a blockage is found, a thin, flexible tube called a stent is sometimes left in the liver to drain bile into the small intestine or a collection bag outside the body. This test is done only if ERCP cannot be done.

- **Laparoscopy:** A surgical procedure to look at the organs inside the abdomen to check for signs of disease. Small incisions (cuts) are made in the wall of the abdomen and alaparoscope (a thin, lighted tube) is inserted into one of the incisions. The laparoscope may have an ultrasound probe at the end in order to bounce high-energy sound waves off internal organs, such as the pancreas. This is called laparoscopic ultrasound. Other instruments may be inserted through the same or other incisions to perform procedures such as taking tissue samples from the pancreas or a sample of fluid from the abdomen to check for cancer.

- **Biopsy:** The removal of cells or tissues so they can be viewed under a microscope by a pathologist to check for signs of cancer. There are several ways to do a biopsy for pancreatic cancer. A fine needle or a core needle may be inserted into the pancreas during an x-ray or ultrasound to remove cells. Tissue may also be removed during a laparoscopy.

Certain factors affect prognosis (chance of recovery) and treatment options.

The prognosis (chance of recovery) and treatment options depend on the following:

- Whether or not the tumor can be removed by surgery.

- The stage of the cancer (the size of the tumor and whether the cancer has spread outside the pancreas to nearby tissues or lymph nodes or to other places in the body).

- The patient's general health.

363

- Whether the cancer has just been diagnosed or has recurred (come back).

Pancreatic cancer can be controlled only if it is found before it has spread, when it can be completely removed by surgery. If the cancer has spread, palliative treatment can improve the patient's quality of life by controlling the symptoms and complications of this disease.

Stages of Pancreatic Cancer

Tests and procedures to stage pancreatic cancer are usually done at the same time as diagnosis.

The process used to find out if cancer has spread within the pancreas or to other parts of the body is called staging. The information gathered from the staging process determines the stage of the disease. It is important to know the stage of the disease in order to plan treatment. The results of some of the tests used to diagnose pancreatic cancer are often also used to stage the disease.

There are three ways that cancer spreads in the body.

Cancer can spread through tissue, the lymph system, and the blood:

- Tissue. The cancer spreads from where it began by growing into nearby areas.
- Lymph system. The cancer spreads from where it began by getting into the lymph system. The cancer travels through the lymph vessels to other parts of the body.
- Blood. The cancer spreads from where it began by getting into the blood. The cancer travels through the blood vessels to other parts of the body.

Cancer may spread from where it began to other parts of the body.

When cancer spreads to another part of the body, it is called metastasis. Cancer cells break away from where they began (the primary tumor) and travel through the lymph system or blood.

- Lymph system. The cancer gets into the lymph system, travels through the lymph vessels, and forms a tumor (metastatic tumor) in another part of the body.

364

- Blood. The cancer gets into the blood, travels through the blood vessels, and forms a tumor (metastatic tumor) in another part of the body.

The metastatic tumor is the same type of cancer as the primary tumor. For example, if pancreatic cancer spreads to the liver, the cancer cells in the liver are actually pancreatic cancer cells. The disease is metastatic pancreatic cancer, not liver cancer.

The following stages are used for pancreatic cancer:

Stage 0 (Carcinoma in Situ)

In stage 0, abnormal cells are found in the lining of the pancreas. These abnormal cells may become cancer and spread into nearby normal tissue. Stage 0 is also called carcinoma in situ.

Stage I

In stage I, cancer has formed and is found in the pancreas only. Stage I is divided into stage IA and stage IB, based on the size of the tumor.

- Stage IA: The tumor is 2 centimeters or smaller.
- Stage IB: The tumor is larger than 2 centimeters.

Stage II

In stage II, cancer may have spread to nearby tissue and organs, and may have spread to lymph nodes near the pancreas. Stage II is divided into stage IIA and stage IIB, based on where the cancer has spread.

- Stage IIA: Cancer has spread to nearby tissue and organs but has not spread to nearby lymph nodes.
- Stage IIB: Cancer has spread to nearby lymph nodes and may have spread to nearby tissue and organs.

Stage III

In stage III, cancer has spread to the major blood vessels near the pancreas and may have spread to nearby lymph nodes.

Stage IV

In stage IV, cancer may be of any size and has spread to distant organs, such as the liver, lung, and peritoneal cavity. It may have also spread to organs and tissues near the pancreas or to lymph nodes.

Treatment Option Overview

There are different types of treatment for patients with pancreatic cancer.

Different types of treatment are available for patients with pancreatic cancer. Some treatments are standard (the currently used treatment), and some are being tested in clinical trials. A treatment clinical trial is a research study meant to help improve current treatments or obtain information on new treatments for patients with cancer. When clinical trials show that a new treatment is better than the standard treatment, the new treatment may become the standard treatment. Patients may want to think about taking part in a clinical trial. Some clinical trials are open only to patients who have not started treatment.

Five types of standard treatment are used:

Surgery

One of the following types of surgery may be used to take out the tumor:

- Whipple procedure: A surgical procedure in which the head of the pancreas, the gallbladder, part of the stomach, part of the small intestine, and the bile duct are removed. Enough of the pancreas is left to produce digestive juices and insulin.

- Total pancreatectomy: This operation removes the whole pancreas, part of the stomach, part of the small intestine, the common bile duct, the gallbladder, the spleen, and nearby lymph nodes.

- Distal pancreatectomy: The body and the tail of the pancreas and usually the spleen are removed.

If the cancer has spread and cannot be removed, the following types of palliative surgery may be done to relieve symptoms and improve quality of life:

- Surgical biliary bypass: If cancer is blocking the small intestine and bile is building up in the gallbladder, a biliary bypass may be done. During this operation, the doctor will cut the gallbladder or bile duct and sew it to the small intestine to create a new pathway around the blocked area.

- Endoscopic stent placement: If the tumor is blocking the bile duct, surgery may be done to put in a stent (a thin tube) to drain bile that has built up in the area. The doctor may place the stent through a catheter that drains to the outside of the body or the stent may go around the blocked area and drain the bile into the small intestine.

- Gastric bypass: If the tumor is blocking the flow of food from the stomach, the stomach may be sewn directly to the small intestine so the patient can continue to eat normally.

Radiation therapy

Radiation therapy is a cancer treatment that uses high-energy x-rays or other types of radiation to kill cancer cells or keep them from growing. There are two types of radiation therapy. External radiation therapy uses a machine outside the body to send radiation toward the cancer. Internal radiation therapy uses a radioactive substance sealed in needles, seeds, wires, or catheters that are placed directly into or near the cancer. The way the radiation therapy is given depends on the type and stage of the cancer being treated.

Chemotherapy

Chemotherapy is a cancer treatment that uses drugs to stop the growth of cancer cells, either by killing the cells or by stopping them from dividing. When chemotherapy is taken by mouth or injected into a vein or muscle, the drugs enter the bloodstream and can reach cancer cells throughout the body (systemic chemotherapy). When chemotherapy is placed directly into the cerebrospinal fluid, an organ, or a body cavity such as the abdomen, the drugs mainly affect cancer cells in those areas (regional chemotherapy). Combination chemotherapy is treatment using more than one anticancer drug. The way the chemotherapy is given depends on the type and stage of the cancer being treated.

Chemoradiation therapy

Chemoradiation therapy combines chemotherapy and radiation therapy to increase the effects of both.

Targeted therapy

Targeted therapy is a type of treatment that uses drugs or other substances to identify and attack specific cancer cells without harming normal cells. Tyrosine kinase inhibitors (TKIs) are targeted therapy drugs that block signals needed for tumors to grow. Erlotinib is a type of TKI used to treat pancreatic cancer.

There are treatments for pain caused by pancreatic cancer.

Pain can occur when the tumor presses on nerves or other organs near the pancreas. When pain medicine is not enough, there are treatments that act on nerves in the abdomen to relieve the pain. The doctor may inject medicine into the area around affected nerves or may cut the nerves to block the feeling of pain. Radiation therapy with or without chemotherapy can also help relieve pain by shrinking the tumor.

Patients with pancreatic cancer have special nutritional needs.

Surgery to remove the pancreas may affect its ability to make pancreatic enzymes that help to digest food. As a result, patients may have problems digesting food and absorbing nutrients into the body. To prevent malnutrition, the doctor may prescribe medicines that replace these enzymes.

New types of treatment are being tested in clinical trials.

Biologic therapy

Biologic therapy is a treatment that uses the patient's immune system to fight cancer. Substances made by the body or made in a laboratory are used to boost, direct, or restore the body's natural defenses against cancer. This type of cancer treatment is also called biotherapy or immunotherapy.

Patients may want to think about taking part in a clinical trial.

For some patients, taking part in a clinical trial may be the best treatment choice. Clinical trials are part of the cancer research process. Clinical trials are done to find out if new cancer treatments are safe and effective or better than the standard treatment.

Many of today's standard treatments for cancer are based on earlier clinical trials. Patients who take part in a clinical trial may receive the standard treatment or be among the first to receive a new treatment.

Patients who take part in clinical trials also help improve the way cancer will be treated in the future. Even when clinical trials do not lead to effective new treatments, they often answer important questions and help move research forward.

Patients can enter clinical trials before, during, or after starting their cancer treatment.

Some clinical trials only include patients who have not yet received treatment. Other trials test treatments for patients whose cancer has not gotten better. There are also clinical trials that test new ways to stop cancer from recurring (coming back) or reduce the side effects of cancer treatment.

Clinical trials are taking place in many parts of the country.

Follow-up tests may be needed

Some of the tests that were done to diagnose the cancer or to find out the stage of the cancer may be repeated. Some tests will be repeated in order to see how well the treatment is working. Decisions about whether to continue, change, or stop treatment may be based on the results of these tests.

Some of the tests will continue to be done from time to time after treatment has ended. The results of these tests can show if your condition has changed or if the cancer has recurred (come back). These tests are sometimes called follow-up tests or check-ups.

Section 23.7

Pancreatic Neuroendocrine Tumors (Islet Cell Tumors)

Text in this section is excerpted from "Pancreatic Neuroendocrine Tumors (Islet Cell Tumors) Treatment," National Cancer Institute at the National Institutes of Health (NIH), March 4, 2015.

General Information About Pancreatic Neuroendocrine Tumors (Islet Cell Tumors)

Pancreatic neuroendocrine tumors form in hormone-making cells (islet cells) of the pancreas.

The pancreas is a gland about 6 inches long that is shaped like a thin pear lying on its side. The wider end of the pancreas is called the head, the middle section is called the body, and the narrow end is called the tail. The pancreas lies behind the stomach and in front of the spine.

There are two kinds of cells in the pancreas:

- **Endocrine pancreas cells** make several kinds of hormones (chemicals that control the actions of certain cells or organs in the body), such as insulin to control blood sugar. They cluster together in many small groups (islets) throughout the pancreas. Endocrine pancreas cells are also called islet cells or islets of Langerhans. Tumors that form in islet cells are called islet cell tumors, pancreatic endocrine tumors, or pancreatic neuroendocrine tumors (pancreatic NETs).

- **Exocrine pancreas cells** make enzymes that are released into the small intestine to help the body digest food. Most of the pancreas is made of ducts with small sacs at the end of the ducts, which are lined with exocrine cells.

Pancreatic neuroendocrine tumors (NETs) may be benign (not cancer) or malignant (cancer). When pancreatic NETs are malignant, they are called pancreatic endocrine cancer or islet cell carcinoma.

Pancreatic NETs are much less common than pancreatic exocrine tumors and have a better prognosis.

Pancreatic NETs may or may not cause signs or symptoms.

Pancreatic NETs may be functional or nonfunctional:

- Functional tumors make extra amounts of hormones, such as gastrin, insulin, and glucagon, that cause signs and symptoms.

- Nonfunctional tumors do not make extra amounts of hormones. Signs and symptoms are caused by the tumor as it spreads and grows. Most nonfunctional tumors are malignant (cancer).

Most pancreatic NETs are functional tumors.

There are different kinds of functional pancreatic NETs.

Pancreatic NETs make different kinds of hormones such as gastrin, insulin, and glucagon. Functional pancreatic NETs include the following:

- **Gastrinoma:** A tumor that forms in cells that make gastrin. Gastrin is a hormone that causes the stomach to release an acid that helps digest food. Both gastrin and stomach acid are increased by gastrinomas. When increased stomach acid, stomach ulcers, and diarrhea are caused by a tumor that makes gastrin, it is called Zollinger-Ellison syndrome. A gastrinoma usually forms in the head of the pancreas and sometimes forms in the small intestine. Most gastrinomas are malignant (cancer).

- **Insulinoma:** A tumor that forms in cells that make insulin. Insulin is a hormone that controls the amount of glucose (sugar) in the blood. It moves glucose into the cells, where it can be used by the body for energy. Insulinomas are usually slow-growing tumors that rarely spread. An insulinoma forms in the head, body, or tail of the pancreas. Insulinomas are usually benign (not cancer).

- **Glucagonoma:** A tumor that forms in cells that make glucagon. Glucagon is a hormone that increases the amount of glucose in the blood. It causes the liver to break down glycogen. Too much glucagon causes hyperglycemia (high blood sugar). A glucagonoma usually forms in the tail of the pancreas. Most glucagonomas are malignant (cancer).

371

- **Other types of tumors**: There are other rare types of functional pancreatic NETs that make hormones, including hormones that control the balance of sugar, salt, and water in the body. These tumors include:
  - VIPomas, which make vasoactive intestinal peptide. VIPoma may also be called Verner-Morrison syndrome.
  - Somatostatinomas, which make somatostatin.

These other types of tumors are grouped together because they are treated in much the same way.

Having certain syndromes can increase the risk of pancreatic NETs.

Anything that increases your risk of getting a disease is called a risk factor. Having a risk factor does not mean that you will get cancer; not having risk factors doesn't mean that you will not get cancer. Talk with your doctor if you think you may be at risk.

Multiple endocrine neoplasia type 1 (MEN1) syndrome is a risk factor for pancreatic NETs.

Different types of pancreatic NETs have different signs and symptoms.

Signs or symptoms can be caused by the growth of the tumor and/or by hormones the tumor makes or by other conditions. Some tumors may not cause signs or symptoms. Check with your doctor if you have any of these problems.

Signs and symptoms of a non-functional pancreatic NET

A non-functional pancreatic NET may grow for a long time without causing signs or symptoms. It may grow large or spread to other parts of the body before it causes signs or symptoms, such as:

- Diarrhea.
- Indigestion.
- A lump in the abdomen.
- Pain in the abdomen or back.
- Yellowing of the skin and whites of the eyes.

Signs and symptoms of a functional pancreatic NET

The signs and symptoms of a functional pancreatic NET depend on the type of hormone being made.

Too much gastrin may cause:

- Stomach ulcers that keep coming back.

- Pain in the abdomen, which may spread to the back. The pain may come and go and it may go away after taking an antacid.

- The flow of stomach contents back into the esophagus (gastro-esophageal reflux).

- Diarrhea.

Too much insulin may cause:

- Low blood sugar. This can cause blurred vision, headache, and feeling lightheaded, tired, weak, shaky, nervous, irritable, sweaty, confused, or hungry.

- Fast heartbeat.

Too much glucagon may cause:

- Skin rash on the face, stomach, or legs.

- High blood sugar. This can cause headaches, frequent urination, dry skin and mouth, or feeling hungry, thirsty, tired, or weak.

- Blood clots. Blood clots in the lung can cause shortness of breath, cough, or pain in the chest. Blood clots in the arm or leg can cause pain, swelling, warmth, or redness of the arm or leg.

- Diarrhea.

- Weight loss for no known reason.

- Sore tongue or sores at the corners of the mouth.

Too much vasoactive intestinal peptide (VIP) may cause:

- Very large amounts of watery diarrhea.

- Dehydration. This can cause feeling thirsty, making less urine, dry skin and mouth, headaches, dizziness, or feeling tired.

- Low potassium level in the blood. This can cause muscle weakness, aching, or cramps, numbness and tingling, frequent urination, fast heartbeat, and feeling confused or thirsty.

- Cramps or pain in the abdomen.
- Weight loss for no known reason.

Too much somatostatin may cause:

- High blood sugar. This can cause headaches, frequent urination, dry skin and mouth, or feeling hungry, thirsty, tired, or weak.
- Diarrhea.
- Steatorrhea (very foul-smelling stool that floats).
- Gallstones.
- Yellowing of the skin and whites of the eyes.
- Weight loss for no known reason.

Lab tests and imaging tests are used to detect (find) and diagnose pancreatic NETs.

The following tests and procedures may be used:

- **Physical exam and history:** An exam of the body to check general signs of health, including checking for signs of disease, such as lumps or anything else that seems unusual. A history of the patient's health habits and past illnesses and treatments will also be taken.
- **Blood chemistry studies:** A procedure in which a blood sample is checked to measure the amounts of certain substances, such as glucose (sugar), released into the blood by organs and tissues in the body. An unusual (higher or lower than normal) amount of a substance can be a sign of disease in the organ or tissue that makes it.
- **Chromogranin A test**: A test in which a blood sample is checked to measure the amount of chromogranin A in the blood. A higher than normal amount of chromogranin A and normal amounts of hormones such as gastrin, insulin, and glucagon can be a sign of a non-functional pancreatic NET.
- **Abdominal CT scan (CAT scan)**: A procedure that makes a series of detailed pictures of the abdomen, taken from different angles. The pictures are made by a computer linked to an x-ray machine. A dye may be injected into a vein or swallowed to help the organs or tissues show up more clearly. This procedure is

also called computed tomography, computerized tomography, or computerized axial tomography.

- **MRI (magnetic resonance imaging)**: A procedure that uses a magnet, radio waves, and a computer to make a series of detailed pictures of areas inside the body. This procedure is also called nuclear magnetic resonance imaging (NMRI).

- **Somatostatin receptor scintigraphy:** A type of radionuclide scan that may be used to find small pancreatic NETs. A small amount of radioactive octreotide (a hormone that attaches to tumors) is injected into a vein and travels through the blood. The radioactive octreotide attaches to the tumor and a special camera that detects radioactivity is used to show where the tumors are in the body. This procedure is also called octreotide scan and SRS.

- **Endoscopic ultrasound (EUS)**: A procedure in which an endoscope is inserted into the body, usually through the mouth or rectum. An endoscope is a thin, tube-like instrument with a light and a lens for viewing. A probe at the end of the endoscope is used to bounce high-energy sound waves (ultrasound) off internal tissues or organs and make echoes. The echoes form a picture of body tissues called a sonogram. This procedure is also called endosonography.

- **Endoscopic retrograde cholangiopancreatography (ERCP)**: A procedure used to x-ray the ducts (tubes) that carry bile from the liver to the gallbladder and from the gallbladder to the small intestine. Sometimes pancreatic cancer causes these ducts to narrow and block or slow the flow of bile, causing jaundice. An endoscope is passed through the mouth, esophagus, and stomach into the first part of the small intestine. An endoscope is a thin, tube-like instrument with a light and a lens for viewing. A catheter (a smaller tube) is then inserted through the endoscope into the pancreatic ducts. A dye is injected through the catheter into the ducts and an x-ray is taken. If the ducts are blocked by a tumor, a fine tube may be inserted into the duct to unblock it. This tube (or stent) may be left in place to keep the duct open. Tissue samples may also be taken and checked under a microscope for signs of cancer.

- **Angiogram:** A procedure to look at blood vessels and the flow of blood. A contrast dye is injected into the blood vessel. As the contrast dye moves through the blood vessel, x-rays are taken to see if there are any blockages.

375

- **Laparotomy:** A surgical procedure in which an incision (cut) is made in the wall of the abdomen to check the inside of the abdomen for signs of disease. The size of the incision depends on the reason the laparotomy is being done. Sometimes organs are removed or tissue samples are taken and checked under a microscope for signs of disease.

- **Intraoperative ultrasound:** A procedure that uses high-energy sound waves (ultrasound) to create images of internal organs or tissues during surgery. A transducer placed directly on the organ or tissue is used to make the sound waves, which create echoes. The transducer receives the echoes and sends them to a computer, which uses the echoes to make pictures called sonograms.

- **Biopsy:** The removal of cells or tissues so they can be viewed under a microscope by a pathologist to check for signs of cancer. There are several ways to do a biopsy for pancreatic NETs. Cells may be removed using a fine or wide needle inserted into the pancreas during an x-ray or ultrasound. Tissue may also be removed during alaparoscopy (a surgical incision made in the wall of the abdomen).

- **Bone scan:** A procedure to check if there are rapidly dividing cells, such as cancer cells, in the bone. A very small amount of radioactive material is injected into a vein and travels through the blood. The radioactive material collects in bones where cancer cells have spread and is detected by a scanner.

Other kinds of lab tests are used to check for the specific type of pancreatic NETs.

The following tests and procedures may be used:

Gastrinoma

- **Fasting serum gastrin test:** A test in which a blood sample is checked to measure the amount of gastrin in the blood. This test is done after the patient has had nothing to eat or drink for at least 8 hours. Conditions other than gastrinoma can cause an increase in the amount of gastrin in the blood.

- **Basal acid output test:** A test to measure the amount of acid made by the stomach. The test is done after the patient has had nothing to eat or drink for at least 8 hours. A tube is inserted through the nose or throat, into the stomach. The stomach contents are removed and four samples of gastric acid are removed through the tube. These samples are used to find out the amount of gastric acid made during the test and the pH level of the gastric secretions.

- **Secretin stimulation test:** If the basal acid output test result is not normal, a secretin stimulation test may be done. The tube is moved into the small intestine and samples are taken from the small intestine after a drug called secretin is injected. Secretin causes the small intestine to make acid. When there is a gastrinoma, the secretin causes an increase in how much gastric acid is made and the level of gastrin in the blood.

- **Somatostatin receptor scintigraphy**: A type of radionuclide scan that may be used to find small pancreatic NETs. A small amount of radioactive octreotide (a hormone that attaches to tumors) is injected into a vein and travels through the blood. The radioactive octreotide attaches to the tumor and a special camera that detects radioactivity is used to show where the tumors are in the body. This procedure is also called octreotide scan and SRS.

Insulinoma

- **Fasting serum glucose and insulin test**: A test in which a blood sample is checked to measure the amounts of glucose (sugar) and insulin in the blood. The test is done after the patient has had nothing to eat or drink for at least 24 hours.

Glucagonoma

Fasting serum glucagon test: A test in which a blood sample is checked to measure the amount of glucagon in the blood. The test is done after the patient has had nothing to eat or drink for at least 8 hours.

Other tumor types

- VIPoma

  - **Serum VIP (vasoactive intestinal peptide) test**: A test in which a blood sample is checked to measure the amount of VIP.

  - **Blood chemistry studies**: A procedure in which a blood sample is checked to measure the amounts of certain substances released into the blood by organs and tissues in the body. An unusual (higher or lower than normal) amount of a substance can be a sign of disease in the organ or tissue that makes it. In VIPoma, there is a lower than normal amount of potassium.

- **Stool analysis:** A stool sample is checked for a higher than normal sodium (salt) and potassium levels.

- Somatostatinoma

  - **Fasting serum somatostatin test**: A test in which a blood sample is checked to measure the amount of somatostatin in the blood. The test is done after the patient has had nothing to eat or drink for at least 8 hours.

  - **Somatostatin receptor scintigraphy**: A type of radionuclide scan that may be used to find small pancreatic NETs. A small amount of radioactive octreotide (a hormone that attaches to tumors) is injected into a vein and travels through the blood. The radioactive octreotide attaches to the tumor and a special camera that detects radioactivity is used to show where the tumors are in the body. This procedure is also called octreotide scan and SRS.

Certain factors affect prognosis (chance of recovery) and treatment options.

Pancreatic NETs can often be cured. The prognosis (chance of recovery) and treatment options depend on the following:

- The type of cancer cell.

- Where the tumor is found in the pancreas.

- Whether the tumor has spread to more than one place in the pancreas or to other parts of the body.

- Whether the patient has MEN1 syndrome.

- The patient's age and general health.

- Whether the cancer has just been diagnosed or has recurred (come back).

Stages of Pancreatic Neuroendocrine Tumors

The plan for cancer treatment depends on where the NET is found in the pancreas and whether it has spread.

The process used to find out if cancer has spread within the pancreas or to other parts of the body is called staging. The results of the tests and procedures used to diagnose pancreatic neuroendocrine tumors (NETs) are also used to find out whether the cancer has spread.

Although there is a standard staging system for pancreatic NETs, it is not used to plan treatment. Treatment of pancreatic NETs is based on the following:

- Whether the cancer is found in one place in the pancreas.
- Whether the cancer is found in several places in the pancreas.
- Whether the cancer has spread to lymph nodes near the pancreas or to other parts of the body such as the liver, lung, peritoneum, or bone.

There are three ways that cancer spreads in the body.

Cancer can spread through tissue, the lymph system, and the blood:

- Tissue. The cancer spreads from where it began by growing into nearby areas.
- Lymph system. The cancer spreads from where it began by getting into the lymph system. The cancer travels through the lymph vessels to other parts of the body.
- Blood. The cancer spreads from where it began by getting into the blood. The cancer travels through the blood vessels to other parts of the body.

Cancer may spread from where it began to other parts of the body.

When cancer spreads to another part of the body, it is called metastasis. Cancer cells break away from where they began (the primary tumor) and travel through the lymph system or blood.

- Lymph system. The cancer gets into the lymph system, travels through the lymph vessels, and forms a tumor (metastatic tumor) in another part of the body.
- Blood. The cancer gets into the blood, travels through the blood vessels, and forms a tumor (metastatic tumor) in another part of the body.

The metastatic tumor is the same type of tumor as the primary tumor. For example, if a pancreatic neuroendocrine tumor spreads to the liver, the tumor cells in the liver are actually neuroendocrine tumor cells. The disease is metastatic pancreatic neuroendocrine tumor, not liver cancer.

Treatment Option Overview

There are different types of treatment for patients with pancreatic NETs.

Different types of treatments are available for patients with pancreatic neuroendocrine tumors (NETs). Some treatments are standard (the currently used treatment), and some are being tested in clinical trials. A treatment clinical trial is a research study meant to help improve current treatments or obtain information on new treatments for patients with cancer. When clinical trials show that a new treatment is better than the standard treatment, the new treatment may become the standard treatment. Patients may want to think about taking part in a clinical trial. Some clinical trials are open only to patients who have not started treatment.

Six types of standard treatment are used:

Surgery

An operation may be done to remove the tumor. One of the following types of surgery may be used:

- Enucleation: Surgery to remove the tumor only. This may be done when cancer occurs in one place in the pancreas.

- Pancreatoduodenectomy: A surgical procedure in which the head of the pancreas, the gallbladder, nearby lymph nodes and part of the stomach, small intestine, and bile duct are removed. Enough of the pancreas is left to make digestive juices and insulin. The organs removed during this procedure depend on the patient's condition. This is also called the Whipple procedure.

- Distal pancreatectomy: Surgery to remove the body and tail of the pancreas. The spleen may also be removed.

- Total gastrectomy: Surgery to remove the whole stomach.

- Parietal cell vagotomy: Surgery to cut the nerve that causes stomach cells to make acid.

- Liver resection: Surgery to remove part or all of the liver.

- Radiofrequency ablation: The use of a special probe with tiny electrodes that kill cancer cells. Sometimes the probe is inserted directly through the skin and only local anesthesia is needed. In other cases, the probe is inserted through an incision in the abdomen. This is done in the hospital with general anesthesia.

- Cryosurgical ablation: A procedure in which tissue is frozen to destroy abnormal cells. This is usually done with a special instrument that contains liquid nitrogen or liquid carbon dioxide. The instrument may be used during surgery or laparoscopy or inserted through the skin. This procedure is also called cryoablation.

Chemotherapy

Chemotherapy is a cancer treatment that uses drugs to stop the growth of cancer cells, either by killing the cells or by stopping them from dividing. When chemotherapy is taken by mouth or injected into a vein or muscle, the drugs enter the bloodstream and can reach cancer cells throughout the body (systemic chemotherapy). When chemotherapy is placed directly into the cerebrospinal fluid, an organ, or a body cavity such as the abdomen, the drugs mainly affect cancer cells in those areas (regional chemotherapy). Combination chemotherapy is the use of more than one anticancer drug. The way the chemotherapy is given depends on the type of the cancer being treated.

Hormone therapy

Hormone therapy is a cancer treatment that removes hormones or blocks their action and stops cancer cells from growing. Hormones are substances made by glands in the body and circulated in the bloodstream. Some hormones can cause certain cancers to grow. If tests show that the cancer cells have places where hormones can attach (receptors), drugs, surgery, or radiation therapy is used to reduce the production of hormones or block them from working.

Hepatic arterial occlusion or chemoembolization

Hepatic arterial occlusion uses drugs, small particles, or other agents to block or reduce the flow of blood to the liver through the hepatic artery (the major blood vessel that carries blood to the liver). This is done to kill cancer cells growing in the liver. The tumor is prevented from getting the oxygen and nutrients it needs to grow. The liver continues to receive blood from the hepatic portal vein, which carries blood from the stomach and intestine.

Chemotherapy delivered during hepatic arterial occlusion is called chemoembolization. The anticancer drug is injected into the hepatic artery through a catheter (thin tube). The drug is mixed with the substance that blocks the artery and cuts off blood flow to the tumor. Most of the anticancer drug is trapped near the tumor and only a small amount of the drug reaches other parts of the body.

The blockage may be temporary or permanent, depending on the substance used to block the artery.

Targeted therapy

Targeted therapy is a type of treatment that uses drugs or other substances to identify and attack specific cancer cells without harming normal cells. Certain types of targeted therapies are being studied in the treatment of pancreatic NETs.

Supportive care

Supportive care is given to lessen the problems caused by the disease or its treatment. Supportive care for pancreatic NETs may include treatment for the following:

- Stomach ulcers may be treated with drug therapy such as:
  - Proton pump inhibitor drugs such as omeprazole, lansoprazole, or pantoprazole.
  - Histamine blocking drugs such as cimetidine, ranitidine, or famotidine.
  - Somatostatin-type drugs such as octreotide.
- Diarrhea may be treated with:
  - Intravenous (IV) fluids with electrolytes such as potassium or chloride.
  - Somatostatin-type drugs such as octreotide.
- Low blood sugar may be treated by having small, frequent meals or with drug therapy to maintain a normal blood sugar level.
- High blood sugar may be treated with drugs taken by mouth or insulin by injection.

Patients may want to think about taking part in a clinical trial.

For some patients, taking part in a clinical trial may be the best treatment choice. Clinical trials are part of the cancer research process. Clinical trials are done to find out if new cancer treatments are safe and effective or better than the standard treatment.

Many of today's standard treatments for cancer are based on earlier clinical trials. Patients who take part in a clinical trial may receive the standard treatment or be among the first to receive a new treatment.

Patients who take part in clinical trials also help improve the way cancer will be treated in the future. Even when clinical trials do not lead to effective new treatments, they often answer important questions and help move research forward.

Patients can enter clinical trials before, during, or after starting their cancer treatment.

Some clinical trials only include patients who have not yet received treatment. Other trials test treatments for patients whose cancer has not gotten better. There are also clinical trials that test new ways to stop cancer from recurring (coming back) or reduce the side effects of cancer treatment.

Clinical trials are taking place in many parts of the country.

Follow-up tests may be needed.

Some of the tests that were done to diagnose the cancer or to find out the stage of the cancer may be repeated. Some tests will be repeated in order to see how well the treatment is working. Decisions about whether to continue, change, or stop treatment may be based on the results of these tests.

Some of the tests will continue to be done from time to time after treatment has ended. The results of these tests can show if your condition has changed or if the cancer has recurred (come back). These tests are sometimes called follow-up tests or check-ups.

Treatment Options for Pancreatic Neuroendocrine Tumors

Gastrinoma

Treatment of gastrinoma may include supportive care and the following:

- For symptoms caused by too much stomach acid, treatment may be a drug that decreases the amount of acid made by the stomach.

- For a single tumor in the head of the pancreas:

  - Surgery to remove the tumor.

  - Surgery to cut the nerve that causes stomach cells to make acid and treatment with a drug that decreases stomach acid.

  - Surgery to remove the whole stomach (rare).

- For a single tumor in the body or tail of the pancreas, treatment is usually surgery to remove the body or tail of the pancreas.

- For several tumors in the pancreas, treatment is usually surgery to remove the body or tail of the pancreas. If tumor remains after surgery, treatment may include either:

  - Surgery to cut the nerve that causes stomach cells to make acid and treatment with a drug that decreases stomach acid; or

  - Surgery to remove the whole stomach (rare).

- For one or more tumors in the duodenum (the part of the small intestine that connects to the stomach), treatment is usually pancreatoduodenectomy (surgery to remove the head of the pancreas, the gallbladder, nearby lymph nodes and part of the stomach, small intestine, and bile duct).

- If no tumor is found, treatment may include the following:

  - Surgery to cut the nerve that causes stomach cells to make acid and treatment with a drug that decreases stomach acid.

  - Surgery to remove the whole stomach (rare).

- If the cancer has spread to the liver, treatment may include:

  - Surgery to remove part or all of the liver.

  - Radiofrequency ablation or cryosurgical ablation.

  - Chemoembolization.

- If cancer has spread to other parts of the body or does not get better with surgery or drugs to decrease stomach acid, treatment may include:

  - Chemotherapy.

  - Hormone therapy.

- If the cancer mostly affects the liver and the patient has severe symptoms from hormones or from the size of tumor, treatment may include:

  - Hepatic arterial occlusion, with or without systemic chemotherapy.

  - Chemoembolization, with or without systemic chemotherapy.

Insulinoma

Treatment of insulinoma may include the following:

- For one small tumor in the head or tail of the pancreas, treatment is usually surgery to remove the tumor.

- For one large tumor in the head of the pancreas that cannot be removed by surgery, treatment is usually pancreatoduodenectomy (surgery to remove the head of the pancreas, the gallbladder, nearby lymph nodes and part of the stomach, small intestine, and bile duct).

- For one large tumor in the body or tail of the pancreas, treatment is usually a distal pancreatectomy (surgery to remove the body and tail of the pancreas).

- For more than one tumor in the pancreas, treatment is usually surgery to remove any tumors in the head of the pancreas and the body and tail of the pancreas.

- For tumors that cannot be removed by surgery, treatment may include the following:

  - Combination chemotherapy.

  - Palliative drug therapy to decrease the amount of insulin made by the pancreas.

  - Hormone therapy.

  - Radiofrequency ablation or cryosurgical ablation.

- For cancer that has spread to lymph nodes or other parts of the body, treatment may include the following:

- Surgery to remove the cancer.

- Radiofrequency ablation or cryosurgical ablation, if the cancer cannot be removed by surgery.

- If the cancer mostly affects the liver and the patient has severe symptoms from hormones or from the size of tumor, treatment may include:

  - Hepatic arterial occlusion, with or without systemic chemotherapy.

  - Chemoembolization, with or without systemic chemotherapy.

Glucagonoma

Treatment may include the following:

- For one small tumor in the head or tail of the pancreas, treatment is usually surgery to remove the tumor.

- For one large tumor in the head of the pancreas that cannot be removed by surgery, treatment is usually pancreatoduo-denectomy (surgery to remove the head of the pancreas, the gallbladder, nearby lymph nodes and part of the stomach, small intestine, and bile duct).

- For more than one tumor in the pancreas, treatment is usually surgery to remove the tumor or surgery to remove the body and tail of the pancreas.

- For tumors that cannot be removed by surgery, treatment may include the following:

  - Combination chemotherapy.

  - Hormone therapy.

  - Radiofrequency ablation or cryosurgical ablation.

- For cancer that has spread to lymph nodes or other parts of the body, treatment may include the following:

  - Surgery to remove the cancer.

  - Radiofrequency ablation or cryosurgical ablation, if the cancer cannot be removed by surgery.

- If the cancer mostly affects the liver and the patient has severe symptoms from hormones or from the size of tumor, treatment may include:

  - Hepatic arterial occlusion, with or without systemic chemotherapy.

  - Chemoembolization, with or without systemic chemotherapy.

Other Pancreatic Neuroendocrine Tumors (Islet Cell Tumors)

For VIPoma, treatment may include the following:

- Fluids and hormone therapy to replace fluids and electrolytes that have been lost from the body.
- Surgery to remove the tumor and nearby lymph nodes.
- Surgery to remove as much of the tumor as possible when the tumor cannot be completely removed or has spread to distant parts of the body. This is palliative therapy to relieve symptoms and improve the quality of life.
- For tumors that have spread to lymph nodes or other parts of the body, treatment may include the following:
  - Surgery to remove the tumor.
  - Radiofrequency ablation or cryosurgical ablation, if the tumor cannot be removed by surgery.
- For tumors that continue to grow during treatment or have spread to other parts of the body, treatment may include the following:
  - Chemotherapy.
  - Targeted therapy.

For somatostatinoma, treatment may include the following:

- Surgery to remove the tumor.
- For cancer that has spread to distant parts of the body, surgery to remove as much of the cancer as possible to relieve symptoms and improve quality of life.
- For tumors that continue to grow during treatment or have spread to other parts of the body, treatment may include the following:
  - Chemotherapy.
  - Targeted therapy.

Treatment of other types of pancreatic neuroendocrine tumors (NETs) may include the following:

- Surgery to remove the tumor.
- For cancer that has spread to distant parts of the body, surgery to remove as much of the cancer as possible or hormone therapy to relieve symptoms and improve quality of life.

- For tumors that continue to grow during treatment or have spread to other parts of the body, treatment may include the following:
- Chemotherapy.
- Targeted therapy.

Recurrent or Progressive Pancreatic Neuroendocrine Tumors (Islet Cell Tumors)

Treatment of pancreatic neuroendocrine tumors (NETs) that continue to grow during treatment or recur (come back) may include the following:

- Surgery to remove the tumor.
- Chemotherapy.
- Hormone therapy.
- Targeted therapy.
- For liver metastases:
  - Regional chemotherapy.
  - Hepatic arterial occlusion or chemoembolization, with or without systemic chemotherapy.
- A clinical trial of a new therapy.

Section 23.8

Small Intestine Cancer

Text in this section is excerpted from "Small Intestine Cancer
Treatment," National Cancer Institute at the National Institutes of
Health (NIH), October 24, 2013.

General Information About Small Intestine Cancer

*Small intestine cancer is a rare disease in which malignant
(cancer) cells form in the tissues of the small intestine.*

The small intestine is part of the body's digestive system, which
also includes the esophagus, stomach, and large intestine. The digestive system removes and processes nutrients (vitamins, minerals,
carbohydrates, fats, proteins, and water) from foods and helps pass
waste material out of the body. The small intestine is a long tube that
connects the stomach to the large intestine. It folds many times to fit
inside the abdomen.

There are five types of small intestine cancer.

The types of cancer found in the small intestine are adenocarcinoma, sarcoma, carcinoid tumors, gastrointestinal stromal tumor, and
lymphoma.

Adenocarcinoma starts in glandular cells in the lining of the small
intestine and is the most common type of small intestine cancer. Most
of these tumors occur in the part of the small intestine near the stomach. They may grow and block the intestine.

Leiomyosarcoma starts in the smooth muscle cells of the small
intestine. Most of these tumors occur in the part of the small intestine
near the large intestine.

*Diet and health history can affect the risk of developing
small intestine cancer.*

Anything that increases your risk of getting a disease is called a
risk factor. Having a risk factor does not mean that you will get cancer;

not having risk factors doesn't mean that you will not get cancer. Talk with your doctor if you think you may be at risk.

Risk factors for small intestine cancer include the following:

- Eating a high-fat diet.
- Having Crohn disease.
- Having celiac disease.
- Having familial adenomatous polyposis (FAP).

Signs and symptoms of small intestine cancer include unexplained weight loss and abdominal pain.

These and other signs and symptoms may be caused by small intestine cancer or by other conditions. Check with your doctor if you have any of the following:

- Pain or cramps in the middle of the abdomen.
- Weight loss with no known reason.
- A lump in the abdomen.
- Blood in the stool.

Tests that examine the small intestine are used to detect (find), diagnose, and stage small intestine cancer.

Procedures that make pictures of the small intestine and the area around it help diagnose small intestine cancer and show how far the cancer has spread. The process used to find out if cancer cells have spread within and around the small intestine is called staging.

In order to plan treatment, it is important to know the type of small intestine cancer and whether the tumor can be removed by surgery. Tests and procedures to detect, diagnose, and stage small intestine cancer are usually done at the same time.

The following tests and procedures may be used:

- **Physical exam and history:** An exam of the body to check general signs of health, including checking for signs of disease, such as lumps or anything else that seems unusual. A history of the patient's health habits and past illnesses and treatments will also be taken.

- **Blood chemistry studies:** A procedure in which a blood sample is checked to measure the amounts of certain substances released into the blood by organs and tissues in the body. An unusual (higher or lower than normal) amount of a substance can be a sign of disease in the organ or tissue that produces it.

- **Liver function tests:** A procedure in which a blood sample is checked to measure the amounts of certain substances released into the blood by the liver. A higher than normal amount of a substance can be a sign of liver disease that may be caused by small intestine cancer.

- **Endoscopy:** A procedure to look at organs and tissues inside the body to check for abnormal areas. There are different types of endoscopy:

  - **Upper endoscopy:** A procedure to look at the inside of the esophagus, stomach, and duodenum (first part of the small intestine, near the stomach). An endoscope is inserted through the mouth and into the esophagus, stomach, and duodenum. An endoscope is a thin, tube-like instrument with a light and alens for viewing. It may also have a tool to remove tissue samples, which are checked under a microscope for signs of cancer.

  - **Capsule endoscopy:** A procedure to look at the inside of the small intestine. A capsule that is about the size of a large pill and contains a light and a tiny wireless camera is swallowed by the patient. The capsule travels through the digestive tract, including the small intestine, and sends many pictures of the inside of the digestive tract to a recorder that is worn around the waist or over the shoulder. The pictures are sent from the recorder to a computer and viewed by the doctor who checks for signs of cancer. The capsule passes out of the body during a bowel movement.

  - **Double balloon endoscopy:** A procedure to look at the inside of the small intestine. A special instrument made up of two tubes (one inside the other) is inserted through the mouth or rectum and into the small intestine. The inside tube (an endoscope with a light and lens for viewing) is moved through part of the small intestine and a balloon at the end of it is inflated to keep the endoscope in place. Next, the outer tube is moved through the small intestine to reach the end of the endoscope, and a balloon at the end of the outer tube is inflated to keep it in place. Then, the balloon at the end of the endoscope is deflated and the endoscope is moved through the next part of the small intestine. These steps are repeated many times as the tubes move through the small intestine. The doctor is able to see the inside of the small intestine through the endoscope and use a tool to remove samples of abnormal tissue. The tissue samples are checked under a microscope for signs of cancer. This procedure may be done if the results of a capsule endoscopy are abnormal. This procedure is also called double balloon enteroscopy.

- **Laparotomy:** A surgical procedure in which an incision (cut) is made in the wall of the abdomen to check the inside of the abdomen for signs of disease. The size of the incision depends on the reason the laparotomy is being done. Sometimes organs or lymph nodes are removed or tissue samples are taken and checked under a microscope for signs of disease.

- **Biopsy:** The removal of cells or tissues so they can be viewed under a microscope to check for signs of cancer. This may be done during an endoscopy or laparotomy. The sample is checked by a pathologist to see if it contains cancer cells.

- **Upper GI series with small bowel follow-through**: A series of x-rays of the esophagus, stomach, and small bowel. The patient drinks a liquid that contains barium (a silver-white metallic compound). The liquid coats the esophagus, stomach, and small bowel. X-rays are taken at different times as the barium travels through the upper GI tract and small bowel.

- **CT scan (CAT scan):** A procedure that makes a series of detailed pictures of areas inside the body, taken from different angles. The pictures are made by a computer linked to an x-ray machine. A dye may be injected into a vein or swallowed to help the organs or tissues show up more clearly. This procedure is also called computed tomography, computerized tomography, or computerized axial tomography.

- **MRI (magnetic resonance imaging)**: A procedure that uses a magnet, radio waves, and a computer to make a series of detailed pictures of areas inside the body. This procedure is also called nuclear magnetic resonance imaging (NMRI).

Certain factors affect prognosis (chance of recovery) and treatment options.

- The prognosis (chance of recovery) and treatment options depend on the following:
- The type of small intestine cancer.
- Whether the cancer is in the inner lining of the small intestine only or has spread into or beyond the wall of the small intestine.
- Whether the cancer has spread to other places in the body, such as the lymph nodes, liver, or peritoneum (tissue that lines the wall of the abdomen and covers most of the organs in the abdomen).
- Whether the cancer can be completely removed by surgery.
- Whether the cancer is newly diagnosed or has recurred.

Stages of Small Intestine Cancer

Tests and procedures to stage small intestine cancer are usually done at the same time as diagnosis.

Staging is used to find out how far the cancer has spread, but treatment decisions are not based on stage.

There are three ways that cancer spreads in the body.

Cancer can spread through tissue, the lymph system, and the blood:

- Tissue. The cancer spreads from where it began by growing into nearby areas.
- Lymph system. The cancer spreads from where it began by getting into the lymph system. The cancer travels through the lymph vessels to other parts of the body.
- Blood. The cancer spreads from where it began by getting into the blood. The cancer travels through the blood vessels to other parts of the body.

Cancer may spread from where it began to other parts of the body.

When cancer spreads to another part of the body, it is called metastasis. Cancer cells break away from where they began (the primary tumor) and travel through the lymph system or blood.

- Lymph system. The cancer gets into the lymph system, travels through the lymph vessels, and forms a tumor (metastatic tumor) in another part of the body.

- Blood. The cancer gets into the blood, travels through the blood vessels, and forms a tumor (metastatic tumor) in another part of the body.

The metastatic tumor is the same type of cancer as the primary tumor. For example, if small intestine cancer spreads to the liver, the cancer cells in the liver are actually small intestine cancer cells. The disease is metastatic small intestine cancer, not liver cancer.

Small intestine cancer is grouped according to whether or not the tumor can be completely removed by surgery.

Treatment depends on whether the tumor can be removed by surgery and if the cancer is being treated as a primary tumor or is metastatic cancer.

Recurrent Small Intestine Cancer

Recurrent small intestine cancer is cancer that has recurred (come back) after it has been treated. The cancer may come back in the small intestine or in other parts of the body.

Treatment Option Overview

There are different types of treatment for patients with small intestine cancer.

Different types of treatments are available for patients with small intestine cancer. Some treatments are standard (the currently used treatment), and some are being tested in clinical trials. A treatment clinical trial is a research study meant to help improve current treatments or obtain information on new treatments for patients with cancer. When clinical trials show that a new treatment is better than the standard treatment, the new treatment may become the standard treatment. Patients may want to think about taking part in a clinical trial. Some clinical trials are open only to patients who have not started treatment.

Three types of standard treatment are used:

Surgery

Surgery is the most common treatment of small intestine cancer. One of the following types of surgery may be done:

- Resection: Surgery to remove part or all of an organ that contains cancer. The resection may include the small intestine and nearby organs (if the cancer has spread). The doctor may remove the section of the small intestine that contains cancer and perform an anastomosis (joining the cut ends of the intestine together). The doctor will usually remove lymph nodes near the small intestine and examine them under a microscope to see whether they contain cancer.

- Bypass: Surgery to allow food in the small intestine to go around (bypass) a tumor that is blocking the intestine but cannot be removed.

Even if the doctor removes all the cancer that can be seen at the time of the surgery, some patients may be given radiation therapy after surgery to kill any cancer cells that are left. Treatment given after the surgery, to lower the risk that the cancer will come back, is called adjuvant therapy.

Radiation therapy

Radiation therapy is a cancer treatment that uses high-energy x-rays or other types of radiation to kill cancer cells or keep them from growing. There are two types of radiation therapy. External radiation therapy uses a machine outside the body to send radiation toward the cancer. Internal radiation therapy uses a radioactive substance sealed in needles, seeds, wires, or catheters that are placed directly into or near the cancer. The way the radiation therapy is given depends on the type and stage of the cancer being treated.

Chemotherapy

Chemotherapy is a cancer treatment that uses drugs to stop the growth of cancer cells, either by killing the cells or by stopping them from dividing. When chemotherapy is taken by mouth or injected into a vein or muscle, the drugs enter the bloodstream and can reach cancer cells throughout the body (systemic chemotherapy). When chemotherapy is placed directly into the cerebrospinal fluid, an organ, or a body cavity such as the abdomen, the drugs mainly affect cancer cells in those areas (regional chemotherapy). The way the chemotherapy is given depends on the type and stage of the cancer being treated.

Biologic therapy

Biologic therapy is a treatment that uses the patient's immune system to fight cancer. Substances made by the body or made in a laboratory are used to boost, direct, or restore the body's natural defenses against cancer. This type of cancer treatment is also called biotherapy or immunotherapy.

Radiation therapy with radiosensitizers

Radiosensitizers are drugs that make tumor cells more sensitive to radiation therapy. Combining radiation therapy with radiosensitizers may kill more tumor cells.

Patients may want to think about taking part in a clinical trial.

For some patients, taking part in a clinical trial may be the best treatment choice. Clinical trials are part of the cancer research process. Clinical trials are done to find out if new cancer treatments are safe and effective or better than the standard treatment.

Many of today's standard treatments for cancer are based on earlier clinical trials. Patients who take part in a clinical trial may receive the standard treatment or be among the first to receive a new treatment.

Patients who take part in clinical trials also help improve the way cancer will be treated in the future. Even when clinical trials do not lead to effective new treatments, they often answer important questions and help move research forward.

Patients can enter clinical trials before, during, or after starting their cancer treatment.

Some clinical trials only include patients who have not yet received treatment. Other trials test treatments for patients whose cancer has not gotten better. There are also clinical trials that test new ways to stop cancer from recurring (coming back) or reduce the side effects of cancer treatment.

Clinical trials are taking place in many parts of the country.

Follow-up tests may be needed.

Some of the tests that were done to diagnose the cancer or to find out the stage of the cancer may be repeated. Some tests will be repeated in order to see how well the treatment is working. Decisions about whether to continue, change, or stop treatment may be based on the results of these tests.

Some of the tests will continue to be done from time to time after treatment has ended. The results of these tests can show if your condition has changed or if the cancer has recurred (come back). These tests are sometimes called follow-up tests or check-ups.

Section 23.9

Colon Cancer

Text in this section is excerpted from "Colon Cancer Treatment,"
National Cancer Institute at the National Institutes of Health (NIH),
April 2, 2015.

General Information About Colon Cancer

Colon cancer is a disease in which malignant (cancer) cells form in the tissues of the colon.

The colon is part of the body's digestive system. The digestive system removes and processes nutrients (vitamins, minerals, carbohydrates, fats, proteins, and water) from foods and helps pass waste material out of the body. The digestive system is made up of the esophagus, stomach, and the small and large intestines. The colon (large bowel) is the first part of the large intestine and is about 5 feet long. Together, the rectum and anal canal make up the last part of the large intestine and are about 6-8 inches long. The anal canal ends at the anus (the opening of the large intestine to the outside of the body).

Gastrointestinal stromal tumors can occur in the colon.

Health history can affect the risk of developing colon cancer.

Anything that increases your chance of getting a disease is called a risk factor. Having a risk factor does not mean that you will get cancer; not having risk factors doesn't mean that you will not get cancer. Talk with your doctor if you think you may be at risk.

Risk factors include the following:

- A family history of cancer of the colon or rectum.

- Certain hereditary conditions, such as familial adenomatous polyposis and hereditary nonpolyposis colon cancer (HNPCC; Lynch Syndrome).

- A history of ulcerative colitis (ulcers in the lining of the large intestine) or Crohn disease.

- A personal history of cancer of the colon, rectum, ovary, endometrium, or breast.

- A personal history of polyps (small areas of bulging tissue) in the colon or rectum.

Signs of colon cancer include blood in the stool or a change in bowel habits.

These and other signs and symptoms may be caused by colon cancer or by other conditions. Check with your doctor if you have any of the following:

- A change in bowel habits.

- Blood (either bright red or very dark) in the stool.

- Diarrhea, constipation, or feeling that the bowel does not empty all the way.

- Stools that are narrower than usual.

- Frequent gas pains, bloating, fullness, or cramps.

- Weight loss for no known reason.

- Feeling very tired.

- Vomiting.

Tests that examine the colon and rectum are used to detect (find) and diagnose colon cancer.

The following tests and procedures may be used:

- **Physical exam and history:** An exam of the body to check general signs of health, including checking for signs of disease, such as lumps or anything else that seems unusual. A history of the patient's health habits and past illnesses and treatments will also be taken.

- **Digital rectal exam:** An exam of the rectum. The doctor or nurse inserts a lubricated, gloved finger into the rectum to feel for lumps or anything else that seems unusual.

- **Fecal occult blood test:** A test to check stool (solid waste) for blood that can only be seen with a microscope. Small samples of stool are placed on special cards and returned to the doctor or laboratory for testing.

- **Barium enema:** A series of x-rays of the lower gastrointestinal tract. A liquid that contains barium (a silver-white metallic compound) is put into the rectum. The barium coats the lower gastrointestinal tract and x-rays are taken. This procedure is also called a lower GI series.

- **Sigmoidoscopy:** A procedure to look inside the rectum and sigmoid (lower) colon for polyps (small areas of bulging tissue), other abnormal areas, or cancer. A sigmoidoscope is inserted through the rectum into the sigmoid colon. A sigmoidoscope is a thin, tube-like instrument with a light and a lens for viewing. It may also have a tool to remove polyps or tissue samples, which are checked under a microscope for signs of cancer.

- **Colonoscopy:** A procedure to look inside the rectum and colon for polyps, abnormal areas, or cancer. A colonoscope is inserted through the rectum into the colon. A colonoscope is a thin, tube-like instrument with a light and a lens for viewing. It may also have a tool to remove polyps or tissue samples, which are checked under a microscope for signs of cancer.

- **Virtual colonoscopy:** A procedure that uses a series of x-rays called computed tomography to make a series of pictures of the colon. A computer puts the pictures together to create detailed images that may show polyps and anything else that seems unusual on the inside surface of the colon. This test is also called colonography or CT colonography.

- **Biopsy:** The removal of cells or tissues so they can be viewed under a microscope by a pathologist to check for signs of cancer.

Certain factors affect prognosis (chance of recovery) and treatment options.

The prognosis (chance of recovery) and treatment options depend on the following:

- The stage of the cancer (whether the cancer is in the inner lining of the colon only or has spread through the colon wall, or has spread to lymph nodes or other places in the body).
- Whether the cancer has blocked or made a hole in the colon.
- Whether there are any cancer cells left after surgery.
- Whether the cancer has recurred.
- The patient's general health.

The prognosis also depends on the blood levels of carcinoembryonic antigen (CEA) before treatment begins. CEA is a substance in the blood that may be increased when cancer is present.

Stages of Colon Cancer

After colon cancer has been diagnosed, tests are done to find out if cancer cells have spread within the colon or to other parts of the body.

The process used to find out if cancer has spread within the colon or to other parts of the body is called staging. The information gathered from the staging process determines the stage of the disease. It is important to know the stage in order to plan treatment.

The following tests and procedures may be used in the staging process:

- **CT scan (CAT scan):** A procedure that makes a series of detailed pictures of areas inside the body, such as the abdomen or chest, taken from different angles. The pictures are made by a computer linked to an x-ray machine. A dye may be injected into a vein or swallowed to help the organs or tissues show up more clearly. This procedure is also called computed tomography, computerized tomography, or computerized axial tomography.

400

- **MRI (magnetic resonance imaging)**: A procedure that uses a magnet, radio waves, and a computer to make a series of detailed pictures of areas inside the colon. A substance called gadolinium is injected into the patient through a vein. The gadolinium collects around the cancer cells so they show up brighter in the picture. This procedure is also called nuclear magnetic resonance imaging (NMRI).

- **PET scan (positron emission tomography scan)**: A procedure to find malignant tumor cells in the body. A small amount of radioactive glucose (sugar) is injected into a vein. The PET scanner rotates around the body and makes a picture of where glucose is being used in the body. Malignant tumor cells show up brighter in the picture because they are more active and take up more glucose than normal cells do.

- **Chest x-ray:** An x-ray of the organs and bones inside the chest. An x-ray is a type of energy beam that can go through the body and onto film, making a picture of areas inside the body.

- **Surgery:** A procedure to remove the tumor and see how far it has spread through the colon.

- **Lymph node biopsy:** The removal of all or part of a lymph node. A pathologist views the tissue under a microscope to look for cancer cells.

- **Complete blood count (CBC):** A procedure in which a sample of blood is drawn and checked for the following:

  - The number of red blood cells, white blood cells, and platelets.

  - The amount of hemoglobin (the protein that carries oxygen) in the red blood cells.

  - The portion of the blood sample made up of red blood cells.

- **Carcinoembryonic antigen (CEA) assay:** A test that measures the level of CEA in the blood. CEA is released into the bloodstream from both cancer cells and normal cells. When found in higher than normal amounts, it can be a sign of colon cancer or other conditions.

There are three ways that cancer spreads in the body.

Cancer can spread through tissue, the lymph system, and the blood:

- Tissue. The cancer spreads from where it began by growing into nearby areas.

- Lymph system. The cancer spreads from where it began by getting into the lymph system. The cancer travels through the lymph vessels to other parts of the body.

- Blood. The cancer spreads from where it began by getting into the blood. The cancer travels through the blood vessels to other parts of the body.

Cancer may spread from where it began to other parts of the body.

When cancer spreads to another part of the body, it is called metastasis. Cancer cells break away from where they began (the primary tumor) and travel through the lymph system or blood.

- Lymph system. The cancer gets into the lymph system, travels through the lymph vessels, and forms a tumor (metastatic tumor) in another part of the body.

- Blood. The cancer gets into the blood, travels through the blood vessels, and forms a tumor (metastatic tumor) in another part of the body.

The metastatic tumor is the same type of cancer as the primary tumor. For example, if colon cancer spreads to the lung, the cancer cells in the lung are actually colon cancer cells. The disease is metastatic colon cancer, not lung cancer.

The following stages are used for colon cancer:

Stage 0 (Carcinoma in Situ)

In stage 0, abnormal cells are found in the mucosa (innermost layer) of the colon wall. These abnormal cells may become cancer and spread. Stage 0 is also called carcinoma in situ.

Stage I

In stage I, cancer has formed in the mucosa (innermost layer) of the colon wall and has spread to the submucosa (layer of tissue under the mucosa). Cancer may have spread to the muscle layer of the colon wall.

Stage II

Stage II colon cancer is divided into stage IIA, stage IIB, and stage IIC.

- Stage IIA: Cancer has spread through the muscle layer of the colon wall to the serosa (outermost layer) of the colon wall.

- Stage IIB: Cancer has spread through the serosa (outermost layer) of the colon wall but has not spread to nearby organs.

- Stage IIC: Cancer has spread through the serosa (outermost layer) of the colon wall to nearby organs.

Stage III

Stage III colon cancer is divided into stage IIIA, stage IIIB, and stage IIIC.

In stage IIIA:

- Cancer has spread through the mucosa (innermost layer) of the colon wall to the submucosa (layer of tissue under the mucosa) and may have spread to the muscle layer of the colon wall. Cancer has spread to at least one but not more than 3 nearby lymph nodes or cancer cells have formed in tissues near the lymph nodes; or

- Cancer has spread through the mucosa (innermost layer) of the colon wall to the submucosa (layer of tissue under the mucosa). Cancer has spread to at least 4 but not more than 6 nearby lymph nodes.

In stage IIIB:

- Cancer has spread through the muscle layer of the colon wall to the serosa (outermost layer) of the colon wall or has spread through the serosa but not to nearby organs. Cancer has spread to at least one but not more than 3 nearby lymph nodes or cancer cells have formed in tissues near the lymph nodes; or

- Cancer has spread to the muscle layer of the colon wall or to the serosa (outermost layer) of the colon wall. Cancer has spread to at least 4 but not more than 6 nearby lymph nodes; or

- Cancer has spread through the mucosa (innermost layer) of the colon wall to the submucosa (layer of tissue under the mucosa) and may have spread to the muscle layer of the colon wall. Cancer has spread to 7 or more nearby lymph nodes.

In stage IIIC:

- Cancer has spread through the serosa (outermost layer) of the colon wall but has not spread to nearby organs. Cancer has spread to at least 4 but not more than 6 nearby lymph nodes; or

- Cancer has spread through the muscle layer of the colon wall to the serosa (outermost layer) of the colon wall or has spread through the serosa but has not spread to nearby organs. Cancer has spread to 7 or more nearby lymph nodes; or

- Cancer has spread through the serosa (outermost layer) of the colon wall and has spread to nearby organs. Cancer has spread to one or more nearby lymph nodes or cancer cells have formed in tissues near the lymph nodes.

Stage IV

Stage IV colon cancer is divided into stage IVA and stage IVB.

- Stage IVA: Cancer may have spread through the colon wall and may have spread to nearby organs or lymph nodes. Cancer has spread to one organ that is not near the colon, such as the liver, lung, or ovary, or to a distant lymph node.

- Stage IVB: Cancer may have spread through the colon wall and may have spread to nearby organs or lymph nodes. Cancer has spread to more than one organ that is not near the colon or into the lining of the abdominal wall.

Treatment Option Overview

There are different types of treatment for patients with colon cancer.

Different types of treatment are available for patients with colon cancer. Some treatments are standard (the currently used treatment), and some are being tested in clinical trials. A treatment clinical trial is a research study meant to help improve current treatments or obtain information on new treatments for patients with cancer. When clinical trials show that a new treatment is better than the standard treatment, the new treatment may become the standard treatment.

Patients may want to think about taking part in a clinical trial. Some clinical trials are open only to patients who have not started treatment.

Six types of standard treatment are used:

Surgery

Surgery (removing the cancer in an operation) is the most common treatment for all stages of colon cancer. A doctor may remove the cancer using one of the following types of surgery:

- Local excision: If the cancer is found at a very early stage, the doctor may remove it without cutting through the abdominal wall. Instead, the doctor may put a tube with a cutting tool through the rectum into the colon and cut the cancer out. This is called a local excision. If the cancer is found in a polyp (a small bulging area of tissue), the operation is called a polypectomy.

- Resection of the colon with anastomosis: If the cancer is larger, the doctor will perform a partial colectomy (removing the cancer and a small amount of healthy tissue around it). The doctor may then perform an anastomosis (sewing the healthy parts of the colon together). The doctor will also usually remove lymph nodes near the colon and examine them under a microscope to see whether they contain cancer.

- Resection of the colon with colostomy: If the doctor is not able to sew the 2 ends of the colon back together, a stoma (an opening) is made on the outside of the body for waste to pass through. This procedure is called a colostomy. A bag is placed around the stoma to collect the waste. Sometimes the colostomy is needed only until the lower colon has healed, and then it can be reversed. If the doctor needs to remove the entire lower colon, however, the colostomy may be permanent.

Even if the doctor removes all the cancer that can be seen at the time of the operation, some patients may be given chemotherapy or radiation therapy after surgery to kill any cancer cells that are left. Treatment given after the surgery, to lower the risk that the cancer will come back, is called adjuvant therapy.

Radiofrequency ablation

Radiofrequency ablation is the use of a special probe with tiny electrodes that kill cancer cells. Sometimes the probe is inserted directly through the skin and only local anesthesia is needed. In other cases, the probe is inserted through an incision in the abdomen. This is done in the hospital with general anesthesia.

Cryosurgery

Cryosurgery is a treatment that uses an instrument to freeze and destroy abnormal tissue. This type of treatment is also called cryotherapy.

Chemotherapy

Chemotherapy is a cancer treatment that uses drugs to stop the growth of cancer cells, either by killing the cells or by stopping them from dividing. When chemotherapy is taken by mouth or injected into a vein or muscle, the drugs enter the bloodstream and can reach cancer cells throughout the body (systemic chemotherapy). When chemotherapy is placed directly into the cerebrospinal fluid, an organ, or a body cavity such as the abdomen, the drugs mainly affect cancer cells in those areas (regional chemotherapy).

Chemoembolization of the hepatic artery may be used to treat cancer that has spread to the liver. This involves blocking the hepatic artery (the main artery that supplies blood to the liver) and injecting anticancer drugs between the blockage and the liver. The liver's arteries then deliver the drugs throughout the liver. Only a small amount of the drug reaches other parts of the body. The blockage may be temporary or permanent, depending on what is used to block the artery. The liver continues to receive some blood from the hepatic portal vein, which carries blood from the stomach and intestine.

The way the chemotherapy is given depends on the type and stage of the cancer being treated.

Radiation therapy

Radiation therapy is a cancer treatment that uses high-energy x-rays or other types of radiation to kill cancer cells or keep them from growing. There are two types of radiation therapy. External radiation therapy uses a machine outside the body to send radiation toward the cancer. Internal radiation therapy uses a radioactive substance sealed in needles, seeds, wires, or catheters that are placed directly into or near the cancer. The way the radiation therapy is given depends on the type and stage of the cancer being treated.

Targeted therapy

Targeted therapy is a type of treatment that uses drugs or other substances to identify and attack specific cancer cells without harming normal cells.

Types of targeted therapies used in the treatment of colon cancer include the following:

- Monoclonal antibodies: Monoclonal antibodies are made in the laboratory from a single type of immune system cell. These antibodies can identify substances on cancer cells or normal substances that may help cancer cells grow. The antibodies attach to the substances and kill the cancer cells, block their growth, or keep them from spreading. Monoclonal antibodies are given by infusion. They may be used alone or to carry drugs, toxins, or radioactive material directly to cancer cells.

- Angiogenesis inhibitors: Angiogenesis inhibitors stop the growth of new blood vessels that tumors need to grow.

Patients may want to think about taking part in a clinical trial.

For some patients, taking part in a clinical trial may be the best treatment choice. Clinical trials are part of the cancer research process. Clinical trials are done to find out if new cancer treatments are safe and effective or better than the standard treatment.

Many of today's standard treatments for cancer are based on earlier clinical trials. Patients who take part in a clinical trial may receive the standard treatment or be among the first to receive a new treatment.

Patients who take part in clinical trials also help improve the way cancer will be treated in the future. Even when clinical trials do not lead to effective new treatments, they often answer important questions and help move research forward.

Patients can enter clinical trials before, during, or after starting their cancer treatment.

Some clinical trials only include patients who have not yet received treatment. Other trials test treatments for patients whose cancer has not gotten better. There are also clinical trials that test new ways to stop cancer from recurring (coming back) or reduce the side effects of cancer treatment.

Clinical trials are taking place in many parts of the country.

Follow-up tests may be needed.

Some of the tests that were done to diagnose the cancer or to find out the stage of the cancer may be repeated. Some tests will be repeated in order to see how well the treatment is working. Decisions about whether to continue, change, or stop treatment may be based on the results of these tests.

Some of the tests will continue to be done from time to time after treatment has ended. The results of these tests can show if your condition has changed or if the cancer has recurred (come back). These tests are sometimes called follow-up tests or check-ups.

Section 23.10

Rectal Cancer

Text in this section is excerpted from "Rectal Cancer Treatment,"
National Cancer Institute at the National Institutes of Health (NIH),
April 2, 2015.

General Information About Rectal Cancer

Rectal cancer is a disease in which malignant (cancer) cells form in the tissues of the rectum.

The rectum is part of the body's digestive system. The digestive system takes in nutrients (vitamins, minerals, carbohydrates, fats, proteins, and water) from foods and helps pass waste material out of the body. The digestive system is made up of the esophagus, stomach, and the small and large intestines. The colon (large bowel) is the first part of the large intestine and is about 5 feet long. Together, the rectum and anal canal make up the last part of the large intestine and are 6-8 inches long. The anal canal ends at the anus (the opening of the large intestine to the outside of the body).

Age and family history can affect the risk of rectal cancer.

Anything that increases your chance of getting a disease is called a risk factor. Having a risk factor does not mean that you will get cancer; not having risk factors doesn't mean that you will not get cancer. Talk with your doctor if you think you may be at risk.

The following are possible risk factors for rectal cancer:

- Being aged 50 or older.
- Having certain hereditary conditions, such as familial adenomatous polyposis (FAP) and hereditary nonpolyposis colon cancer (HNPCC or Lynch syndrome).
- Having a personal history of any of the following:
  - Colorectal cancer.
  - Polyps (small pieces of bulging tissue) in the colon or rectum.
  - Cancer of the ovary, endometrium, or breast.
- Having a parent, brother, sister, or child with a history of colorectal cancer or polyps.

Signs of rectal cancer include a change in bowel habits or blood in the stool.

These and other signs and symptoms may be caused by rectal cancer or by other conditions. Check with your doctor if you have any of the following:

- Blood (either bright red or very dark) in the stool.
- A change in bowel habits.
  - Diarrhea.
  - Constipation.
  - Feeling that the bowel does not empty completely.
  - Stools that are narrower or have a different shape than usual.
- General abdominal discomfort (frequent gas pains, bloating, fullness, or cramps).
- Change in appetite.

- Weight loss for no known reason.

- Feeling very tired.

Tests that examine the rectum and colon are used to detect (find) and diagnose rectal cancer.

Tests used to diagnose rectal cancer include the following:

- **Physical exam and history:** An exam of the body to check general signs of health, including checking for signs of disease, such as lumps or anything else that seems unusual. A history of the patient's health habits and past illnesses and treatments will also be taken.

- **Digital rectal exam (DRE)**: An exam of the rectum. The doctor or nurse inserts a lubricated, gloved finger into the lower part of the rectum to feel for lumps or anything else that seems unusual. In women, the vagina may also be examined.

- **Colonoscopy:** A procedure to look inside the rectum and colon for polyps (small pieces of bulging tissue), abnormal areas, or cancer. A colonoscope is a thin, tube-like instrument with a light and a lens for viewing. It may also have a tool to remove polyps or tissue samples, which are checked under a microscope for signs of cancer.

- **Biopsy:** The removal of cells or tissues so they can be viewed under a microscope to check for signs of cancer. Tumor tissue that is removed during the biopsy may be checked to see if the patient is likely to have the gene mutation that causes HNPCC. This may help to plan treatment. The following tests may be used:

  - **Reverse-transcription polymerase chain reaction (RT-PCR) test**: A laboratory test in which cells in a sample of tissue are studied using chemicals to look for certain changes in the structure or function of genes.

  - **Immunohistochemistry:** A test that uses antibodies to check for certain antigens in a sample of tissue. The antibody is usually linked to a radioactive substance or a dye that causes the tissue to light up under a microscope. This type of test may be used to tell the difference between different types of cancer.

- **Carcinoembryonic antigen (CEA) assay:** A test that measures the level of CEA in the blood. CEA is released into the

410

bloodstream from both cancer cells and normal cells. When found in higher than normal amounts, it can be a sign of rectal cancer or other conditions.

Certain factors affect prognosis (chance of recovery) and treatment options.

The prognosis (chance of recovery) and treatment options depend on the following:

- The stage of the cancer (whether it affects the inner lining of the rectum only, involves the whole rectum, or has spread to lymph nodes, nearby organs, or other places in the body).

- Whether the tumor has spread into or through the bowel wall.

- Where the cancer is found in the rectum.

- Whether the bowel is blocked or has a hole in it.

- Whether all of the tumor can be removed by surgery.

- The patient's general health.

- Whether the cancer has just been diagnosed or has recurred (come back).

Stages of Rectal Cancer

After rectal cancer has been diagnosed, tests are done to find out if cancer cells have spread within the rectum or to other parts of the body.

The process used to find out whether cancer has spread within the rectum or to other parts of the body is called staging. The information gathered from the staging process determines the stage of the disease. It is important to know the stage in order to plan treatment.

The following tests and procedures may be used in the staging process:

- **Chest x-ray:** An x-ray of the organs and bones inside the chest. An x-ray is a type of energy beam that can go through the body and onto film, making a picture of areas inside the body.

- **Colonoscopy:** A procedure to look inside the rectum and colon for polyps (small pieces of bulging tissue). abnormal areas, or cancer. A colonoscope is a thin, tube-like instrument with a light and a lens for viewing. It may also have a tool to remove polyps or tissue samples, which are checked under a microscope for signs of cancer.

- **CT scan (CAT scan)**: A procedure that makes a series of detailed pictures of areas inside the body, such as the abdomen, pelvis, or chest, taken from different angles. The pictures are made by a computer linked to an x-ray machine. A dye may be injected into a vein or swallowed to help the organs or tissues show up more clearly. This procedure is also called computed tomography, computerized tomography, or computerized axial tomography.

- **MRI (magnetic resonance imaging)**: A procedure that uses a magnet, radio waves, and a computer to make a series of detailed pictures of areas inside the body. This procedure is also called nuclear magnetic resonance imaging (NMRI).

- **PET scan (positron emission tomography scan)**: A procedure to find malignant tumor cells in the body. A small amount of radioactive glucose (sugar) is injected into a vein. The PET scanner rotates around the body and makes a picture of where glucose is being used in the body. Malignant tumor cells show up brighter in the picture because they are more active and take up more glucose than normal cells do.

- **Endorectal ultrasound:** A procedure used to examine the rectum and nearby organs. An ultrasound transducer (probe) is inserted into the rectum and used to bounce high-energy sound waves (ultrasound) off internal tissues or organs and make echoes. The echoes form a picture of body tissues called a sonogram. The doctor can identify tumors by looking at the sonogram. This procedure is also called transrectal ultrasound.

There are three ways that cancer spreads in the body.

Cancer can spread through tissue, the lymph system, and the blood:

- Tissue. The cancer spreads from where it began by growing into nearby areas.

- Lymph system. The cancer spreads from where it began by getting into the lymph system. The cancer travels through the lymph vessels to other parts of the body.

- Blood. The cancer spreads from where it began by getting into the blood. The cancer travels through the blood vessels to other parts of the body.

Cancer may spread from where it began to other parts of the body.

When cancer spreads to another part of the body, it is called metastasis. Cancer cells break away from where they began (the primary tumor) and travel through the lymph system or blood.

- Lymph system. The cancer gets into the lymph system, travels through the lymph vessels, and forms a tumor (metastatic tumor) in another part of the body.

- Blood. The cancer gets into the blood, travels through the blood vessels, and forms a tumor (metastatic tumor) in another part of the body.

The metastatic tumor is the same type of cancer as the primary tumor. For example, if rectal cancer spreads to the lung, the cancer cells in the lung are actually rectal cancer cells. The disease is metastatic rectal cancer, not lung cancer.

The following stages are used for rectal cancer:

Stage 0 (Carcinoma in Situ)

In stage 0, abnormal cells are found in the mucosa (innermost layer) of the rectum wall. These abnormal cells may become cancer and spread. Stage 0 is also called carcinoma in situ.

Stage I

In stage I, cancer has formed in the mucosa (innermost layer) of the rectum wall and has spread to the submucosa (layer of tissue under the mucosa). Cancer may have spread to the muscle layer of the rectum wall.

Stage II

Stage II rectal cancer is divided into stage IIA, stage IIB, and stage IIC.

- Stage IIA: Cancer has spread through the muscle layer of the rectum wall to the serosa (outermost layer) of the rectum wall.

- Stage IIB: Cancer has spread through the serosa (outermost layer) of the rectum wall but has not spread to nearby organs.

- Stage IIC: Cancer has spread through the serosa (outermost layer) of the rectum wall to nearby organs.

Stage III

Stage III rectal cancer is divided into stage IIIA, stage IIIB, and stage IIIC.

In stage IIIA:

- Cancer has spread through the mucosa (innermost layer) of the rectum wall to the submucosa (layer of tissue under the mucosa) and may have spread to the muscle layer of the rectum wall. Cancer has spread to at least one but not more than 3 nearby lymph nodes or cancer cells have formed in tissues near the lymph nodes; or

- Cancer has spread through the mucosa (innermost layer) of the rectum wall to the submucosa (layer of tissue under the mucosa). Cancer has spread to at least 4 but not more than 6 nearby lymph nodes.

In stage IIIB:

- Cancer has spread through the muscle layer of the rectum wall to the serosa (outermost layer) of the rectum wall or has spread through the serosa but not to nearby organs. Cancer has spread to at least one but not more than 3 nearby lymph nodes or cancer cells have formed in tissues near the lymph nodes; or

- Cancer has spread to the muscle layer of the rectum wall or to the serosa (outermost layer) of the rectum wall. Cancer has spread to at least 4 but not more than 6 nearby lymph nodes; or

- Cancer has spread through the mucosa (innermost layer) of the rectum wall to the submucosa (layer of tissue under the mucosa) and may have spread to the muscle layer of the rectum wall. Cancer has spread to 7 or more nearby lymph nodes.

In stage IIIC:

- Cancer has spread through the serosa (outermost layer) of the rectum wall but has not spread to nearby organs. Cancer has spread to at least 4 but not more than 6 nearby lymph nodes; or

- Cancer has spread through the muscle layer of the rectum wall to the serosa (outermost layer) of the rectum wall or has spread

through the serosa but has not spread to nearby organs. Cancer
has spread to 7 or more nearby lymph nodes; or

- Cancer has spread through the serosa (outermost layer) of the
  rectum wall and has spread to nearby organs. Cancer has spread
  to one or more nearby lymph nodes or cancer cells have formed
  in tissues near the lymph nodes.

Stage IV

Stage IV rectal cancer is divided into stage IVA and stage IVB.

- Stage IVA: Cancer may have spread through the rectum wall
  and may have spread to nearby organs or lymph nodes. Cancer
  has spread to one organ that is not near the rectum, such as the
  liver, lung, or ovary, or to a distant lymph node.

- Stage IVB: Cancer may have spread through the rectum wall
  and may have spread to nearby organs or lymph nodes. Cancer
  has spread to more than one organ that is not near the rectum
  or into the lining of the abdominal wall.

Treatment Options Overview

*There are different types of treatment for patients with rectal
cancer.*

Different types of treatment are available for patients with rectal
cancer. Some treatments are standard (the currently used treatment),
and some are being tested in clinical trials. A treatment clinical trial is
a research study meant to help improve current treatments or obtain
information on new treatments for patients with cancer. When clinical trials show that a new treatment is better than the standard
treatment, the new treatment may become the standard treatment.
Patients may want to think about taking part in a clinical trial. Some
clinical trials are open only to patients who have not started treatment.

Four types of standard treatment are used:

Surgery

Surgery is the most common treatment for all stages of rectal cancer.
The cancer is removed using one of the following types of surgery:

- Polypectomy: If the cancer is found in a polyp (a small piece of
  bulging tissue), the polyp is often removed during a colonoscopy.

- Local excision: If the cancer is found on the inside surface of the rectum and has not spread into the wall of the rectum, the cancer and a small amount of surrounding healthy tissue is removed.

- Resection: If the cancer has spread into the wall of the rectum, the section of the rectum with cancer and nearby healthy tissue is removed. Sometimes the tissue between the rectum and the abdominal wall is also removed. The lymph nodes near the rectum are removed and checked under a microscope for signs of cancer.

- Radiofrequency ablation: The use of a special probe with tiny electrodes that kill cancer cells. Sometimes the probe is inserted directly through the skin and only local anesthesia is needed. In other cases, the probe is inserted through an incision in the abdomen. This is done in the hospital with general anesthesia.

- Cryosurgery: A treatment that uses an instrument to freeze and destroy abnormal tissue. This type of treatment is also called cryotherapy.

- Pelvic exenteration: If the cancer has spread to other organs near the rectum, the lower colon, rectum, and bladder are removed. In women, the cervix, vagina, ovaries, and nearby lymph nodes may be removed. In men, the prostate may be removed. Artificial openings (stoma) are made for urine and stool to flow from the body to a collection bag.

After the cancer is removed, the surgeon will either:

- do an anastomosis (sew the healthy parts of the rectum together, sew the remaining rectum to the colon, or sew the colon to the anus);

- make a stoma (an opening) from the rectum to the outside of the body for waste to pass through. This procedure is done if the cancer is too close to the anus and is called a colostomy. A bag is placed around the stoma to collect the waste. Sometimes the colostomy is needed only until the rectum has healed, and then it can be reversed. If the entire rectum is removed, however, the colostomy may be permanent.

Radiation therapy and/or chemotherapy may be given before surgery to shrink the tumor, make it easier to remove the cancer, and help with bowel control after surgery. Treatment given before surgery is called neoadjuvant therapy. Even if all the cancer that can be seen at the time of the operation is removed, some patients may be given radiation therapy and/or chemotherapy after surgery to kill any cancer cells that are left. Treatment given after the surgery, to lower the risk that the cancer will come back, is called adjuvant therapy.

Radiation therapy

Radiation therapy is a cancer treatment that uses high-energy x-rays or other types of radiation to kill cancer cells. There are two types of radiation therapy. External radiation therapy uses a machine outside the body to send radiation toward the cancer. Internal radiation therapy uses a radioactive substance sealed in needles, seeds, wires, or catheters that are placed directly into or near the cancer. The way the radiation therapy is given depends on the type and stage of the cancer being treated.

Short-course preoperative radiation therapy is used in some types of rectal cancer. This treatment uses fewer and lower doses of radiation than standard treatment, followed by surgery several days after the last dose.

Chemotherapy

Chemotherapy is a cancer treatment that uses drugs to stop the growth of cancer cells, either by killing the cells or by stopping the cells from dividing. When chemotherapy is taken by mouth or injected into a vein or muscle, the drugs enter the bloodstream and can reach cancer cells throughout the body (systemic chemotherapy). When chemotherapy is placed directly in the cerebrospinal fluid, an organ, or a body cavity such as the abdomen, the drugs mainly affect cancer cells in those areas (regional chemotherapy).

Chemoembolization of the hepatic artery is a type of regional chemotherapy that may be used to treat cancer that has spread to the liver. This is done by blocking the hepatic artery (the main artery that supplies blood to the liver) and injecting anticancer drugs between the blockage and the liver. The liver's arteries then carry the drugs into the liver. Only a small amount of the drug reaches other parts of the body. The blockage may be temporary or permanent, depending on what is used to block the artery. The liver continues to receive some blood from the hepatic portal vein, which carries blood from the stomach and intestine.

The way the chemotherapy is given depends on the type and stage of the cancer being treated.

Targeted therapy

Targeted therapy is a type of treatment that uses drugs or other substances to identify and attack specific cancer cells without harming normal cells. Monoclonal antibody therapy is a type of targeted therapy being used for the treatment of rectal cancer.

Monoclonal antibody therapy uses antibodies made in the laboratory from a single type of immune system cell. These antibodies can identify substances on cancer cells or normal substances that may help cancer cells grow. The antibodies attach to the substances and kill the cancer cells, block their growth, or keep them from spreading. Monoclonal antibodies are given by infusion. They may be used alone or to carry drugs, toxins, or radioactive material directly to cancer cells.

Bevacizumab is a monoclonal antibody that binds to a protein called vascular endothelial growth factor (VEGF). This may prevent the growth of new blood vessels that tumors need to grow. Cetuximab and panitumumab are types of monoclonal antibodies that bind to a protein called epidermal growth factor receptor (EGFR) on the surface of some types of cancer cells. This may stop cancer cells from growing and dividing.

Patients may want to think about taking part in a clinical trial.

For some patients, taking part in a clinical trial may be the best treatment choice. Clinical trials are part of the cancer research process. Clinical trials are done to find out if new cancer treatments are safe and effective or better than the standard treatment.

Many of today's standard treatments for cancer are based on earlier clinical trials. Patients who take part in a clinical trial may receive the standard treatment or be among the first to receive a new treatment.

Patients who take part in clinical trials also help improve the way cancer will be treated in the future. Even when clinical trials do not lead to effective new treatments, they often answer important questions and help move research forward.

Patients can enter clinical trials before, during, or after starting their cancer treatment.

Some clinical trials only include patients who have not yet received treatment. Other trials test treatments for patients whose cancer has

not gotten better. There are also clinical trials that test new ways to stop cancer from recurring (coming back) or reduce the side effects of cancer treatment.

Clinical trials are taking place in many parts of the country.

Follow-up tests may be needed.

Some of the tests that were done to diagnose the cancer or to find out the stage of the cancer may be repeated. Some tests will be repeated in order to see how well the treatment is working. Decisions about whether to continue, change, or stop treatment may be based on the results of these tests.

Some of the tests will continue to be done from time to time after treatment has ended. The results of these tests can show if your condition has changed or if the cancer has recurred (come back). These tests are sometimes called follow-up tests or check-ups.

After treatment for rectal cancer, a blood test to measure amounts of carcinoembryonic antigen (a substance in the blood that may be increased when cancer is present) may be done to see if the cancer has come back.

Treatment Options by Stage

Stage 0 (Carcinoma in Situ)

Treatment of stage 0 may include the following:

- Simple polypectomy.
- Local excision.
- Resection (when the tumor is too large to remove by local excision).

For more specific results, refine the search by using other search features, such as the location of the trial, the type of treatment, or the name of the drug. Talk with your doctor about clinical trials that may be right for you.

Stage I Rectal Cancer

Treatment of stage I rectal cancer may include the following:

- Local excision.
- Resection.
- Resection with radiation therapy and chemotherapy after surgery.

For more specific results, refine the search by using other search features, such as the location of the trial, the type of treatment, or the name of the drug. Talk with your doctor about clinical trials that may be right for you.

Stages II and III Rectal Cancer

Treatment of stage II and stage III rectal cancer may include the following:

- Surgery.
- Chemotherapy combined with radiation therapy, followed by surgery.
- Short-course radiation therapy followed by surgery and chemotherapy.
- Resection followed by chemotherapy combined with radiation therapy.
- A clinical trial of a new treatment.

For more specific results, refine the search by using other search features, such as the location of the trial, the type of treatment, or the name of the drug. Talk with your doctor about clinical trials that may be right for you.

Stage IV and Recurrent Rectal Cancer

Treatment of stage IV and recurrent rectal cancer may include the following:

- Surgery with or without chemotherapy or radiation therapy.
- Systemic chemotherapy with or without targeted therapy, such as bevacizumab,cetuximab, or panitumumab.
- Chemotherapy to control the growth of the tumor.
- Radiation therapy, chemotherapy, or a combination of both, as palliative therapy to relieve symptoms and improve the quality of life.
- Placement of a stent to help keep the rectum open if it is partly blocked by the tumor, as palliative therapy to relieve symptoms and improve the quality of life.
- A clinical trial of a new anticancer drug.

Treatment of rectal cancer that has spread to other organs depends on where the cancer has spread.

- Treatment for areas of cancer that have spread to the liver includes the following:

  - Surgery to remove the tumor. Chemotherapy may be given before surgery, to shrink the tumor.

  - Cryosurgery or radiofrequency ablation.

  - Chemoembolization and/or systemic chemotherapy.

  - A clinical trial of chemoembolization combined with radiation therapy to the tumors in the liver.

Section 23.11

Anal Cancer

Text in this section is excerpted from "Anal Cancer Treatment,"
National Cancer Institute at the National Institutes of Health (NIH),
May 12, 2015.

General Information About Anal Cancer

Anal cancer is a disease in which malignant (cancer) cells form in the tissues of the anus.

The anus is the end of the large intestine, below the rectum, through which stool (solid waste) leaves the body. The anus is formed partly from the outer skin layers of the body and partly from the intestine. Two ring-like muscles, called sphincter muscles, open and close the anal opening and let stool pass out of the body. The anal canal, the part of the anus between the rectum and the anal opening, is about 1–1½ inches long.

The skin around the outside of the anus is called the perianal area. Tumors in this area are skin tumors, not anal cancer.

Being infected with the human papillomavirus (HPV) increases the risk of developing anal cancer.

Risk factors include the following:

- Being infected with human papillomavirus (HPV).
- Having many sexual partners.
- Having receptive anal intercourse (anal sex).
- Being older than 50 years.
- Frequent anal redness, swelling, and soreness.
- Having anal fistulas (abnormal openings).
- Smoking cigarettes.

Signs of anal cancer include bleeding from the anus or rectum or a lump near the anus.

These and other signs and symptoms may be caused by anal cancer or by other conditions. Check with your doctor if you have any of the following:

- Bleeding from the anus or rectum.
- Pain or pressure in the area around the anus.
- Itching or discharge from the anus.
- A lump near the anus.
- A change in bowel habits.

Tests that examine the rectum and anus are used to detect (find) and diagnose anal cancer.

The following tests and procedures may be used:

- **Physical exam and history:** An exam of the body to check general signs of health, including checking for signs of disease, such as lumps or anything else that seems unusual. A history of the patient's health habits and past illnesses and treatments will also be taken.

- **Digital rectal examination (DRE):** An exam of the anus and rectum. The doctor or nurse inserts a lubricated, gloved finger into the lower part of the rectum to feel for lumps or anything else that seems unusual.

- **Anoscopy**: An exam of the anus and lower rectum using a short, lighted tube called an anoscope.

- **Proctoscopy:** An exam of the rectum using a short, lighted tube called a proctoscope.

- **Endo-anal or endorectal ultrasound:** A procedure in which an ultrasound transducer (probe) is inserted into the anus or rectum and used to bounce high-energy sound waves (ultrasound) off internal tissues or organs and make echoes. The echoes form a picture of body tissues called a sonogram.

- **Biopsy:** The removal of cells or tissues so they can be viewed under a microscope by a pathologist to check for signs of cancer. If an abnormal area is seen during the anoscopy, a biopsy may be done at that time.

Certain factors affect the prognosis (chance of recovery) and treatment options.

The prognosis (chance of recovery) depends on the following:

- The size of the tumor.

- Where the tumor is in the anus.

- Whether the cancer has spread to the lymph nodes.

The treatment options depend on the following:

- The stage of the cancer.

- Where the tumor is in the anus.

- Whether the patient has human immunodeficiency virus (HIV).

- Whether cancer remains after initial treatment or has recurred.

Stages of Anal Cancer

After anal cancer has been diagnosed, tests are done to find out if cancer cells have spread within the anus or to other parts of the body.

The process used to find out if cancer has spread within the anus or to other parts of the body is called staging. The information gathered from the staging process determines the stage of the disease. It is important to know the stage in order to plan treatment. The following tests may be used in the staging process:

- **CT scan (CAT scan):** A procedure that makes a series of detailed pictures of areas inside the body, such as the abdomen or chest, taken from different angles. The pictures are made by a computer linked to an x-ray machine. A dye may be injected into a vein or swallowed to help the organs or tissues show up more clearly. This procedure is also called computed tomography, computerized tomography, or computerized axial tomography. For anal cancer, a CT scan of the pelvis and abdomen may be done.

- **Chest x-ray:** An x-ray of the organs and bones inside the chest. An x-ray is a type of energy beam that can go through the body and onto film, making a picture of areas inside the body.

- **MRI (magnetic resonance imaging):** A procedure that uses a magnet, radio waves, and a computer to make a series of detailed pictures of areas inside the body. This procedure is also called nuclear magnetic resonance imaging (NMRI).

- **PET scan (positron emission tomography scan):** A procedure to find malignant tumor cells in the body. A small amount of radioactive glucose (sugar) is injected into a vein. The PET scanner rotates around the body and makes a picture of where glucose is being used in the body. Malignant tumor cells show up brighter in the picture because they are more active and take up more glucose than normal cells do.

There are three ways that cancer spreads in the body.

Cancer can spread through tissue, the lymph system, and the blood:

- Tissue. The cancer spreads from where it began by growing into nearby areas.

- Lymph system. The cancer spreads from where it began by getting into the lymph system. The cancer travels through the lymph vessels to other parts of the body.

- Blood. The cancer spreads from where it began by getting into the blood. The cancer travels through the blood vessels to other parts of the body.

Cancer may spread from where it began to other parts of the body.

When cancer spreads to another part of the body, it is called metastasis. Cancer cells break away from where they began (the primary tumor) and travel through the lymph system or blood.

- Lymph system. The cancer gets into the lymph system, travels through the lymph vessels, and forms a tumor (metastatic tumor) in another part of the body.

- Blood. The cancer gets into the blood, travels through the blood vessels, and forms a tumor (metastatic tumor) in another part of the body.

The metastatic tumor is the same type of cancer as the primary tumor. For example, if anal cancer spreads to the lung, the cancer cells in the lung are actually anal cancer cells. The disease is metastatic anal cancer, not lung cancer.

The following stages are used for anal cancer:

Stage 0 (Carcinoma in Situ)

In stage 0, abnormal cells are found in the innermost lining of the anus. These abnormal cells may become cancer and spread into nearby normal tissue. Stage 0 is also called carcinoma in situ.

Stage I

In stage I, cancer has formed and the tumor is 2 centimeters or smaller.

Stage II

In stage II, the tumor is larger than 2 centimeters.

Stage IIIA

In stage IIIA, the tumor may be any size and has spread to either:

- lymph nodes near the rectum; or
- nearby organs, such as the vagina, urethra, and bladder.

Stage IIIB

In stage IIIB, the tumor may be any size and has spread:

- to nearby organs and to lymph nodes near the rectum; or
- to lymph nodes on one side of the pelvis and/or groin, and may have spread to nearby organs; or
- to lymph nodes near the rectum and in the groin, and/or to lymph nodes on both sides of the pelvis and/or groin, and may have spread to nearby organs.

Stage IV

In stage IV, the tumor may be any size and cancer may have spread to lymph nodes or nearby organs and has spread to distant parts of the body.

Treatment Option Overview

There are different types of treatment for patients with anal cancer.

Different types of treatments are available for patients with anal cancer. Some treatments are standard (the currently used treatment), and some are being tested in clinical trials. A treatment clinical trial is a research study meant to help improve current treatments or obtain information on new treatments for patients with cancer. When clinical trials show that a new treatment is better than the standard treatment, the new treatment may become the standard treatment. Patients may want to think about taking part in a clinical trial. Some clinical trials are open only to patients who have not started treatment.

Three types of standard treatment are used:

Radiation therapy

Radiation therapy is a cancer treatment that uses high-energy x-rays or other types of radiation to kill cancer cells. There are two types of radiation therapy. External radiation therapy uses a machine outside the body to send radiation toward the cancer. Internal radiation therapy uses a radioactive substance sealed in needles, seeds, wires, or catheters that are placed directly into or near the cancer. The way the radiation therapy is given depends on the type and stage of the cancer being treated.

Chemotherapy

Chemotherapy is a cancer treatment that uses drugs to stop the growth of cancer cells, either by killing the cells or by stopping the cells from dividing. When chemotherapy is taken by mouth or injected into a vein or muscle, the drugs enter the bloodstream and can reach cancer cells throughout the body (systemic chemotherapy). When chemotherapy is placed directly into the cerebrospinal fluid, an organ, or a body cavity such as the abdomen, the drugs mainly affect cancer cells in those areas (regional chemotherapy). The way the chemotherapy is given depends on the type and stage of the cancer being treated.

Surgery

- Local resection: A surgical procedure in which the tumor is cut from the anus along with some of the healthy tissue around it. Local resection may be used if the cancer is small and has not spread. This procedure may save the sphincter muscles so the patient can still control bowel movements. Tumors that form in the lower part of the anus can often be removed with local resection.

- Abdominoperineal resection: A surgical procedure in which the anus, the rectum, and part of the sigmoid colon are removed through an incision made in the abdomen. The doctor sews the end of the intestine to an opening, called a stoma, made in the surface of the abdomen so body waste can be collected in a disposable bag outside of the body. This is called a colostomy. Lymph nodes that contain cancer may also be removed during this operation.

Having the human immunodeficiency virus can affect treatment of anal cancer.

Cancer therapy can further damage the already weakened immune systems of patients who have the human immunodeficiency virus (HIV). For this reason, patients who have anal cancer and HIV are usually treated with lower doses of anticancer drugs and radiation than patients who do not have HIV.

New types of treatment are being tested in clinical trials.

Radiosensitizers

Radiosensitizers are drugs that make tumor cells more sensitive to radiation therapy. Combining radiation therapy with radiosensitizers may kill more tumor cells.

Patients may want to think about taking part in a clinical trial.

For some patients, taking part in a clinical trial may be the best treatment choice. Clinical trials are part of the cancer research process. Clinical trials are done to find out if new cancer treatments are safe and effective or better than the standard treatment.

Many of today's standard treatments for cancer are based on earlier clinical trials. Patients who take part in a clinical trial may receive the standard treatment or be among the first to receive a new treatment.

Patients who take part in clinical trials also help improve the way cancer will be treated in the future. Even when clinical trials do not lead to effective new treatments, they often answer important questions and help move research forward.

Patients can enter clinical trials before, during, or after starting their cancer treatment.

Some clinical trials only include patients who have not yet received treatment. Other trials test treatments for patients whose cancer has not gotten better. There are also clinical trials that test new ways to stop cancer from recurring (coming back) or reduce the side effects of cancer treatment.

Clinical trials are taking place in many parts of the country.

Follow-up tests may be needed.

Some of the tests that were done to diagnose the cancer or to find out the stage of the cancer may be repeated. Some tests will be repeated in order to see how well the treatment is working. Decisions about whether to continue, change, or stop treatment may be based on the results of these tests.

Some of the tests will continue to be done from time to time after treatment has ended. The results of these tests can show if your condition has changed or if the cancer has recurred (come back). These tests are sometimes called follow-up tests or check-ups.

Treatment Options by Stage

Stage 0 (Carcinoma in Situ)

Treatment of stage 0 is usually local resection.

Stage I Anal Cancer

Treatment of stage I anal cancer may include the following:

- Local resection.
- External-beam radiation therapy with or without chemotherapy. If cancer remains after treatment, more chemotherapy and radiation therapy may be given to avoid the need for a permanent colostomy.
- Internal radiation therapy.
- Abdominoperineal resection, if cancer remains or comes back after treatment with radiation therapy and chemotherapy.
- Internal radiation therapy for cancer that remains after treatment with external-beam radiation therapy.

Patients who have had treatment that saves the sphincter muscles may receive follow-up exams every 3 months for the first 2 years, including rectal exams with endoscopy and biopsy, as needed.

Stage II Anal Cancer

Treatment of stage II anal cancer may include the following:

- Local resection.
- External-beam radiation therapy with chemotherapy. If cancer remains after treatment, more chemotherapy and radiation therapy may be given to avoid the need for a permanent colostomy.
- Internal radiation therapy.
- Abdominoperineal resection, if cancer remains or comes back after treatment with radiation therapy and chemotherapy.
- A clinical trial of new treatment options.

429

Patients who have had treatment that saves the sphincter muscles may receive follow-up exams every 3 months for the first 2 years, including rectal exams with endoscopy and biopsy, as needed.

Stage IIIA Anal Cancer

Treatment of stage IIIA anal cancer may include the following:

- External-beam radiation therapy with chemotherapy. If cancer remains after treatment, more chemotherapy and radiation therapy may be given to avoid the need for a permanent colostomy.

- Internal radiation therapy.

- Abdominoperineal resection, if cancer remains or comes back after treatment with chemotherapy and radiation therapy.

- A clinical trial of new treatment options.

Stage IIIB Anal Cancer

Treatment of stage IIIB anal cancer may include the following:

- External-beam radiation therapy with chemotherapy.

- Local resection or abdominoperineal resection, if cancer remains or comes back after treatment with chemotherapy and radiation therapy. Lymph nodes may also be removed.

- A clinical trial of new treatment options.

Stage IV Anal Cancer

Treatment of stage IV anal cancer may include the following:

- Surgery as palliative therapy to relieve symptoms and improve the quality of life.

- Radiation therapy as palliative therapy.

- Chemotherapy with radiation therapy as palliative therapy.

- A clinical trial of new treatment options.

Chapter 24

Genito-Urinary Cancers

Chapter Contents

Section 24.1

Urethral Cancer

Text in this section is excerpted from "Urethral Cancer Treatment,"
National Cancer Institute at the National Institutes of Health (NIH),
October 22, 2014.

General Information About Urethral Cancer

Urethral cancer is a disease in which malignant (cancer) cells form in the tissues of the urethra.

The urethra is the tube that carries urine from the bladder to outside the body. In women, the urethra is about 1½ inches long and is just above the vagina. In men, the urethra is about 8 inches long, and goes through the prostate gland and the penis to the outside of the body. In men, the urethra also carries semen.

Urethral cancer is a rare cancer that occurs more often in men than in women.

There are different types of urethral cancer that begin in cells that line the urethra.

These cancers are named for the types of cells that become malignant (cancer):

- Squamous cell carcinoma is the most common type of urethral cancer. It forms in cells in the part of the urethra near the bladder in women, and in the lining of the urethra in the penis in men.

- Transitional cell carcinoma forms in the area near the urethral opening in women, and in the part of the urethra that goes through the prostate gland in men.

- Adenocarcinoma forms in the glands that are around the urethra in both men and women.

Urethral cancer can metastasize (spread) quickly to tissues around the urethra and is often found in nearby lymph nodes by the time it is diagnosed.

A history of bladder cancer can affect the risk of urethral cancer.

Anything that increases your chance of getting a disease is called a risk factor. Having a risk factor does not mean that you will get cancer; not having risk factors doesn't mean that you will not get cancer. Talk with your doctor if you think you may be at risk. Risk factors for urethral cancer include the following:

- Having a history of bladder cancer.
- Having conditions that cause chronic inflammation in the urethra, including:
  - Sexually transmitted diseases (STDs), including human papillomavirus (HPV), especially HPV type 16.
  - Frequent urinary tract infections (UTIs).

Signs of urethral cancer include bleeding or trouble with urination.

These and other signs and symptoms may be caused by urethral cancer or by other conditions. There may be no signs or symptoms in the early stages. Check with your doctor if you have any of the following:

- Trouble starting the flow of urine.
- Weak or interrupted ("stop-and-go") flow of urine.
- Frequent urination, especially at night.
- Incontinence.
- Discharge from the urethra.
- Bleeding from the urethra or blood in the urine.
- A lump or thickness in the perineum or penis.
- A painless lump or swelling in the groin.

Tests that examine the urethra and bladder are used to detect (find) and diagnose urethral cancer.

The following tests and procedures may be used:

- **Physical exam and history:** An exam of the body to check general signs of health, including checking for signs of disease, such as lumps or anything else that seems unusual. A history of the patient's health habits and past illnesses and treatments will also be taken.

- **Pelvic exam:** An exam of the vagina, cervix, uterus, fallopian tubes, ovaries, and rectum. The doctor or nurse inserts one or two lubricated, gloved fingers of one hand into the vagina and places the other hand over the lower abdomen to feel the size, shape, and position of the uterus and ovaries. A speculum is also inserted into the vagina and the doctor or nurse looks at the vagina and cervix for signs of disease.

- **Digital rectal exam:** An exam of the rectum. The doctor or nurse inserts a lubricated, gloved finger into the lower part of the rectum to feel for lumps or anything else that seems unusual.

- **Urine cytology:** Examination of urine under a microscope to check for abnormal cells.

- **Urinalysis:** A test to check the color of urine and its contents, such as sugar, protein, blood, and white blood cells. If white blood cells (a sign of infection) are found, a urine culture is usually done to find out what type of infection it is.

- **Blood chemistry studies:** A procedure in which a blood sample is checked to measure the amounts of certain substances released into the blood by organs and tissues in the body. An unusual (higher or lower than normal) amount of a substance can be a sign of disease in the organ or tissue that makes it.

- **Complete blood count (CBC):** A procedure in which a sample of blood is drawn and checked for the following:
  - The number of red blood cells, white blood cells, and platelets.
  - The amount of hemoglobin (the protein that carries oxygen) in the red blood cells.
  - The portion of the blood sample made up of red blood cells.

- **CT scan (CAT scan):** A procedure that makes a series of detailed pictures of areas inside the body, such as the pelvis and abdomen, taken from different angles. The pictures are made by a computer linked to an x-ray machine. A dye may be injected into a vein or swallowed to help the organs or tissues show up more clearly. This procedure is also called computed tomography, computerized tomography, or computerized axial tomography.

- **Ureteroscopy:** A procedure to look inside the ureter and renal pelvis to check for abnormal areas. A ureteroscope is a thin, tube-like instrument with a light and a lens for viewing. The ureteroscope is inserted through the urethra into the bladder, ureter, and renal pelvis. A tool may be inserted through the ureteroscope to take tissue samples to be checked under a microscope for signs of disease.

- **Biopsy:** The removal of cell or tissue samples from the urethra, bladder, and, sometimes, the prostate gland. The samples are viewed under a microscope by a pathologist to check for signs of cancer.

Certain factors affect prognosis (chance of recovery) and treatment options.

The prognosis (chance of recovery) and treatment options depend on the following:

- Where the cancer formed in the urethra.

- Whether the cancer has spread through the mucosa lining the urethra to nearby tissue, to lymph nodes, or to other parts of the body.

- Whether the patient is a male or female.

- The patient's general health.

- Whether the cancer has just been diagnosed or has recurred (come back).

Stages of Urethral Cancer

After urethral cancer has been diagnosed, tests are done to find out if cancer cells have spread within the urethra or to other parts of the body.

The process used to find out if cancer has spread within the urethra or to other parts of the body is called staging. The information gathered from the staging process determines the stage of the disease. It is important to know the stage in order to plan treatment.

The following procedures may be used in the staging process:

- **Chest x-ray:** An x-ray of the organs and bones inside the chest. An x-ray is a type of energy beam that can go through the body and onto film, making a picture of areas inside the body.

- **CT scan (CAT scan) of the pelvis and abdomen:** A procedure that makes a series of detailed pictures of the pelvis and abdomen, taken from different angles. The pictures are made by a computer linked to an x-ray machine. A dye may be injected into a vein or swallowed to help the organs or tissues show up more clearly. This procedure is also called computed tomography, computerized tomography, or computerized axial tomography.

- **MRI (magnetic resonance imaging):** A procedure that uses a magnet, radio waves, and a computer to make a series of detailed pictures of the urethra, nearby lymph nodes, and other soft tissue and bones in the pelvis. A substance called gadolinium is injected into the patient through a vein. The gadolinium collects around the cancer cells so they show up brighter in the picture. This procedure is also called nuclear magnetic resonance imaging (NMRI).

- **Urethrography:** A series of x-rays of the urethra. An x-ray is a type of energy beam that can go through the body and onto film, making a picture of areas inside the body. A dye is injected through the urethra into the bladder. The dye coats the bladder and urethra and x-rays are taken to see if the urethra is blocked and if cancer has spread to nearby tissue.

There are three ways that cancer spreads in the body.

Cancer can spread through tissue, the lymph system, and the blood:

- Tissue. The cancer spreads from where it began by growing into nearby areas.

- Lymph system. The cancer spreads from where it began by getting into the lymph system. The cancer travels through the lymph vessels to other parts of the body.

- Blood. The cancer spreads from where it began by getting into the blood. The cancer travels through the blood vessels to other parts of the body.

Cancer may spread from where it began to other parts of the body.

When cancer spreads to another part of the body, it is called metastasis. Cancer cells break away from where they began (the primary tumor) and travel through the lymph system or blood.

- Lymph system. The cancer gets into the lymph system, travels through the lymph vessels, and forms a tumor (metastatic tumor) in another part of the body.

- Blood. The cancer gets into the blood, travels through the blood vessels, and forms a tumor (metastatic tumor) in another part of the body.

The metastatic tumor is the same type of cancer as the primary tumor. For example, if urethral cancer spreads to the lung, the cancer cells in the lung are actually urethral cancer cells. The disease is metastatic urethral cancer, not lung cancer.

Urethral cancer is staged and treated based on the part of the urethra that is affected.

Urethral cancer is staged and treated based on the part of the urethra that is affected and how deeply the tumor has spread into tissue around the urethra. Urethral cancer can be described as distal or proximal.

Distal urethral cancer

In distal urethral cancer, the cancer usually has not spread deeply into the tissue. In women, the part of the urethra that is closest to the outside of the body (about ½ inch) is affected. In men, the part of the urethra that is in the penis is affected.

Proximal urethral cancer

Proximal urethral cancer affects the part of the urethra that is not the distal urethra. In women and men, proximal urethral cancer usually has spread deeply into tissue.

Bladder and/or prostate cancer may occur at the same time as urethral cancer.

In men, cancer that forms in the proximal urethra (the part of the urethra that passes through the prostate to the bladder) may occur at the same time as cancer of the bladder and/or prostate. Sometimes this occurs at diagnosis and sometimes it occurs later.

Treatment Option Overview

There are different types of treatment for patients with urethral cancer.

Different types of treatments are available for patients with urethral cancer. Some treatments are standard (the currently used treatment), and some are being tested in clinical trials. A treatment clinical trial is a research study meant to help improve current treatments or obtain information on new treatments for patients with cancer. When clinical trials show that a new treatment is better than the standard treatment, the new treatment may become the standard treatment. Patients may want to think about taking part in a clinical trial. Some clinical trials are open only to patients who have not started treatment.

Four types of standard treatment are used:

Surgery

Surgery to remove the cancer is the most common treatment for cancer of the urethra. One of the following types of surgery may be done:

- Open excision: Removal of the cancer by surgery.

- Transurethral resection (TUR): Surgery to remove the cancer using a special tool inserted into the urethra.

- Electroresection with fulguration: Surgery to remove the cancer by electric current. A lighted tool with a small wire loop on the end is used to remove the cancer or to burn the tumor away with high-energy electricity.

- Laser surgery: A surgical procedure that uses a laser beam (a narrow beam of intense light) as a knife to make bloodless cuts in tissue or to remove or destroy tissue.

- Lymph node dissection: Lymph nodes in the pelvis and groin may be removed.

- Cystourethrectomy: Surgery to remove the bladder and the urethra.

- Cystoprostatectomy: Surgery to remove the bladder and the prostate.

- Anterior exenteration: Surgery to remove the urethra, the bladder, and the vagina. Plastic surgery may be done to rebuild the vagina.

- Partial penectomy: Surgery to remove the part of the penis surrounding the urethra where cancer has spread. Plastic surgery may be done to rebuild the penis.

- Radical penectomy: Surgery to remove the entire penis. Plastic surgery may be done to rebuild the penis.

If the urethra is removed, the surgeon will make a new way for the urine to pass from the body. This is called urinary diversion. If the bladder is removed, the surgeon will make a new way for urine to be stored and passed from the body. The surgeon may use part of the small intestine to make a tube that passes urine through an opening (stoma). This is called an ostomy or urostomy. If a patient has an ostomy, a disposable bag to collect urine is worn under clothing. The surgeon may also use part of the small intestine to make a new storage pouch (continent reservoir) inside the body where the urine can collect. A tube (catheter) is then used to drain the urine through a stoma.

Even if the doctor removes all the cancer that can be seen at the time of the surgery, some patients may be given chemotherapy or radiation therapy after surgery to kill any cancer cells that are left. Treatment given after the surgery, to lower the risk that the cancer will come back, is called adjuvant therapy.

Radiation therapy

Radiation therapy is a cancer treatment that uses high-energy x-rays or other types of radiation to kill cancer cells. There are two types of radiation therapy. External radiation therapy uses a machine outside the body to send radiation toward the cancer. Internal radiation therapy uses a radioactive substance sealed in needles, seeds, wires, or catheters that are placed directly into or near the cancer. The way the radiation therapy is given depends on the type of cancer and where the cancer formed in the urethra.

Chemotherapy

Chemotherapy is a cancer treatment that uses drugs to stop the growth of cancer cells, either by killing the cells or by stopping the cells from dividing. When chemotherapy is taken by mouth or injected into a vein or muscle, the drugs enter the bloodstream and can reach cancer cells throughout the body (systemic chemotherapy). When chemotherapy is placed directly into the cerebrospinal fluid, an organ, or a body cavity such as the abdomen, the drugs mainly affect cancer cells in those areas (regional chemotherapy). The way the chemotherapy is given depends on the type of cancer and where the cancer formed in the urethra.

Active surveillance

Active surveillance is following a patient's condition without giving any treatment unless there are changes in test results. It is used to find early signs that the condition is getting worse. In active surveillance, patients are given certain exams and tests, including biopsies, on a regular schedule.

Patients may want to think about taking part in a clinical trial.

For some patients, taking part in a clinical trial may be the best treatment choice. Clinical trials are part of the cancer research process. Clinical trials are done to find out if new cancer treatments are safe and effective or better than the standard treatment.

Many of today's standard treatments for cancer are based on earlier clinical trials. Patients who take part in a clinical trial may receive the standard treatment or be among the first to receive a new treatment.

Patients who take part in clinical trials also help improve the way cancer will be treated in the future. Even when clinical trials do not lead to effective new treatments, they often answer important questions and help move research forward.

Patients can enter clinical trials before, during, or after starting their cancer treatment.

Some clinical trials only include patients who have not yet received treatment. Other trials test treatments for patients whose cancer has not gotten better. There are also clinical trials that test new ways to stop cancer from recurring (coming back) or reduce the side effects of cancer treatment.

Clinical trials are taking place in many parts of the country.

Follow-up tests may be needed.

Some of the tests that were done to diagnose the cancer or to find out the stage of the cancer may be repeated. Some tests will be repeated in order to see how well the treatment is working. Decisions about whether to continue, change, or stop treatment may be based on the results of these tests.

Some of the tests will continue to be done from time to time after treatment has ended. The results of these tests can show if your condition has changed or if the cancer has recurred (come back). These tests are sometimes called follow-up tests or check-ups.

Section 24.2

Bladder Cancer

Text in this section is excerpted from "Bladder Cancer Treatment,"
National Cancer Institute at the National Institutes of Health (NIH),
May 29, 2015.

General Information About Bladder Cancer

*Bladder cancer is a disease in which malignant (cancer)
cells form in the tissues of the bladder.*

The bladder is a hollow organ in the lower part of the abdomen. It is shaped like a small balloon and has a muscular wall that allows it to get larger or smaller to store urine made by the kidneys. There are two kidneys, one on each side of the backbone, above the waist. Tiny tubules in the kidneys filter and clean the blood. They take out waste products and make urine. The urine passes from each kidney through a long tube called a ureter into the bladder. The bladder holds the urine until it passes through the urethra and leaves the body.

There are three types of bladder cancer that begin in cells in the lining of the bladder. These cancers are named for the type of cells that become malignant (cancerous):

- Transitional cell carcinoma: Cancer that begins in cells in the innermost tissue layer of the bladder. These cells are able to stretch when the bladder is full and shrink when it is emptied. Most bladder cancers begin in the transitional cells. Transitional cell carcinoma can be low-grade or high-grade:

  - Low-grade transitional cell carcinoma often recurs (comes back) after treatment, but rarely spreads into the muscle layer of the bladder or to other parts of the body.

  - High-grade transitional cell carcinoma often recurs (comes back) after treatment and often spreads into the muscle layer of the bladder, to other parts of the body, and to lymph

441

nodes. Almost all deaths from bladder cancer are due to high-grade disease.

- Squamous cell carcinoma: Cancer that begins in squamous cells, which are thin, flat cells that may form in the bladder after long-term infection or irritation.

- Adenocarcinoma: Cancer that begins in glandular (secretory) cells that are found in the lining of the bladder. This is a very rare type of bladder cancer.

Cancer that is in the lining of the bladder is called superficial bladder cancer. Cancer that has spread through the lining of the bladder and invades the muscle wall of the bladder or has spread to nearby organs and lymph nodes is called invasive bladder cancer.

Smoking can affect the risk of bladder cancer.

Anything that increases your chance of getting a disease is called a risk factor. Having a risk factor does not mean that you will get cancer; not having risk factors doesn't mean that you will not get cancer. Talk to your doctor if you think you may be at risk for bladder cancer. Risk factors for bladder cancer include:

- Using tobacco, especially smoking cigarettes.

- Having a family history of bladder cancer.

- Having certain changes in the genes that are linked to bladder cancer.

- Being exposed to certain chemicals in the workplace.

- Past treatment with certain anticancer drugs, such as cyclophosphamide or ifosfamide, or radiation therapy to the pelvis.

- Taking Aristolochia fangchi, a Chinese herb.

- Drinking well water that has high levels of arsenic.

- Drinking water that has been treated with chlorine.

- Having a history of bladder infections, including bladder infections caused by Schistosoma haematobium.

- Using urinary catheters for a long time.

Signs and symptoms of bladder cancer include blood in the urine and pain during urination.

These and other signs and symptoms may be caused by bladder cancer or by other conditions. Check with your doctor if you have any of the following:

- Blood in the urine (slightly rusty to bright red in color).
- Frequent urination.
- Pain during urination.
- Lower back pain.

Tests that examine the urine and bladder are used to help detect (find) and diagnose bladder cancer.

The following tests and procedures may be used:

- **Physical exam and history:** An exam of the body to check general signs of health, including checking for signs of disease, such as lumps or anything else that seems unusual. A history of the patient's health habits and past illnesses and treatments will also be taken.

- **Internal exam:** An exam of the vagina and/or rectum. The doctor inserts lubricated, gloved fingers into the vagina and/or rectum to feel for lumps.

- **Urinalysis:** A test to check the color of urine and its contents, such as sugar, protein, red blood cells, and white blood cells.

- **Urine cytology:** A laboratory test in which a sample of urine is checked under a microscope for abnormal cells.

- **Cystoscopy:** A procedure to look inside the bladder and urethra to check for abnormal areas. A cystoscope is inserted through the urethra into the bladder. A cystoscope is a thin, tube-like instrument with a light and a lens for viewing. It may also have a tool to remove tissue samples, which are checked under a microscope for signs of cancer.

- **Intravenous pyelogram (IVP):** A series of x-rays of the kidneys, ureters, and bladder to find out if cancer is present in these organs. A contrast dye is injected into a vein. As the contrast dye moves through the kidneys, ureters, and bladder, x-rays are taken to see if there are any blockages.

- **Biopsy:** The removal of cells or tissues so they can be viewed under a microscope by a pathologist to check for signs of cancer. A biopsy for bladder cancer is usually done during cystoscopy. It may be possible to remove the entire tumor during biopsy.

Certain factors affect prognosis (chance of recovery) and treatment options.

The prognosis (chance of recovery) depends on the following:

- The stage of the cancer (whether it is superficial or invasive bladder cancer, and whether it has spread to other places in the body). Bladder cancer in the early stages can often be cured.
- The type of bladder cancer cells and how they look under a microscope.
- Whether there is carcinoma in situ in other parts of the bladder.
- The patient's age and general health.

If the cancer is superficial, prognosis also depends on the following:

- How many tumors there are.
- The size of the tumors.
- Whether the tumor has recurred (come back) after treatment. Treatment options depend on the stage of bladder cancer.

Stages of Bladder Cancer

After bladder cancer has been diagnosed, tests are done to find out if cancer cells have spread within the bladder or to other parts of the body.

The process used to find out if cancer has spread within the bladder lining and muscle or to other parts of the body is called staging. The information gathered from the staging process determines the stage of the disease. It is important to know the stage in order to plan treatment. The following tests and procedures may be used in the staging process:

- **CT scan (CAT scan):** A procedure that makes a series of detailed pictures of areas inside the body, taken from different angles. The pictures are made by a computer linked to an x-ray

machine. A dye may be injected into a vein or swallowed to help the organs or tissues show up more clearly. This procedure is also called computed tomography, computerized tomography, or computerized axial tomography. To stage bladder cancer, the CT scan may take pictures of the chest, abdomen, and pelvis.

- **MRI (magnetic resonance imaging):** A procedure that uses a magnet, radio waves, and a computer to make a series of detailed pictures of areas inside the body. This procedure is also called nuclear magnetic resonance imaging (NMRI).

- **Chest x-ray:** An x-ray of the organs and bones inside the chest. An x-ray is a type of energy beam that can go through the body and onto film, making a picture of areas inside the body.

- **Bone scan:** A procedure to check if there are rapidly dividing cells, such as cancer cells, in the bone. A very small amount of radioactive material is injected into a vein and travels through the bloodstream. The radioactive material collects in the bones and is detected by a scanner.

There are three ways that cancer spreads in the body.

Cancer can spread through tissue, the lymph system, and the blood:

- Tissue. The cancer spreads from where it began by growing into nearby areas.

- Lymph system. The cancer spreads from where it began by getting into the lymph system. The cancer travels through the lymph vessels to other parts of the body.

- Blood. The cancer spreads from where it began by getting into the blood. The cancer travels through the blood vessels to other parts of the body.

Cancer may spread from where it began to other parts of the body.

When cancer spreads to another part of the body, it is called metastasis. Cancer cells break away from where they began (the primary tumor) and travel through the lymph system or blood.

- Lymph system. The cancer gets into the lymph system, travels through the lymph vessels, and forms a tumor (metastatic tumor) in another part of the body.

- Blood. The cancer gets into the blood, travels through the blood vessels, and forms a tumor (metastatic tumor) in another part of the body.

The metastatic tumor is the same type of cancer as the primary tumor. For example, if bladder cancer spreads to the bone, the cancer cells in the bone are actually bladder cancer cells. The disease is metastatic bladder cancer, not bone cancer.

The following stages are used for bladder cancer:

Stage 0 (Papillary Carcinoma and Carcinoma in Situ)

In stage 0, abnormal cells are found in tissue lining the inside of the bladder. These abnormal cells may become cancer and spread into nearby normal tissue. Stage 0 is divided into stage 0a and stage 0is, depending on the type of the tumor:

- Stage 0 is also called papillary carcinoma, which may look like tiny mushrooms growing from the lining of the bladder.
- Stage 0 is also called carcinoma in situ, which is a flat tumor on the tissue lining the inside of the bladder.

Stage I

In stage I, cancer has formed and spread to the layer of connective tissue next to the inner lining of the bladder.

Stage II

In stage II, cancer has spread to the layers of muscle tissue of the bladder.

Stage III

In stage III, cancer has spread from the bladder to the layer of fat surrounding it and may have spread to the reproductive organs (prostate, seminal vesicles, uterus, or vagina).

Stage IV

In stage IV, one or more of the following is true:

- Cancer has spread from the bladder to the wall of the abdomen or pelvis.

- Cancer has spread to one or more lymph nodes.

- Cancer has spread to other parts of the body, such as the lung, bone, or liver.

Treatment Option Overview

There are different types of treatment for patients with bladder cancer.

Different types of treatment are available for patients with bladder cancer. Some treatments are standard (the currently used treatment), and some are being tested in clinical trials. A treatment clinical trial is a research study meant to help improve current treatments or obtain information on new treatments for patients with cancer. When clinical trials show that a new treatment is better than the standard treatment, the new treatment may become the standard treatment. Patients may want to think about taking part in a clinical trial. Some clinical trials are open only to patients who have not started treatment.

Four types of standard treatment are used:

Surgery

One of the following types of surgery may be done:

- Transurethral resection (TUR) with fulguration: Surgery in which a cystoscope (a thin lighted tube) is inserted into the bladder through the urethra. A tool with a small wire loop on the end is then used to remove the cancer or to burn the tumor away with high-energy electricity. This is known as fulguration.

- Radical cystectomy: Surgery to remove the bladder and any lymph nodes and nearby organs that contain cancer. This surgery may be done when the bladder cancer invades the muscle wall, or when superficial cancer involves a large part of the bladder. In men, the nearby organs that are removed are the prostate and the seminal vesicles. In women, the uterus, the ovaries, and part of the vagina are removed. Sometimes, when the cancer has spread outside the bladder and cannot be completely removed, surgery to remove only the bladder may be done to reduce urinary symptoms caused by the cancer. When the bladder must be removed, the surgeon creates another way for urine to leave the body.

- Partial cystectomy: Surgery to remove part of the bladder. This surgery may be done for patients who have a low-grade tumor that has invaded the wall of the bladder but is limited to one area of the bladder. Because only a part of the bladder is removed, patients are able to urinate normally after recovering from this surgery. This is also called segmental cystectomy.

- Urinary diversion: Surgery to make a new way for the body to store and pass urine.

Even if the doctor removes all the cancer that can be seen at the time of the surgery, some patients may be given chemotherapy after surgery to kill any cancer cells that are left. Treatment given after surgery, to lower the risk that the cancer will come back, is called adjuvant therapy.

Radiation therapy

Radiation therapy is a cancer treatment that uses high-energy x-rays or other types of radiation to kill cancer cells or keep them from growing. There are two types of radiation therapy. External radiation therapy uses a machine outside the body to send radiation toward the cancer. Internal radiation therapy uses a radioactive substance sealed in needles, seeds, wires, or catheters that are placed directly into or near the cancer. The way the radiation therapy is given depends on the type and stage of the cancer being treated.

Chemotherapy

Chemotherapy is a cancer treatment that uses drugs to stop the growth of cancer cells, either by killing the cells or by stopping them from dividing. When chemotherapy is taken by mouth or injected into a vein or muscle, the drugs enter the bloodstream and can reach cancer cells throughout the body (systemic chemotherapy). When chemotherapy is placed directly into the cerebrospinal fluid, an organ, or a body cavity such as the abdomen, the drugs mainly affect cancer cells in those areas (regional chemotherapy). For bladder cancer, regional chemotherapy may be intravesical (put into the bladder through a tube inserted into the urethra). The way the chemotherapy is given depends on the type and stage of the cancer being treated. Combination chemotherapy is treatment using more than one anticancer drug.

Biologic therapy

Biologic therapy is a treatment that uses the patient's immune system to fight cancer. Substances made by the body or made in a laboratory are used to boost, direct, or restore the body's natural defenses against cancer. This type of cancer treatment is also called biotherapy or immunotherapy.

Bladder cancer may be treated with an intravesical biologic therapy called BCG (bacillus Calmette-Guérin). The BCG is given in a solution that is placed directly into the bladder using a catheter (thin tube).

Patients may want to think about taking part in a clinical trial.

For some patients, taking part in a clinical trial may be the best treatment choice. Clinical trials are part of the cancer research process. Clinical trials are done to find out if new cancer treatments are safe and effective or better than the standard treatment.

Many of today's standard treatments for cancer are based on earlier clinical trials. Patients who take part in a clinical trial may receive the standard treatment or be among the first to receive a new treatment.

Patients who take part in clinical trials also help improve the way cancer will be treated in the future. Even when clinical trials do not lead to effective new treatments, they often answer important questions and help move research forward.

Patients can enter clinical trials before, during, or after starting their cancer treatment.

Some clinical trials only include patients who have not yet received treatment. Other trials test treatments for patients whose cancer has not gotten better. There are also clinical trials that test new ways to stop cancer from recurring (coming back) or reduce the side effects of cancer treatment.

Clinical trials are taking place in many parts of the country.

Follow-up tests may be needed.

Some of the tests that were done to diagnose the cancer or to find out the stage of the cancer may be repeated. Some tests will be repeated in order to see how well the treatment is working. Decisions about whether to continue, change, or stop treatment may be based on the results of these tests.

Some of the tests will continue to be done from time to time after treatment has ended. The results of these tests can show if your condition has changed or if the cancer has recurred (come back). These tests are sometimes called follow-up tests or check-ups.

Bladder cancer often recurs (comes back), even when the cancer is superficial. Surveillance of the urinary tract to check for recurrence is standard after a diagnosis of bladder cancer. Surveillance is closely watching a patient's condition but not giving any treatment unless there are changes in test results that show the condition is getting worse. During active surveillance, certain exams and tests are done on a regular schedule. Surveillance may include ureteroscopy and imaging tests.

Section 24.3

Penile Cancer

Text in this section is excerpted from "Penile Cancer Treatment,"
National Cancer Institute at the National Institutes of Health (NIH),
April 2, 2015.

General Information About Penile Cancer

Penile cancer is a disease in which malignant (cancer) cells form in the tissues of the penis.

The penis is a rod-shaped male reproductive organ that passes sperm and urine from the body. It contains two types of erectile tissue (spongy tissue with blood vessels that fill with blood to make an erection):

- Corpora cavernosa: The two columns of erectile tissue that form most of the penis.

- Corpus spongiosum: The single column of erectile tissue that forms a small portion of the penis. The corpus spongiosum surrounds the urethra (the tube through which urine and sperm pass from the body).

The erectile tissue is wrapped in connective tissue and covered with skin. The glans (head of the penis) is covered with loose skin called the foreskin.

Human papillomavirus infection may increase the risk of developing penile cancer.

Anything that increases your chance of getting a disease is called a risk factor. Having a risk factor does not mean that you will get cancer; not having risk factors doesn't mean that you will not get cancer. Talk with your doctor if you think you may be at risk. Risk factors for penile cancer include the following:

Circumcision may help prevent infection with the human papillomavirus (HPV). A circumcision is an operation in which the doctor removes part or all of the foreskin from the penis. Many boys are circumcised shortly after birth. Men who were not circumcised at birth may have a higher risk of developing penile cancer.

Other risk factors for penile cancer include the following:

- Being age 60 or older.
- Having phimosis (a condition in which the foreskin of the penis cannot be pulled back over the glans).
- Having poor personal hygiene.
- Having many sexual partners.
- Using tobacco products.

Signs of penile cancer include sores, discharge, and bleeding.

These and other signs may be caused by penile cancer or by other conditions. Check with your doctor if you have any of the following:

- Redness, irritation, or a sore on the penis.
- A lump on the penis.

Tests that examine the penis are used to detect (find) and diagnose penile cancer.

The following tests and procedures may be used:

- **Physical exam and history:** An exam of the body to check general signs of health, including checking the penis for signs of disease, such as lumps or anything else that seems unusual.

451

A history of the patient's health habits and past illnesses and treatments will also be taken.

- **Biopsy:** The removal of cells or tissues so they can be viewed under a microscope by a pathologist to check for signs of cancer. The tissue sample is removed during one of the following procedures:

  - Fine-needle aspiration (FNA) biopsy: The removal of tissue or fluid using a thin needle.

  - Incisional biopsy: The removal of part of a lump or a sample of tissue that doesn't look normal.

  - Excisional biopsy: The removal of an entire lump or area of tissue that doesn't look normal.

Certain factors affect prognosis (chance of recovery) and treatment options.

The prognosis (chance of recovery) and treatment options depend on the following:

- The stage of the cancer.
- The location and size of the tumor.
- Whether the cancer has just been diagnosed or has recurred (come back).

Stages of Penile Cancer

After penile cancer has been diagnosed, tests are done to find out if cancer cells have spread within the penis or to other parts of the body.

The process used to find out if cancer has spread within the penis or to other parts of the body is called staging. The information gathered from the staging process determines the stage of the disease. It is important to know the stage in order to plan treatment.

The following tests and procedures may be used in the staging process:

- **CT scan (CAT scan):** A procedure that makes a series of detailed pictures of areas inside the body, taken from different angles. The pictures are made by a computer linked to an x-ray machine. A dye may be injected into a vein or swallowed to help the organs or tissues show up more clearly. This procedure is also called computed tomography, computerized tomography, or computerized axial tomography.

- **MRI (magnetic resonance imaging):** A procedure that uses a magnet, radio waves, and a computer to make a series of detailed pictures of areas inside the body. A substance called gadolinium is injected into a vein. The gadolinium collects around the cancer cells so they show up brighter in the picture. This procedure is also called nuclear magnetic resonance imaging (NMRI).

- **Ultrasound exam:** A procedure in which high-energy sound waves (ultrasound) are bounced off internal tissues or organs and make echoes. The echoes form a picture of body tissues called a sonogram.

- **Chest x-ray:** An x-ray of the organs and bones inside the chest. An x-ray is a type of energy beam that can go through the body and onto film, making a picture of areas inside the body.

- **Biopsy:** The removal of cells or tissues so they can be viewed under a microscope by a pathologist to check for signs of cancer. The tissue sample is removed during one of the following procedures:

  - **Sentinel lymph node biopsy:** The removal of the sentinel lymph node during surgery. The sentinel lymph node is the first lymph node to receive lymphatic drainage from a tumor. It is the first lymph node the cancer is likely to spread to from the tumor. A radioactive substance and/or blue dye is injected near the tumor. The substance or dye flows through the lymph ducts to the lymph nodes. The first lymph node to receive the substance or dye is removed. A pathologist views the tissue under a microscope to look for cancer cells. If cancer cells are not found, it may not be necessary to remove more lymph nodes.

  - **Lymph node dissection:** A procedure to remove one or more lymph nodes during surgery. A sample of tissue is checked under a microscope for signs of cancer. This procedure is also called a lymphadenectomy.

There are three ways that cancer spreads in the body.

Cancer can spread through tissue, the lymph system, and the blood:

- Tissue. The cancer spreads from where it began by growing into nearby areas.

- Lymph system. The cancer spreads from where it began by getting into the lymph system. The cancer travels through the lymph vessels to other parts of the body.

- Blood. The cancer spreads from where it began by getting into the blood. The cancer travels through the blood vessels to other parts of the body.

Cancer may spread from where it began to other parts of the body.

When cancer spreads to another part of the body, it is called metastasis. Cancer cells break away from where they began (the primary tumor) and travel through the lymph system or blood.

- Lymph system. The cancer gets into the lymph system, travels through the lymph vessels, and forms a tumor (metastatic tumor) in another part of the body.

- Blood. The cancer gets into the blood, travels through the blood vessels, and forms a tumor (metastatic tumor) in another part of the body.

The metastatic tumor is the same type of cancer as the primary tumor. For example, if penile cancer spreads to the lung, the cancer cells in the lung are actually penile cancer cells. The disease is metastatic penile cancer, not lung cancer.

The following stages are used for penile cancer:

Stage 0 (Carcinoma in Situ)

In stage 0, abnormal cells or growths that look like warts are found on the surface of the skin of the penis. These abnormal cells or growths may become cancer and spread into nearby normal tissue. Stage 0 is also called carcinoma in situ.

Stage I

In stage I, cancer has formed and spread to connective tissue just under the skin of the penis. Cancer has not spread to lymph vessels or blood vessels. The tumor cells look a lot like normal cells under a microscope.

Stage II

In stage II, cancer has spread:

- to connective tissue just under the skin of the penis. Also, cancer has spread to lymph vessels or blood vessels or the tumor cells may look very different from normal cells under a microscope; or

- through connective tissue to erectile tissue (spongy tissue that fills with blood to make an erection); or

- beyond erectile tissue to the urethra.

Stage III

Stage III is divided into stage IIIA and stage IIIB.

In stage IIIA, cancer has spread to one lymph node in the groin. Cancer has also spread:

- to connective tissue just under the skin of the penis. Also, cancer may have spread to lymph vessels or blood vessels or the tumor cells may look very different from normal cells under a microscope; or

- through connective tissue to erectile tissue (spongy tissue that fills with blood to make an erection); or

- beyond erectile tissue to the urethra.

In stage IIIB, cancer has spread to more than one lymph node on one side of the groin or to lymph nodes on both sides of the groin. Cancer has also spread:

- to connective tissue just under the skin of the penis. Also, cancer may have spread to lymph vessels or blood vessels or the tumor cells may look very different from normal cells under a micro-scope; or

- through connective tissue to erectile tissue (spongy tissue that fills with blood to make an erection); or

- beyond erectile tissue to the urethra.

Stage IV

In stage IV, cancer has spread:

- to tissues near the penis such as the prostate, and may have spread to lymph nodes in the groin or pelvis; or

- to one or more lymph nodes in the pelvis, or cancer has spread from the lymph nodes to the tissues around the lymph nodes; or

- to distant parts of the body.

Treatment Option Overview

There are different types of treatment for patients with penile cancer.

Different types of treatments are available for patients with penile cancer. Some treatments are standard (the currently used treatment), and some are being tested in clinical trials. A treatment clinical trial is a research study meant to help improve current treatments or obtain information on new treatments for patients with cancer. When clinical trials show that a new treatment is better than the standard treatment, the new treatment may become the standard treatment. Patients may want to think about taking part in a clinical trial. Some clinical trials are open only to patients who have not started treatment.

Three types of standard treatment are used:

Surgery

Surgery is the most common treatment for all stages of penile cancer. A doctor may remove the cancer using one of the following operations:

- Mohs microsurgery: A procedure in which the tumor is cut from the skin in thin layers. During the surgery, the edges of the tumor and each layer of tumor removed are viewed through a microscope to check for cancer cells. Layers continue to be removed until no more cancer cells are seen. This type of surgery removes as little normal tissue as possible and is often used to remove cancer on the skin. It is also called Mohs surgery.

- Laser surgery: A surgical procedure that uses a laser beam (a narrow beam of intense light) as a knife to make bloodless cuts in tissue or to remove a surface lesion such as a tumor.

- Cryosurgery: A treatment that uses an instrument to freeze and destroy abnormal tissue. This type of treatment is also called cryotherapy.

- Circumcision: Surgery to remove part or all of the foreskin of the penis.

- Wide local excision: Surgery to remove only the cancer and some normal tissue around it.

- Amputation of the penis: Surgery to remove part or all of the penis. If part of the penis is removed, it is a partial penectomy. If all of the penis is removed, it is a total penectomy.

Lymph nodes in the groin may be taken out during surgery.

Even if the doctor removes all the cancer that can be seen at the time of the surgery, some patients may be given chemotherapy or radiation therapy after surgery to kill any cancer cells that are left. Treatment given after the surgery, to lower the risk that the cancer will come back, is called adjuvant therapy.

Radiation therapy

Radiation therapy is a cancer treatment that uses high-energy x-rays or other types of radiation to kill cancer cells or keep them from growing. There are two types of radiation therapy. External radiation therapy uses a machine outside the body to send radiation toward the cancer. Internal radiation therapy uses a radioactive substance sealed in needles, seeds, wires, or catheters that are placed directly into or near the cancer. The way the radiation therapy is given depends on the type and stage of the cancer being treated.

Chemotherapy

Chemotherapy is a cancer treatment that uses drugs to stop the growth of cancer cells, either by killing the cells or by stopping them from dividing. When chemotherapy is taken by mouth or injected into a vein or muscle, the drugs enter the bloodstream and can reach cancer cells throughout the body (systemic chemotherapy). When chemotherapy is placed directly onto the skin (topical chemotherapy) or into the cerebrospinal fluid, an organ, or a body cavity such as the abdomen, the drugs mainly affect cancer cells in those areas (regional chemotherapy). The way the chemotherapy is given depends on the type and stage of the cancer being treated.

Topical chemotherapy may be used to treat stage 0 penile cancer.

New types of treatment are being tested in clinical trials.

Biologic therapy

Biologic therapy is a treatment that uses the patient's immune system to fight cancer. Substances made by the body or made in a laboratory are used to boost, direct, or restore the body's natural defenses against cancer. This type of cancer treatment is also called biotherapy or immunotherapy. Topical biologic therapy may be used to treat stage 0 penile cancer.

Radiosensitizers

Radiosensitizers are drugs that make tumor cells more sensitive to radiation therapy. Combining radiation therapy with radiosensitizers helps kill more tumor cells.

Sentinel lymph node biopsy followed by surgery

Sentinel lymph node biopsy is the removal of the sentinel lymph node during surgery. The sentinel lymph node is the first lymph node to receive lymphatic drainage from a tumor. It is the first lymph node the cancer is likely to spread to from the tumor. A radioactive substance and/or blue dye is injected near the tumor. The substance or dye flows through the lymph ducts to the lymph nodes. The first lymph node to receive the substance or dye is removed. A pathologist views the tissue under a microscope to look for cancer cells. If cancer cells are not found, it may not be necessary to remove more lymph nodes. After the sentinel lymph node biopsy, the surgeon removes the cancer.

Patients may want to think about taking part in a clinical trial.

For some patients, taking part in a clinical trial may be the best treatment choice. Clinical trials are part of the cancer research process. Clinical trials are done to find out if new cancer treatments are safe and effective or better than the standard treatment.

Many of today's standard treatments for cancer are based on earlier clinical trials. Patients who take part in a clinical trial may receive the standard treatment or be among the first to receive a new treatment.

Patients who take part in clinical trials also help improve the way cancer will be treated in the future. Even when clinical trials do not lead to effective new treatments, they often answer important questions and help move research forward.

Patients can enter clinical trials before, during, or after starting their cancer treatment.

Some clinical trials only include patients who have not yet received treatment. Other trials test treatments for patients whose cancer has not gotten better. There are also clinical trials that test new ways to stop cancer from recurring (coming back) or reduce the side effects of cancer treatment.

Clinical trials are taking place in many parts of the country.

Follow-up tests may be needed.

Some of the tests that were done to diagnose the cancer or to find out the stage of the cancer may be repeated. Some tests will be repeated in order to see how well the treatment is working. Decisions about whether to continue, change, or stop treatment may be based on the results of these tests.

Some of the tests will continue to be done from time to time after treatment has ended. The results of these tests can show if your condition has changed or if the cancer has recurred (come back). These tests are sometimes called follow-up tests or check-ups.

Section 24.4

Testicular Cancer

Text in this section is excerpted from "Testicular Cancer Treatment,"
National Cancer Institute at the National Institutes of Health (NIH),
December 31, 2014.

General Information About Testicular Cancer

Testicular cancer is a disease in which malignant (cancer) cells form in the tissues of one or both testicles.

The testicles are 2 egg-shaped glands located inside the scrotum (a
sac of loose skin that lies directly below the penis). The testicles are
held within the scrotum by the spermatic cord, which also contains
the vas deferens and vessels and nerves of the testicles.

The testicles are the male sex glands and produce testosterone
and sperm. Germ cells within the testicles produce immature sperm
that travel through a network of tubules (tiny tubes) and larger tubes
into the epididymis (a long coiled tube next to the testicles) where the
sperm mature and are stored.

Almost all testicular cancers start in the germ cells. The two main
types of testicular germ cell tumors are seminomas and nonseminomas. These 2 types grow and spread differently and are treated differently. Nonseminomas tend to grow and spread more quickly than
seminomas. Seminomas are more sensitive to radiation. A testicular
tumor that contains both seminoma and nonseminoma cells is treated
as a nonseminoma.

Testicular cancer is the most common cancer in men 20 to 35 years old.

Health history can affect the risk of testicular cancer.

Anything that increases the chance of getting a disease is called a
risk factor. Having a risk factor does not mean that you will get cancer; not having risk factors doesn't mean that you will not get cancer.
Talk with your doctor if you think you may be at risk. Risk factors for
testicular cancer include:

- Having had an undescended testicle.

- Having had abnormal development of the testicles.

- Having a personal history of testicular cancer.

- Having a family history of testicular cancer (especially in a father or brother).

- Being white.

Signs and symptoms of testicular cancer include swelling or discomfort in the scrotum.

These and other signs and symptoms may be caused by testicular cancer or by other conditions. Check with your doctor if you have any of the following:

- A painless lump or swelling in either testicle.

- A change in how the testicle feels.

- A dull ache in the lower abdomen or the groin.

- A sudden build-up of fluid in the scrotum.

- Pain or discomfort in a testicle or in the scrotum.

Tests that examine the testicles and blood are used to detect (find) and diagnose testicular cancer.

The following tests and procedures may be used:

- **Physical exam and history:** An exam of the body to check general signs of health, including checking for signs of disease, such as lumps or anything else that seems unusual. The testicles will be examined to check for lumps, swelling, or pain. A history of the patient's health habits and past illnesses and treatments will also be taken.

- **Ultrasound exam:** A procedure in which high-energy sound waves (ultrasound) are bounced off internal tissues or organs and make echoes. The echoes form a picture of body tissues called a sonogram.

- **Serum tumor marker test:** A procedure in which a sample of blood is examined to measure the amounts of certain substances released into the blood by organs, tissues, or tumor cells in the body. Certain substances are linked to specific types of cancer when found in increased levels in the blood. These are called

461

tumor markers. The following tumor markers are used to detect testicular cancer:

- Alpha-fetoprotein (AFP).
- Beta-human chorionic gonadotropin (β-hCG).

Tumor marker levels are measured before inguinal orchiectomy and biopsy, to help diagnose testicular cancer.

- **Inguinal orchiectomy:** A procedure to remove the entire testicle through an incision in the groin. A tissue sample from the testicle is then viewed under a microscope to check for cancer cells. (The surgeon does not cut through the scrotum into the testicle to remove a sample of tissue for biopsy, because if cancer is present, this procedure could cause it to spread into the scrotum and lymph nodes. It's important to choose a surgeon who has experience with this kind of surgery.) If cancer is found, the cell type (seminoma or nonseminoma) is determined in order to help plan treatment.

Certain factors affect prognosis (chance of recovery) and treatment options.

The prognosis (chance of recovery) and treatment options depend on the following:

- Stage of the cancer (whether it is in or near the testicle or has spread to other places in the body, and blood levels of AFP, β-hCG, and LDH).
- Type of cancer.
- Size of the tumor.
- Number and size of retroperitoneal lymph nodes.

Testicular cancer can usually be cured in patients who receive adjuvant chemotherapy or radiation therapy after their primary treatment.

Treatment for testicular cancer can cause infertility.

Certain treatments for testicular cancer can cause infertility that may be permanent. Patients who may wish to have children should consider sperm banking before having treatment. Sperm banking is the process of freezing sperm and storing it for later use.

Stages of Testicular Cancer

After testicular cancer has been diagnosed, tests are done to find out if cancer cells have spread within the testicles or to other parts of the body.

The process used to find out if cancer has spread within the testicles or to other parts of the body is called staging. The information gathered from the staging process determines the stage of the disease. It is important to know the stage in order to plan treatment.

The following tests and procedures may be used in the staging process:

- **Chest x-ray:** An x-ray of the organs and bones inside the chest. An x-ray is a type of energy beam that can go through the body and onto film, making a picture of areas inside the body.

- **CT scan (CAT scan):** A procedure that makes a series of detailed pictures of areas inside the body, taken from different angles. The pictures are made by a computer linked to an x-ray machine. A dye may be injected into a vein or swallowed to help the organs or tissues show up more clearly. This procedure is also called computed tomography, computerized tomography, or computerized axial tomography.

- **PET scan (positron emission tomography scan):** A procedure to find malignant tumor cells in the body. A small amount of radioactive glucose (sugar) is injected into a vein. The PET scanner rotates around the body and makes a picture of where glucose is being used in the body. Malignant tumor cells show up brighter in the picture because they are more active and take up more glucose than normal cells do.

- **MRI (magnetic resonance imaging):** A procedure that uses a magnet, radio waves, and a computer to make a series of detailed pictures of areas inside the body. This procedure is also called nuclear magnetic resonance imaging (NMRI).

- **Abdominal lymph node dissection:** A surgical procedure in which lymph nodes in the abdomen are removed and a sample of tissue is checked under a microscope for signs of cancer. This procedure is also called lymphadenectomy. For patients with nonseminoma, removing the lymph nodes may help stop the spread of disease. Cancer cells in the lymph nodes of seminoma patients can be treated with radiation therapy.

463

- **Serum tumor marker test:** A procedure in which a sample of blood is examined to measure the amounts of certain substances released into the blood by organs, tissues, or tumor cells in the body. Certain substances are linked to specific types of cancer when found in increased levels in the blood. These are called tumor markers. The following 3 tumor markers are used in staging testicular cancer:

  - Alpha-fetoprotein (AFP)

  - Beta-human chorionic gonadotropin (β-hCG).

  - Lactate dehydrogenase (LDH).

Tumor marker levels are measured again, after inguinal orchiectomy and biopsy, in order to determine the stage of the cancer. This helps to show if all of the cancer has been removed or if more treatment is needed. Tumor marker levels are also measured during follow-up as a way of checking if the cancer has come back.

There are three ways that cancer spreads in the body.

Cancer can spread through tissue, the lymph system, and the blood:

- Tissue. The cancer spreads from where it began by growing into nearby areas.

- Lymph system. The cancer spreads from where it began by getting into the lymph system. The cancer travels through the lymph vessels to other parts of the body.

- Blood. The cancer spreads from where it began by getting into the blood. The cancer travels through the blood vessels to other parts of the body.

Cancer may spread from where it began to other parts of the body.

When cancer spreads to another part of the body, it is called metastasis. Cancer cells break away from where they began (the primary tumor) and travel through the lymph system or blood.

- Lymph system. The cancer gets into the lymph system, travels through the lymph vessels, and forms a tumor (metastatic tumor) in another part of the body.

- Blood. The cancer gets into the blood, travels through the blood vessels, and forms a tumor (metastatic tumor) in another part of the body.

The metastatic tumor is the same type of cancer as the primary tumor. For example, if testicular cancer spreads to the lung, the cancer cells in the lung are actually testicular cancer cells. The disease is metastatic testicular cancer, not lung cancer.

The following stages are used for testicular cancer:

Stage 0 (Testicular Intraepithelial Neoplasia)

In stage 0, abnormal cells are found in the tiny tubules where the sperm cells begin to develop. These abnormal cells may become cancer and spread into nearby normal tissue. All tumor marker levels are normal. Stage 0 is also called testicular intraepithelial neoplasia and intratubular germ cell neoplasia.

Stage I

In stage I, cancer has formed. Stage I is divided into stage IA, stage IB, and stage IS and is determined after an inguinal orchiectomy is done.

- In stage IA, cancer is in the testicle and epididymis and may have spread to the inner layer of the membrane surrounding the testicle. All tumor marker levels are normal.

- In stage IB, cancer:

  - is in the testicle and the epididymis and has spread to the blood vessels or lymph vessels in the testicle; or

  - has spread to the outer layer of the membrane surrounding the testicle; or

  - is in the spermatic cord or the scrotum and may be in the blood vessels or lymph vessels of the testicle.

All tumor marker levels are normal.
In stage IS, cancer is found anywhere within the testicle, spermatic cord, or the scrotum and either:

- all tumor marker levels are slightly above normal; or

- one or more tumor marker levels are moderately above normal or high.

Stage II

Stage II is divided into stage IIA, stage IIB, and stage IIC and is determined after an inguinal orchiectomy is done.

- In stage IIA, cancer:
  - is anywhere within the testicle, spermatic cord, or scrotum; and
  - has spread to up to 5 lymph nodes in the abdomen, none larger than 2 centimeters.

  All tumor marker levels are normal or slightly above normal.

- In stage IIB, cancer is anywhere within the testicle, spermatic cord, or scrotum; and either:
  - has spread to up to 5 lymph nodes in the abdomen; at least one of the lymph nodes is larger than 2 centimeters, but none are larger than 5 centimeters; or
  - has spread to more than 5 lymph nodes; the lymph nodes are not larger than 5 centimeters.

  All tumor marker levels are normal or slightly above normal.

- In stage IIC, cancer:
  - is anywhere within the testicle, spermatic cord, or scrotum; and
  - has spread to a lymph node in the abdomen that is larger than 5 centimeters.

  All tumor marker levels are normal or slightly above normal.

Stage III

Stage III is divided into stage IIIA, stage IIIB, and stage IIIC and is determined after an inguinal orchiectomy is done.

- In stage IIIA, cancer:
  - is anywhere within the testicle, spermatic cord, or scrotum; and
  - may have spread to one or more lymph nodes in the abdomen; and

- has spread to distant lymph nodes or to the lungs.

Tumor marker levels may range from normal to slightly above normal.

- In stage IIIB, cancer:
  - is anywhere within the testicle, spermatic cord, or scrotum; and
  - may have spread to one or more lymph nodes in the abdomen, to distant lymph nodes, or to the lungs.
  - The level of one or more tumor markers is moderately above normal.
- In stage IIIC, cancer:
  - is anywhere within the testicle, spermatic cord, or scrotum; and
  - may have spread to one or more lymph nodes in the abdomen, to distant lymph nodes, or to the lungs.
  - The level of one or more tumor markers is high.

  or

Cancer:

- is anywhere within the testicle, spermatic cord, or scrotum; and
- may have spread to one or more lymph nodes in the abdomen; and
- has not spread to distant lymph nodes or the lung but has spread to other parts of the body.

  Tumor marker levels may range from normal to high.

Section 24.5

Prostate Cancer

Text in this section is excerpted from "Prostate Cancer Treatment,"
National Cancer Institute at the National Institutes of Health (NIH),
April 16, 2015.

General Information About Prostate Cancer

*Prostate cancer is a disease in which malignant (cancer)
cells form in the tissues of the prostate.*

The prostate is a gland in the male reproductive system. It lies just
below the bladder (the organ that collects and empties urine) and in front
of the rectum (the lower part of the intestine). It is about the size of a walnut and surrounds part of the urethra (the tube that empties urine from
the bladder). The prostate gland makes fluid that is part of the semen.

Prostate cancer is found mainly in older men. In the U.S., about 1
out of 5 men will be diagnosed with prostate cancer.

*Signs of prostate cancer include a weak flow of urine or
frequent urination.*

These and other signs and symptoms may be caused by prostate
cancer or by other conditions. Check with your doctor if you have any
of the following:

- Weak or interrupted ("stop-and-go") flow of urine.
- Sudden urge to urinate.
- Frequent urination (especially at night).
- Trouble starting the flow of urine.
- Trouble emptying the bladder completely.
- Pain or burning while urinating.
- Blood in the urine or semen.
- A pain in the back, hips, or pelvis that doesn't go away.

- Shortness of breath, feeling very tired, fast heartbeat, dizziness, or pale skin caused by anemia.

Other conditions may cause the same symptoms. As men age, the prostate may get bigger and block the urethra or bladder. This may cause trouble urinating or sexual problems. The condition is called benign prostatic hyperplasia (BPH), and although it is not cancer, surgery may be needed. The symptoms of benign prostatic hyperplasia or of other problems in the prostate may be like symptoms of prostate cancer.

Tests that examine the prostate and blood are used to detect (find) and diagnose prostate cancer.

The following tests and procedures may be used:

- **Physical exam and history:** An exam of the body to check general signs of health, including checking for signs of disease, such as lumps or anything else that seems unusual. A history of the patient's health habits and past illnesses and treatments will also be taken.

- **Digital rectal exam (DRE):** An exam of the rectum. The doctor or nurse inserts a lubricated, gloved finger into the rectum and feels the prostate through the rectal wall for lumps or abnormal areas.

- **Prostate-specific antigen (PSA) test:** A test that measures the level of PSA in the blood. PSA is a substance made by the prostate that may be found in an increased amount in the blood of men who have prostate cancer. PSA levels may also be high in men who have an infection or inflammation of the prostate or BPH (an enlarged, but noncancerous, prostate).

- **Transrectal ultrasound:** A procedure in which a probe that is about the size of a finger is inserted into the rectum to check the prostate. The probe is used to bounce high-energy sound waves (ultrasound) off internal tissues or organs and make echoes. The echoes form a picture of body tissues called a sonogram. Transrectal ultrasound may be used during a biopsy procedure.

- **Transrectal magnetic resonance imaging (MRI):** A procedure that uses a strong magnet, radio waves, and a computer to make a series of detailed pictures of areas inside the body. A probe that gives off radio waves is inserted into the rectum near the prostate. This helps the MRI machine make clearer pictures of the prostate and nearby tissue. A transrectal MRI is done to find out if the cancer has spread outside the prostate into nearby tissues. This procedure is also called nuclear magnetic resonance imaging (NMRI).

- **Biopsy:** The removal of cells or tissues so they can be viewed under a microscope by a pathologist. The pathologist will check the tissue sample to see if there are cancer cells and find out the Gleason score. The Gleason score ranges from 2-10 and describes how likely it is that a tumor will spread. The lower the number, the less likely the tumor is to spread.

A transrectal biopsy is used to diagnose prostate cancer. A transrectal biopsy is the removal of tissue from the prostate by inserting a thin needle through the rectum and into the prostate. This procedure is usually done using transrectal ultrasound to help guide where samples of tissue are taken from. A pathologist views the tissue under a microscope to look for cancer cells.

Certain factors affect prognosis (chance of recovery) and treatment options.

The prognosis (chance of recovery) and treatment options depend on the following:

- The stage of the cancer (level of PSA, Gleason score, grade of the tumor, how much of the prostate is affected by the cancer, and whether the cancer has spread to other places in the body).
- The patient's age.
- Whether the cancer has just been diagnosed or has recurred (come back).

Treatment options also may depend on the following:

- Whether the patient has other health problems.
- The expected side effects of treatment.
- Past treatment for prostate cancer.
- The wishes of the patient.

Most men diagnosed with prostate cancer do not die of it.

Stages of Prostate Cancer

After prostate cancer has been diagnosed, tests are done to find out if cancer cells have spread within the prostate or to other parts of the body.

The process used to find out if cancer has spread within the prostate or to other parts of the body is called staging. The information gathered from the staging process determines the stage of the disease. It is important to know the stage in order to plan treatment. The results of the tests used to diagnose prostate cancer are often also used to stage the disease. In prostate cancer, staging tests may not be done unless the patient has symptoms or signs that the cancer has spread, such as bone pain, a high PSA level, or a high Gleason score.

The following tests and procedures also may be used in the staging process:

- **Bone scan:** A procedure to check if there are rapidly dividing cells, such as cancer cells, in the bone. A very small amount of radioactive material is injected into a vein and travels through the bloodstream. The radioactive material collects in the bones and is detected by a scanner.

- **MRI (magnetic resonance imaging):** A procedure that uses a magnet, radio waves, and a computer to make a series of detailed pictures of areas inside the body. This procedure is also called nuclear magnetic resonance imaging (NMRI).

- **CT scan (CAT scan):** A procedure that makes a series of detailed pictures of areas inside the body, taken from different angles. The pictures are made by a computer linked to an x-ray machine. A dye may be injected into a vein or swallowed to help the organs or tissues show up more clearly. This procedure is also called computed tomography, computerized tomography, or computerized axial tomography.

- **Pelvic lymphadenectomy:** A surgical procedure to remove the lymph nodes in the pelvis. A pathologist views the tissue under a microscope to look for cancer cells.

- **Seminal vesicle biopsy:** The removal of fluid from the seminal vesicles (glands that make semen) using a needle. A pathologist views the fluid under a microscope to look for cancer cells.

- **ProstaScint scan:** A procedure to check for cancer that has spread from the prostate to other parts of the body, such as the lymph nodes. A very small amount of radioactive material is injected into a vein and travels through the bloodstream. The radioactive material attaches to prostate cancer cells and is detected by a scanner. The radioactive material shows up as a bright spot on the picture in areas where there are a lot of prostate cancer cells.

The stage of the cancer is based on the results of the staging and diagnostic tests, including the prostate-specific antigen (PSA) test and the Gleason score. The tissue samples removed during the biopsy are used to find out the Gleason score. The Gleason score ranges from 2-10 and describes how different the cancer cells look from normal cells and how likely it is that the tumor will spread. The lower the number, the less likely the tumor is to spread.

There are three ways that cancer spreads in the body.

Cancer can spread through tissue, the lymph system, and the blood:

- Tissue. The cancer spreads from where it began by growing into nearby areas.

- Lymph system. The cancer spreads from where it began by getting into the lymph system. The cancer travels through the lymph vessels to other parts of the body.

- Blood. The cancer spreads from where it began by getting into the blood. The cancer travels through the blood vessels to other parts of the body.

Cancer may spread from where it began to other parts of the body.

When cancer spreads to another part of the body, it is called metastasis. Cancer cells break away from where they began (the primary tumor) and travel through the lymph system or blood.

- Lymph system. The cancer gets into the lymph system, travels through the lymph vessels, and forms a tumor (metastatic tumor) in another part of the body.

- Blood. The cancer gets into the blood, travels through the blood vessels, and forms a tumor (metastatic tumor) in another part of the body.

472

The metastatic tumor is the same type of cancer as the primary tumor. For example, if prostate cancer spreads to the bone, the cancer cells in the bone are actually prostate cancer cells. The disease is metastatic prostate cancer, not bone cancer.

Denosumab, a monoclonal antibody, may be used to prevent bone metastases.

The following stages are used for prostate cancer:

Stage I

In stage I, cancer is found in the prostate only. The cancer:

- is found by needle biopsy (done for a high PSA level) or in a small amount of tissue during surgery for other reasons (such as benign prostatic hyperplasia). The PSA level is lower than 10 and the Gleason score is 6 or lower; or

- is found in one-half or less of one lobe of the prostate. The PSA level is lower than 10 and the Gleason score is 6 or lower; or

- cannot be felt during a digital rectal exam and cannot be seen in imaging tests. Cancer is found in one-half or less of one lobe of the prostate. The PSA level and the Gleason score are not known.

Stage II

In stage II, cancer is more advanced than in stage I, but has not spread outside the prostate. Stage II is divided into stages IIA and IIB.

In stage IIA, cancer:

- is found by needle biopsy (done for a high PSA level) or in a small amount of tissue during surgery for other reasons (such as benign prostatic hyperplasia). The PSA level is lower than 20 and the Gleason score is 7; or

- is found by needle biopsy (done for a high PSA level) or in a small amount of tissue during surgery for other reasons (such as benign prostatic hyperplasia). The PSA level is at least 10 but lower than 20 and the Gleason score is 6 or lower; or

- is found in one-half or less of one lobe of the prostate. The PSA level is at least 10 but lower than 20 and the Gleason score is 6 or lower; or

- is found in one-half or less of one lobe of the prostate. The PSA level is lower than 20 and the Gleason score is 7; or

- is found in more than one-half of one lobe of the prostate.

In stage IIB, cancer:

- is found in opposite sides of the prostate. The PSA can be any level and the Gleason score can range from 2 to 10; or

- cannot be felt during a digital rectal exam and cannot be seen in imaging tests. The PSA level is 20 or higher and the Gleason score can range from 2 to 10; or

- cannot be felt during a digital rectal exam and cannot be seen in imaging tests. The PSA can be any level and the Gleason score is 8 or higher.

Stage III

In stage III, cancer has spread beyond the outer layer of the prostate and may have spread to the seminal vesicles. The PSA can be any level and the Gleason score can range from 2 to 10.

Stage IV

In stage IV, the PSA can be any level and the Gleason score can range from 2 to 10. Also, cancer:

- has spread beyond the seminal vesicles to nearby tissue or organs, such as the rectum, bladder, or pelvic wall; or

- may have spread to the seminal vesicles or to nearby tissue or organs, such as the rectum, bladder, or pelvic wall. Cancer has spread to nearby lymph nodes; or

- has spread to distant parts of the body, which may include lymph nodes or bones. Prostate cancer often spreads to the bones.

Treatment Option Overview

There are different types of treatment for patients with prostate cancer.

Different types of treatment are available for patients with prostate cancer. Some treatments are standard (the currently used treatment), and some are being tested in clinical trials. A treatment clinical trial is a research study meant to help improve current treatments or obtain information on new treatments for patients with cancer. When clinical trials show that a new treatment is better than the standard treatment, the new treatment may become the standard treatment. Patients may want to think about taking part in a clinical trial. Some clinical trials are open only to patients who have not started treatment.

Seven types of standard treatment are used:

Watchful waiting or active surveillance

Watchful waiting and active surveillance are treatments used for older men who do not have signs or symptoms or have other medical conditions and for men whose prostate cancer is found during a screening test.

Watchful waiting is closely monitoring a patient's condition without giving any treatment until signs or symptoms appear or change. Treatment is given to relieve symptoms and improve quality of life.

Active surveillance is closely following a patient's condition without giving any treatment unless there are changes in test results. It is used to find early signs that the condition is getting worse. In active surveillance, patients are given certain exams and tests, including digital rectal exam, PSA test, transrectal ultrasound, and transrectal needle biopsy, to check if the cancer is growing. When the cancer begins to grow, treatment is given to cure the cancer.

Other terms that are used to describe not giving treatment to cure prostate cancer right after diagnosis are observation, watch and wait, and expectant management.

Surgery

Patients in good health whose tumor is in the prostate gland only may be treated with surgery to remove the tumor. The following types of surgery are used:

- Radical prostatectomy: A surgical procedure to remove the prostate, surrounding tissue, and seminal vesicles. There are two types of radical prostatectomy:

- Retropubic prostatectomy: A surgical procedure to remove the prostate through an incision (cut) in the abdominal wall. Removal of nearby lymph nodes may be done at the same time.

- Perineal prostatectomy: A surgical procedure to remove the prostate through an incision (cut) made in the perineum (area between the scrotum and anus). Nearby lymph nodes may also be removed through a separate incision in the abdomen.

- Pelvic lymphadenectomy: A surgical procedure to remove the lymph nodes in the pelvis. A pathologist views the tissue under a microscope to look for cancer cells. If the lymph nodes contain cancer, the doctor will not remove the prostate and may recommend other treatment.

- Transurethral resection of the prostate (TURP): A surgical procedure to remove tissue from the prostate using a resectoscope (a thin, lighted tube with a cutting tool) inserted through the urethra. This procedure is done to treat benign prostatic hypertrophy and it is sometimes done to relieve symptoms caused by a tumor before other cancer treatment is given. TURP may also be done in men whose tumor is in the prostate only and who cannot have a radical prostatectomy.

In some cases, nerve-sparing surgery can be done. This type of surgery may save the nerves that control erection. However, men with large tumors or tumors that are very close to the nerves may not be able to have this surgery.

Possible problems after prostate cancer surgery include the following:

- Impotence.

- Leakage of urine from the bladder or stool from the rectum.

- Shortening of the penis (1 to 2 centimeters). The exact reason for this is not known.

- Inguinal hernia (bulging of fat or part of the small intestine through weak muscles into the groin). Inguinal hernia may occur more often in men treated with radical prostatectomy than in men who have some other types of prostate surgery, radiation therapy, or prostate biopsy alone. It is most likely to occur within the first 2 years after radical prostatectomy.

Radiation therapy

Radiation therapy is a cancer treatment that uses high-energy x-rays or other types of radiation to kill cancer cells or keep them from growing. There are different types of radiation therapy:

- External radiation therapy uses a machine outside the body to send radiation toward the cancer. Conformal radiation is a type of external radiation therapy that uses a computer to create a 3-dimensional (3-D) picture of the tumor. The radiation beams are shaped to fit the tumor.

- Internal radiation therapy uses a radioactive substance sealed in needles, seeds, wires, or catheters that are placed directly into or near the cancer. In early-stage prostate cancer, the radioactive seeds are placed in the prostate using needles that are inserted through the skin between the scrotum and rectum. The placement of the radioactive seeds in the prostate is guided by images from transrectal ultrasound or computed tomography (CT). The needles are removed after the radioactive seeds are placed in the prostate.

- Alpha emitter radiation therapy uses a radioactive substance to treat prostate cancer that has spread to the bone. A radioactive substance called radium-223 is injected into a vein and travels through the bloodstream. The radium-223 collects in areas of bone with cancer and kills the cancer cells.

The way the radiation therapy is given depends on the type and stage of the cancer being treated.

Men treated with radiation therapy for prostate cancer have an increased risk of having bladder and/or gastrointestinal cancer.

Radiation therapy can cause impotence and urinary problems.

Hormone therapy

Hormone therapy is a cancer treatment that removes hormones or blocks their action and stops cancer cells from growing. Hormones are substances made by glands in the body and circulated in the bloodstream. In prostate cancer, male sex hormones can cause prostate cancer to grow. Drugs, surgery, or other hormones are used to reduce the amount of male hormones or block them from working.

Hormone therapy for prostate cancer may include the following:

- Luteinizing hormone-releasing hormone agonists can stop the testicles from making testosterone. Examples are leuprolide, goserelin, and buserelin.

- Antiandrogens can block the action of androgens (hormones that promote male sex characteristics), such as testosterone.

477

Examples are flutamide, bicalutamide, enzalutamide, and nilutamide.

- Drugs that can prevent the adrenal glands from making androgens include ketoconazole and aminoglutethimide.

- Orchiectomy is a surgical procedure to remove one or both testicles, the main source of male hormones, such as testosterone, to decrease the amount of hormone being made.

- Estrogens (hormones that promote female sex characteristics) can prevent the testicles from making testosterone. However, estrogens are seldom used today in the treatment of prostate cancer because of the risk of serious side effects.

Hot flashes, impaired sexual function, loss of desire for sex, and weakened bones may occur in men treated with hormone therapy. Other side effects include diarrhea, nausea, and itching.

Chemotherapy

Chemotherapy is a cancer treatment that uses drugs to stop the growth of cancer cells, either by killing the cells or by stopping them from dividing. When chemotherapy is taken by mouth or injected into a vein or muscle, the drugs enter the bloodstream and can reach cancer cells throughout the body (systemic chemotherapy). When chemotherapy is placed directly into the cerebrospinal fluid, an organ, or a body cavity such as the abdomen, the drugs mainly affect cancer cells in those areas (regional chemotherapy). The way the chemotherapy is given depends on the type and stage of the cancer being treated.

Biologic therapy

Biologic therapy is a treatment that uses the patient's immune system to fight cancer. Substances made by the body or made in a laboratory are used to boost, direct, or restore the body's natural defenses against cancer. Sipuleucel-T is a type of biologic therapy used to treat prostate cancer that has metastasized (spread to other parts of the body).

Bisphosphonate therapy

Bisphosphonate drugs, such as clodronate or zoledronate, reduce bone disease when cancer has spread to the bone. Men who are treated with antiandrogen therapy or orchiectomy are at an increased risk of bone loss. In these men, bisphosphonate drugs lessen the risk of bone fracture (breaks). The use of bisphosphonate drugs to prevent or slow the growth of bone metastases is being studied in clinical trials.

There are treatments for bone pain caused by bone metastases or hormone therapy.

Prostate cancer that has spread to the bone and certain types of hormone therapy can weaken bones and lead to bone pain. Treatments for bone pain include the following:

- Pain medicine.
- External radiation therapy.
- Strontium-89 (a radioisotope).
- Targeted therapy with a monoclonal antibody, such as denosumab.
- Bisphosphonate therapy.
- Corticosteroids.

New types of treatment are being tested in clinical trials.

Cryosurgery

Cryosurgery is a treatment that uses an instrument to freeze and destroy prostate cancer cells. Ultrasound is used to find the area that will be treated. This type of treatment is also called cryotherapy.

Cryosurgery can cause impotence and leakage of urine from the bladder or stool from the rectum.

High-intensity focused ultrasound

High-intensity focused ultrasound is a treatment that uses ultrasound (high-energy sound waves) to destroy cancer cells. To treat prostate cancer, an endorectal probe is used to make the sound waves.

Proton beam radiation therapy

Proton beam radiation therapy is a type of high-energy, external radiation therapy that targets tumors with streams of protons (small,

479

positively charged particles). This type of radiation therapy is being studied in the treatment of prostate cancer.

Patients may want to think about taking part in a clinical trial.

For some patients, taking part in a clinical trial may be the best treatment choice. Clinical trials are part of the cancer research process. Clinical trials are done to find out if new cancer treatments are safe and effective or better than the standard treatment.

Many of today's standard treatments for cancer are based on earlier clinical trials. Patients who take part in a clinical trial may receive the standard treatment or be among the first to receive a new treatment.

Patients who take part in clinical trials also help improve the way cancer will be treated in the future. Even when clinical trials do not lead to effective new treatments, they often answer important questions and help move research forward.

Patients can enter clinical trials before, during, or after starting their cancer treatment.

Some clinical trials only include patients who have not yet received treatment. Other trials test treatments for patients whose cancer has not gotten better. There are also clinical trials that test new ways to stop cancer from recurring (coming back) or reduce the side effects of cancer treatment.

Clinical trials are taking place in many parts of the country.

Follow-up tests may be needed.

Some of the tests that were done to diagnose the cancer or to find out the stage of the cancer may be repeated. Some tests will be repeated in order to see how well the treatment is working. Decisions about whether to continue, change, or stop treatment may be based on the results of these tests.

Some of the tests will continue to be done from time to time after treatment has ended. The results of these tests can show if your condition has changed or if the cancer has recurred (come back). These tests are sometimes called follow-up tests or check-ups.

Chapter 25

Gynecological Cancer

Chapter Contents

Section 25.1

Ovarian Epithelial, Fallopian Tube, and Primary Peritoneal Cancer

Text in this section is excerpted from "Ovarian Epithelial,
Fallopian Tube, and Primary Peritoneal Cancer Treatment,"
National Cancer Institute at the National Institutes of Health
(NIH), April 2, 2015.

General Information About Ovarian Epithelial, Fallopian Tube, and Primary Peritoneal Cancer

Ovarian epithelial cancer, fallopian tube cancer, and primary peritoneal cancer are diseases in which malignant (cancer) cells form in the tissue covering the ovary or lining the fallopian tube or peritoneum.

The ovaries are a pair of organs in the female reproductive system. They are in the pelvis, one on each side of the uterus (the hollow, pear-shaped organ where a fetus grows). Each ovary is about the size and shape of an almond. The ovaries make eggs and female hormones (chemicals that control the way certain cells or organs work).

The fallopian tubes are a pair of long, slender tubes, one on each side of the uterus. Eggs pass from the ovaries, through the fallopian tubes, to the uterus. Cancer sometimes begins at the end of the fallopian tube near the ovary and spreads to the ovary.

The peritoneum is the tissue that lines the abdominal wall and covers organs in the abdomen. Primary peritoneal cancer is cancer that forms in the peritoneum and has not spread there from another part of the body. Cancer sometimes begins in the peritoneum and spreads to the ovary.

Ovarian epithelial cancer is one type of cancer that affects the ovary.

Ovarian epithelial cancer, fallopian tube cancer, and primary peritoneal cancer are treated the same way.

Women who have a family history of ovarian cancer are at an increased risk of ovarian cancer.

Anything that increases your risk of getting a disease is called a risk factor. Having a risk factor does not mean that you will get cancer; not having risk factors doesn't mean that you will not get cancer. Talk with your doctor if you think you may be at risk.

Women who have one first-degree relative (mother, daughter, or sister) with a history of ovarian cancer have an increased risk of ovarian cancer. This risk is higher in women who have one first-degree relative and one second-degree relative (grandmother or aunt) with a history of ovarian cancer. This risk is even higher in women who have two or more first-degree relatives with a history of ovarian cancer.

Some ovarian, fallopian tube, and primary peritoneal cancers are caused by inherited gene mutations (changes).

The genes in cells carry the hereditary information that is received from a person's parents. Hereditary ovarian cancer makes up about 5% to 10% of all cases of ovarian cancer. Three hereditary patterns have been identified: ovarian cancer alone, ovarian and breast cancers, and ovarian and colon cancers.

Fallopian tube cancer and peritoneal cancer may also be caused by certain inherited gene mutations.

There are tests that can detect mutated genes. These genetic tests are sometimes done for members of families with a high risk of cancer.

Women with an increased risk of ovarian cancer may consider surgery to lessen the risk.

Some women who have an increased risk of ovarian cancer may choose to have a risk-reducing oophorectomy (the removal of healthy ovaries so that cancer cannot grow in them). In high-risk women, this procedure has been shown to greatly decrease the risk of ovarian cancer.

Signs and symptoms of ovarian, fallopian tube, or peritoneal cancer include pain or swelling in the abdomen.

Ovarian, fallopian tube, or peritoneal cancer may not cause early signs or symptoms. When signs or symptoms do appear, the cancer is often advanced. Signs and symptoms may include the following:

- Pain, swelling, or a feeling of pressure in the abdomen or pelvis.

- Vaginal bleeding that is heavy or irregular, especially after menopause.

- Vaginal discharge that is clear, white, or colored with blood.

- A lump in the pelvic area.

- Gastrointestinal problems, such as gas, bloating, or constipation.

These signs and symptoms also may be caused by other conditions and not by ovarian, fallopian tube, or peritoneal cancer. If the signs or symptoms get worse or do not go away on their own, check with your doctor so that any problem can be diagnosed and treated as early as possible.

Women with ovarian cancer should think about taking part in a clinical trial.

Tests that examine the ovaries and pelvic area are used to detect (find) and diagnose ovarian, fallopian tube, and peritoneal cancer.

The following tests and procedures may be used:

- **Physical exam and history:** An exam of the body to check general signs of health, including checking for signs of disease, such as lumps or anything else that seems unusual. A history of the patient's health habits and past illnesses and treatments will also be taken.

- **Pelvic exam:** An exam of the vagina, cervix, uterus, fallopian tubes, ovaries, and rectum. The doctor or nurse inserts one or two lubricated, gloved fingers of one hand into the vagina and the other hand is placed over the lower abdomen to feel the size, shape, and position of the uterus and ovaries. A speculum is also inserted into the vagina and the doctor or nurse looks at the vagina and cervix for signs of disease. A Pap test or Pap smear of the cervix is usually done. The doctor or nurse also inserts a lubricated, gloved finger into the rectum to feel for lumps or abnormal areas.

- **Ultrasound exam:** A procedure in which high-energy sound waves (ultrasound) are bounced off internal tissues or organs in the abdomen, and make echoes. The echoes form a picture of body tissues called a sonogram. The picture can be printed to be looked at later.

Some patients may have a transvaginal ultrasound.

- **CA 125 assay:** A test that measures the level of CA 125 in the blood. CA 125 is a substance released by cells into the bloodstream. An increased CA 125 level can be a sign of cancer or another condition such as endometriosis.

- **CT scan (CAT scan):** A procedure that makes a series of detailed pictures of areas inside the body, taken from different angles. The pictures are made by a computer linked to an x-ray machine. A dye may be injected into a vein or swallowed to help the organs or tissues show up more clearly. This procedure is also called computed tomography, computerized tomography, or computerized axial tomography.

- **PET scan (positron emission tomography scan):** A procedure to find malignant tumor cells in the body. A very small amount of radioactive glucose (sugar) is injected into a vein. The PET scanner rotates around the body and makes a picture of where glucose is being used in the body. Malignant tumor cells show up brighter in the picture because they are more active and take up more glucose than normal cells do.

- **MRI (magnetic resonance imaging):** A procedure that uses a magnet, radio waves, and a computer to make a series of detailed pictures of areas inside the body. This procedure is also called nuclear magnetic resonance imaging (NMRI).

- **Chest x-ray:** An x-ray of the organs and bones inside the chest. An x-ray is a type of energy beam that can go through the body and onto film, making a picture of areas inside the body.

- **Biopsy:** The removal of cells or tissues so they can be viewed under a microscope by a pathologist to check for signs of cancer. The tissue is usually removed during surgery to remove the tumor.

Certain factors affect treatment options and prognosis (chance of recovery).

The prognosis (chance of recovery) and treatment options depend on the following:

- The stage and grade of the cancer.
- The type and size of the tumor.

485

- Whether all of the tumor can be removed by surgery.

- Whether the patient has swelling of the abdomen.

- The patient's age and general health.

- Whether the cancer has just been diagnosed or has recurred (come back).

Stages of Ovarian Epithelial, Fallopian Tube, and Primary Peritoneal Cancer

After ovarian, fallopian tube, or peritoneal cancer has been diagnosed, tests are done to find out if cancer cells have spread within the ovaries or to other parts of the body.

The process used to find out whether cancer has spread within the organ or to other parts of the body is called staging. The information gathered from the staging process determines the stage of the disease. It is important to know the stage in order to plan treatment. The results of the tests used to diagnose cancer are often also used to stage the disease.

There are three ways that cancer spreads in the body.

Cancer can spread through tissue, the lymph system, and the blood:

- Tissue. The cancer spreads from where it began by growing into nearby areas.

- Lymph system. The cancer spreads from where it began by getting into the lymph system. The cancer travels through the lymph vessels to other parts of the body.

- Blood. The cancer spreads from where it began by getting into the blood. The cancer travels through the blood vessels to other parts of the body.

Cancer may spread from where it began to other parts of the body.

When cancer spreads to another part of the body, it is called metastasis. Cancer cells break away from where they began (the primary tumor) and travel through the lymph system or blood.

- Lymph system. The cancer gets into the lymph system, travels through the lymph vessels, and forms a tumor (metastatic tumor) in another part of the body.

- Blood. The cancer gets into the blood, travels through the blood vessels, and forms a tumor (metastatic tumor) in another part of the body.

The metastatic tumor is the same type of cancer as the primary tumor. For example, if ovarian epithelial cancer spreads to the lung, the cancer cells in the lung are actually ovarian epithelial cancer cells. The disease is metastatic ovarian epithelial cancer, not lung cancer.

The following stages are used for ovarian epithelial, fallopian tube, and primary peritoneal cancer:

Stage I

In stage I, cancer is found in one or both ovaries or fallopian tubes. Stage I is divided into stage IA, stage IB, and stage IC.

- Stage IA: Cancer is found inside a single ovary or fallopian tube.

- Stage IB: Cancer is found inside both ovaries or fallopian tubes.

- Stage IC: Cancer is found inside one or both ovaries or fallopian tubes and one of the following is true:

  - cancer is also found on the outside surface of one or both ovaries or fallopian tubes; or

  - the capsule (outer covering) of the ovary has ruptured (broken open); or

  - cancer cells are found in the fluid of the peritoneal cavity (the body cavity that contains most of the organs in the abdomen) or in washings of the peritoneum (tissue lining the peritoneal cavity).

Stage II

In stage II, cancer is found in one or both ovaries or fallopian tubes and has spread into other areas of the pelvis or primary peritoneal cancer is found within the pelvis. Stage II ovarian epithelial and fallopian tube cancers are divided into stage IIA and stage IIB.

- Stage IIA: Cancer has spread from where it first formed to the uterus and/or the fallopian tubes and/or the ovaries.

- Stage IIB: Cancer has spread from the ovary or fallopian tube to organs in the peritoneal cavity (the space that contains the abdominal organs).

Stage III

In stage III, cancer is found in one or both ovaries or fallopian tubes, or is primary peritoneal cancer, and has spread outside the pelvis to other parts of the abdomen and/or to nearby lymph nodes. Stage III is divided into stage IIIA, stage IIIB, and stage IIIC.

- In stage IIIA, one of the following is true:

  - Cancer has spread to lymph nodes in the area outside or behind the peritoneum only; or

  - Cancer cells that can be seen only with a microscope have spread to the surface of the peritoneum outside the pelvis. Cancer may have spread to nearby lymph nodes.

- Stage IIIB: Cancer has spread to the peritoneum outside the pelvis and the cancer in the peritoneum is 2 centimeters or smaller. Cancer may have spread to lymph nodes behind the peritoneum.

- Stage IIIC: Cancer has spread to the peritoneum outside the pelvis and the cancer in the peritoneum is larger than 2 centimeters. Cancer may have spread to lymph nodes behind the peritoneum or to the surface of the liver or spleen.

Stage IV

In stage IV, cancer has spread beyond the abdomen to other parts of the body. Stage IV is divided into stage IVA and stage IVB.

- Stage IVA: Cancer cells are found in extra fluid that builds up around the lungs.

- Stage IVB: Cancer has spread to organs and tissues outside the abdomen, including lymph nodes in the groin.

Ovarian epithelial, fallopian tube, and primary peritoneal cancers are grouped for treatment as early or advanced cancer.

Stage I ovarian epithelial and fallopian tube cancers are treated as early cancers.

Stages II, III, and IV ovarian epithelial, fallopian tube, and primary peritoneal cancers are treated as advanced cancers.

Treatment Option Overview

There are different types of treatment for patients with ovarian epithelial cancer.

Different types of treatment are available for patients with ovarian epithelial cancer. Some treatments are standard, and some are being tested in clinical trials. A treatment clinical trial is a research study meant to help improve current treatments or obtain information on new treatments for patients with cancer. When clinical trials show that a new treatment is better than the treatment currently used as standard treatment, the new treatment may become the standard treatment. Patients may want to think about taking part in a clinical trial. Some clinical trials are open only to patients who have not started treatment.

Four kinds of standard treatment are used.

Surgery

Most patients have surgery to remove as much of the tumor as possible. Different types of surgery may include:

- Hysterectomy: Surgery to remove the uterus and, sometimes, the cervix. When only the uterus is removed, it is called a partial hysterectomy. When both the uterus and the cervix are removed, it is called a total hysterectomy. If the uterus and cervix are taken out through the vagina, the operation is called a vaginal hysterectomy. If the uterus and cervix are taken out through a large incision (cut) in the abdomen, the operation is called a total abdominal hysterectomy. If the uterus and cervix are taken out through a small incision (cut) in the abdomen using a laparoscope, the operation is called a total laparoscopic hysterectomy.

- Unilateral salpingo-oophorectomy: A surgical procedure to remove one ovary and one fallopian tube.

- Bilateral salpingo-oophorectomy: A surgical procedure to remove both ovaries and both fallopian tubes.

- Omentectomy: A surgical procedure to remove the omentum (tissue in the peritoneum that contains blood vessels, nerves, lymph vessels, and lymph nodes).

489

- Lymph node biopsy: The removal of all or part of a lymph node. A pathologist views the tissue under a microscope to look for cancer cells.

Radiation therapy

Radiation therapy is a cancer treatment that uses high-energy x-rays or other types of radiation to kill cancer cells or keep them from growing. There are two types of radiation therapy. External radiation therapy uses a machine outside the body to send radiation toward the cancer. Internal radiation therapy uses a radioactive substance sealed in needles, seeds, wires, or catheters that are placed directly into or near the cancer. The way the radiation therapy is given depends on the type and stage of the cancer being treated.

Some women receive a treatment called intraperitoneal radiation therapy, in which radioactive liquid is put directly in the abdomen through a catheter.

Chemotherapy

Chemotherapy is a cancer treatment that uses drugs to stop the growth of cancer cells, either by killing the cells or by stopping them from dividing. When chemotherapy is taken by mouth or injected into a vein or muscle, the drugs enter the bloodstream and can reach cancer cells throughout the body (systemic chemotherapy). When chemotherapy is placed directly into the cerebrospinal fluid, an organ, or a body cavity such as the abdomen, the drugs mainly affect cancer cells in those areas (regional chemotherapy).

A type of regional chemotherapy used to treat ovarian cancer is intraperitoneal (IP) chemotherapy. In IP chemotherapy, the anticancer drugs are carried directly into the peritoneal cavity (the space that contains the abdominal organs) through a thin tube.

Treatment with more than one anticancer drug is called combination chemotherapy.

The way the chemotherapy is given depends on the type and stage of the cancer being treated.

Targeted therapy

Targeted therapy is a type of treatment that uses drugs or other substances to identify and attack specific cancer cells without harming normal cells.

Monoclonal antibody therapy is a type of targeted therapy that uses antibodies made in the laboratory, from a single type of immune system cell. These antibodies can identify substances on cancer cells or normal substances that may help cancer cells grow. The antibodies attach to the substances and kill the cancer cells, block their growth, or keep them from spreading. Monoclonal antibodies are given by infusion. They may be used alone or to carry drugs, toxins, or radioactive material directly to cancer cells.

Bevacizumab is a monoclonal antibody that may be used with chemotherapy to treat ovarian epithelial cancer, fallopian tube cancer, or primary peritoneal cancer that has recurred (come back).

Other types of targeted therapy are being studied in the treatment of ovarian epithelial cancer. PARP inhibitors are targeted therapy drugs that block DNA repair and may cause cancer cells to die. PARP inhibitor therapy is being studied in treating ovarian epithelial cancer that remains after chemotherapy.

New types of treatment are being tested in clinical trials.

Biologic therapy

Biologic therapy is a treatment that uses the patient's immune system to fight cancer. Substances made by the body or made in a laboratory are used to boost, direct, or restore the body's natural defenses against cancer. This type of cancer treatment is also called biotherapy or immunotherapy.

Patients may want to think about taking part in a clinical trial.

For some patients, taking part in a clinical trial may be the best treatment choice. Clinical trials are part of the cancer research process. Clinical trials are done to find out if new cancer treatments are safe and effective or better than the standard treatment.

Many of today's standard treatments for cancer are based on earlier clinical trials. Patients who take part in a clinical trial may receive the standard treatment or be among the first to receive a new treatment.

Patients who take part in clinical trials also help improve the way cancer will be treated in the future. Even when clinical trials do not lead to effective new treatments, they often answer important questions and help move research forward.

Patients can enter clinical trials before, during, or after starting their cancer treatment.

Some clinical trials only include patients who have not yet received treatment. Other trials test treatments for patients whose cancer has not gotten better. There are also clinical trials that test new ways to stop cancer from recurring (coming back) or reduce the side effects of cancer treatment.

Clinical trials are taking place in many parts of the country.

Follow-up tests may be needed.

Some of the tests that were done to diagnose the cancer or to find out the stage of the cancer may be repeated. Some tests will be repeated in order to see how well the treatment is working. Decisions about whether to continue, change, or stop treatment may be based on the results of these tests.

Some of the tests will continue to be done from time to time after treatment has ended. The results of these tests can show if your condition has changed or if the cancer has recurred (come back). These tests are sometimes called follow-up tests or check-ups.

Section 25.2

Ovarian Low Malignant Potential Tumors

Text in this section is excerpted from "Ovarian Low Malignant Potential Tumors Treatment," National Cancer Institute at the National Institutes of Health (NIH), July 12, 2014.

General Information About Ovarian Low Malignant Potential Tumors

Ovarian low malignant potential tumor is a disease in which abnormal cells form in the tissue covering the ovary.

Ovarian low malignant potential tumors have abnormal cells that may become cancer, but usually do not. This disease usually remains in the ovary. When disease is found in one ovary, the other ovary should also be checked carefully for signs of disease.

The ovaries are a pair of organs in the female reproductive system. They are in the pelvis, one on each side of the uterus (the hollow, pear-shaped organ where a fetus grows). Each ovary is about the size and shape of an almond. The ovaries make eggs and female hormones.

Signs and symptoms of ovarian low malignant potential tumor include pain or swelling in the abdomen.

Ovarian low malignant potential tumor may not cause early signs or symptoms. If you do have signs or symptoms, they may include the following:

- Pain or swelling in the abdomen.
- Pain in the pelvis.
- Gastrointestinal problems, such as gas, bloating, or constipation.

These signs and symptoms may be caused by other conditions. If they get worse or do not go away on their own, check with your doctor.

Tests that examine the ovaries are used to detect (find), diagnose, and stage ovarian low malignant potential tumor.

The following tests and procedures may be used:

- **Physical exam and history:** An exam of the body to check general signs of health, including checking for signs of disease, such as lumps or anything else that seems unusual. A history of the patient's health habits and past illnesses and treatments will also be taken.

- **Pelvic exam:** An exam of the vagina, cervix, uterus, fallopian tubes, ovaries, and rectum. The doctor or nurse inserts one or two lubricated, gloved fingers of one hand into the vagina and places the other hand over the lower abdomen to feel the size, shape, and position of the uterus and ovaries. A speculum is also inserted into the vagina and the doctor or nurse looks at the vagina and cervix for signs of disease. A Pap test of the cervix is usually done. The doctor or nurse also inserts a lubricated, gloved finger into the rectum to feel for lumps or abnormal areas.

- **Ultrasound exam:** A procedure in which high-energy sound waves (ultrasound) are bounced off internal tissues or organs

493

and make echoes. The echoes form a picture of body tissues called a sonogram. The picture can be printed to be looked at later.

Other patients may have a transvaginal ultrasound.

- **CT scan (CAT scan):** A procedure that makes a series of detailed pictures of areas inside the body, taken from different angles. The pictures are made by a computer linked to an x-ray machine. A dye may be injected into a vein or swallowed to help the organs or tissues show up more clearly. This procedure is also called computed tomography, computerized tomography, or computerized axial tomography.

- **CA 125 assay:** A test that measures the level of CA 125 in the blood. CA 125 is a substance released by cells into the bloodstream. An increased CA 125 level is sometimes a sign of cancer or other condition.

- **Chest x-ray:** An x-ray of the organs and bones inside the chest. An x-ray is a type of energy beam that can go through the body and onto film, making a picture of areas inside the body.

- **Biopsy:** The removal of cells or tissues so they can be viewed under a microscope by a pathologist to check for signs of cancer. The tissue is usually removed during surgery to remove the tumor.

Certain factors affect prognosis (chance of recovery) and treatment options.

The prognosis (chance of recovery) and treatment options depend on the following:

- The stage of the disease (whether it affects part of the ovary, involves the whole ovary, or has spread to other places in the body).

- What type of cells make up the tumor.

- The size of the tumor.

- The patient's general health.

Patients with ovarian low malignant potential tumors have a good prognosis, especially when the tumor is found early.

494

Stages of Ovarian Low Malignant Potential Tumors

After ovarian low malignant potential tumor has been diagnosed, tests are done to find out if abnormal cells have spread within the ovary or to other parts of the body.

The process used to find out whether abnormal cells have spread within the ovary or to other parts of the body is called staging. The information gathered from the staging process determines the stage of the disease. It is important to know the stage in order to plan treatment. Certain tests or procedures are used for staging. Staging laparotomy (a surgical incision made in the wall of the abdomen to remove ovarian tissue) may be used. Most patients are diagnosed with stage I disease.

The following stages are used for ovarian low malignant potential tumor:

Stage I

In stage I, the tumor is found in one or both ovaries. Stage I is divided into stage IA, stage IB, and stage IC.

Stage IA: The tumor is found inside a single ovary.

Stage IB: The tumor is found inside both ovaries.

Stage IC: The tumor is found inside one or both ovaries and one of the following is true:

- tumor cells are found on the outside surface of one or both ovaries; or

- the capsule (outer covering) of the ovary has ruptured (broken open); or

- tumor cells are found in the fluid of the peritoneal cavity (the body cavity that contains most of the organs in the abdomen) or in washings of the peritoneum (tissue lining the peritoneal cavity).

Stage II

In stage II, the tumor is found in one or both ovaries and has spread into other areas of the pelvis. Stage II is divided into stage IIA, stage IIB, and stage IIC.

- Stage IIA: The tumor has spread to the uterus and/or fallopian tubes (the long slender tubes through which eggs pass from the ovaries to the uterus).

- Stage IIB: The tumor has spread to other tissue within the pelvis.

- Stage IIC: The tumor is found inside one or both ovaries and has spread to the uterus and/or fallopian tubes, or to other tissue within the pelvis. Also, one of the following is true:

  - tumor cells are found on the outside surface of one or both ovaries; or

  - the capsule (outer covering) of the ovary has ruptured (broken open); or

  - tumor cells are found in the fluid of the peritoneal cavity (the body cavity that contains most of the organs in the abdomen) or in washings of the peritoneum (tissue lining the peritoneal cavity).

Stage III

In stage III, the tumor is found in one or both ovaries and has spread outside the pelvis to other parts of the abdomen and/or nearby lymph nodes. Stage III is divided into stage IIIA, stage IIIB, and stage IIIC.

Stage IIIA: The tumor is found in the pelvis only, but tumor cells that can be seen only with a microscope have spread to the surface of the peritoneum (tissue that lines the abdominal wall and covers most of the organs in the abdomen), the small intestines, or the tissue that connects the small intestines to the wall of the abdomen.

Stage IIIB: The tumor has spread to the peritoneum and the tumor in the peritoneum is 2 centimeters or smaller.

Stage IIIC: The tumor has spread to the peritoneum and the tumor in the peritoneum is larger than 2 centimeters and/or has spread to lymph nodes in the abdomen.

The spread of tumor cells to the surface of the liver is also considered stage III disease.

Stage IV

In stage IV, tumor cells have spread beyond the abdomen to other parts of the body, such as the lungs or tissue inside the liver.

Tumor cells in the fluid around the lungs is also considered stage IV disease.

Ovarian low malignant potential tumors almost never reach stage IV.

Treatment Option Overview

There are different types of treatment for patients with ovarian low malignant potential tumor.

Different types of treatment are available for patients with ovarian low malignant potential tumor. Some treatments are standard (the currently used treatment), and some are being tested in clinical trials. A treatment clinical trial is a research study meant to help improve current treatments or obtain information on new treatments for patients with cancer, tumors, and related conditions. When clinical trials show that a new treatment is better than the standard treatment, the new treatment may become the standard treatment. Patients may want to think about taking part in a clinical trial. Some clinical trials are open only to patients who have not started treatment.

Two types of standard treatment are used:

Surgery

The type of surgery (removing the tumor in an operation) depends on the size and spread of the tumor and the woman's plans for having children. Surgery may include the following:

- Unilateral salpingo-oophorectomy: Surgery to remove one ovary and one fallopian tube.

- Bilateral salpingo-oophorectomy: Surgery to remove both ovaries and both fallopian tubes.

- Total hysterectomy and bilateral salpingo-oophorectomy: Surgery to remove the uterus, cervix, and both ovaries and fallopian tubes. If the uterus and cervix are taken out through the vagina, the operation is called a vaginal hysterectomy. If the uterus and cervix are taken out through a large incision (cut) in the abdomen, the operation is called a total abdominal hysterectomy. If the uterus and cervix are taken out through a small incision (cut) in the abdomen using a laparoscope, the operation is called a total laparoscopic hysterectomy.

- Partial oophorectomy: Surgery to remove part of one ovary or part of both ovaries.

- Omentectomy: Surgery to remove the omentum (a piece of the tissue lining the abdominal wall).

Even if the doctor removes all disease that can be seen at the time of the operation, the patient may be given chemotherapy after surgery to kill any tumor cells that are left. Treatment given after the surgery, to lower the risk that the tumor will come back, is called adjuvant therapy.

Chemotherapy

Chemotherapy is a cancer treatment that uses drugs to stop the growth of cancer cells, either by killing the cells or by stopping them from dividing. When chemotherapy is taken by mouth or injected into a vein or muscle, the drugs enter the bloodstream and can reach cancer cells throughout the body (systemic chemotherapy). When chemotherapy is placed directly into the cerebrospinal fluid, an organ, or a body cavity such as the abdomen, the drugs mainly affect cancer cells in those areas (regional chemotherapy). The way the chemotherapy is given depends on the type and stage of the cancer being treated.

Patients may want to think about taking part in a clinical trial.

For some patients, taking part in a clinical trial may be the best treatment choice. Clinical trials are part of the medical research process. Clinical trials are done to find out if new treatments are safe and effective or better than the standard treatment.

Many of today's standard treatments for disease are based on earlier clinical trials. Patients who take part in a clinical trial may receive the standard treatment or be among the first to receive a new treatment.

Patients who take part in clinical trials also help improve the way diseases will be treated in the future. Even when clinical trials do not lead to effective new treatments, they often answer important questions and help move research forward.

Patients can enter clinical trials before, during, or after starting their treatment.

Some clinical trials only include patients who have not yet received treatment. Other trials test treatments for patients whose disease has not gotten better. There are also clinical trials that test new ways to stop a disease from recurring (coming back) or reduce the side effects of treatment.

Clinical trials are taking place in many parts of the country.

Follow-up tests may be needed.

Some of the tests that were done to diagnose the disease may be repeated. Some tests will be repeated in order to see how well the treatment is working. Decisions about whether to continue, change, or stop treatment may be based on the results of these tests. This is sometimes called re-staging.

Some of the tests will continue to be done from time to time after treatment has ended. The results of these tests can show if your condition has changed or if the disease has recurred (come back). These tests are sometimes called follow-up tests or check-ups.

Section 25.3

Endometrial Cancer

Text in this section is excerpted from "Endometrial Cancer Treatment," National Cancer Institute at the National Institutes of Health (NIH), April 6, 2015.

General Information About Endometrial Cancer

Endometrial cancer is a disease in which malignant (cancer) cells form in the tissues of the endometrium.

The endometrium is the lining of the uterus, a hollow, muscular organ in a woman's pelvis. The uterus is where a fetus grows. In most nonpregnant women, the uterus is about 3 inches long. The lower, narrow end of the uterus is the cervix, which leads to the vagina.

Cancer of the endometrium is different from cancer of the muscle of the uterus, which is called sarcoma of the uterus.

Obesity, high blood pressure, and diabetes mellitus may increase the risk of endometrial cancer.

Anything that increases your risk of getting a disease is called a risk factor. Having a risk factor does not mean that you will get cancer; not having risk factors doesn't mean that you will not get cancer. Talk with your doctor if you think you may be at risk. Risk factors for endometrial cancer include the following:

- Being obese.
- Having high blood pressure.
- Having diabetes mellitus.

Taking tamoxifen for breast cancer or taking estrogen alone (without progesterone) can increase the risk of endometrial cancer.

Endometrial cancer may develop in breast cancer patients who have been treated with tamoxifen. A patient taking this drug should have a pelvic exam every year and report any vaginal bleeding (other than menstrual bleeding) as soon as possible. Women taking estrogen (a hormone that can affect the growth of some cancers) alone have an increased risk of endometrial cancer. Taking estrogen combined with progesterone (another hormone) does not increase a woman's risk of this cancer.

Signs and symptoms of endometrial cancer include unusual vaginal discharge or pain in the pelvis.

These and other signs and symptoms may be caused by endometrial cancer or by other conditions. Check with your doctor if you have any of the following:

- Bleeding or discharge not related to menstruation (periods).
- Difficult or painful urination.
- Pain during sexual intercourse.
- Pain in the pelvic area.

Tests that examine the endometrium are used to detect (find) and diagnose endometrial cancer.

Because endometrial cancer begins inside the uterus, it does not usually show up in the results of a Pap test. For this reason, a sample of endometrial tissue must be removed and checked under a microscope to look for cancer cells. One of the following procedures may be used:

- **Endometrial biopsy:** The removal of tissue from the endometrium (inner lining of the uterus) by inserting a thin, flexible tube through the cervix and into the uterus. The tube is used to gently scrape a small amount of tissue from the endometrium and then remove the tissue samples. A pathologist views the tissue under a microscope to look for cancer cells.

- **Dilatation and curettage:** A procedure to remove samples of tissue from the inner lining of the uterus. The cervix is dilated and a curette (spoon-shaped instrument) is inserted into the uterus to remove tissue. The tissue samples are checked under a microscope for signs of disease. This procedure is also called a D&C.

Other tests and procedures used to diagnose endometrial cancer include the following:

- **Physical exam and history:** An exam of the body to check general signs of health, including checking for signs of disease, such as lumps or anything else that seems unusual. A history of the patient's health habits and past illnesses and treatments will also be taken.

- **Transvaginal ultrasound exam:** A procedure used to examine the vagina, uterus, fallopian tubes, and bladder. An ultrasound transducer (probe) is inserted into the vagina and used to bounce high-energy sound waves (ultrasound) off internal tissues or organs and make echoes. The echoes form a picture of body tissues called a sonogram. The doctor can identify tumors by looking at the sonogram.

- **CT scan (CAT scan):** A procedure that makes a series of detailed pictures of areas inside the body, taken from different angles. The pictures are made by a computer linked to an x-ray machine. A dye may be injected into a vein or swallowed to help the organs or tissues show up more clearly. This procedure is also called computed tomography, computerized tomography, or computerized axial tomography.

Certain factors affect prognosis (chance of recovery) and treatment options.

The prognosis (chance of recovery) and treatment options depend on the following:

- The stage of the cancer (whether it is in the endometrium only, involves the whole uterus, or has spread to other places in the body).

- How the cancer cells look under a microscope.

- Whether the cancer cells are affected by progesterone.

Endometrial cancer is highly curable.

Stages of Endometrial Cancer

After endometrial cancer has been diagnosed, tests are done to find out if cancer cells have spread within the uterus or to other parts of the body.

The process used to find out whether the cancer has spread within the uterus or to other parts of the body is called staging. The information gathered from the staging process determines the stage of the disease. It is important to know the stage in order to plan treatment. Certain tests and procedures are used in the staging process. A hysterectomy (an operation in which the uterus is removed) will usually be done to help find out how far the cancer has spread.

The following procedures may be used in the staging process:

- **Pelvic exam:** An exam of the vagina, cervix, uterus, fallopian tubes, ovaries, and rectum. The doctor or nurse inserts one or two lubricated, gloved fingers of one hand into the vagina and the other hand is placed over the lower abdomen to feel the size, shape, and position of the uterus and ovaries. A speculum is also inserted into the vagina and the doctor or nurse looks at the vagina and cervix for signs of disease. A Pap test or Pap smear of the cervix is usually done. The doctor or nurse also inserts a lubricated, gloved finger into the rectum to feel for lumps or abnormal areas.

- **Chest x-ray:** An x-ray of the organs and bones inside the chest. An x-ray is a type of energy beam that can go through the body and onto film, making a picture of areas inside the body.

- **MRI (magnetic resonance imaging):** A procedure that uses a magnet, radio waves, and a computer to make a series of detailed pictures of areas inside the body. This procedure is also called nuclear magnetic resonance imaging (NMRI).

- **PET scan (positron emission tomography scan):** A procedure to find malignant tumor cells in the body. A small amount of radioactive glucose (sugar) is injected into a vein. The PET scanner rotates around the body and makes a picture of where glucose is being used in the body. Malignant tumor cells show up brighter in the picture because they are more active and take up more glucose than normal cells do.

There are three ways that cancer spreads in the body.

Cancer can spread through tissue, the lymph system, and the blood:

- Tissue. The cancer spreads from where it began by growing into nearby areas.

- Lymph system. The cancer spreads from where it began by getting into the lymph system. The cancer travels through the lymph vessels to other parts of the body.

- Blood. The cancer spreads from where it began by getting into the blood. The cancer travels through the blood vessels to other parts of the body.

Cancer may spread from where it began to other parts of the body.

When cancer spreads to another part of the body, it is called metastasis. Cancer cells break away from where they began (the primary tumor) and travel through the lymph system or blood.

- Lymph system. The cancer gets into the lymph system, travels through the lymph vessels, and forms a tumor (metastatic tumor) in another part of the body.

- Blood. The cancer gets into the blood, travels through the blood vessels, and forms a tumor (metastatic tumor) in another part of the body.

The metastatic tumor is the same type of cancer as the primary tumor. For example, if endometrial cancer spreads to the lung, the cancer cells in the lung are actually endometrial cancer cells. The disease is metastatic endometrial cancer, not lung cancer.

The following stages are used for endometrial cancer:

Stage I

In stage I, cancer is found in the uterus only. Stage I is divided into stages IA and IB, based on how far the cancer has spread.

- Stage IA: Cancer is in the endometrium only or less than halfway through the myometrium (muscle layer of the uterus).

- Stage IB: Cancer has spread halfway or more into the myometrium.

Stage II

In stage II, cancer has spread into connective tissue of the cervix, but has not spread outside the uterus.

Stage III

In stage III, cancer has spread beyond the uterus and cervix, but has not spread beyond the pelvis. Stage III is divided into stages IIIA, IIIB, and IIIC, based on how far the cancer has spread within the pelvis.

- Stage IIIA: Cancer has spread to the outer layer of the uterus and/or to the fallopian tubes, ovaries, and ligaments of the uterus.

- Stage IIIB: Cancer has spread to the vagina or to the parametrium (connective tissue and fat around the uterus).

- Stage IIIC: Cancer has spread to lymph nodes in the pelvis and/or around the aorta (largest artery in the body, which carries blood away from the heart).

Stage IV

In stage IV, cancer has spread beyond the pelvis. Stage IV is divided into stages IVA and IVB, based on how far the cancer has spread.

- Stage IVA: Cancer has spread to the bladder and/or bowel wall.

- Stage IVB: Cancer has spread to other parts of the body beyond the pelvis, including the abdomen and/or lymph nodes in the groin.

Treatment Option Overview

There are different types of treatment for patients with endometrial cancer.

Different types of treatment are available for patients with endometrial cancer. Some treatments are standard (the currently used treatment), and some are being tested in clinical trials. A treatment clinical trial is a research study meant to help improve current treatments or obtain information on new treatments for patients with cancer. When clinical trials show that a new treatment is better than the standard treatment, the new treatment may become the standard treatment. Patients may want to think about taking part in a clinical trial. Some clinical trials are open only to patients who have not started treatment.

Five types of standard treatment are used:

Surgery

Surgery (removing the cancer in an operation) is the most common treatment for endometrial cancer. The following surgical procedures may be used:

- Total hysterectomy: Surgery to remove the uterus, including the cervix. If the uterus and cervix are taken out through the vagina, the operation is called a vaginal hysterectomy. If the uterus and cervix are taken out through a large incision (cut) in the abdomen, the operation is called a total abdominal hysterectomy. If the uterus and cervix are taken out through a small incision (cut) in the abdomen using a laparoscope, the operation is called a total laparoscopic hysterectomy.

- Bilateral salpingo-oophorectomy: Surgery to remove both ovaries and both fallopian tubes.

- Radical hysterectomy: Surgery to remove the uterus, cervix, and part of the vagina. The ovaries, fallopian tubes, or nearby lymph nodes may also be removed.

Even if the doctor removes all the cancer that can be seen at the time of the surgery, some patients may be given radiation therapy or hormone treatment after surgery to kill any cancer cells that are left. Treatment given after the surgery, to lower the risk that the cancer will come back, is called adjuvant therapy.

Radiation therapy

Radiation therapy is a cancer treatment that uses high-energy x-rays or other types of radiation to kill cancer cells or keep them from growing. There are two types of radiation therapy. External radiation therapy uses a machine outside the body to send radiation toward the cancer. Internal radiation therapy uses a radioactive substance sealed in needles, seeds, wires, or catheters that are placed directly into or near the cancer. The way the radiation therapy is given depends on the type and stage of the cancer being treated.

Chemotherapy

Chemotherapy is a cancer treatment that uses drugs to stop the growth of cancer cells, either by killing the cells or by stopping the cells from dividing. When chemotherapy is taken by mouth or injected into a vein or muscle, the drugs enter the bloodstream and can reach cancer cells throughout the body (systemic chemotherapy). When chemotherapy is placed directly into the cerebrospinal fluid, an organ, or a body cavity such as the abdomen, the drugs mainly affect cancer cells in those areas (regional chemotherapy). The way the chemotherapy is given depends on the type and stage of the cancer being treated.

Hormone therapy

Hormone therapy is a cancer treatment that removes hormones or blocks their action and stops cancer cells from growing. Hormones are substances made by glands in the body and circulated in the bloodstream. Some hormones can cause certain cancers to grow. If tests show that the cancer cells have places where hormones can attach (receptors), drugs, surgery, or radiation therapy is used to reduce the production of hormones or block them from working.

Biologic therapy

Biologic therapy is a treatment that uses the patient's immune system to fight cancer. Substances made by the body or made in a laboratory are used to boost, direct, or restore the body's natural defenses against cancer. This type of cancer treatment is also called biotherapy or immunotherapy.

New types of treatment are being tested in clinical trials.

Targeted therapy

Targeted therapy is a type of treatment that uses drugs or other substances to identify and attack specific cancer cells without harming normal cells. Monoclonal antibodies and tyrosine kinase inhibitors are two types of targeted therapy being studied in the treatment of endometrial cancer.

Monoclonal antibody therapy is a cancer treatment that uses antibodies made in the laboratory from a single type of immune system cell. These antibodies can identify substances on cancer cells or normal substances that may help cancer cells grow. The antibodies attach to the substances and kill the cancer cells, block their growth, or keep them from spreading. Monoclonal antibodies are given by infusion. They may be used alone or to carry drugs, toxins, or radioactive material directly to cancer cells.

Tyrosine kinase inhibitors are targeted therapy drugs that block signals needed for tumors to grow. Tyrosine kinase inhibitors may be used with other anticancer drugs as adjuvant therapy.

Patients may want to think about taking part in a clinical trial.

For some patients, taking part in a clinical trial may be the best treatment choice. Clinical trials are part of the cancer research process. Clinical trials are done to find out if new cancer treatments are safe and effective or better than the standard treatment.

Many of today's standard treatments for cancer are based on earlier clinical trials. Patients who take part in a clinical trial may receive the standard treatment or be among the first to receive a new treatment.

Patients who take part in clinical trials also help improve the way cancer will be treated in the future. Even when clinical trials do not lead to effective new treatments, they often answer important questions and help move research forward.

Patients can enter clinical trials before, during, or after starting their cancer treatment.

Some clinical trials only include patients who have not yet received treatment. Other trials test treatments for patients whose cancer has

not gotten better. There are also clinical trials that test new ways to stop cancer from recurring (coming back) or reduce the side effects of cancer treatment.

Clinical trials are taking place in many parts of the country.

Follow-up tests may be needed.

Some of the tests that were done to diagnose the cancer or to find out the stage of the cancer may be repeated. Some tests will be repeated in order to see how well the treatment is working. Decisions about whether to continue, change, or stop treatment may be based on the results of these tests.

Some of the tests will continue to be done from time to time after treatment has ended. The results of these tests can show if your condition has changed or if the cancer has recurred (come back). These tests are sometimes called follow-up tests or check-ups.

Section 25.4

Gestational Trophoblastic Disease

Text in this section is excerpted from "Gestational Trophoblastic Disease Treatment," National Cancer Institute at the National Institutes of Health (NIH), May 29, 2015.

General Information About Gestational Trophoblastic Disease

Gestational trophoblastic disease (GTD) is a group of rare diseases in which abnormal trophoblast cells grow inside the uterus after conception.

In gestational trophoblastic disease (GTD), a tumor develops inside the uterus from tissue that forms after conception (the joining of sperm and egg). This tissue is made of trophoblast cells and normally surrounds the fertilized egg in the uterus. Trophoblast cells help connect the fertilized egg to the wall of the uterus and form part of the placenta (the organ that passes nutrients from the mother to the fetus).

Sometimes there is a problem with the fertilized egg and trophoblast cells. Instead of a healthy fetus developing, a tumor forms. Until there are signs or symptoms of the tumor, the pregnancy will seem like a normal pregnancy.

Most GTD is benign (not cancer) and does not spread, but some types become malignant (cancer) and spread to nearby tissues or distant parts of the body.

Gestational trophoblastic disease (GTD) is a general term that includes different types of disease:

- Hydatidiform Moles (HM)

  - Complete HM.

  - Partial HM.

- Gestational Trophoblastic Neoplasia (GTN)

  - Invasive moles.

  - Choriocarcinomas.

  - Placental-site trophoblastic tumors (PSTT; very rare).

  - Epithelioid trophoblastic tumors (ETT; even more rare).

Hydatidiform mole (HM) is the most common type of GTD.

HMs are slow-growing tumors that look like sacs of fluid. An HM is also called a molar pregnancy. The cause of hydatidiform moles is not known.

HMs may be complete or partial:

- A complete HM forms when sperm fertilizes an egg that does not contain the mother's DNA. The egg has DNA from the father and the cells that were meant to become the placenta are abnormal.

- A partial HM forms when sperm fertilizes a normal egg and there are two sets of DNA from the father in the fertilized egg. Only part of the fetus forms and the cells that were meant to become the placenta are abnormal.

Most hydatidiform moles are benign, but they sometimes become cancer. Having one or more of the following risk factors increases the risk that a hydatidiform mole will become cancer:

- A pregnancy before 20 or after 35 years of age.

- A very high level of beta human chorionic gonadotropin (β-hCG), a hormone made by the body during pregnancy.

509

- A large tumor in the uterus.

- An ovarian cyst larger than 6 centimeters.

- High blood pressure during pregnancy.

- An overactive thyroid gland (extra thyroid hormone is made).

- Severe nausea and vomiting during pregnancy.

- Trophoblastic cells in the blood, which may block small blood vessels.

- Serious blood clotting problems caused by the HM.

Gestational trophoblastic neoplasia (GTN) is a type of gestational trophoblastic disease (GTD) that is almost always malignant.

Gestational trophoblastic neoplasia (GTN) includes the following:

Invasive moles

Invasive moles are made up of trophoblast cells that grow into the muscle layer of the uterus. Invasive moles are more likely to grow and spread than a hydatidiform mole. Rarely, a complete or partial HM may become an invasive mole. Sometimes an invasive mole will disappear without treatment.

Choriocarcinomas

A choriocarcinoma is a malignant tumor that forms from trophoblast cells and spreads to the muscle layer of the uterus and nearby blood vessels. It may also spread to other parts of the body, such as the brain, lungs, liver, kidney, spleen, intestines, pelvis, or vagina. A choriocarcinoma is more likely to form in women who have had any of the following:

- Molar pregnancy, especially with a complete hydatidiform mole.

- Normal pregnancy.

- Tubal pregnancy (the fertilized egg implants in the fallopian tube rather than the uterus).

- Miscarriage.

Placental-site trophoblastic tumors

A placental-site trophoblastic tumor (PSTT) is a rare type of gestational trophoblastic neoplasia that forms where the placenta attaches to the uterus. The tumor forms from trophoblast cells and spreads into the muscle of the uterus and into blood vessels. It may also spread to the lungs, pelvis, or lymph nodes. A PSTT grows very slowly and signs or symptoms may appear months or years after a normal pregnancy.

Epithelioid trophoblastic tumors

An epithelioid trophoblastic tumor (ETT) is a very rare type of gestational trophoblastic neoplasia that may be benign or malignant. When the tumor is malignant, it may spread to the lungs.

Age and a previous molar pregnancy affect the risk of GTD.

Anything that increases your risk of getting a disease is called a risk factor. Having a risk factor does not mean that you will get cancer; not having risk factors doesn't mean that you will not get cancer. Talk to your doctor if you think you may be at risk. Risk factors for GTD include the following:

- Being pregnant when you are younger than 20 or older than 35 years of age.
- Having a personal history of hydatidiform mole.

Signs of GTD include abnormal vaginal bleeding and a uterus that is larger than normal.

These and other signs and symptoms may be caused by gestational trophoblastic disease or by other conditions. Check with your doctor if you have any of the following:

- Vaginal bleeding not related to menstruation.
- A uterus that is larger than expected during pregnancy.
- Pain or pressure in the pelvis.
- Severe nausea and vomiting during pregnancy.
- High blood pressure with headache and swelling of feet and hands early in the pregnancy.
- Vaginal bleeding that continues for longer than normal after delivery.
- Fatigue, shortness of breath, dizziness, and a fast or irregular heartbeat caused by anemia.

GTD sometimes causes an overactive thyroid. Signs and symptoms of an overactive thyroid include the following:

- Fast or irregular heartbeat.
- Shakiness.
- Sweating.
- Frequent bowel movements.
- Trouble sleeping.
- Feeling anxious or irritable.
- Weight loss.

Tests that examine the uterus are used to detect (find) and diagnose gestational trophoblastic disease.

The following tests and procedures may be used:

- **Physical exam and history:** An exam of the body to check general signs of health, including checking for signs of disease, such as lumps or anything else that seems unusual. A history of the patient's health habits and past illnesses and treatments will also be taken.

- **Pelvic exam:** An exam of the vagina, cervix, uterus, fallopian tubes, ovaries, and rectum. A speculum is inserted into the vagina and the doctor or nurse looks at the vagina and cervix for signs of disease. A Pap test of the cervix is usually done. The doctor or nurse also inserts one or two lubricated, gloved fingers of one hand into the vagina and places the other hand over the lower abdomen to feel the size, shape, and position of the uterus and ovaries. The doctor or nurse also inserts a lubricated, gloved finger into the rectum to feel for lumps or abnormal areas.

- **Ultrasound exam of the pelvis:** A procedure in which high-energy sound waves (ultrasound) are bounced off internal tissues or organs in the pelvis and make echoes. The echoes form a picture of body tissues called a sonogram. Sometimes a transvaginal ultrasound (TVUS) will be done. For TVUS, an ultrasound transducer (probe) is inserted into the vagina to make the sonogram.

- **Lumbar puncture:** A procedure used to collect cerebrospinal fluid (CSF) from the spinal column. This is done by placing a needle into the spinal column. The CSF is checked for signs of cancer. This procedure is also called an LP or spinal tap.

- **Blood chemistry studies:** A procedure in which a blood sample is checked to measure the amounts of certain substances released into the blood by organs and tissues in the body. An unusual (higher or lower than normal) amount of a substance can be a sign of disease in the organ or tissue that makes it. Blood is also tested to check the liver, kidney, and bone marrow.

- **Serum tumor marker test:** A procedure in which a sample of blood is checked to measure the amounts of certain substances made by organs, tissues, or tumor cells in the body. Certain substances are linked to specific types of cancer when found in increased levels in the body. These are called tumor markers. For GTD, the blood is checked for the level of beta human chorionic gonadotropin (β-hCG), a hormone that is made by the body during pregnancy. β-hCG in the blood of a woman who is not pregnant may be a sign of GTD.

- **Urinalysis:** A test to check the color of urine and its contents, such as sugar, protein, blood, bacteria, and the level of β-hCG.

Certain factors affect prognosis (chance of recovery) and treatment options.

Gestational trophoblastic disease usually can be cured. Treatment and prognosis depend on the following:

- The type of GTD.
- Whether the tumor has spread to the uterus, lymph nodes, or distant parts of the body.
- The number of tumors and where they are in the body.
- The size of the largest tumor.
- The level of β-hCG in the blood.
- How soon the tumor was diagnosed after the pregnancy began.
- Whether GTD occurred after a molar pregnancy, miscarriage, or normal pregnancy.
- Previous treatment for gestational trophoblastic neoplasia.

Treatment options also depend on whether the woman wishes to become pregnant in the future.

Stages of Gestational Trophoblastic Tumors and Neoplasia

After gestational trophoblastic neoplasia has been diagnosed, tests are done to find out if cancer has spread from where it started to other parts of the body.

The process used to find out the extent or spread of cancer is called staging, The information gathered from the staging process helps determine the stage of disease. For GTN, stage is one of the factors used to plan treatment.

The following tests and procedures may be done to help find out the stage of the disease:

Chest x-ray: An x-ray of the organs and bones inside the chest. An x-ray is a type of energy beam that can go through the body onto film, making pictures of areas inside the body.

CT scan (CAT scan): A procedure that makes a series of detailed pictures of areas inside the body, taken from different angles. The pictures are made by a computer linked to an x-ray machine. A dye may be injected into a vein or swallowed to help the organs or tissues show up more clearly. This procedure is also called computed tomography, computerized tomography, or computerized axial tomography.

MRI (magnetic resonance imaging) with gadolinium: A procedure that uses a magnet, radio waves, and a computer to make a series of detailed pictures of areas inside the body, such as brain and spinal cord. A substance called gadolinium is injected into a vein. The gadolinium collects around the cancer cells so they show up brighter in the picture. This procedure is also called nuclear magnetic resonance imaging (NMRI).

There are three ways that cancer spreads in the body.

Cancer can spread through tissue, the lymph system, and the blood:

- Tissue. The cancer spreads from where it began by growing into nearby areas.

- Lymph system. The cancer spreads from where it began by getting into the lymph system. The cancer travels through the lymph vessels to other parts of the body.

- Blood. The cancer spreads from where it began by getting into the blood. The cancer travels through the blood vessels to other parts of the body.

Cancer may spread from where it began to other parts of the body.

When cancer spreads to another part of the body, it is called metastasis. Cancer cells break away from where they began (the primary tumor) and travel through the lymph system or blood.

- Lymph system. The cancer gets into the lymph system, travels through the lymph vessels, and forms a tumor (metastatic tumor) in another part of the body.

- Blood. The cancer gets into the blood, travels through the blood vessels, and forms a tumor (metastatic tumor) in another part of the body.

The metastatic tumor is the same type of cancer as the primary tumor. For example, if choriocarcinoma spreads to the lung, the cancer cells in the lung are actually choriocarcinoma cells. The disease is metastatic choriocarcinoma, not lung cancer.

There is no staging system for hydatidiform moles.

Hydatidiform moles (HM) are found in the uterus only and do not spread to other parts of the body.

The following stages are used for GTN:

Stage I

In stage I, the tumor is in the uterus only.

Stage II

In stage II, cancer has spread outside of the uterus to the ovary, fallopian tube, vagina, and/or the ligaments that support the uterus.

Stage III

In stage III, cancer has spread to the lung.

Stage IV

In stage IV, cancer has spread to distant parts of the body other than the lungs.

The treatment of gestational trophoblastic neoplasia is based on the type of disease, stage, or risk group.

Invasive moles and choriocarcinomas are treated based on risk groups. The stage of the invasive mole or choriocarcinoma is one factor used to determine risk group. Other factors include the following:

- The age of the patient when the diagnosis is made.

- Whether the GTN occurred after a molar pregnancy, miscarriage, or normal pregnancy.

- How soon the tumor was diagnosed after the pregnancy began.

- The level of beta human chorionic gonadotropin (β-hCG) in the blood.

- The size of the largest tumor.

- Where the tumor has spread to and the number of tumors in the body.

- How many chemotherapy drugs the tumor has been treated with (for recurrent or resistant tumors).

There are two risk groups for invasive moles and choriocarcinomas: low risk and high risk. Patients with low-risk disease usually receive less aggressive treatment than patients with high-risk disease.

Placental-site trophoblastic tumor (PSTT) and epithelioid trophoblastic tumor (ETT) treatments depend on the stage of disease.

Treatment Option Overview

There are different types of treatment for patients with gestational trophoblastic disease.

Different types of treatment are available for patients with gestational trophoblastic disease. Some treatments are standard (the currently used treatment), and some are being tested in clinical trials. Before starting treatment, patients may want to think about taking part in a clinical trial. A treatment clinical trial is a research study meant to help improve current treatments or obtain information on new treatments for patients with cancer. When clinical trials show that a new treatment is better than the standard treatment, the new treatment may become the standard treatment.

Three types of standard treatment are used:

Surgery

The doctor may remove the cancer using one of the following operations:

- Dilatation and curettage (D&C) with suction evacuation: A surgical procedure to remove abnormal tissue and parts of the inner lining of the uterus. The cervix is dilated and the material inside the uterus is removed with a small vacuum-like device. The walls of the uterus are then gently scraped with a curette (spoon-shaped instrument) to remove any material that may remain in the uterus. This procedure may be used for molar pregnancies.

- Hysterectomy: Surgery to remove the uterus, and sometimes the cervix. If the uterus and cervix are taken out through the vagina, the operation is called a vaginal hysterectomy. If the uterus and cervix are taken out through a large incision (cut) in the abdomen, the operation is called a total abdominal hysterectomy. If the uterus and cervix are taken out through a small incision (cut) in the abdomen using a laparoscope, the operation is called a total laparoscopic hysterectomy.

Chemotherapy

Chemotherapy is a cancer treatment that uses drugs to stop the growth of cancer cells, either by killing the cells or by stopping them from dividing. When chemotherapy is taken by mouth or injected into a vein or muscle, the drugs enter the bloodstream and can reach cancer cells throughout the body (systemic chemotherapy). When chemotherapy is placed directly into the cerebrospinal fluid, an organ, or a body cavity such as the abdomen, the drugs mainly affect cancer cells in those areas (regional chemotherapy). The way the chemotherapy is given depends on the type and stage of the cancer being treated, or whether the tumor is low-risk or high-risk.

Combination chemotherapy is treatment using more than one anti-cancer drug.

Even if the doctor removes all the cancer that can be seen at the time of the surgery, some patients may be given chemotherapy after surgery to kill any tumor cells that are left. Treatment given after the surgery, to lower the risk that the cancer will come back, is called adjuvant therapy.

517

Radiation therapy

Radiation therapy is a cancer treatment that uses high-energy x-rays or other types of radiation to kill cancer cells or keep them from growing. There are two types of radiation therapy. External radiation therapy uses a machine outside the body to send radiation toward the cancer. Internal radiation therapy uses a radioactive substance sealed in needles, seeds, wires, or catheters that are placed directly into or near the cancer. The way the radiation therapy is given depends on the type of cancer being treated.

Patients may want to think about taking part in a clinical trial.

For some patients, taking part in a clinical trial may be the best treatment choice. Clinical trials are part of the cancer research process. Clinical trials are done to find out if new cancer treatments are safe and effective or better than the standard treatment.

Many of today's standard treatments for cancer are based on earlier clinical trials. Patients who take part in a clinical trial may receive the standard treatment or be among the first to receive a new treatment.

Patients who take part in clinical trials also help improve the way cancer will be treated in the future. Even when clinical trials do not lead to effective new treatments, they often answer important questions and help move research forward.

Patients can enter clinical trials before, during, or after starting their cancer treatment.

Some clinical trials only include patients who have not yet received treatment. Other trials test treatments for patients whose cancer has not gotten better. There are also clinical trials that test new ways to stop cancer from recurring (coming back) or reduce the side effects of cancer treatment.

Clinical trials are taking place in many parts of the country.

Some of the tests that were done to diagnose the cancer or to find out the stage of the cancer may be repeated. Some tests will be repeated in order to see how well the treatment is working. Decisions about whether to continue, change, or stop treatment may be based on the results of these tests.

Some of the tests will continue to be done from time to time after treatment has ended. The results of these tests can show if your condition has changed or if the cancer has recurred (come back). These tests are sometimes called follow-up tests or check-ups.

Blood levels of beta human chorionic gonadotropin (β-hCG) will be checked for up to 6 months after treatment has ended. This is because a β-hCG level that is higher than normal may mean that the tumor has not responded to treatment or it has become cancer.

Treatment Options for Gestational Trophoblastic Disease

Hydatidiform Moles

Treatment of a hydatidiform mole may include the following:

* Surgery (Dilatation and curettage with suction evacuation) to remove the tumor.

After surgery, beta human chorionic gonadotropin (β-hCG) blood tests are done every week until the β-hCG level returns to normal. Patients also have follow-up doctor visits monthly for up to 6 months. If the level of β-hCG does not return to normal or increases, it may mean the hydatidiform mole was not completely removed and it has become cancer. Pregnancy causes β-hCG levels to increase, so your doctor will ask you not to become pregnant until follow-up is finished.

Gestational Trophoblastic Neoplasia

Low-risk Gestational Trophoblastic Neoplasia

Treatment of low-risk gestational trophoblastic neoplasia (GTN) (invasive mole or choriocarcinoma) may include the following:

* Chemotherapy with one or more anticancer drugs. Treatment is given until the beta human chorionic gonadotropin (β-hCG) level is normal for at least 3 weeks after treatment ends.

If the level of β-hCG in the blood does not return to normal or the tumor spreads to distant parts of the body, chemotherapy regimens used for high-risk metastatic GTN are given.

High-risk Metastatic Gestational Trophoblastic Neoplasia

Treatment of high-risk metastatic gestational trophoblastic neoplasia (invasive mole or choriocarcinoma) may include the following:

- Combination chemotherapy.

- Intrathecal chemotherapy and radiation therapy to the brain (for cancer that has spread to the lung, to keep it from spreading to the brain).

- High-dose chemotherapy or intrathecal chemotherapy and/or radiation therapy to the brain (for cancer that has spread to the brain).

Treatment of stage I placental-site gestational trophoblastic tumors and epithelioid trophoblastic tumors may include the following:

- Surgery to remove the uterus.

Treatment of stage II placental-site gestational trophoblastic tumors and epithelioid trophoblastic tumors may include the following:

- Surgery to remove the tumor, which may be followed by combination chemotherapy.

Treatment of stage III and IV placental-site gestational trophoblastic tumors and epithelioid trophoblastic tumors may include following:

- Combination chemotherapy.

- Surgery to remove cancer that has spread to other places, such as the lung or abdomen.

Recurrent or Resistant Gestational Trophoblastic Neoplasia

Treatment of recurrent or resistant gestational trophoblastic tumor may include the following:

- Chemotherapy with one or more anticancer drugs for tumors previously treated with surgery.

- Combination chemotherapy for tumors previously treated with chemotherapy.

- Surgery for tumors that do not respond to chemotherapy.

Section 25.5

Cervical Cancer

Text in this section is excerpted from "Cervical Cancer Treatment,"
National Cancer Institute at the National Institutes of Health (NIH),
May 29, 2015.

General Information About Cervical Cancer

*Cervical cancer is a disease in which malignant (cancer)
cells form in the tissues of the cervix.*

The cervix is the lower, narrow end of the uterus (the hollow, pear-shaped organ where a fetus grows). The cervix leads from the uterus to the vagina (birth canal).

Cervical cancer usually develops slowly over time. Before cancer appears in the cervix, the cells of the cervix go through changes known as dysplasia, in which abnormal cells begin to appear in the cervical tissue. Over time, the abnormal cells may become cancer cells and start to grow and spread more deeply into the cervix and to surrounding areas.

Cervical cancer in children is rare.

*Human papillomavirus (HPV) infection is the major risk
factor for cervical cancer.*

Anything that increases your risk of getting a disease is called a risk factor. Having a risk factor does not mean that you will get cancer; not having risk factors doesn't mean that you will not get cancer. Talk with your doctor if you think you may be at risk.

Infection of the cervix with human papillomavirus (HPV) is almost always the cause of cervical cancer. Not all women with HPV infection, however, will develop cervical cancer. Women who do not regularly have tests to detect HPV or abnormal cells in the cervix are at increased risk of cervical cancer. There are two vaccines to prevent HPV in girls and young women who do not have HPV.

Other possible risk factors include the following:

- Giving birth to many children.
- Having many sexual partners.
- Having first sexual intercourse at a young age.
- Smoking cigarettes.
- Using oral contraceptives ("the Pill").

There are usually no signs or symptoms of early cervical cancer but it can be detected early with regular check-ups.

Early cervical cancer may not cause signs or symptoms. Women should have regular check-ups, including tests to check for HPV or abnormal cells in the cervix. The prognosis (chance of recovery) is better when the cancer is found early.

Signs and symptoms of cervical cancer include vaginal bleeding and pelvic pain.

These and other signs and symptoms may be caused by cervical cancer or by other conditions. Check with your doctor if you have any of the following:

- Vaginal bleeding (including bleeding after sexual intercourse).
- Unusual vaginal discharge.
- Pelvic pain.
- Pain during sexual intercourse.

Tests that examine the cervix are used to detect (find) and diagnose cervical cancer.

The following procedures may be used:

- **Physical exam and history:** An exam of the body to check general signs of health, including checking for signs of disease, such as lumps or anything else that seems unusual. A history of the patient's health habits and past illnesses and treatments will also be taken.
- **Pelvic exam:** An exam of the vagina, cervix, uterus, fallopian tubes, ovaries, and rectum. A speculum is inserted into the

vagina and the doctor or nurse looks at the vagina and cervix for signs of disease. A Pap test of the cervix is usually done. The doctor or nurse also inserts one or two lubricated, gloved fingers of one hand into the vagina and places the other hand over the lower abdomen to feel the size, shape, and position of the uterus and ovaries. The doctor or nurse also inserts a lubricated, gloved finger into the rectum to feel for lumps or abnormal areas.

- **Pap test:** A procedure to collect cells from the surface of the cervix and vagina. A piece of cotton, a brush, or a small wooden stick is used to gently scrape cells from the cervix and vagina. The cells are viewed under a microscope to find out if they are abnormal. This procedure is also called a Pap smear.

- **Human papillomavirus (HPV) test:** A laboratory test used to check DNA or RNA for certain types of HPV infection. Cells are collected from the cervix and DNA or RNA from the cells is checked to find out if an infection is caused by a type of HPV that is linked to cervical cancer. This test may be done using the sample of cells removed during a Pap test. This test may also be done if the results of a Pap test show certain abnormal cervical cells.

- **Endocervical curettage:** A procedure to collect cells or tissue from the cervical canal using a curette (spoon-shaped instrument). Tissue samples are taken and checked under a microscope for signs of cancer. This procedure is sometimes done at the same time as a colposcopy.

- **Colposcopy:** A procedure in which a colposcope (a lighted, magnifying instrument) is used to check the vagina and cervix for abnormal areas. Tissue samples may be taken using a curette (spoon-shaped instrument) or a brush and checked under a microscope for signs of disease.

- **Biopsy:** If abnormal cells are found in a Pap test, the doctor may do a biopsy. A sample of tissue is cut from the cervix and viewed under a microscope by a pathologist to check for signs of cancer. A biopsy that removes only a small amount of tissue is usually done in the doctor's office. A woman may need to go to a hospital for a cervical cone biopsy (removal of a larger, cone-shaped sample of cervical tissue).

Certain factors affect prognosis (chance of recovery) and treatment options.

The prognosis (chance of recovery) depends on the following:

- The stage of the cancer (the size of the tumor and whether it affects part of the cervix or the whole cervix, or has spread to the lymph nodes or other places in the body).
- The type of cervical cancer.
- The patient's age and general health.
- Whether the patient has a certain type of human papillomavirus (HPV).
- Whether the patient has human immunodeficiency virus (HIV).
- Whether the cancer has just been diagnosed or has recurred (come back).

Treatment options depend on the following:

- The stage of the cancer.
- The type of cervical cancer.
- The patient's desire to have children.
- The patient's age.

Treatment of cervical cancer during pregnancy depends on the stage of the cancer and the stage of the pregnancy. For cervical cancer found early or for cancer found during the last trimester of pregnancy, treatment may be delayed until after the baby is born. For more information, see the section on Cervical Cancer During Pregnancy.

Stages of Cervical Cancer

After cervical cancer has been diagnosed, tests are done to find out if cancer cells have spread within the cervix or to other parts of the body.

The process used to find out if cancer has spread within the cervix or to other parts of the body is called staging. The information gathered from the staging process determines the stage of the disease. It is important to know the stage in order to plan treatment.

The following tests and procedures may be used in the staging process:

- **CT scan (CAT scan):** A procedure that makes a series of detailed pictures of areas inside the body, taken from different angles. The pictures are made by a computer linked to an x-ray machine. A dye may be injected into a vein or swallowed to help the organs or tissues show up more clearly. This procedure is also called computed tomography, computerized tomography, or computerized axial tomography.

- **PET scan (positron emission tomography scan):** A procedure to find malignant tumor cells in the body. A small amount of radioactive glucose (sugar) is injected into a vein. The PET scanner rotates around the body and makes a picture of where glucose is being used in the body. Malignant tumor cells show up brighter in the picture because they are more active and take up more glucose than normal cells do.

- **MRI (magnetic resonance imaging):** A procedure that uses a magnet, radio waves, and a computer to make a series of detailed pictures of areas inside the body. This procedure is also called nuclear magnetic resonance imaging (NMRI).

- **Ultrasound exam:** A procedure in which high-energy sound waves (ultrasound) are bounced off internal tissues or organs and make echoes. The echoes form a picture of body tissues called a sonogram. This picture can be printed to be looked at later.

- **Chest x-ray:** An x-ray of the organs and bones inside the chest. An x-ray is a type of energy beam that can go through the body and onto film, making a picture of areas inside the body.

- **Cystoscopy:** A procedure to look inside the bladder and urethra to check for abnormal areas. A cystoscope is inserted through the urethra into the bladder. A cystoscope is a thin, tube-like instrument with a light and a lens for viewing. It may also have a tool to remove tissue samples, which are checked under a microscope for signs of cancer.

- **Laparoscopy:** A surgical procedure to look at the organs inside the abdomen to check for signs of disease. Small incisions (cuts) are made in the wall of the abdomen and a laparoscope (a thin, lighted tube) is inserted into one of the incisions. Other instruments may be inserted through the same or other incisions to perform procedures such as removing organs or taking tissue samples to be checked under a microscope for signs of disease.

- **Pretreatment surgical staging:** Surgery (an operation) is done to find out if the cancer has spread within the cervix or to other parts of the body. In some cases, the cervical cancer can be removed at the same time. Pretreatment surgical staging is usually done only as part of a clinical trial.

The results of these tests are viewed together with the results of the original tumor biopsy to determine the cervical cancer stage.

There are three ways that cancer spreads in the body.

Cancer can spread through tissue, the lymph system, and the blood:

- Tissue. The cancer spreads from where it began by growing into nearby areas.

- Lymph system. The cancer spreads from where it began by getting into the lymph system. The cancer travels through the lymph vessels to other parts of the body.

- Blood. The cancer spreads from where it began by getting into the blood. The cancer travels through the blood vessels to other parts of the body.

Cancer may spread from where it began to other parts of the body.

When cancer spreads to another part of the body, it is called metastasis. Cancer cells break away from where they began (the primary tumor) and travel through the lymph system or blood.

- Lymph system. The cancer gets into the lymph system, travels through the lymph vessels, and forms a tumor (metastatic tumor) in another part of the body.

- Blood. The cancer gets into the blood, travels through the blood vessels, and forms a tumor (metastatic tumor) in another part of the body.

The metastatic tumor is the same type of cancer as the primary tumor. For example, if cervical cancer spreads to the lung, the cancer cells in the lung are actually cervical cancer cells. The disease is metastatic cervical cancer, not lung cancer.

The following stages are used for cervical cancer:

Carcinoma in Situ (Stage 0)

In carcinoma in situ (stage 0), abnormal cells are found in the inner-most lining of the cervix. These abnormal cells may become cancer and spread into nearby normal tissue.

Stage I

In stage I, cancer is found in the cervix only.

Stage I is divided into stages IA and IB, based on the amount of cancer that is found.

- Stage IA:

A very small amount of cancer that can only be seen with a micro-scope is found in the tissues of the cervix.

Stage IA is divided into stages IA1 and IA2, based on the size of the tumor.

- In stage IA1, the cancer is not more than 3 millimeters deep and not more than 7 millimeters wide.

- In stage IA2, the cancer is more than 3 but not more than 5 millimeters deep, and not more than 7 millimeters wide.

- Stage IB:

Stage IB is divided into stages IB1 and IB2, based on the size of the tumor.

- In stage IB1:
    - the cancer can only be seen with a microscope and is more than 5 millimeters deep and more than 7 millimeters wide; or
    - the cancer can be seen without a microscope and is not more than 4 centimeters.

- In stage IB2, the cancer can be seen without a microscope and is more than 4 centimeters.

Stage II

In stage II, cancer has spread beyond the uterus but not to the pelvic wall (the tissues that line the part of the body between the hips) or to the lower third of the vagina.

Stage II is divided into stages IIA and IIB, based on how far the cancer has spread.

- Stage IIA: Cancer has spread beyond the cervix to the upper two thirds of the vagina but not to tissues around the uterus. Stage IIA is divided into stages IIA1 and IIA2, based on the size of the tumor.

  - In stage IIA1, the tumor can be seen without a microscope and is not more than 4 centimeters.

  - In stage IIA2, the tumor can be seen without a microscope and is more than 4 centimeters.

- Stage IIB: Cancer has spread beyond the cervix to the tissues around the uterus.

Stage III

In stage III, cancer has spread to the lower third of the vagina, and/or to the pelvic wall, and/or has caused kidney problems.

Stage III is divided into stages IIIA and IIIB, based on how far the cancer has spread.

- Stage IIIA:

Cancer has spread to the lower third of the vagina but not to the pelvic wall.

- Stage IIIB:

Cancer has spread to the pelvic wall; or

- the tumor has become large enough to block the ureters (tubes that connect the kidneys to the bladder) and has caused the kidneys to get bigger or stop working.

Stage IV

In stage IV, cancer has spread to the bladder, rectum, or other parts of the body.

Stage IV is divided into stages IVA and IVB, based on where the cancer has spread.

- **Stage IVA:**

Cancer has spread to nearby organs, such as the bladder or rectum.

• Stage IVB:

Cancer has spread to other parts of the body, such as the liver, lungs, bones, or distant lymph nodes.

Treatment Option Overview

There are different types of treatment for patients with cervical cancer.

Different types of treatment are available for patients with cervical cancer. Some treatments are standard (the currently used treatment), and some are being tested in clinical trials. A treatment clinical trial is a research study meant to help improve current treatments or obtain information on new treatments for patients with cancer. When clinical trials show that a new treatment is better than the standard treatment, the new treatment may become the standard treatment. Patients may want to think about taking part in a clinical trial. Some clinical trials are open only to patients who have not started treatment.

Four types of standard treatment are used:

Surgery

Surgery (removing the cancer in an operation) is sometimes used to treat cervical cancer. The following surgical procedures may be used:

• Conization: A procedure to remove a cone-shaped piece of tissue from the cervix and cervical canal. A pathologist views the tissue under a microscope to look for cancer cells. Conization may be used to diagnose or treat a cervical condition. This procedure is also called a cone biopsy.

Conization may be done using one of the following procedures:

• Cold-knife conization: A surgical procedure that uses a scalpel (sharp knife) to remove abnormal tissue or cancer.

• Loop electrosurgical excision procedure (LEEP): A surgical procedure that uses electrical current passed through a thin wire loop as a knife to remove abnormal tissue or cancer.

• Laser surgery: A surgical procedure that uses a laser beam (a narrow beam of intense light) as a knife to make bloodless cuts in tissue or to remove a surface lesion such as a tumor.

The type of conization procedure used depends on where the cancer cells are in the cervix and the type of cervical cancer.

- Total hysterectomy: Surgery to remove the uterus, including the cervix. If the uterus and cervix are taken out through the vagina, the operation is called a vaginal hysterectomy. If the uterus and cervix are taken out through a large incision (cut) in the abdomen, the operation is called a total abdominal hysterectomy. If the uterus and cervix are taken out through a small incision in the abdomen using a laparoscope, the operation is called a total laparoscopic hysterectomy.

- Radical hysterectomy: Surgery to remove the uterus, cervix, part of the vagina, and a wide area of ligaments and tissues around these organs. The ovaries, fallopian tubes, or nearby lymph nodes may also be removed.

- Modified radical hysterectomy: Surgery to remove the uterus, cervix, upper part of the vagina, and ligaments and tissues that closely surround these organs. Nearby lymph nodes may also be removed. In this type of surgery, not as many tissues and/or organs are removed as in a radical hysterectomy.

- Radical trachelectomy: Surgery to remove the cervix, nearby tissue and lymph nodes, and the upper part of the vagina. The uterus and ovaries are not removed.

- Bilateral salpingo-oophorectomy: Surgery to remove both ovaries and both fallopian tubes.

- Pelvic exenteration: Surgery to remove the lower colon, rectum, and bladder. The cervix, vagina, ovaries, and nearby lymph nodes are also removed. Artificial openings (stoma) are made for urine and stool to flow from the body to a collection bag. Plastic surgery may be needed to make an artificial vagina after this operation.

Radiation therapy

Radiation therapy is a cancer treatment that uses high-energy x-rays or other types of radiation to kill cancer cells or keep them from growing. There are two types of radiation therapy. External radiation therapy uses a machine outside the body to send radiation toward the cancer. Internal radiation therapy uses a radioactive substance sealed in needles, seeds, wires, or catheters that are placed directly into or near the cancer. The way the radiation therapy is given depends on the type and stage of the cancer being treated.

Intensity-modulated radiation therapy (IMRT) is a type of 3-dimensional (3-D) radiation therapy that uses a computer to make pictures of the size and shape of the tumor. Thin beams of radiation of different intensities (strengths) are aimed at the tumor from many angles. This type of radiation therapy causes less damage to healthy tissue near the tumor.

Chemotherapy

Chemotherapy is a cancer treatment that uses drugs to stop the growth of cancer cells, either by killing the cells or by stopping them from dividing. When chemotherapy is taken by mouth or injected into a vein or muscle, the drugs enter the bloodstream and can reach cancer cells throughout the body (systemic chemotherapy). When chemotherapy is placed directly into the cerebrospinal fluid, an organ, or a body cavity such as the abdomen, the drugs mainly affect cancer cells in those areas (regional chemotherapy). The way the chemotherapy is given depends on the type and stage of the cancer being treated.

Targeted therapy

Targeted therapy is a type of treatment that uses drugs or other substances to identify and attack specific cancer cells without harming normal cells.

Monoclonal antibody therapy is a type of targeted therapy that uses antibodies made in the laboratory from a single type of immune system cell. These antibodies can identify substances on cancer cells or normal substances that may help cancer cells grow. The antibodies attach to the substances and kill the cancer cells, block their growth, or keep them from spreading. Monoclonal antibodies are given by infusion. They may be used alone or to carry drugs, toxins, or radioactive material directly to cancer cells.

Bevacizumab is a monoclonal antibody that binds to a protein called vascular endothelial growth factor (VEGF) and may prevent the growth of new blood vessels that tumors need to grow. Bevacizumab is used to treat cervical cancer that has metastasized (spread to other parts of the body) and recurrent cervical cancer.

Patients may want to think about taking part in a clinical trial.

For some patients, taking part in a clinical trial may be the best treatment choice. Clinical trials are part of the cancer research process.

Clinical trials are done to find out if new cancer treatments are safe and effective or better than the standard treatment.

Many of today's standard treatments for cancer are based on earlier clinical trials. Patients who take part in a clinical trial may receive the standard treatment or be among the first to receive a new treatment.

Patients who take part in clinical trials also help improve the way cancer will be treated in the future. Even when clinical trials do not lead to effective new treatments, they often answer important questions and help move research forward.

Patients can enter clinical trials before, during, or after starting their cancer treatment.

Some clinical trials only include patients who have not yet received treatment. Other trials test treatments for patients whose cancer has not gotten better. There are also clinical trials that test new ways to stop cancer from recurring (coming back) or reduce the side effects of cancer treatment.

Clinical trials are taking place in many parts of the country.

Follow-up tests may be needed.

Some of the tests that were done to diagnose the cancer or to find out the stage of the cancer may be repeated. Some tests will be repeated in order to see how well the treatment is working. Decisions about whether to continue, change, or stop treatment may be based on the results of these tests.

Some of the tests will continue to be done from time to time after treatment has ended. The results of these tests can show if your condition has changed or if the cancer has recurred (come back). These tests are sometimes called follow-up tests or check-ups.

Your doctor will ask if you have any of the following signs or symptoms, which may mean the cancer has come back:

- Pain in the abdomen, back, or leg.
- Swelling in the leg.
- Trouble urinating.
- Cough.
- Feeling tired.

For cervical cancer, follow-up tests are usually done every 3 to 4 months for the first 2 years, followed by check-ups every 6 months. The check-up includes a current health history and exam of the body to check for signs and symptoms of recurrent cervical cancer and for late effects of treatment.

Section 25.6

Vaginal Cancer

Text in this section is excerpted from "Vaginal Cancer Treatment," National Cancer Institute at the National Institutes of Health (NIH), November 14, 2014.

General Information About Vaginal Cancer

Vaginal cancer is a disease in which malignant (cancer) cells form in the vagina.

The vagina is the canal leading from the cervix (the opening of uterus) to the outside of the body. At birth, a baby passes out of the body through the vagina (also called the birth canal).

Vaginal cancer is not common. There are two main types of vaginal cancer:

- Squamous cell carcinoma: Cancer that forms in squamous cells, the thin, flat cells lining the vagina. Squamous cell vaginal cancer spreads slowly and usually stays near the vagina, but may spread to the lungs, liver, or bone. This is the most common type of vaginal cancer.

- Adenocarcinoma: Cancer that begins in glandular (secretory) cells. Glandular cells in the lining of the vagina make and release fluids such as mucus. Adenocarcinoma is more likely than squamous cell cancer to spread to the lungs and lymph nodes. A rare type of adenocarcinoma is linked to being exposed to diethylstilbestrol (DES) before birth. Adenocarcinomas that are not linked with being exposed to DES are most common in women after menopause.

Age and being exposed to the drug DES (diethylstilbestrol) before birth affect a woman's risk of vaginal cancer.

Anything that increases your risk of getting a disease is called a risk factor. Having a risk factor does not mean that you will get cancer; not having risk factors doesn't mean that you will not get cancer. Talk with your doctor if you think you may be at risk. Risk factors for vaginal cancer include the following:

- Being aged 60 or older.

- Being exposed to DES while in the mother's womb. In the 1950s, the drug DES was given to some pregnant women to prevent miscarriage (premature birth of a fetus that cannot survive). Women who were exposed to DES before birth have an increased risk of vaginal cancer. Some of these women develop a rare form of vaginal cancer called clear cell adenocarcinoma.

- Having human papilloma virus (HPV) infection.

- Having a history of abnormal cells in the cervix or cervical cancer.

- Having a history of abnormal cells in the uterus or cancer of the uterus.

- Having had a hysterectomy for health problems that affect the uterus.

Signs and symptoms of vaginal cancer include pain or abnormal vaginal bleeding.

Vaginal cancer often does not cause early signs or symptoms. It may be found during a routine pelvic exam and Pap test. Signs and symptoms may be caused by vaginal cancer or by other conditions. Check with your doctor if you have any of the following:

- Bleeding or discharge not related to menstrual periods.

- Pain during sexual intercourse.

- Pain in the pelvic area.

- A lump in the vagina.

- Pain when urinating.
- Constipation.

Tests that examine the vagina and other organs in the pelvis are used to detect (find) and diagnose vaginal cancer.

The following tests and procedures may be used:

- **Physical exam and history:** An exam of the body to check general signs of health, including checking for signs of disease, such as lumps or anything else that seems unusual. A history of the patient's health habits and past illnesses and treatments will also be taken.

- **Pelvic exam:** An exam of the vagina, cervix, uterus, fallopian tubes, ovaries, and rectum. The doctor or nurse inserts one or two lubricated, gloved fingers of one hand into the vagina and places the other hand over the lower abdomen to feel the size, shape, and position of the uterus and ovaries. A speculum is also inserted into the vagina and the doctor or nurse looks at the vagina and cervix for signs of disease. A Pap test or Pap smear of the cervix is usually done. The doctor or nurse also inserts a lubricated, gloved finger into the rectum to feel for lumps or abnormal areas.

- **Pap test:** A procedure to collect cells from the surface of the cervix and vagina. A piece of cotton, a brush, or a small wooden stick is used to gently scrape cells from the cervix and vagina. The cells are viewed under a microscope to find out if they are abnormal. This procedure is also called a Pap smear.

- **Colposcopy:** A procedure in which a colposcope (a lighted, magnifying instrument) is used to check the vagina and cervix for abnormal areas. Tissue samples may be taken using a curette (spoon-shaped instrument) and checked under a microscope for signs of disease.

- **Biopsy:** The removal of cells or tissues from the vagina and cervix so they can be viewed under a microscope by a pathologist to check for signs of cancer. If a Pap test shows abnormal cells in the vagina, a biopsy may be done during a colposcopy.

Certain factors affect prognosis (chance of recovery) and treatment options.

The prognosis (chance of recovery) depends on the following:

- The stage of the cancer (whether it is in the vagina only or has spread to other areas).

- The size of the tumor.

- The grade of tumor cells (how different they look from normal cells under a microscope).

- Where the cancer is within the vagina.

- Whether there are signs or symptoms at diagnosis.

- The patient's age and general health.

- Whether the cancer has just been diagnosed or has recurred (come back).

When found in early stages, vaginal cancer can often be cured.

Treatment options depend on the following:

- The stage and size of the cancer.

- Whether the cancer is close to other organs that may be damaged by treatment.

- Whether the tumor is made up of squamous cells or is an adenocarcinoma.

- Whether the patient has a uterus or has had a hysterectomy.

- Whether the patient has had past radiation treatment to the pelvis.

Stages of Vaginal Cancer

After vaginal cancer has been diagnosed, tests are done to find out if cancer cells have spread within the vagina or to other parts of the body.

The process used to find out if cancer has spread within the vagina or to other parts of the body is called staging. The information gathered from the staging process determines the stage of the disease. It is important to know the stage in order to plan treatment. The following procedures may be used in the staging process:

- **Chest x-ray:** An x-ray of the organs and bones inside the chest. An x-ray is a type of energy beam that can go through the body and onto film, making a picture of areas inside the body.

- **CT scan (CAT scan):** A procedure that makes a series of detailed pictures of areas inside the body, taken from different

536

angles. The pictures are made by a computer linked to an x-ray machine. A dye may be injected into a vein or swallowed to help the organs or tissues show up more clearly. This procedure is also called computed tomography, computerized tomography, or computerized axial tomography.

- **MRI (magnetic resonance imaging):** A procedure that uses a magnet, radio waves, and a computer to make a series of detailed pictures of areas inside the body. This procedure is also called nuclear magnetic resonance imaging (NMRI).

- **PET scan (positron emission tomography scan):** A procedure to find malignant tumor cells in the body. A small amount of radioactive glucose (sugar) is injected into a vein. The PET scanner rotates around the body and makes a picture of where glucose is being used in the body. Malignant tumor cells show up brighter in the picture because they are more active and take up more glucose than normal cells do.

- **Cystoscopy:** A procedure to look inside the bladder and urethra to check for abnormal areas. A cystoscope is inserted through the urethra into the bladder. A cystoscope is a thin, tube-like instrument with a light and a lens for viewing. It may also have a tool to remove tissue samples, which are checked under a microscope for signs of cancer.

- **Ureteroscopy:** A procedure to look inside the ureters to check for abnormal areas. A ureteroscope is inserted through the bladder and into the ureters. A ureteroscope is a thin, tube-like instrument with a light and a lens for viewing. It may also have a tool to remove tissue to be checked under a microscope for signs of disease. A ureteroscopy and cystoscopy may be done during the same procedure.

- **Proctoscopy:** A procedure to look inside the rectum to check for abnormal areas. A proctoscope is inserted through the rectum. A proctoscope is a thin, tube-like instrument with a light and a lens for viewing. It may also have a tool to remove tissue to be checked under a microscope for signs of disease.

- **Biopsy:** A biopsy may be done to find out if cancer has spread to the cervix. A sample of tissue is removed from the cervix and viewed under a microscope. A biopsy that removes only a small amount of tissue is usually done in the doctor's office. A cone biopsy (removal of a larger, cone-shaped piece of tissue from the cervix and cervical canal) is usually done in the hospital. A biopsy of the vulva may also be done to see if cancer has spread there.

There are three ways that cancer spreads in the body.

Cancer can spread through tissue, the lymph system, and the blood:

- Tissue. The cancer spreads from where it began by growing into nearby areas.

- Lymph system. The cancer spreads from where it began by getting into the lymph system. The cancer travels through the lymph vessels to other parts of the body.

- Blood. The cancer spreads from where it began by getting into the blood. The cancer travels through the blood vessels to other parts of the body.

Cancer may spread from where it began to other parts of the body.

When cancer spreads to another part of the body, it is called metastasis. Cancer cells break away from where they began (the primary tumor) and travel through the lymph system or blood.

- Lymph system. The cancer gets into the lymph system, travels through the lymph vessels, and forms a tumor (metastatic tumor) in another part of the body.

- Blood. The cancer gets into the blood, travels through the blood vessels, and forms a tumor (metastatic tumor) in another part of the body.

The metastatic tumor is the same type of cancer as the primary tumor. For example, if vaginal cancer spreads to the lung, the cancer cells in the lung are actually vaginal cancer cells. The disease is metastatic vaginal cancer, not lung cancer.

In vaginal intraepithelial neoplasia (VAIN), abnormal cells are found in tissue lining the inside of the vagina.

These abnormal cells are not cancer. Vaginal intraepithelial neoplasia (VAIN) is grouped based on how deep the abnormal cells are in the tissue lining the vagina:

- VAIN 1: Abnormal cells are found in the outermost one third of the tissue lining the vagina.

- VAIN 2: Abnormal cells are found in the outermost two-thirds of the tissue lining the vagina.

- VAIN 3: Abnormal cells are found in more than two-thirds of the tissue lining the vagina. When abnormal cells are found throughout the tissue lining, it is called carcinoma in situ.

VAIN may become cancer and spread into the vaginal wall. VAIN is sometimes called stage 0.

The following stages are used for vaginal cancer:

Stage I

In stage I, cancer is found in the vaginal wall only.

Stage II

In stage II, cancer has spread through the wall of the vagina to the tissue around the vagina. Cancer has not spread to the wall of the pelvis.

Stage III

In stage III, cancer has spread to the wall of the pelvis.

Stage IV

Stage IV is divided into stage IVA and stage IVB:

- Stage IVA: Cancer may have spread to one or more of the following areas:

  - The lining of the bladder.

  - The lining of the rectum.

  - Beyond the area of the pelvis that has the bladder, uterus, ovaries, and cervix.

- Stage IVB: Cancer has spread to parts of the body that are not near the vagina, such as the lung or bone.

Treatment Option Overview

There are different types of treatment for patients with vaginal cancer.

Different types of treatments are available for patients with vaginal cancer. Some treatments are standard (the currently used treatment), and some are being tested in clinical trials. A treatment clinical trial is a research study meant to help improve current treatments or obtain information on new treatments for patients with cancer. When clinical trials show that a new treatment is better than the standard treatment, the new treatment may become the standard treatment. Patients may want to think about taking part in a clinical trial. Some clinical trials are open only to patients who have not started treatment.

Three types of standard treatment are used:

Surgery

Surgery is the most common treatment of vaginal cancer. The following surgical procedures may be used:

- Laser surgery: A surgical procedure that uses a laser beam (a narrow beam of intense light) as a knife to make bloodless cuts in tissue or to remove a surface lesion such as a tumor.

- Wide local excision: A surgical procedure that takes out the cancer and some of the healthy tissue around it.

- Vaginectomy: Surgery to remove all or part of the vagina.

- Total hysterectomy: Surgery to remove the uterus, including the cervix. If the uterus and cervix are taken out through the vagina, the operation is called a vaginal hysterectomy. If the uterus and cervix are taken out through a large incision (cut) in the abdomen, the operation is called a total abdominal hysterectomy. If the uterus and cervix are taken out through a small incision in the abdomen using a laparoscope, the operation is called a total laparoscopic hysterectomy.

- Lymph node dissection: A surgical procedure in which lymph nodes are removed and a sample of tissue is checked under a microscope for signs of cancer. This procedure is also called lymphadenectomy. If the cancer is in the upper vagina, the pelvic lymph nodes may be removed. If the cancer is in the lower vagina, lymph nodes in the groin may be removed.

- Pelvic exenteration: Surgery to remove the lower colon, rectum, bladder, cervix, vagina, and ovaries. Nearby lymph nodes are also removed. Artificial openings (stoma) are made for urine and stool to flow from the body into a collection bag.

Skin grafting may follow surgery, to repair or reconstruct the vagina. Skin grafting is a surgical procedure in which skin is moved from one part of the body to another. A piece of healthy skin is taken from a part of the body that is usually hidden, such as the buttock or thigh, and used to repair or rebuild the area treated with surgery.

Even if the doctor removes all the cancer that can be seen at the time of the surgery, some patients may be given radiation therapy after surgery to kill any cancer cells that are left. Treatment given after the surgery, to lower the risk that the cancer will come back, is called adjuvant therapy.

Radiation therapy

Radiation therapy is a cancer treatment that uses high-energy x-rays or other types of radiation to kill cancer cells or keep them from growing. There are two types of radiation therapy. External radiation therapy uses a machine outside the body to send radiation toward the cancer. Internal radiation therapy uses a radioactive substance sealed in needles, seeds, wires, or catheters that are placed directly into or near the cancer. The way the radiation therapy is given depends on the type and stage of the cancer being treated.

Chemotherapy

Chemotherapy is a cancer treatment that uses drugs to stop the growth of cancer cells, either by killing the cells or by stopping them from dividing. When chemotherapy is taken by mouth or injected into a vein or muscle, the drugs enter the bloodstream and can affect cancer cells throughout the body (systemic chemotherapy). When chemotherapy is placed directly into the cerebrospinal fluid, an organ, or a body cavity such as the abdomen, the drugs mainly affect cancer cells in those areas (regional chemotherapy). The way the chemotherapy is given depends on the type and stage of the cancer being treated.

Topical chemotherapy for squamous cell vaginal cancer may be applied to the vagina in a cream or lotion.

New types of treatment are being tested in clinical trials.

Radiosensitizers

Radiosensitizers are drugs that make tumor cells more sensitive to radiation therapy. Combining radiation therapy with radiosensitizers may kill more tumor cells.

Patients may want to think about taking part in a clinical trial.

For some patients, taking part in a clinical trial may be the best treatment choice. Clinical trials are part of the cancer research process. Clinical trials are done to find out if new cancer treatments are safe and effective or better than the standard treatment.

Many of today's standard treatments for cancer are based on earlier clinical trials. Patients who take part in a clinical trial may receive the standard treatment or be among the first to receive a new treatment.

Patients who take part in clinical trials also help improve the way cancer will be treated in the future. Even when clinical trials do not lead to effective new treatments, they often answer important questions and help move research forward.

Patients can enter clinical trials before, during, or after starting their cancer treatment.

Some clinical trials only include patients who have not yet received treatment. Other trials test treatments for patients whose cancer has not gotten better. There are also clinical trials that test new ways to stop cancer from recurring (coming back) or reduce the side effects of cancer treatment.

Clinical trials are taking place in many parts of the country.

Follow-up tests may be needed.

Some of the tests that were done to diagnose the cancer or to find out the stage of the cancer may be repeated. Some tests will be repeated in order to see how well the treatment is working. Decisions about whether to continue, change, or stop treatment may be based on the results of these tests.

Treatment Options by Stage

Vaginal Intraepithelial Neoplasia (VAIN)

Treatment of vaginal intraepithelial neoplasia (VAIN) 1 is usually watchful waiting.

Treatment of VAIN 2 and 3 may include the following:

- Watchful waiting.
- Laser surgery.
- Wide local excision, with or without a skin graft.
- Partial or total vaginectomy, with or without a skin graft.
- Topical chemotherapy.
- Internal radiation therapy.
- A clinical trial of a new topical chemotherapy drug.

Stage I Vaginal Cancer

Treatment of stage I squamous cell vaginal cancer may include the following:

- Internal radiation therapy.
- External radiation therapy, especially for large tumors or the lymph nodes near tumors in the lower part of the vagina.
- Wide local excision or vaginectomy with vaginal reconstruction. Radiation therapy may be given after the surgery.
- Vaginectomy and lymph node dissection, with or without vaginal reconstruction. Radiation therapy may be given after the surgery.

Treatment of stage I vaginal adenocarcinoma may include the following:

- Vaginectomy, hysterectomy, and lymph node dissection. This may be followed by vaginal reconstruction and/or radiation therapy.
- Internal radiation therapy. External radiation therapy may also be given to the lymph nodes near tumors in the lower part of the vagina.

- A combination of therapies that may include wide local excision with or without lymph node dissection and internal radiation therapy.

Stage II Vaginal Cancer

Treatment of stage II vaginal cancer is the same for squamous cell cancer and adenocarcinoma. Treatment may include the following:

- Both internal and external radiation therapy to the vagina. External radiation therapy may also be given to the lymph nodes near tumors in the lower part of the vagina.

- Vaginectomy or pelvic exenteration. Internal and/or external radiation therapy may also be given.

Stage III Vaginal Cancer

Treatment of stage III vaginal cancer is the same for squamous cell cancer and adenocarcinoma. Treatment may include the following:

- External radiation therapy. Internal radiation therapy may also be given.

- Surgery (rare) followed by external radiation therapy. Internal radiation therapy may also be given.

Stage IVA Vaginal Cancer

Treatment of stage IVA vaginal cancer is the same for squamous cell cancer and adenocarcinoma. Treatment may include the following:

- External radiation therapy and/or internal radiation therapy.

- Surgery (rare) followed by external radiation therapy and/or internal radiation therapy.

Stage IVB Vaginal Cancer

Treatment of stage IVB vaginal cancer is the same for squamous cell cancer and adenocarcinoma. Treatment may include the following:

- Radiation therapy as palliative therapy, to relieve symptoms and improve the quality of life. Chemotherapy may also be given.

- A clinical trial of anticancer drugs and/or radiosensitizers.

Although no anticancer drugs have been shown to help patients with stage IVB vaginal cancer live longer, they are often treated with regimens used for cervical cancer.

Section 25.7

Vulvar Cancer

Text in this section is excerpted from "Vulvar Cancer Treatment," National Cancer Institute at the National Institutes of Health (NIH), July 23, 2014.

General Information About Vulvar Cancer

Vulvar cancer is a rare disease in which malignant (cancer) cells form in the tissues of the vulva.

Vulvar cancer forms in a woman's external genitalia. The vulva includes:

- Inner and outer lips of the vagina.

- Clitoris (sensitive tissue between the lips).

- Opening of the vagina and its glands.

- Mons pubis (the rounded area in front of the pubic bones that becomes covered with hair at puberty).

- Perineum (the area between the vulva and the anus).

Vulvar cancer most often affects the outer vaginal lips. Less often, cancer affects the inner vaginal lips, clitoris, or vaginal glands.
Vulvar cancer usually forms slowly over a number of years. Abnormal cells can grow on the surface of the vulvar skin for a long time. This condition is called vulvar intraepithelial neoplasia (VIN). Because it is possible for VIN to become vulvar cancer, it is very important to get treatment.

Having vulvar intraepithelial neoplasia or HPV infection can affect the risk of vulvar cancer.

Anything that increases your risk of getting a disease is called a risk factor. Having a risk factor does not mean that you will get cancer; not having risk factors doesn't mean that you will not get cancer. Talk with your doctor if you think you may be at risk. Risk factors for vulvar cancer include the following:

- Having vulvar intraepithelial neoplasia (VIN).
- Having human papillomavirus (HPV) infection.
- Having a history of genital warts.

Other possible risk factors include the following:

- Having many sexual partners.
- Having first sexual intercourse at a young age.
- Having a history of abnormal Pap tests (Pap smears).

Signs of vulvar cancer include bleeding or itching.

Vulvar cancer often does not cause early signs or symptoms. Signs and symptoms may be caused by vulvar cancer or by other conditions. Check with your doctor if you have any of the following:

- A lump or growth on the vulva.
- Changes in the vulvar skin, such as color changes or growths that look like a wart or ulcer.
- Itching in the vulvar area, that does not go away.
- Bleeding not related to menstruation (periods).
- Tenderness in the vulvar area.

Tests that examine the vulva are used to detect (find) and diagnose vulvar cancer.

The following tests and procedures may be used:

- **Physical exam and history:** An exam of the body to check general signs of health, including checking the vulva for signs of disease, such as lumps or anything else that seems unusual. A history of the patient's health habits and past illnesses and treatments will also be taken.

- **Biopsy:** The removal of samples of cells or tissues from the vulva so they can be viewed under a microscope by a pathologist to check for signs of cancer.

Certain factors affect prognosis (chance of recovery) and treatment options.

The prognosis (chance of recovery) and treatment options depend on the following:

- The stage of the cancer.

- The patient's age and general health.

- Whether the cancer has just been diagnosed or has recurred (come back).

Stages of Vulvar Cancer

After vulvar cancer has been diagnosed, tests are done to find out if cancer cells have spread within the vulva or to other parts of the body.

The process used to find out if cancer has spread within the vulva or to other parts of the body is called staging. The information gathered from the staging process determines the stage of the disease. It is important to know the stage in order to plan treatment. The following tests and procedures may be used in the staging process:

- **Pelvic exam:** An exam of the vagina, cervix, uterus, fallopian tubes, ovaries, and rectum. The doctor or nurse inserts one or two lubricated, gloved fingers of one hand into the vagina and places the other hand over the lower abdomen to feel the size, shape, and position of the uterus and ovaries. A speculum is also inserted into the vagina and the doctor or nurse looks at the vagina and cervix for signs of disease. A Pap test or Pap smear of the cervix is usually done. The doctor or nurse also inserts a lubricated, gloved finger into the rectum to feel for lumps or abnormal areas.

- **Colposcopy:** A procedure in which a colposcope (a lighted, magnifying instrument) is used to check the vagina and cervix for abnormal areas. Tissue samples may be taken using a curette (spoon-shaped instrument) and checked under a microscope for signs of disease.

- **Cystoscopy:** A procedure to look inside the bladder and urethra to check for abnormal areas. A cystoscope is inserted through the urethra into the bladder. A cystoscope is a thin, tube-like instrument with a light and a lens for viewing. It may also have a tool to remove tissue samples, which are checked under a microscope for signs of cancer.

- **Proctoscopy:** A procedure to look inside the rectum and anus to check for abnormal areas. A proctoscope is inserted into the anus and rectum. A proctoscope is a thin, tube-like instrument with a light and a lens for viewing. It may also have a tool to remove tissue samples, which are checked under a microscope for signs of cancer.

- **X-rays:** An x-ray is a type of energy beam that can go through the body and onto film, making a picture of areas inside the body. To stage vulvar cancer, x-rays may be taken of the organs and bones inside the chest, and the pelvic bones.

- **Intravenous pyelogram (IVP):** A series of x-rays of the kidneys, ureters, and bladder to find out if cancer has spread to these organs. A contrast dye is injected into a vein. As the contrast dye moves through the kidneys, ureters and bladder, x-rays are taken to see if there are any blockages. This procedure is also called intravenous urography.

- **CT scan (CAT scan):** A procedure that makes a series of detailed pictures of areas inside the body, taken from different angles. The pictures are made by a computer linked to an x-ray machine. A dye may be injected into a vein or swallowed to help the organs or tissues show up more clearly. This procedure is also called computed tomography, computerized tomography, or computerized axial tomography.

- **MRI (magnetic resonance imaging):** A procedure that uses a magnet, radio waves, and a computer to make a series of detailed pictures of areas inside the body. This procedure is also called nuclear magnetic resonance imaging (NMRI).

- **PET scan (positron emission tomography scan):** A procedure to find malignant tumor cells in the body. A small amount of radioactive glucose (sugar) is injected into a vein. The PET scanner rotates around the body and makes a picture of where glucose is being used in the body. Malignant tumor cells show up brighter in the picture because they are more active and take up more glucose than normal cells do.

- **Sentinel lymph node biopsy:** The removal of the sentinel lymph node during surgery. The sentinel lymph node is the first lymph node to receive lymphatic drainage from a tumor. It is the first lymph node the cancer is likely to spread to from the tumor. A radioactive substance and/or blue dye is injected near the tumor. The substance or dye flows through the lymph ducts to the lymph nodes. The first lymph node to receive the substance or dye is removed. A pathologist views the tissue under a microscope to look for cancer cells. If cancer cells are not found, it may not be necessary to remove more lymph nodes. Sentinel lymph node biopsy may be done during surgery to remove the tumor for early-stage vulvar cancer.

There are three ways that cancer spreads in the body.

Cancer can spread through tissue, the lymph system, and the blood:

- Tissue. The cancer spreads from where it began by growing into nearby areas.

- Lymph system. The cancer spreads from where it began by getting into the lymph system. The cancer travels through the lymph vessels to other parts of the body.

- Blood. The cancer spreads from where it began by getting into the blood. The cancer travels through the blood vessels to other parts of the body.

Cancer may spread from where it began to other parts of the body.

When cancer spreads to another part of the body, it is called metastasis. Cancer cells break away from where they began (the primary tumor) and travel through the lymph system or blood.

- Lymph system. The cancer gets into the lymph system, travels through the lymph vessels, and forms a tumor (metastatic tumor) in another part of the body.

- Blood. The cancer gets into the blood, travels through the blood vessels, and forms a tumor (metastatic tumor) in another part of the body.

The metastatic tumor is the same type of cancer as the primary tumor. For example, if vulvar cancer spreads to the lung, the cancer cells in the lung are actually vulvar cancer cells. The disease is metastatic vulvar cancer, not lung cancer.

In vulvar intraepithelial neoplasia (VIN), abnormal cells are found on the surface of the vulvar skin.

These abnormal cells are not cancer. Vulvar intraepithelial neoplasia (VIN) may become cancer and spread into nearby tissue. VIN is sometimes called stage 0 or carcinoma in situ.

The following stages are used for vulvar cancer:

Stage I

In stage I, cancer has formed. The tumor is found only in the vulva or perineum (area between the rectum and the vagina). Stage I is divided into stages IA and IB.

- In stage IA, the tumor is 2 centimeters or smaller and has spread 1 millimeter or less into the tissue of the vulva. Cancer has not spread to the lymph nodes.

- In stage IB, the tumor is larger than 2 centimeters or has spread more than 1 millimeter into the tissue of the vulva. Cancer has not spread to the lymph nodes.

Stage II

In stage II, the tumor is any size and has spread into the lower part of the urethra, the lower part of the vagina, or the anus. Cancer has not spread to the lymph nodes.

Stage III

In stage III, the tumor is any size and may have spread into the lower part of the urethra, the lower part of the vagina, or the anus. Cancer has spread to one or more nearby lymph nodes. Stage III is divided into stages IIIA, IIIB, and IIIC.

- In stage IIIA, cancer is found in 1 or 2 lymph nodes that are smaller than 5 millimeters or in one lymph node that is 5 millimeters or larger.

- In stage IIIB, cancer is found in 2 or more lymph nodes that are 5 millimeters or larger, or in 3 or more lymph nodes that are smaller than 5 millimeters.

- In stage IIIC, cancer is found in lymph nodes and has spread to the outside surface of the lymph nodes.

Stage IV

In stage IV, the tumor has spread into the upper part of the urethra, the upper part of the vagina, or to other parts of the body. Stage IV is divided into stages IVA and IVB.

- In stage IVA:

  - cancer has spread into the lining of the upper urethra, the upper vagina, the bladder, or the rectum, or has attached to the pelvic bone; or

  - cancer has spread to nearby lymph nodes and the lymph nodes are not moveable or have formed an ulcer.

- In stage IVB, cancer has spread to lymph nodes in the pelvis or to other parts of the body.

Treatment Option Overview

There are different types of treatment for patients with vulvar cancer.

Different types of treatments are available for patients with vulvar cancer. Some treatments are standard (the currently used treatment), and some are being tested in clinical trials. A treatment clinical trial is a research study meant to help improve current treatments or obtain information on new treatments for patients with cancer. When clinical trials show that a new treatment is better than the standard treatment, the new treatment may become the standard treatment. Patients may want to think about taking part in a clinical trial. Some clinical trials are open only to patients who have not started treatment.

Four types of standard treatment are used:

Surgery

Surgery is the most common treatment for vulvar cancer. The goal of surgery is to remove all the cancer without any loss of the woman's sexual function. One of the following types of surgery may be done:

- Laser surgery: A surgical procedure that uses a laser beam (a narrow beam of intense light) as a knife to make bloodless cuts in tissue or to remove a surface lesion such as a tumor.

- Wide local excision: A surgical procedure to remove the cancer and some of the normal tissue around the cancer.

- Radical local excision: A surgical procedure to remove the cancer and a large amount of normal tissue around it. Nearby lymph nodes in the groin may also be removed.

- Ultrasound surgical aspiration (USA): A surgical procedure to break the tumor up into small pieces using very fine vibrations. The small pieces of tumor are washed away and removed by suction. This procedure causes less damage to nearby tissue.

- Vulvectomy: A surgical procedure to remove part or all of the vulva:

  - Skinning vulvectomy: The top layer of vulvar skin where the cancer is found is removed. Skin grafts from other parts of the body may be needed to cover the area where the skin was removed.

  - Modified radical vulvectomy: Surgery to remove part of the vulva. Nearby lymph nodes may also be removed.

  - Radical vulvectomy: Surgery to remove the entire vulva. Nearby lymph nodes are also removed.

- Pelvic exenteration: A surgical procedure to remove the lower colon, rectum, and bladder. The cervix, vagina, ovaries, and nearby lymph nodes are also removed. Artificial openings (stoma) are made for urine and stool to flow from the body into a collection bag.

Even if the doctor removes all the cancer that can be seen at the time of the surgery, some patients may have chemotherapy or radiation therapy after surgery to kill any cancer cells that are left. Treatment given after the surgery, to lower the risk that the cancer will come back, is called adjuvant therapy.

Radiation therapy

Radiation therapy is a cancer treatment that uses high-energy x-rays or other types of radiation to kill cancer cells. There are two types of radiation therapy. External radiation therapy uses a machine outside the body to send radiation toward the cancer. Internal radiation therapy uses a radioactive substance sealed in needles, seeds, wires, or catheters that are placed directly into or near the cancer. The way the radiation therapy is given depends on the type and stage of the cancer being treated.

Chemotherapy

Chemotherapy is a cancer treatment that uses drugs to stop the growth of cancer cells, either by killing the cells or by stopping the cells from dividing. When chemotherapy is taken by mouth or injected into a vein or muscle, the drugs enter the bloodstream and can reach cancer cells throughout the body (systemic chemotherapy). When chemotherapy is placed directly into the cerebrospinal fluid, an organ, a body cavity such as the abdomen, or onto the skin, the drugs mainly affect cancer cells in those areas (regional chemotherapy). The way the chemotherapy is given depends on the type and stage of the cancer being treated.

Topical chemotherapy for vulvar cancer may be applied to the skin in a cream or lotion.

Biologic therapy

Biologic therapy is a treatment that uses the patient's immune system to fight cancer. Substances made by the body or made in a laboratory are used to boost, direct, or restore the body's natural defenses against cancer. This type of cancer treatment is also called biotherapy or immunotherapy.

Imiquimod is a biologic therapy that may be used to treat vulvar lesions and is applied to the skin in a cream.

Patients may want to think about taking part in a clinical trial.

For some patients, taking part in a clinical trial may be the best treatment choice. Clinical trials are part of the cancer research process. Clinical trials are done to find out if new cancer treatments are safe and effective or better than the standard treatment.

Many of today's standard treatments for cancer are based on earlier clinical trials. Patients who take part in a clinical trial may receive the standard treatment or be among the first to receive a new treatment.

Patients who take part in clinical trials also help improve the way cancer will be treated in the future. Even when clinical trials do not lead to effective new treatments, they often answer important questions and help move research forward.

Patients can enter clinical trials before, during, or after starting their cancer treatment.

Some clinical trials only include patients who have not yet received treatment. Other trials test treatments for patients whose cancer has not gotten better. There are also clinical trials that test new ways to stop cancer from recurring (coming back) or reduce the side effects of cancer treatment.

Clinical trials are taking place in many parts of the country.

Follow-up tests may be needed.

Some of the tests that were done to diagnose the cancer or to find out the stage of the cancer may be repeated. Some tests will be repeated in order to see how well the treatment is working. Decisions about whether to continue, change, or stop treatment may be based on the results of these tests.

Some of the tests will continue to be done from time to time after treatment has ended. The results of these tests can show if your condition has changed or if the cancer has recurred (come back). These tests are sometimes called follow-up tests or check-ups.

It is important to have regular follow-up exams to check for recurrent vulvar cancer.

Chapter 26

Germ Cell Cancer

Chapter Contents

Section 26.1

Childhood Extracranial Germ Cell Tumor

Text in this section is excerpted from "Childhood Extracranial Germ
Cell Tumors Treatment," National Cancer Institute at the National
Institutes of Health (NIH), April 10, 2015.

General Information About Childhood Extracranial Germ Cell Tumors

Childhood extracranial germ cell tumors form from germ cells in parts of the body other than the brain.

A germ cell is a type of cell that forms as a fetus (unborn baby)
develops. These cells later become sperm in the testicles or eggs in
the ovaries. Sometimes while the fetus is forming, germ cells travel to
parts of the body where they should not be and grow into a germ cell
tumor. The tumor may form before or after birth.

Extracranial germ cell tumors are most common in teenagers 15
to 19 years of age.

This section is about germ cell tumors that form in parts of the
body that are extracranial (outside the brain). Extracranial germ cell
tumors usually form in the following areas of the body:

- Testicles.

- Ovaries.

- Sacrum or coccyx (bottom part of the spine).

- Retroperitoneum (the back wall of the abdomen).

- Mediastinum (area between the lungs).

Extracranial germ cell tumors are most common in teenagers 15
to 19 years of age.

Childhood extracranial germ cell tumors may be benign or malignant.

Extracranial germ cell tumors may be benign (non-cancer) or malignant (cancer).

There are three types of extracranial germ cell tumors.

Extracranial germ cell tumors are grouped into mature teratomas, immature teratomas, and malignant germ cell tumors:

Mature Teratomas

Mature teratomas are the most common type of extracranial germ cell tumor. Mature teratomas are benign tumors and not likely to become cancer. They usually occur in the sacrum or coccyx (bottom part of the spine) in newborns or in the ovaries of girls at the start of puberty. The cells of mature teratomas look almost like normal cells under a microscope. Some mature teratomas release enzymes or hormones that cause signs and symptoms of disease.

Immature Teratomas

Immature teratomas also usually occur in the sacrum or coccyx (bottom part of the spine) in newborns or the ovaries of girls at the start of puberty. Immature teratomas have cells that look very different from normal cells under a microscope. Immature teratomas may be cancer. They often have several different types of tissue in them, such as hair, muscle, and bone. Some immature teratomas release enzymes or hormones that cause signs and symptoms of disease.

Malignant Germ Cell Tumors

Malignant germ cell tumors are cancer. There are two main types of malignant germ cell tumors:

- Germinomas: Tumors that make a hormone called beta-human chorionic gonadotropin (β-hCG). There are three types of germinomas.
  - Dysgerminomas form in the ovary in girls.
  - Seminomas form in the testicle in boys.
  - Germinomas form in areas of the body that are not the ovary or testicle.
- Nongerminomas: There are four types of nongerminomas.
  - Yolk sac tumors make a hormone called alpha-fetoprotein (AFP). They can form in the ovary, testicle, or other areas of the body.

557

- Choriocarcinomas make a hormone called beta-human chorionic gonadotropin (β-hCG). They can form in the ovary, testicle, or other areas of the body.

- Embryonal carcinomas may make a hormone called β-hCG and/or a hormone called AFP. They can form in the testicle or other parts of the body, but not in the ovary.

- Mixed germ cell tumors are made up of both malignant germ cell tumor and teratoma. They can form in the ovary, testicle, or other areas of the body.

Childhood extracranial germ cell tumors are grouped as gonadal or extragonadal.

Malignant extracranial germ cell tumors are gonadal or extragonadal.

Gonadal Germ Cell Tumors

Gonadal germ cell tumors form in the testicles in boys or ovaries in girls.

Testicular Germ Cell Tumors

Testicular germ cell tumors are divided into two main types, seminoma and nonseminoma.

- Seminomas make a hormone called beta-human chorionic gonadotropin (β-hCG).

- Nonseminomas are usually large and cause signs or symptoms. They tend to grow and spread more quickly than seminomas.

Testicular germ cell tumors usually occur before the age of 4 years or in teenagers and young adults. Testicular germ cell tumors in teenagers and young adults are different from those that form in early childhood.

Boys older than 14 years with testicular germ cell tumors are treated in pediatric cancer centers, but the treatment is much like the treatment used in adults.

Ovarian germ cell tumors

Ovarian germ cell tumors are more common in teenage girls and young women. Most ovarian germ cell tumors are benign teratomas.

Sometimes immature teratomas, dysgerminomas, yolk sac tumors, and mixed germ cell tumors (cancer) occur.

Extragonadal Extracranial Germ Cell Tumors

Extragonadal extracranial germ cell tumors form in areas other than the brain, testicles, or ovaries.

Most extragonadal extracranial germ cell tumors form along the midline of the body. This includes the following:

- Sacrum (the large, triangle-shaped bone in the lower spine that forms part of the pelvis).

- Coccyx (the small bone at the bottom of the spine, also called the tailbone).

- Mediastinum (the area between the lungs).

- Back of the abdomen.

- Neck.

In younger children, extragonadal extracranial germ cell tumors usually occur at birth or in early childhood. Most of these tumors are teratomas in the sacrum or coccyx.

In older children, teenagers, and young adults, extragonadal extracranial germ cell tumors are often in the mediastinum.

The cause of most childhood extracranial germ cell tumors is unknown.

Having certain inherited disorders can increase the risk of an extracranial germ cell tumor.

Anything that increases your risk of getting a disease is called a risk factor. Having a risk factor does not mean that you will get cancer; not having risk factors doesn't mean that you will not get cancer. Talk with your child's doctor if you think your child may be at risk.

Possible risk factors for extracranial germ cell tumors include the following:

- Having certain genetic syndromes:

- Klinefelter syndrome may increase the risk of germ cell tumors in the mediastinum.

- Swyer syndrome may increase the risk of germ cell tumors in the testicles or ovaries.

- Turner syndrome may increase the risk of germ cell tumors in the ovaries.

- Having an undescended testicle may increase the risk of developing a testicular germ cell tumors.

Signs of childhood extracranial germ cell tumors depend on the type of tumor and where it is in the body.

Different tumors may cause the following signs and symptoms. Other conditions may cause these same signs and symptoms. Check with a doctor if your child has any of the following:

- A lump in the abdomen or lower back.

- A painless lump in the testicle.

- Pain in the abdomen.

- Fever.

- Constipation.

- In females, no menstrual periods.

- In females, unusual vaginal bleeding.

Imaging studies and blood tests are used to detect (find) and diagnose childhood extracranial germ cell tumors.

The following tests and procedures may be used:

- **Physical exam and history:** An exam of the body to check general signs of health, including checking for signs of disease, such as lumps or anything else that seems unusual. The testicles may be checked for lumps, swelling, or pain. A history of the patient's health habits and past illnesses and treatments will also be taken.

- **Serum tumor marker test:** A procedure in which a sample of blood is checked to measure the amounts of certain substances released into the blood by organs, tissues, or tumor cells in the body. Certain substances are linked to specific types of cancer when found in increased levels in the blood. These are called tumor markers.

Most malignant germ cell tumors release tumor markers. The following tumor markers are used to detect extracranial germ cell tumors:

- Alpha-fetoprotein (AFP).

- Beta-human chorionic gonadotropin (β-hCG).

For testicular germ cell tumors, blood levels of the tumor markers help show if the tumor is a seminoma or nonseminoma.

- **Blood chemistry studies:** A procedure in which a blood sample is checked to measure the amounts of certain substances released into the blood by organs and tissues in the body. An unusual (higher or lower than normal) amount of a substance can be a sign of disease in the organ or tissue that makes it.

- **Chest x-ray:** An x-ray of the organs and bones inside the chest. An x-ray is a type of energy beam that can go through the body and onto film, making a picture of areas inside the body.

- **CT scan (CAT scan):** A procedure that makes a series of detailed pictures of areas inside the body, taken from different angles. The pictures are made by a computer linked to an x-ray machine. A dye may be injected into a vein or swallowed to help the organs or tissues show up more clearly. This procedure is also called computed tomography, computerized tomography, or computerized axial tomography.

- **MRI (magnetic resonance imaging):** A procedure that uses a magnet, radio waves, and a computer to make a series of detailed pictures of areas inside the body. This procedure is also called nuclear magnetic resonance imaging (NMRI).

- **Ultrasound exam:** A procedure in which high-energy sound waves (ultrasound) are bounced off internal tissues or organs and make echoes. The echoes form a picture of body tissues called a sonogram. The picture can be printed to be looked at later.

- **Biopsy:** The removal of cells or tissues so they can be viewed under a microscope by a pathologist to check for signs of cancer. In some cases, the tumor is removed during surgery and then a biopsy is done.

The following tests may be done on the sample of tissue that is removed:

- **Cytogenetic analysis:** A laboratory test in which cells in a sample of tissue are viewed under a microscope to look for certain changes in the chromosomes.

- **Immunohistochemistry:** A test that uses antibodies to check for certain antigens in a sample of tissue. The antibody is usually linked to a radioactive substance or a dye that causes the tissue to light up under a microscope. This type of test may be used to tell the difference between different types of cancer.

Certain factors affect prognosis (chance of recovery) and treatment options.

The prognosis (chance of recovery) and treatment options depend on the following:

- The type of germ cell tumor.

- Where the tumor first began to grow.

- The stage of the cancer (whether it has spread to nearby areas or to other places in the body).

- Whether the tumor can be completely removed by surgery.

- The patient's age and general health.

- Whether the cancer has just been diagnosed or has recurred (come back).

The prognosis for childhood extracranial germ cell tumors, especially ovarian germ cell tumors, is good.

Stages of Childhood Extracranial Germ Cell Tumors

After a childhood extracranial germ cell tumor has been diagnosed, tests are done to find out if cancer cells have spread from where the tumor started to nearby areas or to other parts of the body.

The process used to find out if cancer has spread from where the tumor started to other parts of the body is called staging. The information gathered from the staging process determines the stage of the disease. It is important to know the stage in order to plan treatment. In some cases, staging may follow surgery to remove the tumor.

The following procedures may be used:

- **MRI (magnetic resonance imaging):** A procedure that uses a magnet, radio waves, and a computer to make a series of detailed pictures of areas inside the body, such as the lymph nodes. This procedure is also called nuclear magnetic resonance imaging.

- **CT scan (CAT scan):** A procedure that makes a series of detailed pictures of areas inside the body, such as the chest or lymph nodes, taken from different angles. The pictures are made by a computer linked to an x-ray machine. A dye may be injected into a vein or swallowed to help the organs or tissues show up more clearly. This procedure is also called computed tomography, computerized tomography, or computerized axial tomography.

- **Bone scan:** A procedure to check if there are rapidly dividing cells, such as cancer cells, in the bone. A very small amount of radioactive material is injected into a vein and travels through the bloodstream. The radioactive material collects in the bones with cancer and is detected by a scanner.

- **Thoracentesis:** The removal of fluid from the space between the lining of the chest and the lung, using a needle. A pathologist views the fluid under a microscope to look for cancer cells.

- **Paracentesis:** The removal of fluid from the space between the lining of the abdomen and the organs in the abdomen, using a needle. A pathologist views the fluid under a microscope to look for cancer cells.

The results from tests and procedures used to detect and diagnose childhood extracranial germ cell tumors may also be used in staging.

There are three ways that cancer spreads in the body.

Cancer can spread through tissue, the lymph system, and the blood:

- Tissue. The cancer spreads from where it began by growing into nearby areas.

- Lymph system. The cancer spreads from where it began by getting into the lymph system. The cancer travels through the lymph vessels to other parts of the body.

- Blood. The cancer spreads from where it began by getting into the blood. The cancer travels through the blood vessels to other parts of the body.

563

Cancer may spread from where it began to other parts of the body.

When cancer spreads to another part of the body, it is called metastasis. Cancer cells break away from where they began (the primary tumor) and travel through the lymph system or blood.

- Lymph system. The cancer gets into the lymph system, travels through the lymph vessels, and forms a tumor (metastatic tumor) in another part of the body.

- Blood. The cancer gets into the blood, travels through the blood vessels, and forms a tumor (metastatic tumor) in another part of the body.

The metastatic tumor is the same type of cancer as the primary tumor. For example, if an extracranial germ cell tumor spreads to the liver, the cancer cells in the liver are actually cancerous germ cells. The disease is metastatic extracranial germ cell tumor, not liver cancer.

The following stages are commonly used for childhood nonseminoma testicular germ cell tumors:

Stage I

In stage I, the cancer is found in the testicle only and is completely removed by surgery.

Stage II

In stage II, the cancer is removed by surgery and some cancer cells remain in the scrotum or cancer that can be seen with a microscope only has spread to the scrotum or spermatic cord. Tumor marker levels do not return to normal after surgery or the tumor marker levels increase.

Stage III

In stage III, the cancer has spread to one or more lymph nodes in the abdomen and is not completely removed by surgery. The cancer that remains after surgery can be seen without a microscope.

Stage IV

In stage IV, the cancer has spread to distant parts of the body such as the liver, brain, bone, or lung.

The following stages may be used for childhood ovarian germ cell tumors:

Stage I

In stage I, the cancer is in the ovary and can be completely removed by surgery and the capsule (outer covering) of the ovary has not ruptured (broken open).

Stage II

In stage II, one of the following is true:

- The cancer is not completely removed by surgery. The remaining cancer can be seen with a microscope only.
- The cancer has spread to the lymph nodes and can be seen with a microscope only.
- The cancer has spread to the capsule (outer covering) of the ovary.

Stage III

In stage III, one of the following is true:

- The cancer is not completely removed by surgery. The remaining cancer can be seen without a microscope.
- The cancer has spread to lymph nodes and the lymph nodes are 2 centimeters or larger. Cancer in the lymph nodes can be seen without a microscope.
- The cancer is found in fluid in the abdomen.

Stage IV

In stage IV, the cancer has spread to the lung, liver, brain, or bone.

Another staging system which may be used for childhood ovarian germ cell tumors is as follows:

Stage I

In stage I, cancer is found in one or both of the ovaries and has not spread. Stage I is divided into stage IA, stage IB, and stage IC.

- Stage IA: Cancer is found in one ovary.

- Stage IB: Cancer is found in both ovaries.

- Stage IC: Cancer is found in one or both ovaries and one of the following is true:

  - cancer is found on the outside surface of one or both ovaries; or

  - the capsule (outer covering) of the tumor has ruptured (broken open); or

  - cancer cells are found in fluid that has collected in the abdomen; or

  - cancer cells are found in washings of the peritoneal cavity (the body cavity that contains most of the organs in the abdomen).

Stage II

In stage II, cancer is found in one or both ovaries and has spread into other areas of the pelvis. Stage II is divided into stage IIA, stage IIB, and stage IIC.

- Stage IIA: Cancer has spread to the uterus and/or the fallopian tubes (the long slender tubes through which eggs pass from the ovaries to the uterus).

- Stage IIB: Cancer has spread to other tissue within the pelvis such as the bladder, rectum, or vagina.

- Stage IIC: Cancer has spread to the uterus and/or fallopian tubes and/or other tissue within the pelvis and one of the following is true:

  - cancer is found on the outside surface of one or both ovaries; or

  - the capsule (outer covering) of the tumor has ruptured (broken open); or

  - cancer cells are found in fluid that has collected in the abdomen; or

  - cancer cells are found in washings of the peritoneal cavity (the body cavity that contains most of the organs in the abdomen).

Stage III

In stage III, cancer is found in one or both ovaries and has spread to other parts of the abdomen. Stage III is divided into stage IIIA, stage IIIB, and stage IIIC:

- Stage IIIA: The tumor is found only in the pelvis only, but cancer cells that can only be seen with a microscope have spread to the surface of the peritoneum (tissue that lines the abdominal wall and covers most of the organs in the abdomen) or to the small bowel.

- Stage IIIB: Cancer has spread to the peritoneum and is 2 centimeters or smaller in diameter.

- Stage IIIC: Cancer has spread to the peritoneum and is larger than 2 centimeters in diameter and/or has spread to lymph nodes in the abdomen.

Cancer that has spread to the surface of the liver is also stage III disease.

Stage IV

In stage IV, cancer is found in one or both ovaries and has metastasized (spread) beyond the abdomen to other parts of the body.

Cancer that has spread to tissues in the liver is also stage IV disease.

The following stages are commonly used for extragonadal extracranial germ cell tumors:

Stage I

In stage I, the cancer is in one place and can be completely removed by surgery. For tumors in the sacrum or coccyx (bottom part of the spine), the sacrum and coccyx are completely removed by surgery. Tumor marker levels return to normal after surgery.

Stage II

In stage II, the cancer has spread to the capsule (outer covering) and/or lymph nodes. The cancer is not completely removed by surgery and the cancer remaining after surgery can be seen with a microscope only. Tumor marker levels do not return to normal after surgery or increase.

Stage III

In stage III, one of the following is true:

- The cancer is not completely removed by surgery. The cancer remaining after surgery can be seen without a microscope.

- The cancer has spread to lymph nodes and is larger than 2 centimeters in diameter.

Stage IV

In stage IV, the cancer has spread to distant parts of the body, including the liver, brain, bone, or lung.

Treatment Options for Childhood Extracranial Germ Cell Tumors

Mature and Immature Teratomas

Treatment of mature teratomas that are not in the sacrum or coccyx (bottom part of the spine) includes the following:

- Surgery to remove the tumor followed by observation.

Treatment of immature teratomas that are not in the sacrum or coccyx includes the following:

- Surgery to remove the tumor followed by observation for stage I tumors.

- Surgery to remove the tumor and combination chemotherapy for stage II–IV tumors. It is not known if chemotherapy will help the patient live longer.

Treatment of immature teratomas that are in the sacrum or coccyx includes the following:

- Surgery (removal of the sacrum and coccyx) followed by observation.

Sometimes a mature or immature teratoma also has malignant cells. The teratoma and malignant cells may need to be treated differently.

Regular follow-up exams with imaging tests and the alpha-fetoprotein (AFP) tumor marker test will be done for at least 3 years.

Malignant Gonadal Germ Cell Tumors

Malignant Testicular Germ Cell Tumors

Treatment of malignant testicular germ cell tumors may include the following:

For boys younger than 15 years:

- Surgery (radical inguinal orchiectomy) followed by observation for stage I tumors.
- Surgery (radical inguinal orchiectomy) followed by combination chemotherapy for stage II-IV tumors. A second surgery may be done to remove any tumor remaining after chemotherapy.

For boys 15 years and older:

Malignant testicular germ cell tumors in boys 15 years and older are treated differently than they are in young boys. Surgery may include removal of lymph nodes in the abdomen.

Malignant Ovarian Germ Cell Tumors

Dysgerminomas

Treatment of stage I dysgerminomas in young girls may include the following:

- Surgery (unilateral salpingo-oophorectomy) followed by observation. Combination chemotherapymay be given if the tumor comes back.
- Treatment of stages II–IV dysgerminomas in young girls may include the following:
- Surgery (unilateral salpingo-oophorectomy) followed by combination chemotherapy.
- Combination chemotherapy to shrink the tumor, followed by surgery (unilateral salpingo-oophorectomy).

Nongerminomas

Treatment of stage I nongerminomas in young girls may include the following:

- Surgery followed by observation.

- Surgery followed by combination chemotherapy.

Treatment of stages II–IV nongerminomas in young girls may include the following:

- Surgery followed by combination chemotherapy. A second surgery may be done to remove any remaining cancer.

- Biopsy followed by combination chemotherapy to shrink the tumor and sometimes surgery for tumors that cannot be removed by surgery when cancer is diagnosed.

The treatment for adolescents and young adults with ovarian germ cell tumor is much like the treatment for adults.

Malignant Extragonadal Extracranial Germ Cell Tumors

Treatment of childhood malignant extragonadal extracranial germ cell tumors may include the following:

- Combination chemotherapy to shrink the tumor followed by surgery to remove the sacrum and coccyx (bottom part of the spine) for tumors that are in the sacrum or coccyx.

- Combination chemotherapy to shrink the tumor followed by surgery to remove tumors that are in the mediastinum.

- Biopsy followed by combination chemotherapy to shrink the tumor and surgery to remove tumors that are in the abdomen.

- Surgery to remove the tumor followed by combination chemotherapy for tumors of the head and neck.

Treatment of malignant extragonadal extracranial germ cell tumors in places not already described includes the following:

- Surgery followed by combination chemotherapy.

Recurrent Childhood Malignant Extracranial Germ Cell Tumors

- There is no standard treatment for recurrent childhood malignant extracranial germ cell tumors. Treatment depends on the following:

  - The type of treatment given when the cancer was diagnosed.

  - How the tumor responded to the initial treatment.

Treatment is usually within a clinical trial and may include the following:

- Surgery followed by combination chemotherapy, for most malignant extracranial germ cell tumors including immature teratomas, malignant testicular germ cell tumors, and malignant ovarian germ cell tumors.

- Surgery for tumors that come back in the sacrum or coccyx (bottom part of the spine), if surgery to remove the sacrum and coccyx was not done when the cancer was diagnosed. Chemotherapy may be given before surgery, to shrink the tumor. If any tumor remains after surgery, radiation therapy may also be given.

- Combination chemotherapy for stage I malignant testicular germ cell tumors and stage I ovarian dysgerminomas.

- High-dose chemotherapy and stem cell transplant.

- Radiation therapy followed by surgery to remove the tumor in the brain for cancer that has spread to the brain.

Section 26.2

Extragonadal Germ Cell Tumor

Text in this section is excerpted from "Extragonadal Germ Cell Tumors Treatment," National Cancer Institute at the National Institutes of Health (NIH), April 2, 2015.

General Information About Extragonadal Germ Cell Tumors

Extragonadal germ cell tumors form from developing sperm or egg cells that travel from the gonads to other parts of the body.

" Extragonadal" means outside of the gonads (sex organs). When cells that are meant to form sperm in the testicles or eggs in the ovaries travel to other parts of the body, they may grow into extragonadal germ cell tumors. These tumors may begin to grow anywhere in the body but usually begin in organs such as the pineal gland in the brain, in the mediastinum, or in the abdomen.

Extragonadal germ cell tumors can be benign (non-cancer) or malignant (cancer). Benign extragonadal germ cell tumors are called benign teratomas. These are more common than malignant extragonadal germ cell tumors and often are very large.

Malignant extragonadal germ cell tumors are divided into two types, nonseminoma and seminoma. Nonseminomas tend to grow and spread more quickly than seminomas. They usually are large and cause signs and symptoms. If untreated, malignant extragonadal germ cell tumors may spread to the lungs, lymph nodes, bones, liver, or other parts of the body.

Age and gender can affect the risk of extragonadal germ cell tumors.

Anything that increases your chance of getting a disease is called a risk factor. Having a risk factor does not mean that you will get cancer; not having risk factors doesn't mean that you will not get cancer. Talk with your doctor if you think you may be at risk. Risk factors for malignant extragonadal germ cell tumors include the following:

- Being male.

- Being age 20 or older.

- Having Klinefelter syndrome.

Signs and symptoms of extragonadal germ cell tumors include breathing problems and chest pain.

Malignant extragonadal germ cell tumors may cause signs and symptoms as they grow into nearby areas. Other conditions may cause the same signs and symptoms. Check with your doctor if you have any of the following:

- Chest pain.

- Breathing problems.

- Cough.

- Fever.

- Headache.

- Change in bowel habits.

- Feeling very tired.

- Trouble walking.

- Trouble in seeing or moving the eyes.

Imaging and blood tests are used to detect (find) and diagnose extragonadal germ cell tumors.

The following tests and procedures may be used:

- **Physical exam and history:** An exam of the body to check general signs of health, including checking for signs of disease, such as lumps or anything else that seems unusual. The testicles may be checked for lumps, swelling, or pain. A history of the patient's health habits and past illnesses and treatments will also be taken.

- **Chest x-ray:** An x-ray of the organs and bones inside the chest. An x-ray is a type of energy beam that can go through the body and onto film, making a picture of areas inside the body.

- **Serum tumor marker test:** A procedure in which a sample of blood is examined to measure the amounts of certain substances released into the blood by organs, tissues, or tumor cells in the body. Certain substances are linked to specific types of cancer when found in increased levels in the blood. These are called tumor markers. The following three tumor markers are used to detect extragonadal germ cell tumor:

  - Alpha-fetoprotein (AFP).

  - Beta-human chorionic gonadotropin (β-hCG).

  - Lactate dehydrogenase (LDH).

Blood levels of the tumor markers help determine if the tumor is a seminoma or nonseminoma.

- **CT scan (CAT scan):** A procedure that makes a series of detailed pictures of areas inside the body, taken from different angles. The pictures are made by a computer linked to an x-ray machine. A dye may be injected into a vein or swallowed to help the organs or tissues show up more clearly. This procedure is also called computed tomography, computerized tomography, or computerized axial tomography.

  Sometimes a CT scan and a PET scan are done at the same time. A PET scan is a procedure to find malignant tumor cells in the

573

body. A small amount of radioactive glucose (sugar) is injected into a vein. The PET scanner rotates around the body and makes a picture of where glucose is being used in the body. Malignant tumor cells show up brighter in the picture because they are more active and take up more glucose than normal cells do. When a PET scan and CT scan are done at the same time, it is called a PET-CT.

- **Biopsy:** The removal of cells or tissues so they can be viewed under a microscope by a pathologist to check for signs of cancer. The type of biopsy used depends on where the extragonadal germ cell tumor is found.

  - **Excisional biopsy:** The removal of an entire lump of tissue.

  - **Incisional biopsy:** The removal of part of a lump or sample of tissue.

  - **Core biopsy:** The removal of tissue using a wide needle.

  - **Fine-needle aspiration (FNA) biopsy:** The removal of tissue or fluid using a thin needle.

Certain factors affect prognosis (chance of recovery) and treatment options.

The prognosis (chance of recovery) and treatment options depend on the following:

- Whether the tumor is nonseminoma or seminoma.
- The size of the tumor and where it is in the body.
- The blood levels of AFP, β-hCG, and LDH.
- Whether the tumor has spread to other parts of the body.
- The way the tumor responds to initial treatment.
- Whether the tumor has just been diagnosed or has recurred (come back).

Stages of Extragonadal Germ Cell Tumors

After an extragonadal germ cell tumor has been diagnosed, tests are done to find out if cancer cells have spread to other parts of the body.

The extent or spread of cancer is usually described as stages. For extragonadal germ cell tumors, prognostic groups are used instead of stages. The tumors are grouped according to how well the cancer is expected to respond to treatment. It is important to know the prognostic group in order to plan treatment.

There are three ways that cancer spreads in the body.

Cancer can spread through tissue, the lymph system, and the blood:

- Tissue. The cancer spreads from where it began by growing into nearby areas.
- Lymph system. The cancer spreads from where it began by getting into the lymph system. The cancer travels through the lymph vessels to other parts of the body.
- Blood. The cancer spreads from where it began by getting into the blood. The cancer travels through the blood vessels to other parts of the body.

Cancer may spread from where it began to other parts of the body.

When cancer spreads to another part of the body, it is called metastasis. Cancer cells break away from where they began (the primary tumor) and travel through the lymph system or blood.

- Lymph system. The cancer gets into the lymph system, travels through the lymph vessels, and forms a tumor (metastatic tumor) in another part of the body.
- Blood. The cancer gets into the blood, travels through the blood vessels, and forms a tumor (metastatic tumor) in another part of the body.

The metastatic tumor is the same type of tumor as the primary tumor. For example, if an extragonadal germ cell tumor spreads to the lung, the tumor cells in the lung are actually cancerous germ cells. The disease is metastatic extragonadal germ cell tumor, not lung cancer.

The following prognostic groups are used for extragonadal germ cell tumors:

Good prognosis

A nonseminoma extragonadal germ cell tumor is in the good prognosis group if:

- the tumor is in the back of the abdomen; and

- the tumor has not spread to organs other than the lungs; and

- the levels of tumor markers AFP and β-hCG are normal and LDH is slightly above normal.

A seminoma extragonadal germ cell tumor is in the good prognosis group if:

- the tumor has not spread to organs other than the lungs; and

- the level of AFP is normal; β-hCG and LDH may be at any level.

Intermediate prognosis

A nonseminoma extragonadal germ cell tumor is in the intermediate prognosis group if:

- the tumor is in the back of the abdomen; and

- the tumor has not spread to organs other than the lungs; and

- the level of any one of the tumor markers (AFP, β-hCG, or LDH) is more than slightly above normal.

A seminoma extragonadal germ cell tumor is in the intermediate prognosis group if:

- the tumor has spread to organs other than the lungs; and

- the level of AFP is normal; β-hCG and LDH may be at any level.

Poor prognosis

A nonseminoma extragonadal germ cell tumor is in the poor prognosis group if:

- the tumor is in the chest; or

- the tumor has spread to organs other than the lungs; or

- the level of any one of the tumor markers (AFP, β-hCG, or LDH) is high.

Seminoma extragonadal germ cell tumor does not have a poor prognosis group.

Treatment Options Overview

There are different types of treatment for patients with extragonadal germ cell tumors.

Different types of treatments are available for patients with extragonadal germ cell tumors. Some treatments are standard (the currently used treatment), and some are being tested in clinical trials. A treatment clinical trial is a research study meant to help improve current treatments or obtain information on new treatments for patients with cancer. When clinical trials show that a new treatment is better than the standard treatment, the new treatment may become the standard treatment. Patients may want to think about taking part in a clinical trial. Some clinical trials are open only to patients who have not started treatment.

Three types of standard treatment are used:

Radiation therapy

Radiation therapy is a cancer treatment that uses high-energy x-rays or other types of radiation to kill cancer cells or keep them from growing. There are two types of radiation therapy. External radiation therapy uses a machine outside the body to send radiation toward the cancer. Internal radiation therapy uses a radioactive substance sealed in needles, seeds, wires, or catheters that are placed directly into or near the cancer. The way the radiation therapy is given depends on the type and stage of the cancer being treated.

Chemotherapy

Chemotherapy is a cancer treatment that uses drugs to stop the growth of cancer cells, either by killing the cells or by stopping them from dividing. When chemotherapy is taken by mouth or injected into a vein or muscle, the drugs enter the bloodstream and can reach cancer cells throughout the body (systemic chemotherapy). When chemotherapy is placed directly in the cerebrospinal fluid, an organ, or a body cavity such as the abdomen, the drugs mainly affect cancer cells in those areas (regional chemotherapy). The way the chemotherapy is given depends on the type and stage of the cancer being treated.

577

Surgery

Patients who have benign tumors or tumor remaining after chemo-therapy or radiation therapy may need to have surgery.

New types of treatment are being tested in clinical trials.

High-dose chemotherapy with stem cell transplant

High-dose chemotherapy with stem cell transplant is a method of giving high doses of chemotherapy and replacing blood -forming cells destroyed by the cancer treatment. Stem cells (immature blood cells) are removed from the blood or bone marrow of the patient or a donor and are frozen and stored. After the chemotherapy is completed, the stored stem cells are thawed and given back to the patient through an infusion. These re-infused stem cells grow into (and restore) the body's blood cells.

Patients may want to think about taking part in a clinical trial.

For some patients, taking part in a clinical trial may be the best treatment choice. Clinical trials are part of the cancer research process. Clinical trials are done to find out if new cancer treatments are safe and effective or better than the standard treatment.

Many of today's standard treatments for cancer are based on earlier clinical trials. Patients who take part in a clinical trial may receive the standard treatment or be among the first to receive a new treatment.

Patients who take part in clinical trials also help improve the way cancer will be treated in the future. Even when clinical trials do not lead to effective new treatments, they often answer important questions and help move research forward.

Patients can enter clinical trials before, during, or after starting their cancer treatment.

Some clinical trials only include patients who have not yet received treatment. Other trials test treatments for patients whose cancer has not gotten better. There are also clinical trials that test new ways to stop cancer from recurring (coming back) or reduce the side effects of cancer treatment.

Clinical trials are taking place in many parts of the country.

Follow-up tests may be needed.

Some of the tests that were done to diagnose the cancer or to find out the stage of the cancer may be repeated. Some tests will be repeated in order to see how well the treatment is working. Decisions about whether to continue, change, or stop treatment may be based on the results of these tests. This is sometimes called re-staging.

Some of the tests will continue to be done from time to time after treatment has ended. The results of these tests can show if your condition has changed or if the cancer has recurred (come back). These tests are sometimes called follow-up tests or check-ups.

After initial treatment for extragonadal germ cell tumors, blood levels of AFP and other tumor markers continue to be checked to find out how well the treatment is working.

Section 26.3

Ovarian Germ Cell Tumor

Text in this section is excerpted from "Ovarian Germ Cell Tumors Treatment," National Cancer Institute at the National Institutes of Health (NIH), May 29, 2015.

General Information About Ovarian Germ Cell Tumors

Ovarian germ cell tumor is a disease in which malignant (cancer) cells form in the germ (egg) cells of the ovary.

Germ cell tumors begin in the reproductive cells (egg or sperm) of the body. Ovarian germ cell tumors usually occur in teenage girls or young women and most often affect just one ovary.

The ovaries are a pair of organs in the female reproductive system. They are in the pelvis, one on each side of the uterus (the hollow, pear-shaped organ where a fetus grows). Each ovary is about the size and shape of an almond. The ovaries make eggs and female hormones

Ovarian germ cell tumor is a general name that is used to describe several different types of cancer. The most common ovarian germ cell tumor is called dysgerminoma.

Signs of ovarian germ cell tumor are swelling of the abdomen or vaginal bleeding after menopause.

Ovarian germ cell tumors can be hard to diagnose (find) early. Often there are no symptoms in the early stages, but tumors may be found during regular gynecologic exams (checkups). Check with your doctor if you have either of the following:

- Swollen abdomen without weight gain in other parts of the body.

- Bleeding from the vagina after menopause (when you are no longer having menstrual periods).

Tests that examine the ovaries, pelvic area, blood, and ovarian tissue are used to detect (find) and diagnose ovarian germ cell tumor.

The following tests and procedures may be used:

- **Physical exam and history:** An exam of the body to check general signs of health, including checking for signs of disease, such as lumps or anything else that seems unusual. A history of the patient's health habits and past illnesses and treatments will also be taken.

- **Pelvic exam:** An exam of the vagina, cervix, uterus, fallopian tubes, ovaries, and rectum. The doctor or nurse inserts one or two lubricated, gloved fingers of one hand into the vagina and the other hand is placed over the lower abdomen to feel the size, shape, and position of the uterus and ovaries. A speculum is also inserted into the vagina and the doctor or nurse looks at the vagina and cervix for signs of disease. A Pap test or Pap smear of the cervix is usually done. The doctor or nurse also inserts a lubricated, gloved finger into the rectum to feel for lumps or abnormal areas.

- **Laparotomy:** A surgical procedure in which an incision (cut) is made in the wall of the abdomen to check the inside of the abdomen for signs of disease. The size of the incision depends on the reason the laparotomy is being done. Sometimes organs are removed or tissue samples are taken and checked under a microscope for signs of disease.

- **CT scan (CAT scan):** A procedure that makes a series of detailed pictures of areas inside the body, taken from different angles. The pictures are made by a computer linked to an x-ray

machine. A dye may be injected into a vein or swallowed to help the organs or tissues show up more clearly. This procedure is also called computed tomography, computerized tomography, or computerized axial tomography.

- **Serum tumor marker test:** A procedure in which a sample of blood is checked to measure the amounts of certain substances released into the blood by organs, tissues, or tumor cells in the body. Certain substances are linked to specific types of cancer when found in increased levels in the blood. These are called tumor markers. An increased level of alpha fetoprotein (AFP) or human chorionic gonadotropin (HCG) in the blood may be a sign of ovarian germ cell tumor.

Certain factors affect prognosis (chance of recovery and treatment options).

The prognosis (chance of recovery) and treatment options depend on the following:

- The type of cancer.
- The size of the tumor.
- The stage of cancer (whether it affects part of the ovary, involves the whole ovary, or has spread to other places in the body).
- The way the cancer cells look under a microscope.
- The patient's general health.

Ovarian germ cell tumors are usually cured if found and treated early.

Stages of Ovarian Germ Cell Tumors

After ovarian germ cell tumor has been diagnosed, tests are done to find out if cancer cells have spread within the ovary or to other parts of the body.

The process used to find out whether cancer has spread within the ovary or to other parts of the body is called staging. The information gathered from the staging process determines the stage of the disease. Unless a doctor is sure the cancer has spread from the ovaries to other parts of the body, an operation called a laparotomy is done to see if the cancer has spread. The doctor must cut into the abdomen and carefully look at all the organs to see if they have cancer in them. The doctor will cut out small pieces of tissue so they can be checked under a microscope for signs of cancer. The doctor may also wash the abdominal cavity with fluid, which is also checked under a microscope to see if it has cancer cells in it. Usually the doctor will remove the cancer and other organs that have cancer in them during the laparotomy. It is important to know the stage in order to plan treatment.

Many of the tests used to diagnose ovarian germ cell tumor are also used for staging. The following tests and procedures may also be used for staging:

- **PET scan (positron emission tomography scan):** A procedure to find malignant tumor cells in the body. A small amount of radioactive glucose (sugar) is injected into a vein. The PET scanner rotates around the body and makes a picture of where glucose is being used in the body. Malignant tumor cells show up brighter in the picture because they are more active and take up more glucose than normal cells do.

- **MRI (magnetic resonance imaging):** A procedure that uses a magnet, radio waves, and a computer to make a series of detailed pictures of areas inside the body. This procedure is also called nuclear magnetic resonance imaging (NMRI).

- **Transvaginal ultrasound exam:** A procedure used to examine the vagina, uterus, fallopian tubes, and bladder. An ultrasound transducer (probe) is inserted into the vagina and used to bounce high-energy sound waves (ultrasound) off internal tissues or organs and make echoes. The echoes form a picture of body tissues called a sonogram. The doctor can identify tumors by looking at the sonogram.

There are three ways that cancer spreads in the body.

Cancer can spread through tissue, the lymph system, and the blood:

- Tissue. The cancer spreads from where it began by growing into nearby areas.

- Lymph system. The cancer spreads from where it began by getting into the lymph system. The cancer travels through the lymph vessels to other parts of the body.

- Blood. The cancer spreads from where it began by getting into the blood. The cancer travels through the blood vessels to other parts of the body.

Cancer may spread from where it began to other parts of the body.

When cancer spreads to another part of the body, it is called metastasis. Cancer cells break away from where they began (the primary tumor) and travel through the lymph system or blood.

- Lymph system. The cancer gets into the lymph system, travels through the lymph vessels, and forms a tumor (metastatic tumor) in another part of the body.
- Blood. The cancer gets into the blood, travels through the blood vessels, and forms a tumor (metastatic tumor) in another part of the body.

The metastatic tumor is the same type of tumor as the primary tumor. For example, if an ovarian germ cell tumor spreads to the liver, the tumor cells in the liver are actually cancerous ovarian germ cells. The disease is metastatic ovarian germ cell tumor, not liver cancer.

The following stages are used for ovarian germ cell tumors:

Stage I

In stage I, cancer is found in one or both ovaries. Stage I is divided into stage IA, stage IB, and stage IC.

- Stage IA: Cancer is found inside a single ovary.
- Stage IB: Cancer is found inside both ovaries.
- Stage IC: Cancer is found inside one or both ovaries and one of the following is true:
  - cancer is also found on the outside surface of one or both ovaries; or
  - the capsule (outer covering) of the ovary has ruptured (broken open); or
  - cancer cells are found in the fluid of the peritoneal cavity (the body cavity that contains most of the organs in the abdomen) or in washings of the peritoneum (tissue lining the peritoneal cavity).

Stage II

In stage II, cancer is found in one or both ovaries and has spread into other areas of the pelvis. Stage II is divided into stage IIA, stage IIB, and stage IIC.

- Stage IIA: Cancer has spread to the uterus and/or fallopian tubes (the long slender tubes through which eggs pass from the ovaries to the uterus).

- Stage IIB: Cancer has spread to other tissue within the pelvis.

- Stage IIC: Cancer is found inside one or both ovaries and has spread to the uterus and/or fallopian tubes, or to other tissue within the pelvis. Also, one of the following is true:

  - cancer is found on the outside surface of one or both ovaries; or

  - the capsule (outer covering) of the ovary has ruptured (broken open); or

  - cancer cells are found in the fluid of the peritoneal cavity (the body cavity that contains most of the organs in the abdomen) or in washings of the peritoneum (tissue lining the peritoneal cavity).

Stage III

In stage III, cancer is found in one or both ovaries and has spread outside the pelvis to other parts of the abdomen and/or nearby lymph nodes. Stage III is divided into stage IIIA, stage IIIB, and stage IIIC.

- Stage IIIA: The tumor is found in the pelvis only, but cancer cells that can be seen only with a microscope have spread to the surface of the peritoneum (tissue that lines the abdominal wall and covers most of the organs in the abdomen), the small intestines, or the tissue that connects the small intestines to the wall of the abdomen.

- Stage IIIB: Cancer has spread to the peritoneum and the cancer in the peritoneum is 2 centimeters or smaller.

- Stage IIIC: Cancer has spread to the peritoneum and the cancer in the peritoneum is larger than 2centimeters and/or cancer has spread to lymph nodes in the abdomen.

Cancer that has spread to the surface of the liver is also considered stage III ovarian cancer.

Stage IV

In stage IV, cancer has spread beyond the abdomen to other parts of the body, such as the lungs or tissue inside the liver.

Cancer cells in the fluid around the lungs is also considered stage IV ovarian cancer.

Treatment Option Overview

There are different types of treatment for patients with ovarian germ cell tumors.

Different types of treatment are available for patients with ovarian germ cell tumor. Some treatments are standard (the currently used treatment), and some are being tested in clinical trials. A treatment clinical trial is a research study meant to help improve current treatments or obtain information on new treatments for patients with cancer. When clinical trials show that a new treatment is better than the standard treatment, the new treatment may become the standard treatment. Patients may want to think about taking part in a clinical trial. Some clinical trials are open only to patients who have not started treatment.

Four types of standard treatment are used:

Surgery

Surgery is the most common treatment of ovarian germ cell tumor. A doctor may take out the cancer using one of the following types of surgery.

- Unilateral salpingo-oophorectomy: A surgical procedure to remove one ovary and one fallopian tube.

- Total hysterectomy: A surgical procedure to remove the uterus, including the cervix. If the uterus and cervix are taken out through the vagina, the operation is called a vaginal hysterectomy. If the uterus and cervix are taken out through a large incision (cut) in the abdomen, the operation is called a total abdominal hysterectomy. If the uterus and cervix are taken out through a small incision (cut) in the abdomen using a laparoscope, the operation is called a total laparoscopic hysterectomy.

- Bilateral salpingo-oophorectomy: A surgical procedure to remove both ovaries and both fallopian tubes.

- Tumor debulking: A surgical procedure in which as much of the tumor as possible is removed. Some tumors may not be able to be completely removed.

Even if the doctor removes all the cancer that can be seen at the time of the operation, some patients may be offered chemotherapy or radiation therapy after surgery to kill any cancer cells that are left. Treatment given after the surgery, to lower the risk that the cancer will come back, is called adjuvant therapy.

After chemotherapy for an ovarian germ cell tumor, a second-look laparotomy may be done. This is similar to the laparotomy that is done to find out the stage of the cancer. Second-look laparotomy is a surgical procedure to find out if tumor cells are left after primary treatment. During this procedure, the doctor will take samples of lymph nodes and other tissues in the abdomen to see if any cancer is left. This procedure is not done for dysgerminomas.

Observation

Observation is closely watching a patient's condition without giving any treatment unless signs or symptoms appear or change.

Chemotherapy

Chemotherapy is a cancer treatment that uses drugs to stop the growth of cancer cells, either by killing the cells or by stopping them from dividing. When chemotherapy is taken by mouth or injected into a vein or muscle, the drugs enter the bloodstream and can reach cancer cells throughout the body (systemic chemotherapy). When chemotherapy is placed directly into the cerebrospinal fluid, an organ, or a body cavity such as the abdomen, the drugs mainly affect cancer cells in those areas (regional chemotherapy). The way the chemotherapy is given depends on the type and stage of the cancer being treated.

Radiation therapy

Radiation therapy is a cancer treatment that uses high-energy x-rays or other types of radiation to kill cancer cells. There are two types of radiation therapy. External radiation therapy uses a machine outside the body to send radiation toward the cancer. Internal radiation therapy uses a radioactive substance sealed in needles, seeds, wires, or catheters that are placed directly into or near the cancer. The way the radiation therapy is given depends on the type and stage of the cancer being treated.

New types of treatment are being tested in clinical trials.

High-dose chemotherapy with bone marrow transplant

High-dose chemotherapy with bone marrow transplant is a method of giving very high doses of chemotherapy and replacing blood -forming cells destroyed by the cancer treatment. Stem cells (immature blood cells) are removed from the bone marrow of the patient or a donor and are frozen and stored. After the chemotherapy is completed, the stored stem cells are thawed and given back to the patient through an infusion. These re-infused stem cells grow into (and restore) the body's blood cells.

New treatment options

Combination chemotherapy (the use of more than one anticancer drug) is being tested in clinical trials.

Patients may want to think about taking part in a clinical trial.

For some patients, taking part in a clinical trial may be the best treatment choice. Clinical trials are part of the cancer research process. Clinical trials are done to find out if new cancer treatments are safe and effective or better than the standard treatment.

Many of today's standard treatments for cancer are based on earlier clinical trials. Patients who take part in a clinical trial may receive the standard treatment or be among the first to receive a new treatment.

Patients who take part in clinical trials also help improve the way cancer will be treated in the future. Even when clinical trials do not lead to effective new treatments, they often answer important questions and help move research forward.

Patients can enter clinical trials before, during, or after starting their cancer treatment.

Some clinical trials only include patients who have not yet received treatment. Other trials test treatments for patients whose cancer has not gotten better. There are also clinical trials that test new ways to stop cancer from recurring (coming back) or reduce the side effects of cancer treatment.

Clinical trials are taking place in many parts of the country.

587

Follow-up tests may be needed.

Some of the tests that were done to diagnose the cancer or to find out the stage of the cancer may be repeated. Some tests will be repeated in order to see how well the treatment is working. Decisions about whether to continue, change, or stop treatment may be based on the results of these tests. This is sometimes called re-staging.

Some of the tests will continue to be done from time to time after treatment has ended. The results of these tests can show if your condition has changed or if the cancer has recurred (come back). These tests are sometimes called follow-up tests or check-ups.

Chapter 27

Musculo-Skeletal Cancer

Chapter Contents

Section 27.1

Bone Cancer

Text in this section is excerpted from "Bone Cancer," National Cancer
Institute at the National Institutes of Health (NIH).

What is bone cancer?

Bone cancer is a malignant (cancerous) tumor of the bone that
destroys normal bone tissue. Not all bone tumors are malignant. In
fact, benign (noncancerous) bone tumors are more common than malignant ones. Both malignant and benign bone tumors may grow and
compress healthy bone tissue, but benign tumors do not spread, do
not destroy bone tissue, and are rarely a threat to life.

Malignant tumors that begin in bone tissue are called primary bone
cancer. Cancer that metastasizes (spreads) to the bones from other parts
of the body, such as the breast, lung, or prostate, is called metastatic
cancer, and is named for the organ or tissue in which it began. Primary
bone cancer is far less common than cancer that spreads to the bones.

Are there different types of primary bone cancer?

Yes. Cancer can begin in any type of bone tissue. Bones are made up
of osteoid (hard or compact), cartilaginous (tough, flexible), and fibrous
(threadlike) tissue, as well as elements of bone marrow (soft, spongy
tissue in the center of most bones).

Common types of primary bone cancer include the following:

- Osteosarcoma, which arises from osteoid tissue in the bone. This
  tumor occurs most often in the knee and upper arm.

- Chondrosarcoma, which begins in cartilaginous tissue. Cartilage
  pads the ends of bones and lines the joints. Chondrosarcoma
  occurs most often in the pelvis (located between the hip bones),
  upper leg, and shoulder. Sometimes a chondrosarcoma contains
  cancerous bone cells. In that case, doctors classify the tumor as
  an osteosarcoma.

- The Ewing Sarcoma Family of Tumors (ESFTs), which usually occur in bone but may also arise in soft tissue (muscle, fat, fibrous tissue, blood vessels, or other supporting tissue). Scientists think that ESFTs arise from elements of primitive nerve tissue in the bone or soft tissue. ESFTs occur most commonly along the backbone and pelvis and in the legs and arms.

- Other types of cancer that arise in soft tissue are called soft tissue sarcomas. They are not bone cancer and are not described in this resource.

What are the possible causes of bone cancer?

Although bone cancer does not have a clearly defined cause, researchers have identified several factors that increase the likelihood of developing these tumors. Osteosarcoma occurs more frequently in people who have had high-dose external radiation therapy or treatment with certain anticancer drugs; children seem to be particularly susceptible. A small number of bone cancers are due to heredity. For example, children who have had hereditary retinoblastoma (an uncommon cancer of the eye) are at a higher risk of developing osteosarcoma, particularly if they are treated with radiation. Additionally, people who have hereditary defects of bones and people with metal implants, which doctors sometimes use to repair fractures, are more likely to develop osteosarcoma. Ewing sarcoma is not strongly associated with any heredity cancer syndromes, congenital childhood diseases, or previous radiation exposure.

How often does bone cancer occur?

Primary bone cancer is rare. It accounts for much less than 1 percent of all cancers. About 2,300 new cases of primary bone cancer are diagnosed in the United States each year. Different types of bone cancer are more likely to occur in certain populations:

- Osteosarcoma occurs most commonly between ages 10 and 19. However, people over age 40 who have other conditions, such as Paget disease (a benign condition characterized by abnormal development of new bone cells), are at increased risk of developing this cancer.

- Chondrosarcoma occurs mainly in older adults (over age 40). The risk increases with advancing age. This disease rarely occurs in children and adolescents.

591

- ESFTs occur most often in children and adolescents under 19 years of age. Boys are affected more often than girls. These tumors are extremely rare in African American children.

What are the symptoms of bone cancer?

Pain is the most common symptom of bone cancer, but not all bone cancers cause pain. Persistent or unusual pain or swelling in or near a bone can be caused by cancer or by other conditions. It is important to see a doctor to determine the cause.

How is bone cancer diagnosed?

To help diagnose bone cancer, the doctor asks about the patient's personal and family medical history. The doctor also performs a physical examination and may order laboratory and other diagnostic tests. These tests may include the following:

- **X-rays,** which can show the location, size, and shape of a bone tumor. If x-rays suggest that an abnormal area may be cancer, the doctor is likely to recommend special imaging tests. Even if x-rays suggest that an abnormal area is benign, the doctor may want to do further tests, especially if the patient is experiencing unusual or persistent pain.

  - A **bone scan**, which is a test in which a small amount of radioactive material is injected into a blood vessel and travels through the bloodstream; it then collects in the bones and is detected by a scanner.

  - A **computed tomography (CT or CAT) scan**, which is a series of detailed pictures of areas inside the body, taken from different angles, that are created by a computer linked to an x-ray machine.

  - A **magnetic resonance imaging (MRI) procedure**, which uses a powerful magnet linked to a computer to create detailed pictures of areas inside the body without using x-rays.

  - A **positron emission tomography (PET) scan**, in which a small amount of radioactive glucose (sugar) is injected into a vein, and a scanner is used to make detailed, computerized pictures of areas inside the body where the glucose is used. Because cancer cells often use more glucose than normal cells, the pictures can be used to find cancer cells in the body.

- An **angiogram**, which is an x-ray of blood vessels.

- **Biopsy** (removal of a tissue sample from the bone tumor) to determine whether cancer is present. The surgeon may perform a needle biopsy or an incisional biopsy. During a needle biopsy, the surgeon makes a small hole in the bone and removes a sample of tissue from the tumor with a needle-like instrument. In an incisional biopsy, the surgeon cuts into the tumor and removes a sample of tissue. Biopsies are best done by an orthopedic oncologist (a doctor experienced in the treatment of bone cancer). A pathologist (a doctor who identifies disease by studying cells and tissues under a microscope) examines the tissue to determine whether it is cancerous.

- **Blood tests** to determine the level of an enzyme called alkaline phosphatase. A large amount of this enzyme is present in the blood when the cells that form bone tissue are very active — when children are growing, when a broken bone is mending, or when a disease or tumor causes production of abnormal bone tissue. Because high levels of alkaline phosphatase are normal in growing children and adolescents, this test is not a completely reliable indicator of bone cancer.

What are the treatment options for bone cancer?

Treatment options depend on the type, size, location, and stage of the cancer, as well as the person's age and general health. Treatment options for bone cancer include surgery, chemotherapy, radiation therapy, and cryosurgery.

- **Surgery** is the usual treatment for bone cancer. The surgeon removes the entire tumor with negative margins (no cancer cells are found at the edge or border of the tissue removed during surgery). The surgeon may also use special surgical techniques to minimize the amount of healthy tissue removed with the tumor.

  Dramatic improvements in surgical techniques and preoperative tumor treatment have made it possible for most patients with bone cancer in an arm or leg to avoid radical surgical procedures (removal of the entire limb). However, most patients who undergo limb-sparing surgery need reconstructive surgery to maximize limb function.

- **Chemotherapy** is the use of anticancer drugs to kill cancer cells. Patients who have bone cancer usually receive a

593

combination of anticancer drugs. However, chemotherapy is not currently used to treat chondrosarcoma.

- **Radiation therapy**, also called radiotherapy, involves the use of high-energy x-rays to kill cancer cells. This treatment may be used in combination with surgery. It is often used to treat chondrosarcoma, which cannot be treated with chemotherapy, as well as ESFTs. It may also be used for patients who refuse surgery.

- **Cryosurgery** is the use of liquid nitrogen to freeze and kill cancer cells. This technique can sometimes be used instead of conventional surgery to destroy the tumor.

Is follow-up treatment necessary? What does it involve?

Yes. Bone cancer sometimes metastasizes, particularly to the lungs, or can recur (come back), either at the same location or in other bones in the body. People who have had bone cancer should see their doctor regularly and should report any unusual symptoms right away. Follow-up varies for different types and stages of bone cancer. Generally, patients are checked frequently by their doctor and have regular blood tests and x-rays. People who have had bone cancer, particularly children and adolescents, have an increased likelihood of developing another type of cancer, such as leukemia, later in life. Regular follow-up care ensures that changes in health are discussed and that problems are treated as soon as possible.

Are clinical trials (research studies) available for people with bone cancer?

Yes. Participation in clinical trials is an important treatment option for many people with bone cancer. To develop new treatments and better ways to use current treatments, NCI, a part of the National Institutes of Health, is sponsoring clinical trials in many hospitals and cancer centers around the country. Clinical trials are a critical step in the development of new methods of treatment. Before any new treatment can be recommended for general use, doctors conduct clinical trials to find out whether the treatment is safe for patients and effective against the disease.

Section 27.2

Ewing Sarcoma

Text in this section is excerpted from "Ewing Sarcoma Treatment,"
National Cancer Institute at the National Institutes of Health (NIH),
January 29, 2015.

General Information About Ewing Sarcoma

Ewing sarcoma is a type of tumor that forms in bone or soft tissue.

Ewing sarcoma is a type of tumor that forms from a certain kind of cell in bone or soft tissue. Other names for Ewing sarcoma are:

- Primitive neuroectodermal tumor.

- Askin tumor (Ewing sarcoma of the chest wall).

- Extraosseous Ewing sarcoma (tumor growing in tissue other than bone).

All of these names may be grouped together and called Ewing sarcoma family of tumors.

Ewing sarcoma may be found in the bones of the legs, arms, feet, hands, chest, pelvis, spine, or skull. Ewing sarcoma also may be found in the soft tissue of the trunk, arms, legs, head and neck, abdominal cavity, or other areas.

Ewing tumors often occur in teenagers and young adults.

Signs and symptoms of Ewing sarcoma include swelling and pain near the tumor.

These and other signs and symptoms may be caused by Ewing sarcoma or by other conditions. Check with your child's doctor if you see any of the following in your child:

- Pain and/or swelling, usually in the arms, legs, chest, back, or pelvis (area between the hips).

- A lump (which may feel soft and warm) in the arms, legs, chest, or pelvis.

- Fever for no known reason.

- A bone that breaks for no known reason.

Tests that examine the bone and soft tissue are used to diagnose and stage Ewing sarcoma.

The following tests and procedures may be used to diagnose or stage Ewing sarcoma:

- **Physical exam and history**

- **MRI (magnetic resonance imaging)**

- **CT scan (CAT scan)**

- **PET scan (positron emission tomography scan).**

- **Bone scan:** A procedure to check if there are rapidly dividing cells, such as cancer cells, in the bone. A very small amount of radioactive material is injected into a vein and travels through the bloodstream. The radioactive material collects in the bones and is detected by a scanner.

- **Bone marrow aspiration and biopsy:** The removal of bone marrow, blood, and a small piece of bone by inserting a hollow needle into the hipbone. Samples are removed from both hip-bones. A pathologist views the bone marrow, blood, and bone under a microscope to see if the cancer has spread.

- **X-ray**

- **Complete blood count (CBC):** A procedure in which a sample of blood is drawn and checked for the following:

    - The number of red blood cells, white blood cells, and platelets.

    - The amount of hemoglobin (the protein that carries oxygen) in the red blood cells.

    - The portion of the blood sample made up of red blood cells.

- **Blood chemistry studies**

A biopsy is done to diagnose Ewing sarcoma.

Tissue samples are removed during an incisional or needle biopsy so they can be viewed under a microscope by a pathologist to check for signs of cancer. It is helpful if the biopsy is done at the same center where treatment will be given.

- **Needle biopsy**
- **Incisional biopsy**
- **Excisional biopsy**

For an incisional or excisional biopsy, the specialists (pathologist, radiation oncologist, and surgeon) who will treat the patient usually work together to decide where the incision should be made. This is done so that the biopsy incision doesn't affect later treatment such as surgery to remove the tumor or radiation therapy.

If there is a chance that the cancer has spread to nearby lymph nodes, one or more lymph nodes may be removed and checked for signs of cancer.

The following tests may be done on the tissue that is removed:

- **Cytogenetic analysis**
- **Immunohistochemistry**
- **Flow cytometry**

Certain factors affect prognosis (chance of recovery) and treatment options.

The prognosis (chance of recovery) depends on certain factors before and after treatment.

Before treatment, prognosis depends on:

- Whether the tumor has spread to distant parts of the body.
- Whether the tumor has spread to nearby lymph nodes.
- Where in the body the tumor started.
- How large the tumor is at diagnosis.
- Whether the tumor has certain gene changes.
- Whether the child is younger than 15 years.
- The patient's gender.
- Whether the child has had treatment for a different cancer before Ewing Sarcoma.
- Whether the tumor has just been diagnosed or has recurred (come back).

After treatment, prognosis is affected by:

- Whether the tumor was completely removed by surgery.

- Whether the tumor responds to chemotherapy or radiation therapy.

- Whether the cancer came back more than two years after the initial treatment.

Treatment options depend on the following:

- Where the tumor is found in the body and how large the tumor is.

- Whether the tumor can be completely removed by surgery.

- The patient's age and general health.

- The effect the treatment will have on the patient's appearance and important body functions.

- Whether the cancer has just been diagnosed or has recurred (come back).

Decisions about surgery may depend on how well the initial treatment with chemotherapy or radiation therapy works.

Stages of Ewing Sarcoma

The results of diagnostic and staging tests are used to find out if cancer cells have spread.

The process used to find out if cancer has spread from where it began to other parts of the body is called staging. There is no standard staging system for Ewing sarcoma. The results of the tests and procedures done to diagnose Ewing sarcoma are used to group the tumors into localized or metastatic.

Ewing sarcoma is described based on whether the cancer has spread from the bone or soft tissue in which the cancer began.

Ewing sarcoma is described as either localized or metastatic.

Localized Ewing sarcoma

The cancer is found in the bone or soft tissue in which it began and may have spread to nearby tissue, including nearby lymph nodes.

598

Metastatic Ewing sarcoma

The cancer has spread from the bone or soft tissue in which it began to other parts of the body. In Ewing tumor of bone, the cancer most often spreads to the lung, other bones, and bone marrow.

There are three ways that cancer spreads in the body.

Cancer can spread through tissue, the lymph system, and the blood:

- Tissue. The cancer spreads from where it began by growing into nearby areas.

- Lymph system. The cancer spreads from where it began by getting into the lymph system. The cancer travels through the lymph vessels to other parts of the body.

- Blood. The cancer spreads from where it began by getting into the blood. The cancer travels through the blood vessels to other parts of the body.

Cancer may spread from where it began to other parts of the body.

When cancer spreads to another part of the body, it is called metastasis. Cancer cells break away from where they began (the primary tumor) and travel through the lymph system or blood.

- Lymph system. The cancer gets into the lymph system, travels through the lymph vessels, and forms a tumor (metastatic tumor) in another part of the body.

- Blood. The cancer gets into the blood, travels through the blood vessels, and forms a tumor (metastatic tumor) in another part of the body.

The metastatic tumor is the same type of cancer as the primary tumor. For example, if Ewing sarcoma spreads to the lung, the cancer cells in the lung are actually Ewing sarcoma cells. The disease is metastatic Ewing sarcoma, not lung cancer.

Treatment Option Overview

There are different types of treatment for children with Ewing sarcoma.

Different types of treatments are available for children with Ewing sarcoma. Some treatments are standard (the currently used treatment), and some are being tested in clinical trials. A treatment clinical trial is a research study meant to help improve current treatments or obtain information on new treatments for patients with cancer. When clinical trials show that a new treatment is better than the standard treatment, the new treatment may become the standard treatment.

Because cancer in children is rare, taking part in a clinical trial should be considered. Some clinical trials are open only to patients who have not started treatment.

Children with Ewing sarcoma should have their treatment planned by a team of health care providers who are experts in treating cancer in children.

Treatment will be overseen by a pediatric oncologist, a doctor who specializes in treating children with cancer. The pediatric oncologist works with other health care providers who are experts in treating children with Ewing sarcoma and who specialize in certain areas of medicine. These may include the following specialists:

- Pediatrician.
- Surgical oncologist or orthopedic oncologist.
- Radiation oncologist.
- Pediatric nurse specialist.
- Social worker.
- Rehabilitation specialist.
- Psychologist.

Some cancer treatments cause side effects months or years after treatment has ended.

Side effects from cancer treatment that begin during or after treatment and continue for months or years are called late effects. Late effects of cancer treatment may include the following:

- Physical problems.
- Changes in mood, feelings, thinking, learning, or memory.
- Second cancers (new types of cancer). Patients treated for Ewing sarcoma have an increased risk of acute myeloid leukemia and

myelodysplastic syndrome. There is also an increased risk of sarcoma in the area treated with radiation therapy.

- Some late effects may be treated or controlled. It is important to talk with your child's doctors about the effects cancer treatment can have on your child.

Three types of standard treatment are used:

Chemotherapy

Chemotherapy is a cancer treatment that uses drugs to stop the growth of cancer cells, either by killing the cells or by stopping them from dividing. When chemotherapy is taken by mouth or injected into a vein or muscle, the drugs enter the bloodstream and can reach cancer cells throughout the body (systemic chemotherapy). When chemotherapy is placed directly into the cerebrospinal fluid, an organ, or a body cavity such as the abdomen, the drugs mainly affect cancer cells in those areas (regional chemotherapy). Combination chemotherapy is treatment using more than one anticancer drug.

The type of chemotherapy given depends on whether the cancer is found only in the place it first formed, has spread to other parts of the body, or has come back after treatment.

Chemotherapy is part of the treatment for all patients with Ewing tumors. It is usually given to kill any tumor cells that have spread to other parts of the body. Chemotherapy may also be given to shrink the tumor before surgery or radiation therapy.

Radiation therapy

Radiation therapy is a cancer treatment that uses high-energy x-rays or other types of radiation to kill cancer cells or keep them from growing. There are two types of radiation therapy. External radiation therapy uses a machine outside the body to send radiation toward the cancer. Internal radiation therapy uses a radioactive substance sealed in needles, seeds, wires, or catheters that are placed directly into or near the cancer.

External radiation therapy is used to treat Ewing sarcoma.

Radiation therapy is used when the tumor cannot be removed by surgery or when surgery to remove the tumor will affect the way the child will look or important body functions. It is used to make the tumor smaller and decrease the amount of tissue that needs to be removed during surgery. It may also be used to treat tumors that have spread to other parts of the body.

Surgery

Surgery is usually done to remove cancer that is left after chemotherapy or radiation therapy. When possible, the whole tumor is removed by surgery. Tissue and bone that are removed may be replaced with a graft, which uses tissue and bone taken from another part of the patient's body or a donor. Sometimes an implant, such as artificial bone, is used.

Even if the doctor removes all of the cancer that can be seen at the time of the operation, chemotherapy or radiation therapy may be given after surgery to kill any cancer cells that are left. Chemotherapy or radiation therapy given after surgery to lower the risk that the cancer will come back is called adjuvant therapy.

New types of treatment are being tested in clinical trials.

Chemotherapy with stem cell transplant

This treatment is a way of giving high doses of chemotherapy to kill cancer cells and then replacing blood -forming cells destroyed by the cancer treatment. Stem cells (immature blood cells) are removed from the bone marrow or blood of the patient or a donor and are frozen and stored. After the chemotherapy is completed, the stored stem cells are thawed and given back to the patient through an infusion. These re-infused stem cells grow into (and restore) the body's blood cells.

Targeted therapy

Targeted therapy is a type of treatment that uses drugs or other substances to identify and attack specific cancer cells without harming normal cells.

Monoclonal antibody therapy is a type of targeted therapy being studied in the treatment of recurrent Ewing sarcoma. Monoclonal antibodies are made in the laboratory, from a single type of immune system cell. These antibodies can identify substances on cancer cells or normal substances that may help cancer cells grow. The antibodies attach to the substances and kill the cancer cells, block their growth, or keep them from spreading. Monoclonal antibodies are given by infusion. They may be used alone or to carry drugs, toxins, or radioactive material directly to cancer cells.

Kinase inhibitor therapy is another type of targeted therapy being studied in the treatment of recurrent Ewing sarcoma. Kinase inhibitors are drugs that block a protein needed for cancer cells to divide.

Patients may want to think about taking part in a clinical trial.

For some patients, taking part in a clinical trial may be the best treatment choice. Clinical trials are part of the cancer research process. Clinical trials are done to find out if new cancer treatments are safe and effective or better than the standard treatment.

Many of today's standard treatments for cancer are based on earlier clinical trials. Patients who take part in a clinical trial may receive the standard treatment or be among the first to receive a new treatment.

Patients who take part in clinical trials also help improve the way cancer will be treated in the future. Even when clinical trials do not lead to effective new treatments, they often answer important questions and help move research forward.

Patients can enter clinical trials before, during, or after starting their cancer treatment.

Some clinical trials only include patients who have not yet received treatment. Other trials test treatments for patients whose cancer has not gotten better. There are also clinical trials that test new ways to stop cancer from recurring (coming back) or reduce the side effects of cancer treatment.

Clinical trials are taking place in many parts of the country.

Follow-up tests may be needed.

Some of the tests that were done to diagnose the cancer or to find out the stage of the cancer may be repeated. Some tests will be repeated in order to see how well the treatment is working. Decisions about whether to continue, change, or stop treatment may be based on the results of these tests. This is sometimes called re-staging.

Some of the tests will continue to be done from time to time after treatment has ended. The results of these tests can show if your child's condition has changed or if the cancer has recurred (come back). These tests are sometimes called follow-up tests or check-ups.

Section 27.3

Osteosarcoma and Malignant Fibrous Histiocytoma of Bone

Text in this section is excerpted from "Osteosarcoma and Malignant Fibrous Histiocytoma of Bone Treatment," National Cancer Institute at the National Institutes of Health (NIH), May 22, 2015.

General Information About Osteosarcoma and Malignant Fibrous Histiocytoma of Bone

Osteosarcoma and malignant fibrous histiocytoma (MFH) of the bone are diseases in which malignant (cancer) cells form in bone.

Osteosarcoma usually starts in osteoblasts, which are a type of bone cell that becomes new bone tissue. Osteosarcoma is most common in teenagers. It commonly forms in the ends of the long bones of the body, which include bones of the arms and legs. In children and teenagers, it often forms in the bones near the knee. Rarely, osteosarcoma may be found in soft tissue or organs in the chest or abdomen.

Osteosarcoma is the most common type of bone cancer. Malignant fibrous histiocytoma (MFH) of bone is a rare tumor of the bone. It is treated like osteosarcoma.

Having past treatment with radiation can increase the risk of osteosarcoma.

Anything that increases your risk of getting a disease is called a risk factor. Having a risk factor does not mean that you will get cancer; not having risk factors doesn't mean that you will not get cancer. Talk with your child's doctor if you think your child may be at risk. Risk factors for osteosarcoma include the following:

- Past treatment with radiation therapy.
- Past treatment with anticancer drugs called alkylating agents.

- Having a certain change in the retinoblastoma gene.
- Having certain conditions, such as the following:
  - Hereditary retinoblastoma.
  - Paget disease.
  - Diamond-Blackfan anemia.
  - Li-Fraumeni syndrome.
  - Rothmund-Thomson syndrome.
  - Bloom syndrome.
  - Werner syndrome.

Signs and symptoms of osteosarcoma and MFH include swelling over a bone or a bony part of the body and joint pain.

These and other signs and symptoms may be caused by osteosarcoma or MFH or by other conditions. Check with a doctor if your child has any of the following:

- Swelling over a bone or bony part of the body.
- Pain in a bone or joint.
- A bone that breaks for no known reason.

Imaging tests are used to detect (find) osteosarcoma and MFH.

Imaging tests are done before the biopsy. The following tests and procedures may be used:

- **Physical exam and history**
- **X-ray**
- **CT scan (CAT scan)**
- **MRI (magnetic resonance imaging)**

A biopsy is done to diagnose osteosarcoma.

Cells and tissues are removed during a biopsy so they can be viewed under a microscope by a pathologist to check for signs of cancer. It is important that the biopsy be done by a surgeon who is an expert in treating cancer of the bone. It is best if that surgeon is also the one who removes the tumor. The biopsy and the surgery to remove the tumor are planned together. The way the biopsy is done affects which type of surgery can be done later.

The type of biopsy that is done will be based on the size of the tumor and where it is in the body. There are two types of biopsy that may be used:

- **Core biopsy**

- **Incisional biopsy**

The following test may be done on the tissue that is removed:

- **Light and electron microscopy:** A laboratory test in which cells in a sample of tissue are viewed under regular and high-powered microscopes to look for certain changes in the cells.

Certain factors affect prognosis (chance of recovery) and treatment options.

The prognosis (chance of recovery) is affected by certain factors before and after treatment.

The prognosis of untreated osteosarcoma and MFH depends on the following:

- Where the tumor is in the body and whether tumors formed in more than one bone.

- The size of the tumor.

- Whether the cancer has spread to other parts of the body and where it has spread.

- The type of tumor (based on how the cancer cells look under a microscope).

- The patient's age and weight at diagnosis.

- Whether the patient has certain genetic diseases.

After osteosarcoma or MFH is treated, prognosis also depends on the following:

- How much of the cancer was killed by chemotherapy.

- How much of the tumor was taken out by surgery.

- Whether chemotherapy is delayed for more than 3 weeks after surgery takes place.

- Whether the cancer has recurred (come back) within 2 years of diagnosis.

Treatment options for osteosarcoma and MFH depend on the following:

- Where the tumor is in the body.

- The size of the tumor.

- The stage of the cancer.

- Whether the bones are still growing.

- The patient's age and general health.

- The desire of the patient and family for the patient to be able to participate in activities such as sports or have a certain appearance.

- Whether the cancer is newly diagnosed or has recurred after treatment.

Stages of Osteosarcoma and Malignant Fibrous Histiocytoma of Bone

After osteosarcoma or malignant fibrous histiocytoma (MFH) has been diagnosed, tests are done to find out if cancer cells have spread to other parts of the body.

The process used to find out if cancer has spread to other parts of the body is called staging. For osteosarcoma and malignant fibrous histiocytoma (MFH), most patients are grouped according to whether cancer is found in only one part of the body or has spread.

The following tests and procedures may be used:

- **X-ray:** An x-ray of the organs, such as the chest, and bones inside the body. An x-ray is a type of energy beam that can go through the body and onto film, making a picture of areas inside the body. X-rays will be taken of the chest and the area where the tumor formed.

- **CT scan (CAT scan):** A procedure that makes a series of detailed pictures of areas inside the body, such as the chest, taken from different angles. The pictures are made by a computer linked to an x-ray machine. A dye may be injected into a vein or swallowed to help the organs or tissues show up more clearly. This procedure is also called computed tomography, computerized tomography, or computerized axial tomography. Pictures will be taken of the chest and the area where the tumor formed.

- **MRI (magnetic resonance imaging):** A procedure that uses a magnet, radio waves, and a computer to make a series of detailed pictures of areas inside the body. This procedure is also called nuclear magnetic resonance imaging (NMRI).

- **Bone scan:** A procedure to check if there are rapidly dividing cells, such as cancer cells, in the bone. A very small amount of radioactive material is injected into a vein and travels through the bloodstream. The radioactive material collects in the bones and is detected by a scanner.

There are three ways that cancer spreads in the body.

Cancer can spread through tissue, the lymph system, and the blood:

- Tissue. The cancer spreads from where it began by growing into nearby areas.

- Lymph system. The cancer spreads from where it began by getting into the lymph system. The cancer travels through the lymph vessels to other parts of the body.

- Blood. The cancer spreads from where it began by getting into the blood. The cancer travels through the blood vessels to other parts of the body.

Cancer may spread from where it began to other parts of the body.

When cancer spreads to another part of the body, it is called metastasis. Cancer cells break away from where they began (the primary tumor) and travel through the lymph system or blood.

- Lymph system. The cancer gets into the lymph system, travels through the lymph vessels, and forms a tumor (metastatic tumor) in another part of the body.

- Blood. The cancer gets into the blood, travels through the blood vessels, and forms a tumor (metastatic tumor) in another part of the body.

The metastatic tumor is the same type of cancer as the primary tumor. For example, if osteosarcoma spreads to the lung, the cancer cells in the lung are actually osteosarcoma cells. The disease is metastatic osteosarcoma, not lung cancer.

Osteosarcoma and MFH are described as either localized or metastatic.

- Localized osteosarcoma or MFH has not spread out of the bone where the cancer started. There may be one or more areas of cancer in the bone that can be removed during surgery.

- Metastatic osteosarcoma or MFH has spread from the bone in which the cancer began to other parts of the body. The cancer most often spreads to the lungs. It may also spread to other bones.

Treatment Option Overview

There are different types of treatment for patients with osteosarcoma or malignant fibrous histiocytoma (MFH) of bone.

Different types of treatment are available for children with osteosarcoma or malignant fibrous histiocytoma (MFH) of bone. Some treatments are standard (the currently used treatment), and some are being tested in clinical trials. A treatment clinical trial is a research study meant to help improve current treatments or obtain information on new treatments for patients with cancer. When clinical trials show that a new treatment is better than the standard treatment, the new treatment may become the standard treatment.

Because cancer in children is rare, taking part in a clinical trial should be considered. Some clinical trials are open only to patients who have not started treatment.

Children with osteosarcoma or MFH should have their treatment planned by a team of health care providers with expertise in treating cancer in children.

Treatment will be overseen by a pediatric oncologist, a doctor who specializes in treating children with cancer. The pediatric oncologist works with other pediatric health care providers who are experts in treating osteosarcoma and MFH and who specialize in certain areas of medicine. These may include the following specialists:

- Pediatrician.

- Orthopedic surgeon.

- Radiation oncologist.

- Rehabilitation specialist.

- Pediatric nurse specialist.

- Social worker.

- Psychologist.

Some cancer treatments cause side effects months or years after treatment has ended.

Side effects from cancer treatment that begin during or after treatment and continue for months or years are called late effects. Late effects of cancer treatment may include the following:

- Physical problems.

- Changes in mood, feelings, thinking, learning, or memory.

- Second cancers (new types of cancer).

Some late effects may be treated or controlled. It is important to talk with your child's doctors about the effects cancer treatment can have on your child.

Four types of standard treatment are used:

Surgery

Surgery to remove the entire tumor will be done when possible. Chemotherapy may be given before surgery to make the tumor smaller. This is called neoadjuvant chemotherapy. Chemotherapy is given so less bone tissue needs to be removed and there are fewer problems after surgery.

The following types of surgery may be done:

- Wide local excision: Surgery to remove the cancer and some healthy tissue around it.

- Limb-sparing surgery: Removal of the tumor in a limb (arm or leg) without amputation, so the use and appearance of the limb is saved. Most patients with osteosarcoma in a limb can be treated with limb-sparing surgery. The tumor is removed by wide local excision. Tissue and bone that are removed may be replaced with a graft using tissue and bone taken from another part of the patient's body, or with an implant such as artificial bone. If a fracture is found at diagnosis or during chemotherapy before surgery, limb-sparing surgery may still be possible in some cases. If the surgeon is not able to remove all of the tumor and enough healthy tissue around it, an amputation may be done.

- Amputation: Surgery to remove part or all of an arm or leg. This may be done when it is not possible to remove all of the tumor in limb-sparing surgery. The patient may be fitted with a prosthesis (artificial limb) after amputation.

- Rotationplasty: Surgery to remove the tumor and the knee joint. The part of the leg that remains below the knee is then attached to the part of the leg that remains above the knee, with the foot facing backward and the ankle acting as a knee. A prosthesis may then be attached to the foot.

Studies have shown that survival is the same whether the first surgery done is a limb-sparing surgery or an amputation.

Even if the doctor removes all the cancer that can be seen at the time of the surgery, patients are also given chemotherapy after surgery to kill any cancer cells that are left in the area where the tumor was removed or that have spread to other parts of the body. Treatment given after the surgery, to lower the risk that the cancer will come back, is called adjuvant therapy.

Chemotherapy

Chemotherapy is a cancer treatment that uses drugs to stop the growth of cancer cells, either by killing the cells or by stopping them from dividing. When chemotherapy is taken by mouth or injected into a vein or muscle, the drugs enter the bloodstream and can reach cancer cells throughout the body (systemic chemotherapy). When chemotherapy is placed directly into the cerebrospinal fluid, an organ, or a body cavity such as the abdomen, the drugs mainly affect cancer cells in those areas (regional chemotherapy). Combination chemotherapy is the use of more than one anticancer drug. The way the chemotherapy is given depends on the type and stage of the cancer being treated.

In the treatment of osteosarcoma and malignant fibrous histiocytosis of bone, chemotherapy is usually given before and after surgery to remove the primary tumor.

Radiation therapy

Radiation therapy is a cancer treatment that uses high-energy x-rays or other types of radiation to kill cancer cells or keep them from growing. There are two types of radiation therapy. External radiation therapy uses a machine outside the body to send radiation toward the cancer. Internal radiation therapy uses a radioactive substance sealed in needles, seeds, wires, or catheters that are placed directly into or near the cancer. The way the radiation therapy is given depends on the type and stage of the cancer being treated.

Osteosarcoma and MFH cells are not killed easily by radiation therapy. It may be used when a small amount of cancer is left after surgery or used together with other treatments.

Samarium

Samarium is a radioactive drug that targets areas where bone cells are growing, such as tumor cells in bone. It helps relieve pain caused by cancer in the bone and it also kills blood cells in the bone marrow. It also is used to treat osteosarcoma that has come back after treatment in a different bone.

Treatment with samarium may be followed by stem cell transplant. Before treatment with samarium, stem cells (immature blood cells) are removed from the blood or bone marrow of the patient and are frozen and stored. After treatment with samarium is complete, the stored stem cells are thawed and given back to the patient through an infusion. These re-infused stem cells grow into (and restore) the body's blood cells.

New types of treatment are being tested in clinical trials.

Targeted therapy

Targeted therapy is a treatment that uses drugs or other substances to find and attack specific cancer cells without harming normal cells. Kinase inhibitor therapy is a type of targeted therapy being studied in clinical trials for osteosarcoma. Kinase inhibitor therapy blocks a protein needed for cancer cells to divide.

Patients may want to think about taking part in a clinical trial.

For some patients, taking part in a clinical trial may be the best treatment choice. Clinical trials are part of the cancer research process. Clinical trials are done to find out if new cancer treatments are safe and effective or better than the standard treatment.

Many of today's standard treatments for cancer are based on earlier clinical trials. Patients who take part in a clinical trial may receive the standard treatment or be among the first to receive a new treatment.

Patients who take part in clinical trials also help improve the way cancer will be treated in the future. Even when clinical trials do not lead to effective new treatments, they often answer important questions and help move research forward.

Patients can enter clinical trials before, during, or after starting their cancer treatment.

Some clinical trials only include patients who have not yet received treatment. Other trials test treatments for patients whose cancer has not gotten better. There are also clinical trials that test new ways to stop cancer from recurring (coming back) or reduce the side effects of cancer treatment.

Clinical trials are taking place in many parts of the country.

Follow-up tests may be needed.

Some of the tests that were done to diagnose the cancer or to find out the stage of the cancer may be repeated. Some tests will be repeated in order to see how well the treatment is working. Decisions about whether to continue, change, or stop treatment may be based on the results of these tests. This is sometimes called re-staging.

Some of the tests will continue to be done from time to time after treatment has ended. The results of these tests can show if your child's condition has changed or if the cancer has recurred (come back). These tests are sometimes called follow-up tests or check-ups.

Section 27.4

Rhabdomyosarcoma, Childhood

Text in this section is excerpted from "Childhood Rhabdomyosarcoma
Treatment," National Cancer Institute at the National Institutes of
Health (NIH), October 8, 2014.

General Information About Childhood Rhabdomyosarcoma

Childhood rhabdomyosarcoma is a disease in which malignant (cancer) cells form in muscle tissue.

Rhabdomyosarcoma is a type of sarcoma. Sarcoma is cancer of soft
tissue (such as muscle), connective tissue (such as tendon or cartilage), or bone. Rhabdomyosarcoma usually begins in muscles that are
attached to bones and that help the body move. Rhabdomyosarcoma is
the most common type of soft tissue sarcoma in children. It can begin
in many places in the body.

There are three main types of rhabdomyosarcoma:

- Embryonal: This type occurs most often in the head and neck
  area or in the genital or urinary organs. It is the most common
  type.

- Alveolar: This type occurs most often in the arms or legs, chest,
  abdomen, genital organs, or anal area. It usually occurs during
  the teen years.

- Anaplastic: This type rarely occurs in children.

Certain genetic conditions increase the risk of childhood rhabdomyosarcoma.

Anything that increases the risk of getting a disease is called a risk
factor. Having a risk factor does not mean that you will get cancer; not
having risk factors doesn't mean that you will not get cancer. Talk with

your child's doctor if you think your child may be at risk. Risk factors for rhabdomyosarcoma include having the following inherited diseases:

- Li-Fraumeni syndrome.
- Pleuropulmonary blastoma.
- Neurofibromatosis type 1 (NF1).
- Beckwith-Wiedemann syndrome.
- Costello syndrome.
- Noonan syndrome.

Children who had a high birth weight or were larger than expected at birth may have an increased risk of embryonal rhabdomyosarcoma. **In most cases, the cause of rhabdomyosarcoma is not known.**

A sign of childhood rhabdomyosarcoma is a lump or swelling that keeps getting bigger.

Signs and symptoms may be caused by childhood rhabdomyo-sarcoma or by other conditions. The signs and symptoms that occur depend on where the cancer forms. Check with your child's doctor if your child has any of the following:

- A lump or swelling that keeps getting bigger or does not go away. It may be painful.
- Bulging of the eye.
- Headache.
- Trouble urinating or having bowel movements.
- Blood in the urine.
- Bleeding in the nose, throat, vagina, or rectum.

Diagnostic tests and a biopsy are used to detect (find) and diagnose childhood rhabdomyosarcoma.

The following tests and procedures may be used:

- **Physical exam and history**
- **X-ray**
- **CT scan (CAT scan**
- **MRI (magnetic resonance imaging)**

- **Bone scan:** A procedure to check if there are rapidly dividing cells, such as cancer cells, in the bone. A very small amount of radioactive material is injected into a vein and travels through the bloodstream. The radioactive material collects in the bones and is detected by a scanner.

- **Bone marrow aspiration and biopsy:** The removal of bone marrow, blood, and a small piece of bone by inserting a hollow needle into the hipbone. Samples are removed from both hipbones. A pathologist views the bone marrow, blood, and bone under a microscope to look for signs of cancer.

- **Lumbar puncture:** A procedure used to collect cerebrospinal fluid (CSF) from the spinal column to check for cancer cells. This is done by placing a needle between two bones in the spine and into the spinal column to remove a sample of CSF. This procedure is also called an LP or spinal tap.

If these tests show there may be a rhabdomyosarcoma, a biopsy is done. A biopsy is the removal of cells or tissues so they can be viewed under a microscope by a pathologist to check for signs of cancer. Because treatment depends on the type of rhabdomyosarcoma, biopsy samples should be checked by a pathologist who has experience in diagnosing rhabdomyosarcoma.

One of the following types of biopsies may be used:

- **Fine-needle aspiration (FNA) biopsy:** The removal of tissue or fluid using a thin needle.

- **Core needle biopsy:** The removal of tissue using a wide needle. This procedure may be guided using ultrasound, CT scan, or MRI.

- **Open biopsy:** The removal of tissue through an incision (cut) made in the skin.

The following tests may be done on the sample of tissue that is removed:

- **Light microscopy:** A laboratory test in which cells in a sample of tissue are viewed under regular and high-powered microscopes to look for certain changes in the cells.

- **Immunohistochemistry:** A test that uses antibodies to check for certain antigens in a sample of tissue. The antibody is usually linked to a radioactive substance or a dye that causes the tissue to light up under a microscope. This type of test may be used to tell the difference between different types of cancer.

- **Immunocytochemistry:** A test that uses antibodies to check for certain antigens in a sample of cells. The antibody is usually linked to a radioactive substance or a dye that causes the cells to light up under a microscope. This type of test may be used to tell the difference between different types of soft tissue sarcoma.

- **Reverse transcription-polymerase chain reaction (RT-PCR) test:** A laboratory test in which cells in a sample of tissue are studied using chemicals to look for certain changes in the structure or function of genes.

- **Cytogenetic analysis:** A laboratory test in which cells in a sample of tissue are viewed under a microscope to look for certain changes in the chromosomes.

Certain factors affect prognosis (chance of recovery) and treatment options.

The prognosis (chance of recovery) and treatment options depend on the following:

- Where in the body the tumor started.

- The width of the tumor when the cancer was diagnosed.

- Whether the tumor has spread to nearby lymph nodes or distant parts of the body.

- Whether there are certain changes in the genes.

- The type of rhabdomyosarcoma.

- Whether the tumor has been completely removed by surgery.

- Whether the tumor responds to radiation therapy.

- The patient's age and general health.

- Whether the tumor has just been diagnosed or has recurred (come back).

For patients with recurrent cancer, prognosis and treatment depend on the following:

- Where in the body the tumor recurred (came back).

- Whether the tumor was treated with radiation therapy.

- The size of the tumor when the cancer was diagnosed.

- How much time passed between the end of cancer treatment and when the cancer recurred.

Stages of Childhood Rhabdomyosarcoma

After childhood rhabdomyosarcoma has been diagnosed, treatment is based on the stage of the cancer and whether all the cancer was removed by surgery.

The process used to find out if cancer has spread within the tissue or to other parts of the body is called staging. It is important to know the stage in order to plan treatment. The doctor will use results of the diagnostic tests to help find out the stage of the disease.

Treatment for childhood rhabdomyosarcoma is based on the stage and the amount of cancer that remains after surgery to remove the tumor. The pathologist will use a microscope to check the tissues, including lymph nodes, removed during surgery, and the edges of the areas where the cancer was removed. This is done to see if all the cancer cells were taken out during the surgery.

There are three ways that cancer spreads in the body.

Cancer can spread through tissue, the lymph system, and the blood:

- Tissue. The cancer spreads from where it began by growing into nearby areas.

- Lymph system. The cancer spreads from where it began by getting into the lymph system. The cancer travels through the lymph vessels to other parts of the body.

- Blood. The cancer spreads from where it began by getting into the blood. The cancer travels through the blood vessels to other parts of the body.

Cancer may spread from where it began to other parts of the body.

When cancer spreads to another part of the body, it is called metastasis. Cancer cells break away from where they began (the primary tumor) and travel through the lymph system or blood.

- Lymph system. The cancer gets into the lymph system, travels through the lymph vessels, and forms a tumor (metastatic tumor) in another part of the body.

- Blood. The cancer gets into the blood, travels through the blood vessels, and forms a tumor (metastatic tumor) in another part of the body.

The metastatic tumor is the same type of cancer as the primary tumor. For example, if rhabdomyosarcoma spreads to the lung, the cancer cells in the lung are actually rhabdomyosarcoma cells. The disease is metastatic rhabdomyosarcoma, not lung cancer.

Staging of childhood rhabdomyosarcoma is done in three parts.

Childhood rhabdomyosarcoma is staged by using three different ways to describe the cancer:

- A staging system.
- A grouping system.
- A risk group.

The staging system is based on the size of the tumor, where it is in the body, and whether it has spread to other parts of the body:

Stage 1

In stage 1, the tumor is any size, has not spread to lymph nodes, and is found in only one of the following "favorable" sites:

- Eye or area around the eye.
- Head and neck (but not in the tissue next to the brain and spinal cord).
- Gallbladder and bile ducts.
- In the testes, vagina, or uterus.

Rhabdomyosarcoma that forms in a "favorable" site has a better prognosis. If the site where cancer occurs is not one of the favorable sites listed above, it is said to be an "unfavorable" site.

Stage 2

In stage 2, cancer is found in an "unfavorable" site (any one area not included in stage 1). The tumor is no larger than 5 centimeters and has not spread to lymph nodes.

Stage 3

In stage 3, cancer is found in an "unfavorable" site (any one area not included in stage 1) and one of the following is true:

- The tumor is no larger than 5 centimeters and cancer has spread to nearby lymph nodes.

- The tumor is larger than 5 centimeters and cancer may have spread to nearby lymph nodes.

Stage 4

In stage 4, the tumor may be any size and cancer may have spread to nearby lymph nodes. Cancer has spread to distant parts of the body, such as the lung, bone marrow, or bone.

The grouping system is based on whether the cancer has spread and whether all the cancer was removed by surgery:

Group I

Cancer was found only in the place where it started and it was completely removed by surgery. Tissue was taken from the edges of where the tumor was removed. The tissue was checked under a microscope by a pathologist and no cancer cells were found.

Group II

Group II is divided into groups IIA, IIB, and IIC.

- IIA: Cancer was removed by surgery but cancer cells were seen when the tissue, taken from the edges of where the tumor was removed, was viewed under a microscope by a pathologist.

- IIB: Cancer had spread to nearby lymph nodes and the cancer and lymph nodes were removed by surgery.

- IIC: Cancer had spread to nearby lymph nodes and the cancer and lymph nodes were removed by surgery. Tissue was taken from the edges of where the tumor was removed. The tissue was checked under a microscope by a pathologist and cancer cells were seen.

Group III

Cancer was partly removed by biopsy or surgery but there is tumor remaining that can be seen with the eye. Cancer has not spread to distant parts of the body.

Group IV

Cancer had spread to distant parts of the body when the cancer was diagnosed.

- Cancer cells are found by an imaging test; and
- there are cancer cells in the fluid around the brain, spinal cord, or lungs, or in fluid in the abdomen; or tumors are found in those areas.

The risk group is based on the staging system and the grouping system.

The risk group describes the chance that rhabdomyosarcoma will recur (come back). Every child treated for rhabdomyosarcoma should receive chemotherapy to decrease the chance cancer will recur. The type of anticancer drug, dose, and the number of treatments given depends on whether the child has low-risk, intermediate-risk, or high-risk rhabdomyosarcoma. The following risk groups are used:

Low-risk childhood rhabdomyosarcoma

Low-risk childhood rhabdomyosarcoma is one of the following:

- An embryonal tumor of any size that is found in a "favorable" site. There may be tumor remaining after surgery that can be seen without a microscope. The cancer may have spread to nearby lymph nodes. The following areas are "favorable" sites:
- Eye or area around the eye.
- Head or neck (but not in the tissue next to the brain and spinal cord).
- Gallbladder and bile ducts.
- In the testes, vagina, or uterus.

- An embryonal tumor of any size that is not found in one of the "favorable" sites listed above. There may be tumor remaining after surgery that can be seen only with a microscope. The cancer may have spread to nearby lymph nodes.

Intermediate-risk childhood rhabdomyosarcoma

Intermediate-risk childhood rhabdomyosarcoma is one of the following:

- An embryonal tumor of any size that is not found in one of the "favorable" sites listed above. There is tumor remaining after surgery, that can be seen with or without a microscope. The cancer may have spread to nearby lymph nodes.

- An alveolar tumor of any size in a "favorable" or "unfavorable" site. There may be tumor remaining after surgery that can be seen with or without a microscope. The cancer may have spread to nearby lymph nodes.

High-risk childhood rhabdomyosarcoma

High-risk childhood rhabdomyosarcoma may be the embryonal type or the alveolar type. It may have spread to nearby lymph nodes and has spread to one or more distant parts of the body.

Treatment Options for Childhood Rhabdomyosarcoma

Previously Untreated Childhood Rhabdomyosarcoma

The treatment of childhood rhabdomyosarcoma often includes surgery, radiation therapy, and chemotherapy. The order that these treatments are given depends on where in the body the tumor started, the size of the tumor, the type of tumor, and whether the tumor has spread to lymph nodes or other parts of the body.

Rhabdomyosarcoma of the brain and head and neck

- For tumors of the brain: Treatment may include surgery to remove the tumor, radiation therapy, and chemotherapy.

- For tumors of the head and neck that are in or near the eye: Treatment may include chemotherapy and radiation therapy. If the tumor remains or comes back after treatment with chemotherapy and radiation therapy, surgery to remove the eye and some tissues around the eye may be needed.

- For tumors of the head and neck that are near the brain and spinal cord but not in or near the eye: Treatment may include radiation therapy and chemotherapy.

- For tumors of the head and neck that cannot be removed by surgery: Treatment may include chemotherapy and radiation therapy.

- For tumors of the larynx (voice box): Treatment may include chemotherapy and radiation therapy. Surgery to remove the larynx is usually not done, so that the voice is not harmed.

Rhabdomyosarcoma of the arms or legs

- Surgery to remove the tumor. If the tumor was not completely removed, a second surgery to remove the tumor may be done.

- For tumors of the hand or foot, radiation therapy and chemotherapy may be given. The tumor may not be removed because the function of the hand or foot would be lessened.

- Lymph node dissection (one or more lymph nodes are removed and a sample of tissue is checked under a microscope for signs of cancer).

- For tumors in the arms, lymph nodes near the tumor and in the armpit area are removed.

- For tumors in the legs, lymph nodes near the tumor and in the groin area are removed.

- Chemotherapy.

- Radiation therapy.

Rhabdomyosarcoma of the chest, abdomen, or pelvis

- For tumors in the chest or abdomen (including the chest wall or abdominal wall): Surgery (wide local excision) may be done. If the tumor is large, chemotherapy, and sometimes radiation therapy, is given to shrink the tumor before surgery.

- For tumors of the pelvis: Surgery (wide local excision) may be done. If the tumor is large, chemotherapy, and sometimes radiation therapy, is given to shrink the tumor before surgery. Some pelvic tumors may be treated with biopsy, rather than wide local excision, followed by radiation therapy.

- For tumors of the diaphragm: A biopsy of the tumor is followed by chemotherapy and radiation therapy to shrink the tumor. Surgery may be done later to remove any remaining cancer cells.

- For tumors of the gallbladder or bile ducts: Surgery is done to remove as much of the tumor as possible, followed by chemotherapy and radiation therapy.

- For tumors of the muscles or tissues around the anus or between the vulva and the anus or the scrotum and the anus: Surgery is done to remove as much of the tumor as possible and some nearby lymph nodes, followed by chemotherapy and radiation therapy.

Rhabdomyosarcoma of the kidney

- Surgery to remove as much of the tumor as possible.

Rhabdomyosarcoma of the bladder and prostate

- For tumors that are only at the top of the bladder: Surgery (wide local excision) is done.

- For tumors of the prostate or bladder (other than the top of the bladder):

- Chemotherapy and radiation therapy are given first to shrink the tumor. If cancer cells remain after chemotherapy and radiation therapy, the tumor is removed by surgery. Surgery may include removal of the prostate, part of the bladder, or pelvic exenteration without removal of the rectum. (This may include removal of the lower colon and bladder. In girls, the cervix, vagina, ovaries, and nearby lymph nodes may be removed).

- Chemotherapy is given first to shrink the tumor. Surgery to remove the tumor, but not the bladder or prostate, is done. Internal radiation therapy may be given after surgery.

Rhabdomyosarcoma of the area near the testicles

- Rhabdomyosarcoma of the testicular area is usually treated with surgery to remove the testicle and spermatic cord.

- The lymph nodes in the back of the abdomen may be checked for cancer, especially if the lymph nodes are enlarged or the child is older than 9 years. Radiation therapy may be given if the tumor cannot be completely removed by surgery. CT scans may be done every 3 months after surgery to see if the cancer is growing in nearby lymph nodes.

Rhabdomyosarcoma of the vulva, vagina, uterus or ovary

- For tumors of the vulva and vagina: Treatment may include chemotherapy followed by surgery to remove the tumor. Internal or external radiation therapy may be given after surgery.

- For tumors of the uterus: Treatment may include chemotherapy with or without radiation therapy. Sometimes surgery may be needed to remove any remaining cancer cells.

- For tumors of the cervix: Treatment may include chemotherapy followed by surgery to remove any remaining tumor.

- For tumors of the ovary: Treatment may include combination chemotherapy followed by surgery to remove any remaining tumor.

Metastatic rhabdomyosarcoma

- Radiation therapy may be given for tumors that have spread to the brain, spinal cord, or lungs.
  Treatment is also given to the site where the tumor first formed.

The following treatment is being studied for rhabdomyosarcoma:

- A clinical trial of immunotherapy.

Recurrent Childhood Rhabdomyosarcoma

Treatment options for recurrent childhood rhabdomyosarcoma are based on many factors, including where in the body the cancer has come back, what type of treatment the patient had before, and the needs of the individual child. Treatment may include one or more of the following:

- Chemotherapy with one or more anticancer drugs.

- Surgery.

- Radiation therapy.

- Clinical trial of new anticancer drugs.

- A clinical trial of high-dose chemotherapy followed by stem cell transplant using the patient's own stem cells.

Section 27.5

Soft Tissue Sarcoma

Text in this section is excerpted from "Adult Soft Tissue Sarcoma Treatment," National Cancer Institute at the National Institutes of Health (NIH), April 2, 2015.

General Information About Adult Soft Tissue Sarcoma

Adult soft tissue sarcoma is a disease in which malignant (cancer) cells form in the soft tissues of the body.

The soft tissues of the body include the muscles, tendons (bands of fiber that connect muscles to bones), fat, blood vessels, lymph vessels, nerves, and tissues around joints. Adult soft tissue sarcomas can form almost anywhere in the body, but are most common in the head, neck, arms, legs, trunk, and abdomen.

There are many types of soft tissue sarcoma. The cells of each type of sarcoma look different under a microscope, based on the type of soft tissue in which the cancer began.

Having certain inherited disorders can increase the risk of adult soft tissue sarcoma.

Anything that increases your risk of getting a disease is called a risk factor. Having a risk factor does not mean that you will get cancer; not having risk factors doesn't mean that you will not get cancer. Talk with your doctor if you think you may be at risk. Risk factors for soft tissue sarcoma include the following inherited disorders:

- Retinoblastoma.

- Neurofibromatosis type 1 (NF1; von Recklinghausen disease).

- Tuberous sclerosis (Bourneville disease).

- Familial adenomatous polyposis (FAP; Gardner syndrome).

- Li-Fraumeni syndrome.

- Werner syndrome (adult progeria).

- Nevoid basal cell carcinoma syndrome (Gorlin syndrome).

Other risk factors for soft tissue sarcoma include the following:

- Past treatment with radiation therapy for certain cancers.

- Being exposed to certain chemicals, such as Thorotrast (thorium dioxide), vinyl chloride, or arsenic.

- Having swelling (lymphedema) in the arms or legs for a long time.

A sign of adult soft tissue sarcoma is a lump or swelling in soft tissue of the body.

A sarcoma may appear as a painless lump under the skin, often on an arm or a leg. Sarcomas that begin in the abdomen may not cause signs or symptoms until they get very big. As the sarcoma grows bigger and presses on nearby organs, nerves, muscles, or blood vessels, signs and symptoms may include:

- Pain.

- Trouble breathing.

Other conditions may cause the same signs and symptoms. Check with your doctor if you have any of these problems.

Adult soft tissue sarcoma is diagnosed with a biopsy.

If your doctor thinks you may have a soft tissue sarcoma, a biopsy will be done. The type of biopsy will be based on the size of the tumor and where it is in the body. There are three types of biopsy that may be used:

- **Incisional biopsy**

- **Core biopsy**

- **Excisional biopsy**

Samples will be taken from the primary tumor, lymph nodes, and other suspicious areas. A pathologist views the tissue under a microscope to look for cancer cells and to find out the grade of the tumor. The grade of a tumor depends on how abnormal the cancer cells look

627

under a microscope and how quickly the cells are dividing. High-grade tumors usually grow and spread more quickly than low-grade tumors.

Because soft tissue sarcoma can be hard to diagnose, patients should ask to have tissue samples checked by a pathologist who has experience in diagnosing soft tissue sarcoma.

The following tests may be done on the tissue that was removed:

- **Immunohistochemistry**
- **Light and electron microscopy**
- **Cytogenetic analysis**
- **FISH (fluorescence in situ hybridization)**
- **Flow cytometry**

Certain factors affect treatment options and prognosis (chance of recovery).

The treatment options and prognosis (chance of recovery) depend on the following:

- The type of soft tissue sarcoma.
- The size, grade, and stage of the tumor.
- How fast the cancer cells are growing and dividing.
- Where the tumor is in the body.
- Whether all of the tumor is removed by surgery.
- The patient's age and general health.
- Whether the cancer has recurred (come back).

Stages of Adult Soft Tissue Sarcoma

After adult soft tissue sarcoma has been diagnosed, tests are done to find out if cancer cells have spread within the soft tissue or to other parts of the body.

The process used to find out if cancer has spread within the soft tissue or to other parts of the body is called staging. Staging of soft tissue sarcoma is also based on the grade and size of the tumor, whether it is superficial (close to the skin's surface) or deep, and whether it has spread to the lymph nodes or other parts of the body. The information gathered from the staging process determines the stage of the disease. It is important to know the stage in order to plan treatment.

The following tests and procedures may be used in the staging process:

- **Physical exam and history**

- **Chest x-ray**

- **Blood chemistry studies**

- **Complete blood count (CBC):** A procedure in which a sample of blood is drawn and checked for the following:

  - The number of red blood cells, white blood cells, and platelets.

  - The amount of hemoglobin (the protein that carries oxygen) in the red blood cells.

  - The portion of the blood sample made up of red blood cells.

- **CT scan (CAT scan**

- **MRI (magnetic resonance imaging**

- **PET scan (positron emission tomography scan)**

   The results of these tests are viewed together with the results of the tumor biopsy to find out the stage of the soft tissue sarcoma before treatment is given. Sometimes chemotherapy or radiation therapy is given as the initial treatment and afterwards the soft tissue sarcoma is staged again.

There are three ways that cancer spreads in the body.

Cancer can spread through tissue, the lymph system, and the blood:

- Tissue. The cancer spreads from where it began by growing into nearby areas.

- Lymph system. The cancer spreads from where it began by getting into the lymph system. The cancer travels through the lymph vessels to other parts of the body.

- Blood. The cancer spreads from where it began by getting into the blood. The cancer travels through the blood vessels to other parts of the body.

Cancer may spread from where it began to other parts of the body.

When cancer spreads to another part of the body, it is called metastasis. Cancer cells break away from where they began (the primary tumor) and travel through the lymph system or blood.

- Lymph system. The cancer gets into the lymph system, travels through the lymph vessels, and forms a tumor (metastatic tumor) in another part of the body.

- Blood. The cancer gets into the blood, travels through the blood vessels, and forms a tumor (metastatic tumor) in another part of the body.

The metastatic tumor is the same type of cancer as the primary tumor. For example, if soft tissue sarcoma spreads to the lung, the cancer cells in the lung are actually soft tissue sarcoma cells. The disease is metastatic soft tissue sarcoma, not lung cancer.

The following stages are used for adult soft tissue sarcoma:

Stage I

Stage I is divided into stages IA and IB:

- In stage IA, the tumor is low-grade (likely to grow and spread slowly) and 5 centimeters or smaller. It may be either superficial (in subcutaneous tissue with no spread into connective tissue or muscle below) or deep (in the muscle and may be in connective or subcutaneous tissue).

- In stage IB, the tumor is low-grade (likely to grow and spread slowly) and larger than 5centimeters. It may be either superficial (in subcutaneous tissue with no spread into connective tissue or muscle below) or deep (in the muscle and may be in connective or subcutaneous tissue).

Stage II

Stage II is divided into stages IIA and IIB:

- In stage IIA, the tumor is mid-grade (somewhat likely to grow and spread quickly) or high-grade (likely to grow and spread quickly) and 5 centimeters or smaller. It may be either superficial (in subcutaneous tissue with no spread into connective tissue or muscle below) or deep (in the muscle and may be in connective or subcutaneous tissue).

- In stage IIB, the tumor is mid-grade (somewhat likely to grow and spread quickly) and larger than 5 centimeters. It may be either superficial (in subcutaneous tissue with no spread into connective tissue or muscle below) or deep (in the muscle and may be in connective or subcutaneous tissue).

Stage III

In stage III, the tumor is either:

- high-grade (likely to grow and spread quickly), larger than 5 centimeters, and either superficial (in subcutaneous tissue with no spread into connective tissue or muscle below) or deep (in the muscle and may be in connective or subcutaneous tissue); or
- any grade, any size, and has spread to nearby lymph nodes.

Stage III cancer that has spread to the lymph nodes is advanced stage III.

Stage IV

In stage IV, the tumor is any grade, any size, and may have spread to nearby lymph nodes. Cancer has spread to distant parts of the body, such as the lungs.

Treatment Option Overview

There are different types of treatment for patients with adult soft tissue sarcoma.

Different types of treatments are available for patients with adult soft tissue sarcoma. Some treatments are standard (the currently used treatment), and some are being tested in clinical trials. A treatment clinical trial is a research study meant to help improve current treatments or obtain information on new treatments for patients with cancer. When clinical trials show that a new treatment is better than the standard treatment, the new treatment may become the standard treatment. Patients may want to think about taking part in a clinical trial. Some clinical trials are open only to patients who have not started treatment.

Three types of standard treatment are used:

Surgery

Surgery is the most common treatment for adult soft tissue sarcoma. For some soft-tissue sarcomas, removal of the tumor in surgery may be the only treatment needed. The following surgical procedures may be used:

- Mohs microsurgery: A procedure in which the tumor is cut from the skin in thin layers. During surgery, the edges of the tumor and each layer of tumor removed are viewed through a microscope to check for cancer cells. Layers continue to be removed until no more cancer cells are seen. This type of surgery removes as little normal tissue as possible and is often used where appearance is important, such as on the skin.

- Wide local excision: Removal of the tumor along with some normal tissue around it. For tumors of the head, neck, abdomen, and trunk, as little normal tissue as possible is removed.

- Limb-sparing surgery: Removal of the tumor in an arm or leg without amputation, so the use and appearance of the limb is saved. Radiation therapy or chemotherapy may be given first to shrink the tumor. The tumor is then removed in a wide local excision. Tissue and bone that are removed may be replaced with a graft using tissue and bone taken from another part of the patient's body, or with an implant such as artificial bone.

- Amputation: Surgery to remove part or all of a limb or appendage, such as an arm or leg. Amputation is rarely used to treat soft tissue sarcoma of the arm or leg.

- Lymphadenectomy: A surgical procedure in which lymph nodes are removed and a sample of tissue is checked under a microscope for signs of cancer. This procedure is also called a lymph node dissection.

Radiation therapy

Radiation therapy is a cancer treatment that uses high-energy x-rays or other types of radiation to kill cancer cells or keep them from growing. There are two types of radiation therapy. External radiation therapy uses a machine outside the body to send radiation toward the cancer. Internal radiation therapy uses a radioactive substance sealed in needles, seeds, wires, or catheters that are placed directly into or near the cancer. The way the radiation therapy is given depends on the type and stage of the cancer being treated.

Chemotherapy

Chemotherapy is a cancer treatment that uses drugs to stop the growth of cancer cells, either by killing the cells or by stopping them from dividing. When chemotherapy is taken by mouth or injected into a vein or muscle, the drugs enter the bloodstream and can reach cancer cells throughout the body (systemic chemotherapy). The way the chemotherapy is given depends on the type and stage of the cancer being treated.

New types of treatment are being tested in clinical trials.

Regional chemotherapy

Clinical trials are studying ways to improve the effect of chemotherapy on tumor cells, including the following:

- Regional hyperthermia therapy: A treatment in which tissue around the tumor is exposed to high temperatures to damage and kill cancer cells or to make cancer cells more sensitive to chemotherapy.

- Isolated limb perfusion: A procedure that sends chemotherapy directly to an arm or leg in which the cancer has formed. The flow of blood to and from the limb is temporarily stopped with a tourniquet, and anticancer drugs are put directly into the blood of the limb. This sends a high dose of drugs to the tumor.

Patients may want to think about taking part in a clinical trial.

For some patients, taking part in a clinical trial may be the best treatment choice. Clinical trials are part of the cancer research process. Clinical trials are done to find out if new cancer treatments are safe and effective or better than the standard treatment.

Many of today's standard treatments for cancer are based on earlier clinical trials. Patients who take part in a clinical trial may receive the standard treatment or be among the first to receive a new treatment.

Patients who take part in clinical trials also help improve the way cancer will be treated in the future. Even when clinical trials do not lead to effective new treatments, they often answer important questions and help move research forward.

Patients can enter clinical trials before, during, or after starting their cancer treatment.

Some clinical trials only include patients who have not yet received treatment. Other trials test treatments for patients whose cancer has not gotten better. There are also clinical trials that test new ways to stop cancer from recurring (coming back) or reduce the side effects of cancer treatment.

Clinical trials are taking place in many parts of the country.

Follow-up tests may be needed.

Some of the tests that were done to diagnose the cancer or to find out the stage of the cancer may be repeated. Some tests will be repeated in order to see how well the treatment is working. Decisions about whether to continue, change, or stop treatment may be based on the results of these tests. This is sometimes called re-staging.

Some of the tests will continue to be done from time to time after treatment has ended. The results of these tests can show if your condition has changed or if the cancer has recurred (come back). These tests are sometimes called follow-up tests or check-ups.

Chapter 28

Skin Cancer

Chapter Contents

Section 28.1

Skin Cancer

Text in this section is excerpted from "Skin Cancer Treatment,"
National Cancer Institute at the National Institutes of Health (NIH),
April 2, 2015.

Skin cancer is a disease in which malignant (cancer) cells form in the tissues of the skin.

The skin is the body's largest organ. It protects against heat, sunlight, injury, and infection. Skin also helps control body temperature and stores water, fat, and vitamin D. The skin has several layers, but the two main layers are the epidermis (upper or outer layer) and the dermis (lower or inner layer). Skin cancer begins in the epidermis, which is made up of three kinds of cells:

• Squamous cells: Thin, flat cells that form the top layer of the epidermis.

• Basal cells: Round cells under the squamous cells.

• Melanocytes: Cells that make melanin and are found in the lower part of the epidermis. Melanin is the pigment that gives skin its natural color. When skin is exposed to the sun, melanocytes make more pigment and cause the skin to darken.

Skin cancer can occur anywhere on the body, but it is most common in skin that is often exposed to sunlight, such as the face, neck, hands, and arms.

There are different types of cancer that start in the skin.

The most common types are basal cell carcinoma and squamous cell carcinoma, which are nonmelanoma skin cancers. Nonmelanoma skin cancers rarely spread to other parts of the body. Melanoma is the rarest form of skin cancer. It is more likely to invade nearby tissues and spread to other parts of the body. Actinic keratosis is a skin condition that sometimes becomes squamous cell carcinoma.

Skin color and being exposed to sunlight can increase the risk of nonmelanoma skin cancer and actinic keratosis.

Anything that increases your chance of getting a disease is called a risk factor. Having a risk factor does not mean that you will get cancer; not having risk factors doesn't mean that you will not get cancer. Talk with your doctor if you think you may be at risk. Risk factors for basal cell carcinoma and squamous cell carcinoma include the following:

- Being exposed to natural sunlight or artificial sunlight (such as from tanning beds) over long periods of time.
- Having a fair complexion, which includes the following:
  - Fair skin that freckles and burns easily, does not tan, or tans poorly.
  - Blue or green or other light-colored eyes.
  - Red or blond hair.
- Having actinic keratosis.
- Past treatment with radiation.
- Having a weakened immune system.
- Having certain changes in the genes that are linked to skin cancer.
- Being exposed to arsenic.
- Risk factors for actinic keratosis include the following:
- Being exposed to natural sunlight or artificial sunlight (such as from tanning beds) over long periods of time.
- Having a fair complexion, which includes the following:
  - Fair skin that freckles and burns easily, does not tan, or tans poorly.
  - Blue or green or other light-colored eyes.
  - Red or blond hair.

Nonmelanoma skin cancer and actinic keratosis often appear as a change in the skin.

Not all changes in the skin are a sign of nonmelanoma skin cancer or actinic keratosis. Check with your doctor if you notice any changes in your skin.

Signs of nonmelanoma skin cancer include the following:

- A sore that does not heal.
- Areas of the skin that are:
  - Raised, smooth, shiny, and look pearly.
  - Firm and look like a scar, and may be white, yellow, or waxy.
  - Raised, and red or reddish-brown.
  - Scaly, bleeding or crusty.

Signs of actinic keratosis include the following:

- A rough, red, pink, or brown, raised, scaly patch on the skin that may be flat or raised.
- Cracking or peeling of the lower lip that is not helped by lip balm or petroleum jelly.

Tests or procedures that examine the skin are used to detect (find) and diagnose nonmelanoma skin cancer and actinic keratosis.

The following procedures may be used:

- **Skin exam**: A doctor or nurse checks the skin for bumps or spots that look abnormal in color, size, shape, or texture.
- **Skin biopsy**: All or part of the abnormal-looking growth is cut from the skin and viewed under a microscope by a pathologist to check for signs of cancer. There are four main types of skin biopsies:
  - **Shave biopsy**: A sterile razor blade is used to "shave-off" the abnormal-looking growth.
  - **Punch biopsy**: A special instrument called a punch or a trephine is used to remove a circle of tissue from the abnormal-looking growth.
  - **Incisional biopsy**: A scalpel is used to remove part of a growth.
  - **Excisional biopsy**: A scalpel is used to remove the entire growth.

Certain factors affect prognosis (chance of recovery) and treatment options.

The prognosis (chance of recovery) depends mostly on the stage of the cancer and the type of treatment used to remove the cancer.

Treatment options depend on the following:

- The stage of the cancer (whether it has spread deeper into the skin or to other places in the body).

- The type of cancer.

- The size of the tumor and what part of the body it affects.

- The patient's general health.

Stages of Skin Cancer

After nonmelanoma skin cancer has been diagnosed, tests are done to find out if cancer cells have spread within the skin or to other parts of the body.

The process used to find out if cancer has spread within the skin or to other parts of the body is called staging. The information gathered from the staging process determines the stage of the disease. It is important to know the stage in order to plan treatment.

The following tests and procedures may be used in the staging process:

- **CT scan (CAT scan):** A procedure that makes a series of detailed pictures of areas inside the body, taken from different angles. The pictures are made by a computer linked to an x-ray machine. A dye may be injected into a vein or swallowed to help the organs or tissues show up more clearly. This procedure is also called computed tomography, computerized tomography, or computerized axial tomography.

- **MRI (magnetic resonance imaging):** A procedure that uses a magnet, radio waves, and a computer to make a series of detailed pictures of areas inside the body. This procedure is also called nuclear magnetic resonance imaging (NMRI).

- **Lymph node biopsy:** For squamous cell carcinoma, the lymph nodes may be removed and checked to see if cancer has spread to them.

There are three ways that cancer spreads in the body.

Cancer can spread through tissue, the lymph system, and the blood:

- Tissue. The cancer spreads from where it began by growing into nearby areas.

- Lymph system. The cancer spreads from where it began by getting into the lymph system. The cancer travels through the lymph vessels to other parts of the body.

- Blood. The cancer spreads from where it began by getting into the blood. The cancer travels through the blood vessels to other parts of the body.

Cancer may spread from where it began to other parts of the body.

When cancer spreads to another part of the body, it is called metastasis. Cancer cells break away from where they began (the primary tumor) and travel through the lymph system or blood.

- Lymph system. The cancer gets into the lymph system, travels through the lymph vessels, and forms a tumor (metastatic tumor) in another part of the body.

- Blood. The cancer gets into the blood, travels through the blood vessels, and forms a tumor (metastatic tumor) in another part of the body.

The metastatic tumor is the same type of cancer as the primary tumor. For example, if skin cancer spreads to the lung, the cancer cells in the lung are actually skin cancer cells. The disease is metastatic skin cancer, not lung cancer.

Staging of nonmelanoma skin cancer depends on whether the tumor has certain "high-risk" features and if the tumor is on the eyelid.

Staging for nonmelanoma skin cancer that is on the eyelid is different from staging for nonmelanoma skin cancer that affects other parts of the body.

The following are high-risk features for nonmelanoma skin cancer that is not on the eyelid:

- The tumor is thicker than 2 millimeters.

- The tumor is described as Clark level IV (has spread into the lower layer of the dermis) or Clark level V (has spread into the layer of fat below the skin).

- The tumor has grown and spread along nerve pathways.

- The tumor began on an ear or on a lip that has hair on it.

- The tumor has cells that look very different from normal cells under a microscope.

The following stages are used for nonmelanoma skin cancer that is not on the eyelid:

Stage 0 (Carcinoma in Situ)

In stage 0, abnormal cells are found in the squamous cell or basal cell layer of the epidermis (topmost layer of the skin). These abnormal cells may become cancer and spread into nearby normal tissue. Stage 0 is also called carcinoma in situ.

Stage I

In stage I, cancer has formed. The tumor is not larger than 2 centimeters at its widest point and may have one high-risk feature.

Stage II

In stage II, the tumor is either:

- larger than 2 centimeters at its widest point; or

- any size and has two or more high-risk features.

Stage III

In stage III:

- The tumor has spread to the jaw, eye socket, or side of the skull. Cancer may have spread to one lymph node on the same side of the body as the tumor. The lymph node is not larger than 3 centimeters.

or

- Cancer has spread to one lymph node on the same side of the body as the tumor. The lymph node is not larger than 3 centimeters and one of the following is true:

- the tumor is not larger than 2 centimeters at its widest point and may have one high-risk feature; or

- the tumor is larger than 2 centimeters at its widest point; or

- the tumor is any size and has two or more high-risk features.

Stage IV

In stage IV, one of the following is true:

- The tumor is any size and may have spread to the jaw, eye socket, or side of the skull. Cancer has spread to one lymph node on the same side of the body as the tumor and the affected node is larger than 3 centimeters but not larger than 6 centimeters, or cancer has spread to more than one lymph node on one or both sides of the body and the affected nodes are not larger than 6 centimeters; or

- The tumor is any size and may have spread to the jaw, eye socket, skull, spine, or ribs. Cancer has spread to one lymph node that is larger than 6 centimeters; or

- The tumor is any size and has spread to the base of the skull, spine, or ribs. Cancer may have spread to the lymph nodes; or

- Cancer has spread to other parts of the body, such as the lung.

The following stages are used for nonmelanoma skin cancer on the eyelid:

Stage 0 (Carcinoma in Situ)

In stage 0, abnormal cells are found in the epidermis (topmost layer of the skin). These abnormal cells may become cancer and spread into nearby normal tissue. Stage 0 is also called carcinoma in situ.

Stage I

Stage I is divided into stages IA, IB, and IC.

- Stage IA: The tumor is 5 millimeters or smaller and has not spread to the connective tissue of the eyelid or to the edge of the eyelid where the lashes are.

- Stage IB: The tumor is larger than 5 millimeters but not larger than 10 millimeters or has spread to the connective tissue of the eyelid or to the edge of the eyelid where the lashes are.

- Stage IC: The tumor is larger than 10 millimeters but not larger than 20 millimeters or has spread through the full thickness of the eyelid.

Stage II

In stage II, one of the following is true:

- The tumor is larger than 20 millimeters.
- The tumor has spread to nearby parts of the eye or eye socket.
- The tumor has spread to spaces around the nerves in the eyelid.

Stage III

Stage III is divided into stages IIIA, IIIB, and IIIC.

- Stage IIIA: To remove all of the tumor, the whole eye and part of the optic nerve must be removed. The bone, muscles, fat, and connective tissue around the eye may also be removed.
- Stage IIIB: The tumor may be anywhere in or near the eye and has spread to nearby lymph nodes.
- Stage IIIC: The tumor has spread to structures around the eye or in the face, or to the brain, and cannot be removed in surgery.

Stage IV

The tumor has spread to distant parts of the body.

Treatment is based on the type of nonmelanoma skin cancer or other skin condition diagnosed:

Basal cell carcinoma

Basal cell carcinoma is the most common type of skin cancer. It usually occurs on areas of the skin that have been in the sun, most often the nose. Often this cancer appears as a raised bump that looks smooth and pearly. Another type looks like a scar and is flat and firm and may be white, yellow, or waxy. Basal cell carcinoma may spread to tissues around the cancer, but it usually does not spread to other parts of the body.

Squamous cell carcinoma

Squamous cell carcinoma occurs on areas of the skin that have been in the sun, such as the ears, lower lip, and the back of the hands. Squamous cell carcinoma may also appear on areas of the skin that have been burned or exposed to chemicals or radiation. Often this cancer appears as a firm red bump. The tumor may feel scaly, bleed, or form a crust. Squamous cell tumors may spread to nearby lymph nodes. Squamous cell carcinoma that has not spread can usually be cured.

Actinic keratosis

Actinic keratosis is a skin condition that is not cancer, but sometimes changes into squamous cell carcinoma. It usually occurs in areas that have been exposed to the sun, such as the face, the back of the hands, and the lower lip. It looks like rough, red, pink, or brown scaly patches on the skin that may be flat or raised, or the lower lip cracks and peels and is not helped by lip balm or petroleum jelly.

Treatment Options for Nonmelanoma Skin Cancer

Basal Cell Carcinoma

Treatment of basal cell carcinoma may include the following:

- Simple excision.
- Mohs micrographic surgery.
- Radiation therapy.
- Electrodesiccation and curettage.
- Cryosurgery.
- Photodynamic therapy.
- Topical chemotherapy.
- Topical biologic therapy with imiquimod.
- Laser surgery.
- Treatment of recurrent basal cell carcinoma is usually Mohs micrographic surgery.

Treatment of basal cell carcinoma that is metastatic or cannot be treated with local therapy is usually chemotherapy or a clinical trial of a new treatment.

Squamous Cell Carcinoma

Treatment of squamous cell carcinoma may include the following:

- Simple excision.
- Mohs micrographic surgery.
- Radiation therapy.
- Electrodesiccation and curettage.
- Cryosurgery.

Treatment of recurrent squamous cell carcinoma may include the following:

- Simple excision.
- Mohs micrographic surgery.
- Radiation therapy.

Treatment of squamous cell carcinoma that is metastatic or cannot be treated with local therapy may include the following:

- Chemotherapy.
- Retinoid therapy and biologic therapy with interferon.
- A clinical trial of a new treatment.

Treatment Options for Actinic Keratosis

Actinic keratosis is not cancer but is treated because it may develop into cancer. Treatment of actinic keratosis may include the following:

- Topical chemotherapy.
- Topical biologic therapy with imiquimod.
- Cryosurgery.
- Electrodesiccation and curettage.
- Dermabrasion.
- Shave excision.
- Photodynamic therapy.
- Laser surgery.

Section 28.2

Melanoma

Text in this section is excerpted from "Melanoma Treatment,"
National Cancer Institute at the National Institutes of Health (NIH),
May 15, 2015.

General Information About Skin Cancer

***Melanoma is a disease in which malignant (cancer) cells
form in melanocytes (cells that color the skin).***

The skin is the body's largest organ. It protects against heat, sunlight, injury, and infection. Skin also helps control body temperature and stores water, fat, and vitamin D. The skin has several layers, but the two main layers are the epidermis (upper or outer layer) and the dermis (lower or inner layer). Skin cancer begins in the epidermis, which is made up of three kinds of cells:

- Squamous cells: Thin, flat cells that form the top layer of the epidermis.

- Basal cells: Round cells under the squamous cells.

- Melanocytes: Cells that make melanin and are found in the lower part of the epidermis. Melanin is the pigment that gives skin its natural color. When skin is exposed to the sun or artificial light, melanocytes make more pigment and cause the skin to darken.

The number of new cases of melanoma has been increasing over the last 40 years. Melanoma is most common in adults, but it is sometimes found in children and adolescents.

There are different types of cancer that start in the skin.

There are two forms of skin cancer: melanoma and nonmelanoma. Melanoma is the rarest form of skin cancer. It is more likely to invade nearby tissues and spread to other parts of the body than other

646

types of skin cancer. When melanoma starts in the skin, it is called cutaneous melanoma. Melanoma may also occur in mucous membranes (thin, moist layers of tissue that cover surfaces such as the lips).

The most common types of skin cancer are basal cell carcinoma and squamous cell carcinoma. They are nonmelanoma skin cancers. Nonmelanoma skin cancers rarely spread to other parts of the body.

Melanoma can occur anywhere on the skin.

In men, melanoma is often found on the trunk (the area from the shoulders to the hips) or the head and neck. In women, melanoma forms most often on the arms and legs.

When melanoma occurs in the eye, it is called intraocular or ocular melanoma.

Unusual moles, exposure to sunlight, and health history can affect the risk of melanoma.

Anything that increases your risk of getting a disease is called a risk factor. Having a risk factor does not mean that you will get cancer; not having risk factors doesn't mean that you will not get cancer. Talk with your doctor if you think you may be at risk.

Risk factors for melanoma include the following:

- Having a fair complexion, which includes the following:

  - Fair skin that freckles and burns easily, does not tan, or tans poorly.

  - Blue or green or other light-colored eyes.

  - Red or blond hair.

- Being exposed to natural sunlight or artificial sunlight (such as from tanning beds) over long periods of time.

- Being exposed to certain factors in the environment (in the air, your home or workplace, and your food and water). Some of the environmental risk factors for melanoma are radiation, solvents, vinyl chloride, and PCBs.

- Having a history of many blistering sunburns, especially as a child or teenager.

- Having several large or many small moles.

- Having a family history of unusual moles (atypical nevus syndrome).

- Having a family or personal history of melanoma.

- Being white.

- Having a weakened immune system.

- Having certain changes in the genes that are linked to melanoma.

Being white or having a fair complexion increases the risk of melanoma, but anyone can have melanoma, including people with dark skin.

Signs of melanoma include a change in the way a mole or pigmented area looks.

These and other signs and symptoms may be caused by melanoma or by other conditions. Check with your doctor if you have any of the following:

- A mole that:
    - changes in size, shape, or color.
    - has irregular edges or borders.
    - is more than one color.
    - is asymmetrical (if the mole is divided in half, the 2 halves are different in size or shape).
    - itches.
    - oozes, bleeds, or is ulcerated (a hole forms in the skin when the top layer of cells breaks down and the tissue below shows through).
- A change in pigmented (colored) skin.
- Satellite moles (new moles that grow near an existing mole).

Tests that examine the skin are used to detect (find) and diagnose melanoma.

If a mole or pigmented area of the skin changes or looks abnormal, the following tests and procedures can help find and diagnose melanoma:

- **Skin exam:** A doctor or nurse checks the skin for moles, birth-marks, or other pigmented areas that look abnormal in color, size, shape, or texture.

- **Biopsy:** A procedure to remove the abnormal tissue and a small amount of normal tissue around it. A pathologist looks at the tissue under a microscope to check for cancer cells. It can be hard to tell the difference between a colored mole and an early melanoma lesion. Patients may want to have the sample of tissue checked by a second pathologist. If the abnormal mole or lesion is cancer, the sample of tissue may also be tested for certain gene changes.

It is important that abnormal areas of the skin not be shaved off or cauterized (destroyed with a hot instrument, an electric current, or a caustic substance) because cancer cells that remain may grow and spread.

Certain factors affect prognosis (chance of recovery) and treatment options.

The prognosis (chance of recovery) and treatment options depend on the following:

- The thickness of the tumor and where it is in the body.

- How quickly the cancer cells are dividing.

- Whether there was bleeding or ulceration of the tumor.

- How much cancer is in the lymph nodes.

- The number of places cancer has spread to in the body.

- The level of lactate dehydrogenase (LDH) in the blood.

- Whether the cancer has certain mutations (changes) in a gene called BRAF.

- The patient's age and general health.

Stages of Melanoma

After melanoma has been diagnosed, tests are done to find out if cancer cells have spread within the skin or to other parts of the body.

The process used to find out whether cancer has spread within the skin or to other parts of the body is called staging. The information gathered from the staging process determines the stage of the disease. It is important to know the stage in order to plan treatment.

The following tests and procedures may be used in the staging process:

- **Physical exam and history:** An exam of the body to check general signs of health, including checking for signs of disease, such as lumps or anything else that seems unusual. A history of the patient's health habits and past illnesses and treatments will also be taken.

- **Lymph node mapping and sentinel lymph node biopsy:** Procedures in which a radioactive substance and/or blue dye is injected near the tumor. The substance or dye flows through lymph ducts to the sentinel node or nodes (the first lymph node or nodes where cancer cells are likely to spread). The surgeon removes only the nodes with the radioactive substance or dye. A pathologist views a sample of tissue under a microscope to check for cancer cells. If no cancer cells are found, it may not be necessary to remove more nodes.

- **CT scan (CAT scan):** A procedure that makes a series of detailed pictures of areas inside the body taken from different angles. The pictures are made by a computer linked to an x-ray machine. A dye may be injected into a vein or swallowed to help the organs or tissues show up more clearly. This procedure is also called computed tomography, computerized tomography, or computerized axial tomography. For melanoma, pictures may be taken of the chest, abdomen, and pelvis.

- **PET scan (positron emission tomography scan):** A procedure to find malignant tumor cells in the body. A small amount of radioactive glucose (sugar) is injected into a vein. The PET scanner rotates around the body and makes a picture of where glucose is being used in the body. Malignant tumor cells show up brighter in the picture because they are more active and take up more glucose than normal cells do.

- **MRI (magnetic resonance imaging) with gadolinium:** A procedure that uses a magnet, radio waves, and a computer to make a series of detailed pictures of areas inside the body, such as the brain. A substance called gadolinium is injected into a vein. The gadolinium collects around the cancer cells so they show up brighter in the picture. This procedure is also called nuclear magnetic resonance imaging (NMRI).

- **Blood chemistry studies:** A procedure in which a blood sample is checked to measure the amounts of certain substances released into the blood by organs and tissues in the body. For melanoma, the blood is checked for an enzyme called lactate dehydrogenase (LDH). LDH levels that are higher than normal may be a sign of melanoma.

The results of these tests are viewed together with the results of the tumor biopsy to find out the stage of the melanoma.

There are three ways that cancer spreads in the body.

Cancer can spread through tissue, the lymph system, and the blood:

- Tissue. The cancer spreads from where it began by growing into nearby areas.

- Lymph system. The cancer spreads from where it began by getting into the lymph system. The cancer travels through the lymph vessels to other parts of the body.

- Blood. The cancer spreads from where it began by getting into the blood. The cancer travels through the blood vessels to other parts of the body.

Cancer may spread from where it began to other parts of the body.

When cancer spreads to another part of the body, it is called metastasis. Cancer cells break away from where they began (the primary tumor) and travel through the lymph system or blood.

- Lymph system. The cancer gets into the lymph system, travels through the lymph vessels, and forms a tumor (metastatic tumor) in another part of the body.

- Blood. The cancer gets into the blood, travels through the blood vessels, and forms a tumor (metastatic tumor) in another part of the body.

The metastatic tumor is the same type of cancer as the primary tumor. For example, if melanoma spreads to the lung, the cancer cells in the lung are actually melanoma cells. The disease is metastatic melanoma, not lung cancer.

651

The method used to stage melanoma is based mainly on the thickness of the tumor and whether cancer has spread to lymph nodes or other parts of the body.

The staging of melanoma depends on the following:

- The thickness of the tumor. The thickness is described using the Breslow scale.

- Whether the tumor is ulcerated (has broken through the skin).

- Whether the tumor has spread to the lymph nodes and if the lymph nodes are joined together (matted).

- Whether the tumor has spread to other parts of the body.

The following stages are used for melanoma:

Stage 0 (Melanoma in Situ)

In stage 0, abnormal melanocytes are found in the epidermis. These abnormal melanocytes may become cancer and spread into nearby normal tissue. Stage 0 is also called melanoma in situ.

Stage I

In stage I, cancer has formed. Stage I is divided into stages IA and IB.

- Stage IA: In stage IA, the tumor is not more than 1 millimeter thick, with no ulceration.

- Stage IB: In stage IB, the tumor is either:

  - not more than 1 millimeter thick and it has ulceration; or

  - more than 1 but not more than 2 millimeters thick, with no ulceration.

Stage II

Stage II is divided into stages IIA, IIB, and IIC.

- Stage IIA: In stage IIA, the tumor is either:

  - more than 1 but not more than 2 millimeters thick, with ulceration; or

  - more than 2 but not more than 4 millimeters thick, with no ulceration.

652

- Stage IIB: In stage IIB, the tumor is either:
  - more than 2 but not more than 4 millimeters thick, with ulceration; or
  - more than 4 millimeters thick, with no ulceration.
- Stage IIC: In stage IIC, the tumor is more than 4 millimeters thick, with ulceration.

Stage III

In stage III, the tumor is any thickness, and has spread to one or more lymph nodes. One or more of the following may also be true:

- Lymph nodes are joined together (matted).
- Cancer is in a lymph vessel between the primary tumor and nearby lymph nodes. The cancer is more than 2 centimeters away from the primary tumor.
- Very small tumors are found on or under the skin, not more than 2 centimeters away from the primary tumor.

Stage IV

In stage IV, the cancer has spread to other places in the body, such as the lung, liver, brain, bone, soft tissue, or gastrointestinal (GI) tract. Cancer may have spread to places in the skin far away from where it first started.

Treatment Option Overview

There are different types of treatment for patients with melanoma.

Different types of treatment are available for patients with melanoma. Some treatments are standard (the currently used treatment), and some are being tested in clinical trials. A treatment clinical trial is a research study meant to help improve current treatments or obtain information on new treatments for patients with cancer. When clinical trials show that a new treatment is better than the standard treatment, the new treatment may become the standard treatment. Patients may want to think about taking part in a clinical trial. Some clinical trials are open only to patients who have not started treatment.

Five types of standard treatment are used:

Surgery

Surgery to remove the tumor is the primary treatment of all stages of melanoma. A wide local excision is used to remove the melanoma and some of the normal tissue around it. Skin grafting (taking skin from another part of the body to replace the skin that is removed) may be done to cover the wound caused by surgery.

It is important to know whether cancer has spread to the lymph nodes. Lymph node mapping and sentinel lymph node biopsy are done to check for cancer in the sentinel lymph node (the first lymph node the cancer is likely to spread to from the tumor) during surgery. A radioactive substance and/or blue dye is injected near the tumor. The substance or dye flows through the lymph ducts to the lymph nodes. The first lymph node to receive the substance or dye is removed. A pathologist views the tissue under a microscope to look for cancer cells. If cancer cells are found, more lymph nodes will be removed and tissue samples will be checked for signs of cancer. This is called a lymphadenectomy.

Even if the doctor removes all the melanoma that can be seen at the time of surgery, some patients may be given chemotherapy after surgery to kill any cancer cells that are left. Chemotherapy given after surgery, to lower the risk that the cancer will come back, is called adjuvant therapy.

Surgery to remove cancer that has spread to the lymph nodes, lung, gastrointestinal (GI) tract, bone, or brain may be done to improve the patient's quality of life by controlling symptoms.

Chemotherapy

Chemotherapy is a cancer treatment that uses drugs to stop the growth of cancer cells, either by killing the cells or by stopping them from dividing. When chemotherapy is taken by mouth or injected into a vein or muscle, the drugs enter the bloodstream and can reach cancer cells throughout the body (systemic chemotherapy). When chemotherapy is placed directly into the cerebrospinal fluid, an organ, or a body cavity such as the abdomen, the drugs mainly affect cancer cells in those areas (regional chemotherapy).

One type of regional chemotherapy is hyper thermic isolated limb perfusion. With this method, anticancer drugs go directly to the arm or leg the cancer is in. The flow of blood to and from the limb is temporarily stopped with a tourniquet. A warm solution with the anticancer drug is put directly into the blood of the limb. This gives a high dose of drugs to the area where the cancer is.

The way the chemotherapy is given depends on the type and stage of the cancer being treated.

Radiation therapy

Radiation therapy is a cancer treatment that uses high-energy x-rays or other types of radiation to kill cancer cells or keep them from growing. There are two types of radiation therapy. External radiation therapy uses a machine outside the body to send radiation toward the cancer. Internal radiation therapy uses a radioactive substance sealed in needles, seeds, wires, or catheters that are placed directly into or near the cancer.

The way the radiation therapy is given depends on the type and stage of the cancer being treated. External radiation therapy is used to treat melanoma.

Biologic therapy

Biologic therapy is a treatment that uses the patient's immune system to fight cancer. Substances made by the body or made in a laboratory are used to boost, direct, or restore the body's natural defenses against cancer. This type of cancer treatment is also called biotherapy or immunotherapy. The following types of biologic therapy are being used or studied in the treatment of melanoma:

- Interferon: Interferon affects the division of cancer cells and can slow tumor growth.

- Interleukin-2 (IL-2): IL-2 boosts the growth and activity of many immune cells, especially lymphocytes (a type of white blood cell). Lymphocytes can attack and kill cancer cells.

- Tumor necrosis factor (TNF) therapy: TNF is a protein made by white blood cells in response to an antigen or infection. TNF is made in the laboratory and used as a treatment to kill cancer cells. It is being studied in the treatment of melanoma.

- Ipilimumab: Ipilimumab is a monoclonal antibody that boosts the body's immune response against melanoma cells. Other monoclonal antibodies are being studied in the treatment of melanoma.

Targeted therapy

Targeted therapy is a type of treatment that uses drugs or other substances to attack cancer cells. Targeted therapies usually cause less harm to normal cells than chemotherapy or radiation therapy. The following types of targeted therapy are used or being studied in the treatment of melanoma:

- Signal transduction inhibitor therapy: Signal transduction inhibitors block signals that are passed from one molecule to another inside a cell. Blocking these signals may kill cancer cells.

  - Vemurafenib, dabrafenib, and trametinib are signal transduction inhibitors used to treat some patients with advanced melanoma or tumors that cannot be removed by surgery. Vemurafenib and dabrafenib block the activity of proteins made by mutant BRAF genes. Trametinib affects the growth and survival of cancer cells.

- Oncolytic virus therapy: A type of targeted therapy that is being studied in the treatment of melanoma. Oncolytic virus therapy uses a virus that infects and breaks down cancer cells but not normal cells. Radiation therapy or chemotherapy may be given after oncolytic virus therapy to kill more cancer cells.

- Monoclonal antibody therapy: Monoclonal antibodies are made in the laboratory from a single type of immune system cell. These antibodies can identify substances on cancer cells or normal substances that may help cancer cells grow. The antibodies attach to the substances and kill the cancer cells, block their growth, or keep them from spreading. Monoclonal antibodies are given by infusion. They may be used alone or to carry drugs, toxins, or radioactive material directly to cancer cells.

  - Pembrolizumab is a monoclonal antibody used to treat patients whose tumor cannot be removed by surgery or has spread to other parts of the body.

- Angiogenesis inhibitors: A type of targeted therapy that is being studied in the treatment of melanoma. Angiogenesis inhibitors block the growth of new blood vessels. In cancer treatment, they may be given to prevent the growth of new blood vessels that tumors need to grow.

Patients may want to think about taking part in a clinical trial.

For some patients, taking part in a clinical trial may be the best treatment choice. Clinical trials are part of the cancer research process. Clinical trials are done to find out if new cancer treatments are safe and effective or better than the standard treatment.

Many of today's standard treatments for cancer are based on earlier clinical trials. Patients who take part in a clinical trial may receive the standard treatment or be among the first to receive a new treatment.

Patients who take part in clinical trials also help improve the way cancer will be treated in the future. Even when clinical trials do not lead to effective new treatments, they often answer important questions and help move research forward.

Patients can enter clinical trials before, during, or after starting their cancer treatment.

Some clinical trials only include patients who have not yet received treatment. Other trials test treatments for patients whose cancer has not gotten better. There are also clinical trials that test new ways to stop cancer from recurring (coming back) or reduce the side effects of cancer treatment.

Clinical trials are taking place in many parts of the country.

Follow-up tests may be needed.

Some of the tests that were done to diagnose the cancer or to find out the stage of the cancer may be repeated. Some tests will be repeated in order to see how well the treatment is working. Decisions about whether to continue, change, or stop treatment may be based on the results of these tests. This is sometimes called re-staging.

Some of the tests will continue to be done from time to time after treatment has ended. The results of these tests can show if your condition has changed or if the cancer has recurred (come back). These tests are sometimes called follow-up tests or check-ups.

Treatment Options by Stage

Stage 0 (Melanoma in Situ)

Treatment of stage 0 is usually surgery to remove the area of abnormal cells and a small amount of normal tissue around it.

Stage I Melanoma

Treatment of stage I melanoma may include the following:

- Surgery to remove the tumor and some of the normal tissue around it. Sometimes lymph node mapping and removal of lymph nodes is also done.

- A clinical trial of new ways to find cancer cells in the lymph nodes.

Stage II Melanoma

Treatment of stage II melanoma may include the following:

- Surgery to remove the tumor and some of the normal tissue around it. Sometimes lymph node mapping and sentinel lymph node biopsy are done to check for cancer in the lymph nodes at the same time as the surgery to remove the tumor. If cancer is found in the sentinel lymph node, more lymph nodes may be removed.

- Surgery followed by biologic therapy with interferon if there is a high risk that the cancer will come back.

- A clinical trial of new types of treatment to be used after surgery.

Stage III Melanoma That Can Be Removed By Surgery

Treatment of stage III melanoma that can be removed by surgery may include the following:

- Surgery to remove the tumor and some of the normal tissue around it. Skin grafting may be done to cover the wound caused by surgery. Sometimes lymph node mapping and sentinel lymph node biopsy are done to check for cancer in the lymph nodes at the same time as the surgery to remove the tumor. If cancer is found in the sentinel lymph node, more lymph nodes may be removed.

- Surgery followed by biologic therapy with interferon if there is a high risk that the cancer will come back.

- A clinical trial of new kinds of treatments to be used after surgery.

- A clinical trial of injections into the tumor, such as oncolytic virus therapy.

Stage III Melanoma That Cannot Be Removed By Surgery, Stage IV Melanoma, and Recurrent Melanoma

Treatment of stage III melanoma that cannot be removed by surgery, stage IV melanoma, and recurrent melanoma may include the following:

- Targeted therapy with vemurafenib or dabrafenib.

- Biologic therapy with interleukin-2 (IL-2), ipilimumab, or pembrolizumab.

- Chemotherapy.

- Palliative therapy to relieve symptoms and improve the quality of life. This may include:

  - Surgery to remove lymph nodes or tumors in the lung, gastrointestinal (GI) tract, bone, or brain.

  - Radiation therapy to the brain, spinal cord, or bone.

Treatments that are being studied in clinical trials for stage III melanoma that cannot be removed by surgery, stage IV melanoma, and recurrent melanoma include the following:

- Biologic therapy agents alone or in combination.

- Targeted therapy with other signal transduction inhibitors.

- Angiogenesis inhibitors.

- Targeted therapy for melanoma with gene mutations.

- Treatment with injections into the tumor, such as oncolytic virus therapy.

- Surgery to remove all known cancer.

- Regional chemotherapy (hyperthermic isolated limb perfusion). Some patients may also have biologic therapy with tumor necrosis factor.

- Systemic chemotherapy.

Section 28.3

Merkel Cell Carcinoma

Text in this section is excerpted from "Merkel Cell Carcinoma
Treatment," National Cancer Institute at the National Institutes of
Health (NIH), May 5, 2015.

General Information About Merkel Cell Carcinoma

*Merkel cell carcinoma is a very rare disease in which
malignant (cancer) cells form in the skin.*

Merkel cells are found in the top layer of the skin. These cells are
very close to the nerve endings that receive the sensation of touch.
Merkel cell carcinoma, also called neuroendocrine carcinoma of the
skin or trabecular cancer, is a very rare type of skin cancer that forms
when Merkel cells grow out of control. Merkel cell carcinoma starts
most often in areas of skin exposed to the sun, especially the head and
neck, as well as the arms, legs, and trunk.

Merkel cell carcinoma tends to grow quickly and to metastasize
(spread) at an early stage. It usually spreads first to nearby lymph
nodes and then may spread to lymph nodes or skin in distant parts of
the body, lungs, brain, bones, or other organs.

*Sun exposure and having a weak immune system can affect
the risk of Merkel cell carcinoma.*

Anything that increases your risk of getting a disease is called a
risk factor. Having a risk factor does not mean that you will get cancer; not having risk factors doesn't mean that you will not get cancer.
Talk with your doctor if you think you may be at risk. Risk factors for
Merkel cell carcinoma include the following:

- Being exposed to a lot of natural sunlight.

- Being exposed to artificial sunlight, such as from tanning beds or
  psoralen and ultraviolet A (PUVA) therapy for psoriasis.

- Having an immune system weakened by disease, such as chronic lymphocytic leukemia or HIV infection.
- Taking drugs that make the immune system less active, such as after an organ transplant.
- Having a history of other types of cancer.
- Being older than 50 years, male, or white.

Merkel cell carcinoma usually appears as a single painless lump on sun-exposed skin.

This and other changes in the skin may be caused by Merkel cell carcinoma or by other conditions. Check with your doctor if you see changes in your skin.

Merkel cell carcinoma usually appears on sun-exposed skin as a single lump that is:

- Fast-growing.
- Painless.
- Firm and dome-shaped or raised.
- Red or violet in color.

Tests and procedures that examine the skin are used to detect (find) and diagnose Merkel cell carcinoma.

The following tests and procedures may be used:

- **Physical exam and history:** An exam of the body to check general signs of health, including checking for signs of disease, such as lumps or anything else that seems unusual. A history of the patient's health habits and past illnesses and treatments will also be taken.
- **Full-body skin exam:** A doctor or nurse checks the skin for bumps or spots that look abnormal in color, size, shape, or texture. The size, shape, and texture of the lymph nodes will also be checked.
- **Skin biopsy:** The removal of skin cells or tissues so they can be viewed under a microscope by a pathologist to check for signs of cancer.

Certain factors affect prognosis (chance of recovery) and treatment options.

The prognosis (chance of recovery) and treatment options depend on the following:

- The stage of the cancer (the size of the tumor and whether it has spread to the lymph nodes or other parts of the body).

- Where the cancer is in the body.

- Whether the cancer has just been diagnosed or has recurred (come back).

- The patient's age and general health.

Prognosis also depends on how deeply the tumor has grown into the skin.

Stages of Merkel Cell Carcinoma

After Merkel cell carcinoma has been diagnosed, tests are done to find out if cancer cells have spread to other parts of the body.

The process used to find out if cancer has spread to other parts of the body is called staging. The information gathered from the staging process determines the stage of the disease. It is important to know the stage in order to plan treatment.

The following tests and procedures may be used in the staging process:

- **CT scan (CAT scan):** A procedure that makes a series of detailed pictures of areas inside the body, taken from different angles. The pictures are made by a computer linked to an x-ray machine. A dye may be injected into a vein or swallowed to help the organs or tissues show up more clearly. A CT scan of the chest and abdomen may be used to check for primary small cell lung cancer, or to find Merkel cell carcinoma that has spread. A CT scan of the head and neck may also be used to find Merkel cell carcinoma that has spread to the lymph nodes. This procedure is also called computed tomography, computerized tomography, or computerized axial tomography.

- **MRI (magnetic resonance imaging):** A procedure that uses a magnet, radio waves, and a computer to make a series of detailed pictures of areas inside the body. This procedure is also called nuclear magnetic resonance imaging (NMRI).

- **PET scan (positron emission tomography scan):** A procedure to find malignant tumor cells in the body. A small amount of radioactive glucose (sugar) is injected into a vein. The PET scanner rotates around the body and makes a picture of where glucose is being used in the body. Malignant tumor cells show up brighter in the picture because they are more active and take up more glucose than normal cells do.

- **Lymph node biopsy:** There are two main types of lymph node biopsy used to stage Merkel cell carcinoma.

  - **Sentinel lymph node biopsy:** The removal of the sentinel lymph node during surgery. The sentinel lymph node is the first lymph node to receive lymphatic drainage from a tumor. It is the first lymph node the cancer is likely to spread to from the tumor. A radioactive substance and/or blue dye is injected near the tumor. The substance or dye flows through the lymph ducts to the lymph nodes. The first lymph node to receive the substance or dye is removed. A pathologist views the tissue under a microscope to look for cancer cells. If cancer cells are not found, it may not be necessary to remove more lymph nodes.

  - **Lymph node dissection**: A surgical procedure in which the lymph nodes are removed and a sample of tissue is checked under a microscope for signs of cancer. For a regional lymph node dissection, some of the lymph nodes in the tumor area are removed. For a radical lymph node dissection, most or all of the lymph nodes in the tumor area are removed. This procedure is also called lymphadenectomy.

- **Immunohistochemistry**: A test that uses antibodies to check for certain antigens in a sample of tissue. The antibody is usually linked to a radioactive substance or a dye that causes the tissue to light up under a microscope. This type of test may be used to tell the difference between different types of cancer.

There are three ways that cancer spreads in the body.

Cancer can spread through tissue, the lymph system, and the blood:

- Tissue. The cancer spreads from where it began by growing into nearby areas.

- Lymph system. The cancer spreads from where it began by getting into the lymph system. The cancer travels through the lymph vessels to other parts of the body.

- Blood. The cancer spreads from where it began by getting into the blood. The cancer travels through the blood vessels to other parts of the body.

Cancer may spread from where it began to other parts of the body.

When cancer spreads to another part of the body, it is called metastasis. Cancer cells break away from where they began (the primary tumor) and travel through the lymph system or blood.

- Lymph system. The cancer gets into the lymph system, travels through the lymph vessels, and forms a tumor (metastatic tumor) in another part of the body.

- Blood. The cancer gets into the blood, travels through the blood vessels, and forms a tumor (metastatic tumor) in another part of the body.

The metastatic tumor is the same type of cancer as the primary tumor. For example, if Merkel cell carcinoma spreads to the liver, the cancer cells in the liver are actually cancerous Merkel cells. The disease is metastatic Merkel cell carcinoma, not liver cancer.

The following stages are used for Merkel cell carcinoma:

Stage 0 (carcinoma in situ)

In stage 0, the tumor is a group of abnormal cells that remain in the place where they first formed and have not spread. These abnormal cells may become cancer and spread to lymph nodes or distant parts of the body.

Stage IA

In stage IA, the tumor is 2 centimeters or smaller at its widest point and no cancer is found when the lymph nodes are checked under a microscope.

Stage IB

In stage IB, the tumor is 2 centimeters or smaller at its widest point and no swollen lymph nodes are found by a physical exam or imaging tests.

Stage IIA

In stage IIA, the tumor is larger than 2 centimeters and no cancer is found when the lymph nodes are checked under a microscope.

Stage IIB

In stage IIB, the tumor is larger than 2 centimeters and no swollen lymph nodes are found by a physical exam or imaging tests.

Stage IIC

In stage IIC, the tumor may be any size and has spread to nearby bone, muscle, connective tissue, or cartilage. It has not spread to lymph nodes or distant parts of the body.

Stage IIIA

In stage IIIA, the tumor may be any size and may have spread to nearby bone, muscle, connective tissue, or cartilage. Cancer is found in the lymph nodes when they are checked under a microscope.

Stage IIIB

In stage IIIB, the tumor may be any size and may have spread to nearby bone, muscle, connective tissue, or cartilage. Cancer has spread to the lymph nodes near the tumor and is found by a physical exam or imaging test. The lymph nodes are removed and cancer is found in the lymph nodes when they are checked under a microscope. There may also be a second tumor, which is either:

- Between the primary tumor and nearby lymph nodes; or

- Farther away from the center of the body than the primary tumor is.

Stage IV

In stage IV, the tumor may be any size and has spread to distant parts of the body, such as the liver, lung, bone, or brain.

Treatment Option Overview

There are different types of treatment for patients with Merkel cell carcinoma.

Different types of treatments are available for patients with Merkel cell carcinoma. Some treatments are standard (the currently used treatment), and some are being tested in clinical trials. A treatment clinical trial is a research study meant to help improve current treatments or obtain information on new treatments for patients with cancer. When clinical trials show that a new treatment is better than the standard treatment, the new treatment may become the standard treatment. Patients may want to think about taking part in a clinical trial. Some clinical trials are open only to patients who have not started treatment.

Three types of standard treatment are used:

Surgery

One or more of the following surgical procedures may be used to treat Merkel cell carcinoma:

- Wide local excision: The cancer is cut from the skin along with some of the tissue around it. A sentinel lymph node biopsy may be done during the wide local excision procedure. If there is cancer in the lymph nodes, a lymph node dissection also may be done.

- Lymph node dissection: A surgical procedure in which the lymph nodes are removed and a sample of tissue is checked under a microscope for signs of cancer. For a regional lymph node dissection, some of the lymph nodes in the tumor area are removed; for a radical lymph node dissection, most or all of the lymph nodes in the tumor area are removed. This procedure is also called lymphadenectomy.

Even if the doctor removes all the cancer that can be seen at the time of the surgery, some patients may be given chemotherapy or radiation therapy after surgery to kill any cancer cells that are left.

Treatment given after the surgery, to lower the risk that the cancer will come back, is called adjuvant therapy.

Radiation therapy

Radiation therapy is a cancer treatment that uses high-energy x-rays or other types of radiation to kill cancer cells. There are two types of radiation therapy. External radiation therapy uses a machine outside the body to send radiation toward the cancer. Internal radiation therapy uses a radioactive substance sealed in needles, seeds, wires, or catheters that are placed directly into or near the cancer. The way the radiation therapy is given depends on the type and stage of the cancer being treated.

Chemotherapy

Chemotherapy is a cancer treatment that uses drugs to stop the growth of cancer cells, either by killing the cells or by stopping the cells from dividing. When chemotherapy is taken by mouth or injected into a vein or muscle, the drugs enter the bloodstream and can reach cancer cells throughout the body (systemic chemotherapy). When chemotherapy is placed directly into the cerebrospinal fluid, an organ, or a body cavity such as the abdomen, the drugs mainly affect cancer cells in those areas (regional chemotherapy). The way the chemotherapy is given depends on the type and stage of the cancer being treated.

Patients may want to think about taking part in a clinical trial.

For some patients, taking part in a clinical trial may be the best treatment choice. Clinical trials are part of the cancer research process. Clinical trials are done to find out if new cancer treatments are safe and effective or better than the standard treatment.

Many of today's standard treatments for cancer are based on earlier clinical trials. Patients who take part in a clinical trial may receive the standard treatment or be among the first to receive a new treatment.

Patients who take part in clinical trials also help improve the way cancer will be treated in the future. Even when clinical trials do not lead to effective new treatments, they often answer important questions and help move research forward.

Patients can enter clinical trials before, during, or after starting their cancer treatment.

Some clinical trials only include patients who have not yet received treatment. Other trials test treatments for patients whose cancer has not gotten better. There are also clinical trials that test new ways to stop cancer from recurring (coming back) or reduce the side effects of cancer treatment.

Clinical trials are taking place in many parts of the country.

Follow-up tests may be needed.

Some of the tests that were done to diagnose the cancer or to find out the stage of the cancer may be repeated. Some tests will be repeated in order to see how well the treatment is working. Decisions about whether to continue, change, or stop treatment may be based on the results of these tests. This is sometimes called re-staging.

Some of the tests will continue to be done from time to time after treatment has ended. The results of these tests can show if your condition has changed or if the cancer has recurred (come back). These tests are sometimes called follow-up tests or check-ups.

Section 28.4

Kaposi Sarcoma

Text in this section is excerpted from "Kaposi Sarcoma Treatment,"
National Cancer Institute at the National Institutes of Health (NIH),
May 12, 2015.

General Information About Kaposi Sarcoma

Kaposi sarcoma is a disease in which malignant tumors (cancer) can form in the skin, mucous membranes, lymph nodes, and other organs.

Kaposi sarcoma is a cancer that causes lesions (abnormal tissue) to grow in the skin; the mucous membranes lining the mouth, nose, and throat; lymph nodes; or other organs. The lesions are usually purple and are made of cancer cells, new blood vessels, red blood cells, and white blood cells. Kaposi sarcoma is different from other cancers in that lesions may begin in more than one place in the body at the same time.

Human herpesvirus-8 (HHV-8) is found in the lesions of all patients with Kaposi sarcoma. This virus is also called Kaposi sarcoma herpesvirus (KSHV). Most people infected with HHV-8 do not get Kaposi sarcoma. Those infected with HHV-8 who are most likely to develop Kaposi sarcoma have immune systems weakened by disease or by drugs given after an organ transplant.

There are several types of Kaposi sarcoma, including:

- Classic Kaposi sarcoma.

- African Kaposi sarcoma.

- Immunosuppressive therapy–related Kaposi sarcoma.

- Epidemic Kaposi sarcoma.

- Non - epidemic Kaposi sarcoma.

Tests that examine the skin, lungs, and gastrointestinal tract are used to detect (find) and diagnose Kaposi sarcoma.

The following tests and procedures may be used:

- **Physical exam and history**: An exam of the body to check general signs of health, including checking skin and lymph nodes for signs of disease, such as lumps or anything else that seems unusual. A history of the patient's health habits and past illnesses and treatments will also be taken.

- **Chest x-ray**: An x-ray of the organs and bones inside the chest. An x-ray is a type of energy beam that can go through the body and onto film, making a picture of areas inside the body. This is used to find Kaposi sarcoma in the lungs.

- **Biopsy**: The removal of cells or tissues so they can be viewed under a microscope by a pathologist to check for signs of cancer.

One of the following types of biopsies may be done to check for Kaposi sarcoma lesions in the skin:

- **Excisional biopsy**: A scalpel is used to remove the entire skin growth.

- **Incisional biopsy**: A scalpel is used to remove part of a skin growth.

- **Core biopsy**: A wide needle is used to remove part of a skin growth.

- **Fine-needle aspiration (FNA) biopsy**: A thin needle is used to remove part of a skin growth.

An endoscopy or bronchoscopy may be done to check for Kaposi sarcoma lesions in the gastrointestinal tract or lungs.

- **Endoscopy for biopsy**: A procedure to look at organs and tissues inside the body to check for abnormal areas. An endoscope is inserted through an incision (cut) in the skin or opening in the body, such as the mouth. An endoscope is a thin, tube-like instrument with a light and a lens for viewing. It may also have a tool to remove tissue or lymph node samples, which are checked under a microscope for signs of disease. This is used to find Kaposi sarcoma lesions in the gastrointestinal tract.

- **Bronchoscopy for biopsy**: A procedure to look inside the trachea and large airways in the lung for abnormal areas. A bronchoscope is inserted through the nose or mouth into the trachea and lungs. A bronchoscope is a thin, tube-like instrument with a light and a lens for viewing. It may also have a tool to remove tissue samples, which are checked under a microscope for signs of disease. This is used to find Kaposi sarcoma lesions in the lungs.

After Kaposi sarcoma has been diagnosed, tests are done to find out if cancer cells have spread to other parts of the body.

The following tests and procedures may be used to find out if cancer has spread to other parts of the body:

- **Blood chemistry studies**: A procedure in which a blood sample is checked to measure the amounts of certain substances released into the blood by organs and tissues in the body. An unusual (higher or lower than normal) amount of a substance can be a sign of disease in the organ or tissue that makes it.

- **CT scan (CAT scan)**: A procedure that makes a series of detailed pictures of areas inside the body, such as the lung, liver, and spleen, taken from different angles. The pictures are made by a computer linked to an x-ray machine. A dye may be injected into a vein or swallowed to help the organs or tissues show up more clearly. This procedure is also called computed tomography, computerized tomography, or computerized axial tomography.

- **PET scan (positron emission tomography scan)**: A procedure to find malignant tumor cells in the body. A small amount of radioactive glucose (sugar) is injected into a vein. The PET scanner rotates around the body and makes a picture of where glucose is being used in the body. Malignant tumor cells show up brighter in the picture because they are more active and take up more glucose than normal cells do. This imaging test checks for signs of cancer in the lung, liver, and spleen.

- **CD34 lymphocyte count**: A procedure in which a blood sample is checked to measure the amount of CD34 cells (a type of white blood cell). A lower than normal amount of CD34 cells can be a sign the immune system is not working well.

Certain factors affect prognosis (chance of recovery) and treatment options.

The prognosis (chance of recovery) and treatment options depend on the following:

- The type of Kaposi sarcoma.
- The general health of the patient, especially the patient's immune system.
- Whether the cancer has just been diagnosed or has recurred (come back).

Classic Kaposi Sarcoma

Classic Kaposi sarcoma is found most often in older men of Italian or Eastern European Jewish origin.

Classic Kaposi sarcoma is a rare disease that gets worse slowly over many years.

Signs of classic Kaposi sarcoma may include slow-growing lesions on the legs and feet.

Patients may have one or more red, purple, or brown skin lesions on the legs and feet, most often on the ankles or soles of the feet. Over time, lesions may form in other parts of the body, such as the stomach, intestines, or lymph nodes. The lesions usually don't cause any symptoms, but may grow in size and number over a period of 10 years or more. Pressure from the lesions may block the flow of lymph and blood in the legs and cause painful swelling. Lesions in the digestive tract may cause gastrointestinal bleeding.

Another cancer may develop.

Some patients with classic Kaposi sarcoma may develop another type of cancer before the Kaposi sarcoma lesions appear or later in life. Most often, this second cancer is non-Hodgkin lymphoma. Frequent follow-up is needed to watch for these second cancers.

African Kaposi Sarcoma

African Kaposi sarcoma is a fairly common form of the disease found in young adult males who live near the equator in Africa. Signs of African Kaposi sarcoma can be the same as classic Kaposi sarcoma. However, African Kaposi sarcoma can also be found in a much more aggressive form that may cause sores on the skin and spread from the skin to the tissues to the bone. Another form of Kaposi sarcoma that is common in young children in Africa does not affect the skin but spreads through the lymph nodes to vital organs, and quickly becomes fatal.

This type of Kaposi sarcoma is not common in the United States.

Immunosuppressive Therapy–related Kaposi Sarcoma

Immunosuppressive therapy–related Kaposi sarcoma is found in patients who have had an organ transplant (for example, a kidney, heart, or liver transplant). These patients take drugs to keep their immune systems from attacking the new organ. When the body's immune system is weakened by these drugs, diseases like Kaposi sarcoma can develop.

Immunosuppressive therapy–related Kaposi sarcoma often affects only the skin, but may also occur in the mucous membranes or certain other organs of the body.

This type of Kaposi sarcoma is also called transplant-related or acquired Kaposi sarcoma.

Epidemic Kaposi Sarcoma

Epidemic Kaposi sarcoma is found in patients who have acquired immunodeficiency syndrome (AIDS).

Epidemic Kaposi sarcoma occurs in patients who have acquired immunodeficiency syndrome (AIDS). AIDS is caused by the human immunodeficiency virus (HIV), which attacks and weakens the immune system. When the body's immune system is weakened by HIV, infections and cancers such as Kaposi sarcoma can develop.

Most cases of epidemic Kaposi sarcoma in the United States have been diagnosed in homosexual or bisexual men infected with HIV.

Signs of epidemic Kaposi sarcoma can include lesions that form in many parts of the body.

The signs of epidemic Kaposi sarcoma can include lesions in different parts of the body, including any of the following:

- Skin.
- Lining of the mouth.
- Lymph nodes.
- Stomach and intestines.
- Lungs and lining of the chest.
- Liver.
- Spleen.

Kaposi sarcoma is sometimes found in the lining of the mouth during a regular dental check-up.

In most patients with epidemic Kaposi sarcoma, the disease will spread to other parts of the body over time. Fever, weight loss, or diarrhea can occur. In the later stages of epidemic Kaposi sarcoma, life-threatening infections are common.

The use of drug therapy called HAART reduces the risk of epidemic Kaposi sarcoma in patients infected with HIV.

HAART (highly active antiretroviral therapy) is a combination of several drugs that block HIV and slow down the development of AIDS and AIDS-related Kaposi sarcoma.

Nonepidemic Gay-related Kaposi Sarcoma

There is a type of nonepidemic Kaposi sarcoma that develops in homosexual men who have no signs or symptoms of HIV infection. This type of Kaposi sarcoma progresses slowly, with new lesions appearing every few years. The lesions are most common on the arms, legs, and genitals, but can develop anywhere on the skin.

This type of Kaposi sarcoma is rare.

Treatment Option Overview

There are different types of treatment for patients with Kaposi sarcoma.

Different types of treatments are available for patients with Kaposi sarcoma. Some treatments are standard (the currently used treatment), and some are being tested in clinical trials. A treatment clinical trial is a research study meant to help improve current treatments or obtain information on new treatments for patients with cancer. When clinical trials show that a new treatment is better than the standard treatment, the new treatment may become the standard treatment. Patients may want to think about taking part in a clinical trial. Some clinical trials are open only to patients who have not started treatment.

Treatment of epidemic Kaposi sarcoma combines treatment for Kaposi sarcoma with treatment for AIDS.

For the treatment of epidemic Kaposi sarcoma, highly active antiretroviral therapy (HAART) is used to slow the progression of AIDS. HAART may be combined with anticancer drugs and medicines that prevent and treat infections.

Four types of standard treatment are used to treat Kaposi sarcoma:

Radiation therapy

Radiation therapy is a cancer treatment that uses high-energy x-rays or other types of radiation to kill cancer cells or keep them from growing. There are two types of radiation therapy. External radiation therapy uses a machine outside the body to send radiation toward the cancer. Internal radiation therapy uses a radioactive substance sealed in needles, seeds, wires, or catheters that are placed directly into or near the cancer. The way the radiation therapy is given depends on the type of cancer being treated.

Certain types of external radiation therapy are used to treat Kaposi sarcoma lesions. Photon radiation therapy treats lesions with high-energy light. Electron beam radiation therapy uses tiny negatively charged particles called electrons.

Surgery

The following surgical procedures may be used for Kaposi sarcoma to treat small, surface lesions:

- Local excision: The cancer is cut from the skin along with a small amount of normal tissue around it.

- Electrodesiccation and curettage: The tumor is cut from the skin with a curette (a sharp, spoon-shaped tool). A needle-shaped electrode is then used to treat the area with an electric current that stops the bleeding and destroys cancer cells that remain around the edge of the wound. The process may be repeated one to three times during the surgery to remove all of the cancer.

- Cryosurgery: A treatment that uses an instrument to freeze and destroy abnormal tissue. This type of treatment is also called cryotherapy.

Chemotherapy

Chemotherapy is a cancer treatment that uses drugs to stop the growth of cancer cells, either by killing the cells or by stopping them from dividing. When chemotherapy is taken by mouth or injected into a vein or muscle, the drugs enter the bloodstream and can reach cancer cells throughout the body (systemic chemotherapy). When chemotherapy is placed directly into the cerebrospinal fluid, an organ, or a body cavity such as the abdomen, the drugs mainly affect cancer cells in those areas (regional chemotherapy). To treat local Kaposi sarcoma lesions, such as in the mouth, anticancer drugs may be injected directly into the lesion (intralesional chemotherapy). Sometimes the chemotherapy is given as a topical agent (applied to the skin as a gel.) The way the chemotherapy is given depends on the type of cancer being treated.

Liposomal chemotherapy uses liposomes (very tiny fat particles) to carry anticancer drugs. Liposomal doxorubicin is used to treat Kaposi sarcoma. The liposomes build up in Kaposi sarcoma tissue more than in healthy tissue, and the doxorubicin is released slowly. This increases the effect of the doxorubicin and causes less damage to healthy tissue.

Biologic therapy

Biologic therapy is a treatment that uses the patient's immune system to fight cancer. Substances made by the body or made in a laboratory are used to boost, direct, or restore the body's natural defenses against cancer. This type of cancer treatment is also called biotherapy or immunotherapy. Interferon alfa is a biologic agent used to treat Kaposi sarcoma.

New types of treatment are being tested in clinical trials.

Targeted therapy

Targeted therapy is a type of treatment that uses drugs or other substances to identify and attack specific cancer cells without harming normal cells. Monoclonal antibody therapy is one type of targeted therapy being studied in the treatment of Kaposi sarcoma.

Monoclonal antibody therapy is a cancer treatment that uses antibodies made in the laboratory from a single type of immune system cell. These antibodies can identify substances on cancer cells or normal substances that may help cancer cells grow. The antibodies attach to the substances and kill the cancer cells, block their growth, or keep them from spreading. Monoclonal antibodies are given by infusion. These may be used alone or to carry drugs, toxins, or radioactive material directly to cancer cells.

Bevacizumab is a monoclonal antibody that is being studied in the treatment of Kaposi sarcoma.

Patients may want to think about taking part in a clinical trial.

For some patients, taking part in a clinical trial may be the best treatment choice. Clinical trials are part of the cancer research process. Clinical trials are done to find out if new cancer treatments are safe and effective or better than the standard treatment.

Many of today's standard treatments for cancer are based on earlier clinical trials. Patients who take part in a clinical trial may receive the standard treatment or be among the first to receive a new treatment.

Patients who take part in clinical trials also help improve the way cancer will be treated in the future. Even when clinical trials do not lead to effective new treatments, they often answer important questions and help move research forward.

Patients can enter clinical trials before, during, or after starting their cancer treatment.

Some clinical trials only include patients who have not yet received treatment. Other trials test treatments for patients whose cancer has not gotten better. There are also clinical trials that test new ways to stop cancer from recurring (coming back) or reduce the side effects of cancer treatment.

Clinical trials are taking place in many parts of the country.

Follow-up tests may be needed.

Some of the tests that were done to diagnose the cancer or to find out the stage of the cancer may be repeated. Some tests will be repeated in order to see how well the treatment is working. Decisions about whether to continue, change, or stop treatment may be based on the results of these tests. This is sometimes called re-staging.

Some of the tests will continue to be done from time to time after treatment has ended. The results of these tests can show if your condition has changed or if the cancer has recurred (come back). These tests are sometimes called follow-up tests or check-ups.

Chapter 29

HIV-Related Cancer

Chapter Contents

679

Section 29.1

AIDS-Related Lymphoma

Text in this section is excerpted from "AIDS-Related Lymphoma
Treatment," National Cancer Institute at the National Institutes of
Health (NIH), May 12, 2015.

General Information About AIDS-Related Lymphoma

*AIDS-related lymphoma is a disease in which malignant
(cancer) cells form in the lymph system of patients who have
acquired immunodeficiency syndrome (AIDS).*

AIDS is caused by the human immunodeficiency virus (HIV), which
attacks and weakens the body's immune system. The immune system
is then unable to fight infection and diseases that invade the body.
People with HIV disease have an increased risk of developing infections, lymphoma, and other types of cancer. A person with HIV disease
who develops certain types of infections or cancer is then diagnosed
with AIDS. Sometimes, people are diagnosed with AIDS and AIDS-
related lymphoma at the same time.

Lymphomas are cancers that affect the white blood cells of the
lymph system, part of the body's immune system. The lymph system
is made up of the following:

- Lymph: Colorless, watery fluid that travels through the lymph
  system and carries white blood cells called lymphocytes.
  Lymphocytes protect the body against infections and the growth
  of tumors.

- Lymph vessels: A network of thin tubes that collect lymph
  from different parts of the body and return it to the
  bloodstream.

- Lymph nodes: Small, bean-shaped structures that filter lymph
  and store white blood cells that help fight infection and disease.
  Lymph nodes are located along the network of lymph vessels
  found throughout the body. Clusters of lymph nodes are found in
  the underarm, pelvis, neck, abdomen, and groin.

- Spleen: An organ that makes lymphocytes, filters the blood, stores blood cells, and destroys old blood cells. The spleen is on the left side of the abdomen near the stomach.
- Thymus: An organ in which lymphocytes grow and multiply. The thymus is in the chest behind the breastbone.
- Tonsils: Two small masses of lymph tissue at the back of the throat. The tonsils make lymphocytes.
- Bone marrow: The soft, spongy tissue in the center of large bones. Bone marrow makes white blood cells, red blood cells, and platelets.

There are many different types of lymphoma.

Lymphomas are divided into two general types: Hodgkin lymphoma and non-Hodgkin lymphoma. Both Hodgkin lymphoma and non-Hodgkin lymphoma may occur in AIDS patients, but non-Hodgkin lymphoma is more common. When a person with AIDS has non-Hodgkin lymphoma, it is called an AIDS-related lymphoma.

AIDS-related lymphomas grow and spread quickly.

Non-Hodgkin lymphomas are grouped by the way their cells look under a microscope. They may be indolent (slow-growing) or aggressive (fast-growing). AIDS-related lymphoma is usually aggressive. There are three main types of AIDS-related lymphoma:

- Diffuse large B-cell lymphoma.
- B-cell immunoblastic lymphoma.
- Small non-cleaved cell lymphoma.

Signs of AIDS-related lymphoma include weight loss, fever, and night sweats.

These and other signs and symptoms may be caused by AIDS-related lymphoma or by other conditions. Check with your doctor if you have any of the following:

- Weight loss or fever for no known reason.
- Night sweats.
- Painless, swollen lymph nodes in the neck, chest, underarm, or groin.
- A feeling of fullness below the ribs.

Tests that examine the body and lymph system are used to help detect (find) and diagnose AIDS-related lymphoma.

The following tests and procedures may be used:

- **Physical exam and history:** An exam of the body to check general signs of health, including checking for signs of disease, such as lumps or anything else that seems unusual. A history of the patient's health habits and past illnesses and treatments will also be taken.

- **Complete blood count (CBC):** A procedure in which a sample of blood is drawn and checked for the following:

  - The number of red blood cells, white blood cells, and platelets.

  - The amount of hemoglobin (the protein that carries oxygen) in the red blood cells.

  - The portion of the sample made up of red blood cells.

- **Lymph node biopsy:** The removal of all or part of a lymph node. A pathologist views the tissue under a microscope to look for cancer cells. One of the following types of biopsies may be done:

  - **Excisional biopsy:** The removal of an entire lymph node.

  - **Incisional biopsy:** The removal of part of a lymph node.

  - **Core biopsy:** The removal of tissue from a lymph node using a wide needle.

  - **Fine-needle aspiration (FNA) biopsy**: The removal of tissue from a lymph node using a thin needle.

- **Bone marrow aspiration and biopsy:** The removal of bone marrow, blood, and a small piece of bone by inserting a hollow needle into the hipbone or breastbone. A pathologist views the bone marrow, blood, and bone under a microscope to look for signs of cancer.

- **HIV test:** A test to measure the level of HIV antibodies in a sample of blood. Antibodies are made by the body when it is invaded by a foreign substance. A high level of HIV antibodies may mean the body has been infected with HIV.

- **Chest x-ray:** An x-ray of the organs and bones inside the chest. An x-ray is a type of energy beam that can go through the body and onto film, making a picture of areas inside the body.

Certain factors affect prognosis (chance of recovery) and treatment options.

The prognosis (chance of recovery) and treatment options depend on the following:

- The stage of the cancer.

- The number of CD4 lymphocytes (a type of white blood cell) in the blood.

- Whether the patient has ever had AIDS-related infections.

- The patient's ability to carry out regular daily activities.

Stages of AIDS-Related Lymphoma

After AIDS-related lymphoma has been diagnosed, tests are done to find out if cancer cells have spread within the lymph system or to other parts of the body.

The process used to find out if cancer cells have spread within the lymph system or to other parts of the body is called staging. The information gathered from the staging process determines the stage of the disease. It is important to know the stage in order to plan treatment, but AIDS-related lymphoma is usually advanced when it is diagnosed. The following tests and procedures may be used in the staging process:

- **Blood chemistry studies:** A procedure in which a blood sample is checked to measure the amounts of certain substances released into the blood by organs and tissues in the body. An unusual (higher or lower than normal) amount of a substance can be a sign of disease in the organ or tissue that makes it. The blood sample will be checked for the level of LDH (lactate dehydrogenase).

- **CT scan (CAT scan):** A procedure that makes a series of detailed pictures of areas inside the body, such as the lung, lymph nodes, and liver, taken from different angles. The pictures are made by a computer linked to an x-ray machine. A dye may be injected into a vein or swallowed to help the organs or tissues show up more clearly. This procedure is also called computed tomography, computerized tomography, or computerized axial tomography.

683

- **PET scan (positron emission tomography scan):** A procedure to find malignant tumor cells in the body. A small amount of radioactive glucose (sugar) is injected into a vein. The PET scanner rotates around the body and makes a picture of where glucose is being used in the body. Malignant tumor cells show up brighter in the picture because they are more active and take up more glucose than normal cells do.

- **MRI (magnetic resonance imaging):** A procedure that uses a magnet, radio waves, and a computer to make a series of detailed pictures of areas inside the body. A substance called gadolinium is injected into the patient through a vein. The gadolinium collects around the cancer cells so they show up brighter in the picture. This procedure is also called nuclear magnetic resonance imaging (NMRI).

- **Lumbar puncture:** A procedure used to collect cerebrospinal fluid from the spinal column. This is done by placing a needle into the spinal column. This procedure is also called an LP or spinal tap. A pathologist views the cerebrospinal fluid under a microscope to look for signs of cancer.

There are three ways that cancer spreads in the body.

Cancer can spread through tissue, the lymph system, and the blood:

- Tissue. The cancer spreads from where it began by growing into nearby areas.

- Lymph system. The cancer spreads from where it began by getting into the lymph system. The cancer travels through the lymph vessels to other parts of the body.

- Blood. The cancer spreads from where it began by getting into the blood. The cancer travels through the blood vessels to other parts of the body.

Stages of AIDS-related lymphoma may include E and S.

AIDS-related lymphoma may be described as follows:

- E: "E" stands for extranodal and means the cancer is found in an area or organ other than the lymph nodes or has spread to tissues beyond, but near, the major lymphatic areas.

- S: "S" stands for spleen and means the cancer is found in the spleen.

The following stages are used for AIDS-related lymphoma:

Stage I

Stage I AIDS-related lymphoma is divided into stage I and stage IE.

- Stage I: Cancer is found in one lymphatic area (lymph node group, tonsils and nearby tissue, thymus, or spleen).
- Stage IE: Cancer is found in one organ or area outside the lymph nodes.

Stage II

Stage II AIDS-related lymphoma is divided into stage II and stage IIE.

- Stage II: Cancer is found in two or more lymph node groups either above or below the diaphragm (the thin muscle below the lungs that helps breathing and separates the chest from the abdomen).
- Stage IIE: Cancer is found in one or more lymph node groups either above or below the diaphragm. Cancer is also found outside the lymph nodes in one organ or area on the same side of the diaphragm as the affected lymph nodes.

Stage III

Stage III AIDS-related lymphoma is divided into stage III, stage IIIE, stage IIIS, and stage IIIE+S.

- Stage III: Cancer is found in lymph node groups above and below the diaphragm (the thin muscle below the lungs that helps breathing and separates the chest from the abdomen).
- Stage IIIE: Cancer is found in lymph node groups above and below the diaphragm and outside the lymph nodes in a nearby organ or area.
- Stage IIIS: Cancer is found in lymph node groups above and below the diaphragm, and in the spleen.
- Stage IIIE+S: Cancer is found in lymph node groups above and below the diaphragm, outside the lymph nodes in a nearby organ or area, and in the spleen.

Stage IV

In stage IV AIDS-related lymphoma, the cancer:

- is found throughout one or more organs that are not part of a lymphatic area (lymph node group, tonsils and nearby tissue, thymus, or spleen) and may be in lymph nodes near those organs; or

- is found in one organ that is not part of a lymphatic area and has spread to organs or lymph nodes far away from that organ; or

- is found in the liver, bone marrow, cerebrospinal fluid (CSF), or lungs (other than cancer that has spread to the lungs from nearby areas).

Patients who are infected with the Epstein-Barr virus or whose AIDS-related lymphoma affects the bone marrow have an increased risk of the cancer spreading to the central nervous system (CNS).

For treatment, AIDS-related lymphomas are grouped based on where they started in the body, as follows:

Peripheral / systemic lymphoma

Lymphoma that starts in lymph nodes or other organs of the lymph system is called peripheral/systemic lymphoma. The lymphoma may spread throughout the body, including to the brain or bone marrow.

Primary CNS lymphoma

Primary CNS lymphoma starts in the central nervous system (brain and spinal cord). Lymphoma that starts somewhere else in the body and spreads to the central nervous system is not primary CNS lymphoma.

Treatment Option Overview

There are different types of treatment for patients with AIDS-related lymphoma.

Different types of treatment are available for patients with AIDS-related lymphoma. Some treatments are standard (the currently used treatment), and some are being tested in clinical trials. A treatment clinical trial is a research study meant to help improve current treatments or obtain information on new treatments for patients with cancer. When clinical trials show that a new treatment is better than the standard treatment, the new treatment may become the standard treatment. Patients may want to think about taking part in a clinical trial. Some clinical trials are open only to patients who have not started treatment.

Treatment of AIDS-related lymphoma combines treatment of the lymphoma with treatment for AIDS.

Patients with AIDS have weakened immune systems and treatment can cause further damage. For this reason, patients who have AIDS-related lymphoma are usually treated with lower doses of drugs than lymphoma patients who do not have AIDS.

Highly-active antiretroviral therapy (HAART) is used to slow progression of HIV (which is a retrovirus). Treatment with HAART may allow some patients to safely receive anticancer drugs in standard or higher doses. Medicine to prevent and treat infections, which can be serious, is also used.

AIDS-related lymphoma usually grows faster than lymphoma that is not AIDS-related and it is more likely to spread to other parts of the body. In general, AIDS-related lymphoma is harder to treat.

Three types of standard treatment are used:

Chemotherapy

Chemotherapy is a cancer treatment that uses drugs to stop the growth of cancer cells, either by killing the cells or by stopping them from dividing. When chemotherapy is taken by mouth or injected into a vein or muscle, the drugs enter the bloodstream and can reach cancer cells throughout the body (systemic chemotherapy). When chemotherapy is placed directly into the cerebrospinal fluid (intrathecal chemotherapy), an organ, or a body cavity such as the abdomen, the drugs mainly affect cancer cells in those areas (regional chemotherapy). Combination chemotherapy is treatment using more than one anticancer drug. The way the chemotherapy is given depends on the type and stage of the cancer being treated.

Intrathecal chemotherapy may be used in patients who are more likely to have lymphoma in the central nervous system (CNS).

Colony-stimulating factors are sometimes given together with chemotherapy. This helps lessen the side effects chemotherapy may have on the bone marrow.

687

Radiation therapy

Radiation therapy is a cancer treatment that uses high-energy x-rays or other types of radiation to kill cancer cells or keep them from growing. There are two types of radiation therapy. External radiation therapy uses a machine outside the body to send radiation toward the cancer. Internal radiation therapy uses a radioactive substance sealed in needles, seeds, wires, or catheters that are placed directly into or near the cancer. The way the radiation therapy is given depends on the type and stage of the cancer being treated.

High-dose chemotherapy with stem cell transplant

High-dose chemotherapy with stem cell transplant is a way of giving high doses of chemotherapy and replacing blood -forming cells destroyed by the cancer treatment. Stem cells (immature blood cells) are removed from the blood or bone marrow of the patient or a donor and are frozen and stored. After the chemotherapy is completed, the stored stem cells are thawed and given back to the patient through an infusion. These re-infused stem cells grow into (and restore) the body's blood cells.

New types of treatment are being tested in clinical trials.

Targeted therapy

Targeted therapy is a type of treatment that uses drugs or other substances to identify and attack specific cancer cells without harming normal cells. Monoclonal antibody therapy is one type of targeted therapy being studied in the treatment of AIDS-related lymphoma.

Monoclonal antibody therapy is a cancer treatment that uses antibodies made in the laboratory from a single type of immune system cell. These antibodies can identify substances on cancer cells or normal substances that may help cancer cells grow. The antibodies attach to the substances and kill the cancer cells, block their growth, or keep them from spreading. Monoclonal antibodies are given by infusion. These may be used alone or to carry drugs, toxins, or radioactive material directly to cancer cells.

Patients may want to think about taking part in a clinical trial.

For some patients, taking part in a clinical trial may be the best treatment choice. Clinical trials are part of the cancer research process.

Clinical trials are done to find out if new cancer treatments are safe and effective or better than the standard treatment.

Many of today's standard treatments for cancer are based on earlier clinical trials. Patients who take part in a clinical trial may receive the standard treatment or be among the first to receive a new treatment.

Patients who take part in clinical trials also help improve the way cancer will be treated in the future. Even when clinical trials do not lead to effective new treatments, they often answer important questions and help move research forward.

Patients can enter clinical trials before, during, or after starting their cancer treatment.

Some clinical trials only include patients who have not yet received treatment. Other trials test treatments for patients whose cancer has not gotten better. There are also clinical trials that test new ways to stop cancer from recurring (coming back) or reduce the side effects of cancer treatment.

Clinical trials are taking place in many parts of the country.

Follow-up tests may be needed.

Some of the tests that were done to diagnose the cancer or to find out the stage of the cancer may be repeated. Some tests will be repeated in order to see how well the treatment is working. Decisions about whether to continue, change, or stop treatment may be based on the results of these tests. This is sometimes called re-staging.

Some of the tests will continue to be done from time to time after treatment has ended. The results of these tests can show if your condition has changed or if the cancer has recurred (come back). These tests are sometimes called follow-up tests or check-ups.

Chapter 30

Cancer of Unknown Primaries

Chapter Contents

Section 30.1

Carcinoma of Unknown Primary

Text in this section is excerpted from "Carcinoma of Unknown
Primary Treatment," National Cancer Institute at the National
Institutes of Health (NIH), April 3, 2015.

General Information About Carcinoma of Unknown Primary

*Carcinoma of unknown primary (CUP) is a rare disease in
which malignant (cancer) cells are found in the body but the
place the cancer began is not known.*

Cancer can form in any tissue of the body. The primary cancer (the
cancer that first formed) can spread to other parts of the body. This
process is called metastasis. Cancer cells usually look like the cells in
the type of tissue in which the cancer began. For example, breast cancer
cells may spread to the lung. Because the cancer began in the breast,
the cancer cells in the lung look like breast cancer cells.

Sometimes doctors find where the cancer has spread but cannot find
where in the body the cancer first began to grow. This type of cancer
is called a cancer of unknown primary (CUP) or occult primary tumor.

Tests are done to find where the primary cancer began and to get
information about where the cancer has spread. When tests are able to
find the primary cancer, the cancer is no longer a CUP and treatment
is based on the type of primary cancer.

Sometimes the primary cancer is never found.

The primary cancer (the cancer that first formed) may not be found
for one of the following reasons:

- The primary cancer is very small and grows slowly.

- The body's immune system killed the primary cancer.

- The primary cancer was removed during surgery for another
  condition and doctors didn't know cancer had formed. For

692

example, a uterus with cancer may be removed during a hyster-ectomy to treat a serious infection.

The signs and symptoms of CUP are different, depending on where the cancer has spread in the body.

Sometimes CUP does not cause any signs or symptoms. Signs and symptoms may be caused by CUP or by other conditions. Check with your doctor if you have any of the following:

- Lump or thickening in any part of the body.
- Pain that is in one part of the body and does not go away.
- A cough that does not go away or hoarseness in the voice.
- Change in bowel or bladder habits, such as constipation, diar-rhea, or frequent urination.
- Unusual bleeding or discharge.
- Fever for no known reason that does not go away.
- Night sweats.
- Weight loss for no known reason or loss of appetite.

Different tests are used to detect (find) cancer.

The following tests and procedures may be used:

- **Physical exam and history:** An exam of the body to check general signs of health, including checking for signs of disease, such as lumps or anything else that seems unusual. A history of the patient's health habits and past illnesses and treatments will also be taken.
- **Urinalysis:** A test to check the color of urine and its contents, such as sugar, protein, blood, and bacteria.
- **Blood chemistry studies:** A procedure in which a blood sample is checked to measure the amounts of certain substances released into the blood by organs and tissues in the body. An unusual (higher or lower than normal) amount of a substance can be a sign of disease in the organ or tissue that makes it.
- **Complete blood count:** A procedure in which a sample of blood is drawn and checked for the following:
  - The number of red blood cells, white blood cells, and platelets.

- The amount of hemoglobin (the protein that carries oxygen) in the red blood cells.

- The portion of the sample made up of red blood cells.

- **Fecal occult blood test:** A test to check stool (solid waste) for blood that can only be seen with a microscope. Small samples of stool are placed on special cards and returned to the doctor or laboratory for testing. Because some cancers bleed, blood in the stool may be a sign of cancer in the colon or rectum.

If tests show there may be cancer, a biopsy is done.

A biopsy is the removal of cells or tissues so they can be viewed under a microscope by a pathologist. The pathologist views the tissue under a microscope to look for cancer cells and to find out the type of cancer. The type of biopsy that is done depends on the part of the body being tested for cancer. One of the following types of biopsies may be used:

- **Excisional biopsy:** The removal of an entire lump of tissue.

- **Incisional biopsy:** The removal of part of a lump or a sample of tissue.

- **Core biopsy:** The removal of tissue using a wide needle.

- **Fine-needle aspiration (FNA) biopsy:** The removal tissue or fluid using a thin needle.

If cancer is found, one or more of the following laboratory tests may be used to study the tissue samples and find out the type of cancer:

- **Histologic study:** A laboratory test in which stains are added to a sample of cancer cells or tissue and viewed under a micro-scope to look for certain changes in the cells. Certain changes in the cells are linked to certain types of cancer.

- **Immunohistochemistry:** A test that uses antibodies to check for certain antigens in a sample of tissue. The antibody is usu-ally linked to a radioactive substance or a dye that causes the tissue to light up under a microscope. This type of test may be used to tell the difference between different types of cancer.

- **Reverse transcription – polymerase chain reaction (RT-PCR) test:** A laboratory test in which cells in a sample of tissue are studied using chemicals to look for certain changes in the genes.

- **Cytogenetic analysis:** A laboratory test in which cells in a sample of tissue are viewed under a microscope to look for certain changes in the chromosomes. Changes in certain chromosomes are linked to certain types of cancer.

- **Light and electron microscopy:** A laboratory test in which cells in a sample of tissue are viewed under regular and high-powered microscopes to look for certain changes in the cells.

When the type of cancer cells or tissue removed is different from the type of cancer cells expected to be found, a diagnosis of CUP may be made.

The cells in the body have a certain look that depends on the type of tissue they come from. For example, a sample of cancer tissue taken from the breast is expected to be made up of breast cells. However, if the sample of tissue is a different type of cell (not made up of breast cells), it is likely that the cells have spread to the breast from another part of the body. In order to plan treatment, doctors first try to find the primary cancer (the cancer that first formed).

Tests and procedures used to find the primary cancer depend on where the cancer has spread.

In some cases, the part of the body where cancer cells are first found helps the doctor decide which diagnostic tests will be most helpful.

- When cancer is found above the diaphragm (the thin muscle under the lungs that helps with breathing), the primary cancer site is likely to be in the upper part of the body, such as in the lung or breast.

- When cancer is found below the diaphragm, the primary cancer site is likely to be in the lower part of the body, such as the pancreas, liver, or other organ in the abdomen.

- Some cancers commonly spread to certain areas of the body. For cancer found in the lymph nodes in the neck, the primary cancer site is likely to be in the head or neck, because head and neck cancers often spread to the lymph nodes in the neck.

The following tests and procedures may be done to find where the cancer first began:

- **CT scan (CAT scan):** A procedure that makes a series of detailed pictures of areas inside the body, such as the chest or abdomen, taken from different angles. The pictures are made by a computer linked to an x-ray machine. A dye may be injected into a vein or swallowed to help the organs or tissues show up more clearly. This procedure is also called computed tomography, computerized tomography, or computerized axial tomography.

- **MRI (magnetic resonance imaging):** A procedure that uses a magnet, radio waves, and a computer to make a series of detailed pictures of areas inside the body. This procedure is also called nuclear magnetic resonance imaging (NMRI).

- **PET scan (positron emission tomography scan):** A procedure to find malignant tumor cells in the body. A small amount of radioactive glucose (sugar) is injected into a vein. The PET scanner rotates around the body and makes a picture of where glucose is being used in the body. Malignant tumor cells show up brighter in the picture because they are more active and take up more glucose than normal cells do.

- **Mammogram**: An x-ray of the breast.

- **Endoscopy**: A procedure to look at organs and tissues inside the body to check for abnormal areas. An endoscope is inserted through an incision (cut) in the skin or opening in the body, such as the mouth. An endoscope is a thin, tube-like instrument with a light and a lens for viewing. It may also have a tool to remove tissue or lymph node samples, which are checked under a microscope for signs of disease. For example, a colonoscopy may be done.

- **Tumor marker test:** A procedure in which a sample of blood, urine, or tissue is checked to measure the amounts of certain substances made by organs, tissues, or tumor cells in the body. Certain substances are linked to specific types of cancer when found in increased levels in the body. These are called tumor markers. The blood may be checked for the levels of CA-125, CgA, alpha-fetoprotein (AFP), beta human chorionic gonadotropin (β-hCG), or prostate-specific antigen (PSA).

Sometimes, none of the tests can find the primary cancer site. In these cases, treatment may be based on what the doctor thinks is the most likely type of cancer.

Certain factors affect prognosis (chance of recovery).

The prognosis (chance of recovery) depends on the following:

- Where the cancer began in the body and where it has spread.
- The number of organs with cancer in them.
- The way the tumor cells look when viewed under a microscope.
- Whether the patient is male or female.
- Whether the cancer has just been diagnosed or has recurred (come back).

For most patients with CUP, current treatments do not cure the cancer. Patients may want to take part in one of the many clinical trials being done to improve treatment. Clinical trials for CUP are taking place in many parts of the country.

Stages of Carcinoma of Unknown Primary

There is no staging system for carcinoma of unknown primary (CUP).

The extent or spread of cancer is usually described as stages. The stage of the cancer is usually used to plan treatment. However, CUP has already spread to other parts of the body when it is found.

The information that is known about the cancer is used to plan treatment.

Doctors use the following types of information to plan treatment:

- The place in the body where the cancer is found, such as the peritoneum or the cervical (neck), axillary (armpit), or inguinal (groin) lymph nodes.
- The type of cancer cell, such as melanoma.
- Whether the cancer cell is poorly differentiated (looks very different from normal cells when viewed under a microscope).
- The signs and symptoms caused by the cancer.
- The results of tests and procedures.

697

- Whether the cancer is newly diagnosed or has recurred (come back).

Treatment Options for Carcinoma of Unknown Primary

Newly Diagnosed Carcinoma of Unknown Primary

Cervical (Neck) Lymph Nodes

Cancer found in cervical (neck) lymph nodes may have spread from a tumor in the head or neck. Treatment of cervical lymph node carcinoma of unknown primary (CUP) may include the following:

- Surgery to remove the tonsils.
- Radiation therapy alone. Intensity-modulated radiation therapy (IMRT) may be used.
- Radiation therapy followed by surgery to remove the lymph nodes.
- Surgery to remove the lymph nodes, with or without radiation therapy.
- A clinical trial of new types of treatment.

Poorly Differentiated Carcinomas

Cancer cells that are poorly differentiated look very different from normal cells. The type of cell they came from is not known. Treatment of poorly differentiated carcinoma of unknown primary, including tumors in the neuroendocrine system (the part of the brain that controls hormone -producing glands throughout the body) may include the following:

- Combination chemotherapy.
- A clinical trial of new types of treatment.

Women with Peritoneal Cancer

Treatment for women who have peritoneal (lining of the abdomen) carcinoma of unknown primary may be the same as for ovarian cancer. Treatment may include the following:

- Chemotherapy.
- A clinical trial of new types of treatment.

Isolated Axillary Lymph Node Metastasis

Cancer found only in the axillary (armpit) lymph nodes may have spread from a tumor in the breast.

Treatment of axillary lymph node metastasis is usually:

- Surgery to remove the lymph nodes.

Treatment also may include one or more of the following:

- Surgery to remove the breast.
- Radiation therapy to the breast.
- Chemotherapy.
- A clinical trial of new types of treatment.

Inguinal Lymph Node Metastasis

Cancer found only in the inguinal (groin) lymph nodes most likely began in the genital, anal, or rectal area. Treatment of inguinal lymph node metastasis may include the following:

- Surgery to remove the cancer and/or lymph nodes in the groin.
- Surgery to remove the cancer and/or lymph nodes in the groin, followed by radiation therapy or chemotherapy.

Melanoma in a Single Lymph Node Area

Treatment of melanoma that is found only in a single lymph node area is usually:

- Surgery to remove the lymph nodes.

Multiple Involvement

There is no standard treatment for carcinoma of unknown primary that is found in several different areas of the body. Treatment may include the following:

- Hormone therapy.
- Internal radiation therapy.
- Chemotherapy with one or more anticancer drugs.
- A clinical trial.

Recurrent Carcinoma of Unknown Primary

Treatment for recurrent carcinoma of unknown primary is usually within a clinical trial. Treatment depends on the following:

- The type of cancer.
- How the cancer was treated before.
- Where the cancer has come back in the body.
- The condition and wishes of the patient.

Chapter 31

Leukemia

Chapter Contents

Section 31.1

Adult Acute Lymphoblastic Leukemia

The text in this section is excerpted from "Adult Acute Lymphoblastic
Leukemia Treatment," National Cancer Institute at the National
Institutes of Health (NIH), April 24, 2015.

General Information About Adult Acute Lymphoblastic Leukemia

*Adult acute lymphoblastic leukemia (ALL) is a type of cancer
in which the bone marrow makes too many lymphocytes (a
type of white blood cell).*

Adult acute lymphoblastic leukemia (ALL; also called acute lymphocytic leukemia) is a cancer of the blood and bone marrow. This type
of cancer usually gets worse quickly if it is not treated.

*Leukemia may affect red blood cells, white blood cells, and
platelets.*

Normally, the bone marrow makes blood stem cells (immature
cells) that become mature blood cells over time. A blood stem cell may
become a myeloid stem cell or a lymphoid stem cell.

A myeloid stem cell becomes one of three types of mature blood cells:

- Red blood cells that carry oxygen and other substances to all tissues of the body.

- Platelets that form blood clots to stop bleeding.

- Granulocytes (white blood cells) that fight infection and disease.

A lymphoid stem cell becomes a lymphoblast cell and then one of three
types of lymphocytes (white blood cells):

- B lymphocytes that make antibodies to help fight infection.

- T lymphocytes that help B lymphocytes make the antibodies that help fight infection.

- Natural killer cells that attack cancer cells and viruses.

In ALL, too many stem cells become lymphoblasts, B lymphocytes, or T lymphocytes. These cells are also called leukemia cells. These leukemia cells are not able to fight infection very well. Also, as the number of leukemia cells increases in the blood and bone marrow, there is less room for healthy white blood cells, red blood cells, and platelets. This may cause infection, anemia, and easy bleeding. The cancer can also spread to the central nervous system (brain and spinal cord).

Previous chemotherapy and exposure to radiation may increase the risk of developing ALL.

Anything that increases your risk of getting a disease is called a risk factor. Having a risk factor does not mean that you will get cancer; not having risk factors doesn't mean that you will not get cancer. Talk with your doctor if you think you may be at risk. Possible risk factors for ALL include the following:

- Being male.
- Being white.
- Being older than 70.
- Past treatment with chemotherapy or radiation therapy.
- Being exposed to radiation from an atomic bomb.
- Having certain genetic disorders, such as Down syndrome.

Signs and symptoms of adult ALL include fever, feeling tired, and easy bruising or bleeding.

The early signs and symptoms of ALL may be like the flu or other common diseases. Check with your doctor if you have any of the following:

- Weakness or feeling tired.
- Fever or night sweats.
- Easy bruising or bleeding.

- Petechiae (flat, pinpoint spots under the skin, caused by bleeding).

- Shortness of breath.

- Weight loss or loss of appetite.

- Pain in the bones or stomach.

- Pain or feeling of fullness below the ribs.

- Painless lumps in the neck, underarm, stomach, or groin.

- Having many infections.

These and other signs and symptoms may be caused by adult acute lymphoblastic leukemia or by other conditions.

Tests that examine the blood and bone marrow are used to detect (find) and diagnose adult ALL.

The following tests and procedures may be used:

- **Physical exam and history:** An exam of the body to check general signs of health, including checking for signs of disease, such as infection or anything else that seems unusual. A history of the patient's health habits and past illnesses and treatments will also be taken.

- **Complete blood count (CBC) with differential:** A procedure in which a sample of blood is drawn and checked for the following:

  - The number of red blood cells and platelets.

  - The number and type of white blood cells.

  - The amount of hemoglobin (the protein that carries oxygen) in the red blood cells.

  - The portion of the blood sample made up of red blood cells.

- **Blood chemistry studies:** A procedure in which a blood sample is checked to measure the amounts of certain substances released into the blood by organs and tissues in the body. An unusual (higher or lower than normal) amount of a substance can be a sign of disease in the organ or tissue that makes it.

- **Peripheral blood smear:** A procedure in which a sample of blood is checked for blast cells, the number and kinds of white blood cells, the number of platelets, and changes in the shape of blood cells.

- **Bone marrow aspiration and biopsy:** The removal of bone marrow, blood, and a small piece of bone by inserting a hollow needle into the hipbone or breastbone. A pathologist views the bone marrow, blood, and bone under a microscope to look for abnormal cells.

The following tests may be done on the samples of blood or bone marrow tissue that are removed:

- **Cytogenetic analysis:** A laboratory test in which the cells in a sample of blood or bone marrow are looked at under a microscope to find out if there are certain changes in the chromosomes in the lymphocytes. For example, sometimes in ALL, part of one chromosome is moved to another chromosome. This is called the Philadelphia chromosome. Other tests, such as fluorescence in situ hybridization (FISH), may also be done to look for certain changes in the chromosomes.

- **Immunophenotyping:** A process used to identify cells, based on the types of antigens or markers on the surface of the cell. This process is used to diagnose the subtype of ALL by comparing the cancer cells to normal cells of the immune system. For example, a cytochemistry study may test the cells in a sample of tissue using chemicals (dyes) to look for certain changes in the sample. A chemical may cause a color change in one type of leukemia cell but not in another type of leukemia cell.

Certain factors affect prognosis (chance of recovery) and treatment options.

The prognosis (chance of recovery) and treatment options depend on the following:

- The age of the patient.
- Whether the cancer has spread to the brain or spinal cord.
- Whether there are certain changes in the genes, including the Philadelphia chromosome.
- Whether the cancer has been treated before or has recurred (come back).

705

Stages of Adult Acute Lymphoblastic Leukemia

Once adult ALL has been diagnosed, tests are done to find out if the cancer has spread to the central nervous system (brain and spinal cord) or to other parts of the body.

The extent or spread of cancer is usually described as stages. It is important to know whether the leukemia has spread outside the blood and bone marrow in order to plan treatment. The following tests and procedures may be used to determine if the leukemia has spread:

- **Chest x-ray:** An x-ray of the organs and bones inside the chest. An x-ray is a type of energy beam that can go through the body and onto film, making a picture of areas inside the body.

- **Lumbar puncture:** A procedure used to collect cerebrospinal fluid from the spinal column. This is done by placing a needle into the spinal column. This procedure is also called an LP or spinal tap.

- **CT scan (CAT scan):** A procedure that makes a series of detailed pictures of the abdomen, taken from different angles. The pictures are made by a computer linked to an x-ray machine. A dye may be injected into a vein or swallowed to help the organs or tissues show up more clearly. This procedure is also called computed tomography, computerized tomography, or computerized axial tomography.

- **MRI (magnetic resonance imaging):** A procedure that uses a magnet, radio waves, and a computer to make a series of detailed pictures of areas inside the body. This procedure is also called nuclear magnetic resonance imaging (NMRI).

There is no standard staging system for adult ALL.

The disease is described as untreated, in remission, or recurrent.

Untreated adult ALL
The ALL is newly diagnosed and has not been treated except to relieve signs and symptoms such as fever, bleeding, or pain.

- The complete blood count is abnormal.

- More than 5% of the cells in the bone marrow are blasts (leukemia cells).

- There are signs and symptoms of leukemia.

Adult ALL in remission

The ALL has been treated.

- The complete blood count is normal.

- 5% or fewer of the cells in the bone marrow are blasts (leukemia cells).

- There are no signs or symptoms of leukemia other than in the bone marrow.

Treatment Option Overview

There are different types of treatment for patients with adult ALL.

Different types of treatment are available for patients with adult acute lymphoblastic leukemia (ALL). Some treatments are standard (the currently used treatment), and some are being tested in clinical trials. A treatment clinical trial is a research study meant to help improve current treatments or obtain information on new treatments for patients with cancer. When clinical trials show that a new treatment is better than the standard treatment, the new treatment may become the standard treatment. Patients may want to think about taking part in a clinical trial. Some clinical trials are open only to patients who have not started treatment.

The treatment of adult ALL usually has two phases.

The treatment of adult ALL is done in phases:

- Remission induction therapy: This is the first phase of treatment. The goal is to kill the leukemia cells in the blood and bone marrow. This puts the leukemia into remission.

- Post-remission therapy: This is the second phase of treatment. It begins once the leukemia is in remission. The goal of post-remission therapy is to kill any remaining leukemia cells that may not be active but could begin to regrow and cause a relapse. This phase is also called remission continuation therapy.

Treatment called central nervous system (CNS) sanctuary therapy is usually given during each phase of therapy. Because standard doses of chemotherapy may not reach leukemia cells in the CNS (brain and spinal cord), the cells are able to "find sanctuary" (hide) in the CNS. High doses of certain anticancer drugs, intrathecal chemotherapy, and radiation therapy to the brain are able to reach leukemia cells in the CNS. They are given to kill the leukemia cells and keep the cancer from recurring (coming back). CNS sanctuary therapy is also called CNS prophylaxis.

Four types of standard treatment are used:

Chemotherapy

Chemotherapy is a cancer treatment that uses drugs to stop the growth of cancer cells, either by killing the cells or by stopping them from dividing. When chemotherapy is taken by mouth or injected into a vein or muscle, the drugs enter the bloodstream and can reach cancer cells throughout the body (systemic chemotherapy). When chemotherapy is placed directly into the cerebrospinal fluid (intrathecal chemotherapy), an organ, or a body cavity such as the abdomen, the drugs mainly affect cancer cells in those areas (regional chemotherapy). Combination chemotherapy is treatment using more than one anticancer drug. The way the chemotherapy is given depends on the type and stage of the cancer being treated.

Intrathecal chemotherapy may be used to treat adult ALL that has spread, or may spread, to the brain and spinal cord. When used to prevent cancer from spreading to the brain and spinal cord, it is called central nervous system (CNS) sanctuary therapy or CNS prophylaxis. Intrathecal chemotherapy is given in addition to chemotherapy by mouth or vein.

Radiation therapy

Radiation therapy is a cancer treatment that uses high-energy x-rays or other types of radiation to kill cancer cells or keep them from growing. There are two types of radiation therapy. External radiation therapy uses a machine outside the body to send radiation toward the cancer. Internal radiation therapy uses a radioactive substance sealed in needles, seeds, wires, or catheters that are placed directly into or near the cancer. External radiation therapy may be used to treat adult ALL that has spread, or may spread, to the brain and spinal cord. When used this way, it is called central nervous system (CNS) sanctuary therapy or CNS prophylaxis.

Chemotherapy with stem cell transplant

Stem cell transplant is a method of giving chemotherapy and replacing blood-forming cells destroyed by the cancer treatment. Stem cells (immature blood cells) are removed from the blood or bone marrow of the patient or a donor and are frozen and stored. After the chemotherapy is completed, the stored stem cells are thawed and given back to the patient through an infusion. These re-infused stem cells grow into (and restore) the body's blood cells.

Targeted therapy

Targeted therapy is a type of treatment that uses drugs or other substances to identify and attack specific cancer cells without harming normal cells.

Targeted therapy drugs called tyrosine kinase inhibitors are used to treat some types of adult ALL. These drugs block the enzyme, tyrosine kinase, that causes stem cells to develop into more white blood cells (blasts) than the body needs. Three of the drugs used are imatinib mesylate (Gleevec), dasatinib, and nilotinib.

New types of treatment are being tested in clinical trials.

Biologic therapy

Biologic therapy is a treatment that uses the patient's immune system to fight cancer. Substances made by the body or made in a laboratory are used to boost, direct, or restore the body's natural defenses against cancer. This type of cancer treatment is also called biotherapy or immunotherapy.

Patients may want to think about taking part in a clinical trial.

For some patients, taking part in a clinical trial may be the best treatment choice. Clinical trials are part of the cancer research process. Clinical trials are done to find out if new cancer treatments are safe and effective or better than the standard treatment.

Many of today's standard treatments for cancer are based on earlier clinical trials. Patients who take part in a clinical trial may receive the standard treatment or be among the first to receive a new treatment.

Patients who take part in clinical trials also help improve the way cancer will be treated in the future. Even when clinical trials do not lead to effective new treatments, they often answer important questions and help move research forward.

Patients can enter clinical trials before, during, or after starting their cancer treatment.

Some clinical trials only include patients who have not yet received treatment. Other trials test treatments for patients whose cancer has not gotten better. There are also clinical trials that test new ways to stop cancer from recurring (coming back) or reduce the side effects of cancer treatment.

Clinical trials are taking place in many part of the country.

Patients with ALL may have late effects after treatment.

Side effects from cancer treatment that begin during or after treatment and continue for months or years are called late effects. Late effects of treatment for ALL may include the risk of second cancers (new types of cancer). Regular follow-up exams are very important for long-term survivors.

Follow-up tests may be needed.

Some of the tests that were done to diagnose the cancer or to find out the stage of the cancer may be repeated. Some tests will be repeated in order to see how well the treatment is working. Decisions about whether to continue, change, or stop treatment may be based on the results of these tests. This is sometimes called re-staging.

Some of the tests will continue to be done from time to time after treatment has ended. The results of these tests can show if your condition has changed or if the cancer has recurred (come back). These tests are sometimes called follow-up tests or check-ups.

Treatment Options for Adult Acute Lymphoblastic Leukemia

Untreated Adult Acute Lymphoblastic Leukemia

Standard treatment of adult acute lymphoblastic leukemia (ALL) during the remission induction phase includes the following:

- Combination chemotherapy.

- Tyrosine kinase inhibitor therapy with imatinib mesylate, in certain patients. Some of these patients will also have combination chemotherapy.

- Supportive care including antibiotics and red blood cell and platelet transfusions.

- CNS prophylaxis therapy including chemotherapy (intrathecal and/or systemic) with or without radiation therapy to the brain.

Adult Acute Lymphoblastic Leukemia in Remission

Standard treatment of adult ALL during the post-remission phase includes the following:

- Chemotherapy.

- Tyrosine kinase inhibitor therapy.

- Chemotherapy with stem cell transplant.

- CNS prophylaxis therapy including chemotherapy (intrathecal and/or systemic) with or without radiation therapy to the brain.

Recurrent Adult Acute Lymphoblastic Leukemia

Standard treatment of recurrent adult ALL may include the following:

- Combination chemotherapy followed by stem cell transplant.

- Low-dose radiation therapy as palliative care to relieve symptoms and improve the quality of life.

- Tyrosine kinase inhibitor therapy with dasatinib for certain patients.

Some of the treatments being studied in clinical trials for recurrent adult ALL include the following:

- A clinical trial of stem cell transplant using the patient's stem cells.

- A clinical trial of biologic therapy.

- A clinical trial of new anticancer drugs.

711

Chapter 32

Lymphoma

Chapter Contents

Section 32.1

Primary CNS Lymphoma

Text in this section is excerpted from "Primary CNS Lymphoma
Treatment," National Cancer Institute at the National Institutes of
Health (NIH), May 28, 2015.

General Information About Primary CNS Lymphoma

*Primary central nervous system (CNS) lymphoma is a
disease in which malignant (cancer) cells form in the lymph
tissue of the brain and / or spinal cord.*

Lymphoma is a disease in which malignant (cancer) cells form in
the lymph system. The lymph system is part of the immune system
and is made up of the lymph, lymph vessels, lymph nodes, spleen,
thymus, tonsils, and bone marrow. Lymphocytes (carried in the
lymph) travel in and out of the central nervous system (CNS). It
is thought that some of these lymphocytes become malignant and
cause lymphoma to form in the CNS. Primary CNS lymphoma can
start in the brain, spinal cord, or meninges (the layers that form
the outer covering of the brain). Because the eye is so close to the
brain, primary CNS lymphoma can also start in the eye (called ocular
lymphoma).

*Having a weakened immune system may increase the risk of
developing primary CNS lymphoma.*

Anything that increases your chance of getting a disease is called a
risk factor. Having a risk factor does not mean that you will get cancer;
not having risk factors doesn't mean that you will not get cancer. Talk
with your doctor if you think you may be at risk.

Primary CNS lymphoma may occur in patients who have acquired
immunodeficiency syndrome (AIDS) or other disorders of the immune
system or who have had a kidney transplant.

Tests that examine the eyes, brain, and spinal cord are used to detect (find) and diagnose primary CNS lymphoma.

The following tests and procedures may be used:

- **Physical exam and history:** An exam of the body to check general signs of health, including checking for signs of disease, such as lumps or anything else that seems unusual. A history of the patient's health habits and past illnesses and treatments will also be taken.

- **Neurological exam:** A series of questions and tests to check the brain, spinal cord, and nerve function. The exam checks a person's mental status, coordination, ability to walk normally, and how well the muscles, senses, and reflexes work. This may also be called a neuro exam or a neurologic exam.

- **Slit-lamp eye exam:** An exam that uses a special microscope with a bright, narrow slit of light to check the outside and inside of the eye.

- **MRI (magnetic resonance imaging):** A procedure that uses a magnet, radio waves, and a computer to make a series of detailed pictures of areas inside the brain and spinal cord. A substance called gadolinium is injected into the patient through a vein. The gadolinium collects around the cancer cells so they show up brighter in the picture. This procedure is also called nuclear magnetic resonance imaging (NMRI).

- **PET scan (positron emission tomography scan):** A procedure to find malignant tumor cells in the body. A small amount of radioactive glucose (sugar) is injected into a vein. The PET scanner rotates around the body and makes a picture of where glucose is being used in the body. Malignant tumor cells show up brighter in the picture because they are more active and take up more glucose than normal cells do.

- **Lumbar puncture:** A procedure used to collect cerebrospinal fluid (the fluid in the spaces around the brain and spinal cord) from the spinal column. This is done by placing a needle into the spinal column. This procedure is also called an LP or spinal tap. Tests to diagnose primary CNS lymphoma may include checking the protein level and for signs of cancer in the cerebrospinal fluid.

- **Stereotactic biopsy:** A biopsy procedure that uses a computer and a 3-dimensional (3-D) scanning device to find a tumor site and guide the removal of tissue so it can be viewed under a microscope to check for signs of cancer.

The following tests may be done on the samples of tissue that are removed:

- **Flow cytometry:** A laboratory test that measures the number of cells in a sample, the percentage of live cells in a sample, and certain characteristics of cells, such as size, shape, and the presence of tumor markers on the cell surface. The cells are stained with a light-sensitive dye, placed in a fluid, and passed in a stream before a laser or other type of light. The measurements are based on how the light-sensitive dye reacts to the light.

- **Immunohistochemistry:** A test that uses antibodies to check for certain antigens in a sample of tissue. The antibody is usually linked to a radioactive substance or a dye that causes the tissue to light up under a microscope. This type of test may be used to tell the difference between different types of cancer.

- **Cytogenetic analysis:** A laboratory test in which cells in a sample of tissue are viewed under a microscope to look for certain changes in the chromosomes. Other tests, such as fluorescence in situ hybridization (FISH), may also be done to look for certain changes in the chromosomes.

- **Complete blood count (CBC) with differential:** A procedure in which a sample of blood is drawn and checked for the following:
    - The number of red blood cells and platelets.
    - The number and type of white blood cells.
    - The amount of hemoglobin (the protein that carries oxygen) in the red blood cells.
    - The portion of the blood sample made up of red blood cells.

- **Blood chemistry studies:** A procedure in which a blood sample is checked to measure the amounts of certain substances released into the blood by organs and tissues in the body. An unusual (higher or lower than normal) amount of a substance can be a sign of disease in the organ or tissue that makes it.

Certain factors affect prognosis (chance of recovery) and treatment options.

The prognosis (chance of recovery) depends on the following:

- The patient's age and general health.
- The level of certain substances in the blood and cerebrospinal fluid (CSF).
- Where the tumor is in the central nervous system.
- Whether the patient has AIDS.

Treatment options depend on the following:

- The stage of the cancer.
- Where the tumor is in the central nervous system.
- The patient's age and general health.
- Whether the cancer has just been diagnosed or has recurred (come back).

Treatment of primary CNS lymphoma works best when the tumor has not spread outside the cerebrum (the largest part of the brain) and the patient is younger than 60 years, able to carry out most daily activities, and does not have AIDS or other diseases that weaken the immune system.

Staging Primary CNS Lymphoma

After primary central nervous system (CNS) lymphoma has been diagnosed, tests are done to find out if cancer cells have spread within the brain and spinal cord or to other parts of the body.

When primary CNS lymphoma continues to grow, it usually does not spread beyond the central nervous system or the eye. The process used to find out if cancer has spread is called staging. It is important to know if cancer has spread to other parts of the body in order to plan treatment. The following tests and procedures may be used in the staging process:

- **CT scan (CAT scan)**: A procedure that makes a series of detailed pictures of areas inside the body, taken from different angles. The pictures are made by a computer linked to an x-ray machine. A dye may be injected into a vein or swallowed to help the organs or tissues show up more clearly. This procedure is also called computed tomography, computerized tomography, or computerized axial tomography. For primary CNS lymphoma, a CT scan is done of the chest, abdomen, and pelvis (the part of the body between the hips).

- **PET scan (positron emission tomography scan)**: A procedure to find malignant tumor cells in the body. A small amount of radioactive glucose (sugar) is injected into a vein. The PET scanner rotates around the body and makes a picture of where glucose is being used in the body. Malignant tumor cells show up brighter in the picture because they are more active and take up more glucose than normal cells do. A PET scan and CT scan may be done at the same time. This is called a PET-CT.

- **MRI (magnetic resonance imaging)**: A procedure that uses a magnet, radio waves, and a computer to make a series of detailed pictures of areas inside the body. This procedure is also called nuclear magnetic resonance imaging (NMRI).

- **Bone marrow aspiration and biopsy:** The removal of bone marrow, blood, and a small piece of bone by inserting a hollow needle into the hipbone or breastbone. A pathologist views the bone marrow, blood, and bone under a microscope to look for signs of cancer.

There are three ways that cancer spreads in the body.

Cancer can spread through tissue, the lymph system, and the blood:

- Tissue. The cancer spreads from where it began by growing into nearby areas.

- Lymph system. The cancer spreads from where it began by getting into the lymph system. The cancer travels through the lymph vessels to other parts of the body.

- Blood. The cancer spreads from where it began by getting into the blood. The cancer travels through the blood vessels to other parts of the body.

Cancer may spread from where it began to other parts of the body.

When cancer spreads to another part of the body, it is called metastasis. Cancer cells break away from where they began (the primary tumor) and travel through the lymph system or blood.

- Lymph system. The cancer gets into the lymph system, travels through the lymph vessels, and forms a tumor (metastatic tumor) in another part of the body.

- Blood. The cancer gets into the blood, travels through the blood vessels, and forms a tumor (metastatic tumor) in another part of the body.

The metastatic tumor is the same type of cancer as the primary tumor. For example, if primary CNS lymphoma spreads to the liver, the cancer cells in the liver are actually lymphoma cells. The disease is metastatic CNS lymphoma, not liver cancer.

There is no standard staging system for primary CNS lymphoma.

Treatment Option Overview

There are different types of treatment for patients with primary CNS lymphoma.

Different types of treatment are available for patients with primary central nervous system (CNS) lymphoma. Some treatments are standard (the currently used treatment), and some are being tested in clinical trials. A treatment clinical trial is a research study meant to help improve current treatments or obtain information on new treatments for patients with cancer. When clinical trials show that a new treatment is better than the standard treatment, the new treatment may become the standard treatment. Patients may want to think about taking part in a clinical trial. Some clinical trials are open only to patients who have not started treatment.

Surgery is not used to treat primary CNS lymphoma.

Three standard treatments are used:

Radiation therapy

Radiation therapy is a cancer treatment that uses high-energy x-rays or other types of radiation to kill cancer cells or keep them from growing. There are two types of radiation therapy. External radiation therapy uses a machine outside the body to send radiation toward the cancer. Internal radiation therapy uses a radioactive substance sealed in needles, seeds, wires, or catheters that are placed directly into or near the cancer. The way the radiation therapy is given depends on the type of cancer being treated.

High-dose radiation therapy to the brain can damage healthy tissue and cause disorders that can affect thinking, learning, problem solving, speech, reading, writing, and memory. Clinical trials have tested the use of chemotherapy alone or before radiation therapy to reduce the damage to healthy brain tissue that occurs with the use of radiation therapy.

Chemotherapy

Chemotherapy is a cancer treatment that uses drugs to stop the growth of cancer cells, either by killing the cells or by stopping them from dividing. When chemotherapy is taken by mouth or injected into a vein or muscle, the drugs enter the bloodstream and can reach cancer cells throughout the body (systemic chemotherapy). When chemotherapy is placed directly into the cerebrospinal fluid (intrathecal chemotherapy), an organ, or a body cavity such as the abdomen, the drugs mainly affect cancer cells in those areas (regional chemotherapy). The way the chemotherapy is given depends on the type of cancer being treated. Primary CNS lymphoma may be treated with intrathecal chemotherapy and/or intraventricular chemotherapy, in which anticancer drugs are placed into the ventricles (fluid -filled cavities) of the brain.

A network of blood vessels and tissue, called the blood-brain barrier, protects the brain from harmful substances. This barrier can also keep anticancer drugs from reaching the brain. In order to treat CNS lymphoma, certain drugs may be used to make openings between cells in the blood-brain barrier. This is called blood-brain barrier disruption. Anticancer drugs infused into the bloodstream may then reach the brain.

Steroid therapy

Steroids are hormones made naturally in the body. They can also be made in a laboratory and used as drugs. Glucocorticoids are steroid drugs that have an anticancer effect in lymphomas.

New types of treatment are being tested in clinical trials.

High-dose chemotherapy with stem cell transplant

High-dose chemotherapy with stem cell transplant is a method of giving high doses of chemotherapy and replacing blood -forming cells destroyed by the cancer treatment. Stem cells (immature blood cells) are removed from the blood or bone marrow of the patient or a donor and are frozen and stored. After the chemotherapy is completed, the stored stem cells are thawed and given back to the patient through an infusion. These re-infused stem cells grow into (and restore) the body's blood cells.

Targeted therapy

Targeted therapy is a type of treatment that uses drugs or other substances to attack cancer cells. Targeted therapies usually cause less harm to normal cells than chemotherapy or radiation therapy do. Monoclonal antibody therapy is one type of targeted therapy being studied in the treatment of primary CNS lymphoma.

Monoclonal antibody therapy is a cancer treatment that uses antibodies made in the laboratory from a single type of immune system cell. These antibodies can identify substances on cancer cells or normal substances that may help cancer cells grow. The antibodies attach to the substances and kill the cancer cells, block their growth, or keep them from spreading. Monoclonal antibodies are given by infusion. They may be used alone or to carry drugs, toxins, or radioactive material directly to cancer cells.

Patients may want to think about taking part in a clinical trial.

For some patients, taking part in a clinical trial may be the best treatment choice. Clinical trials are part of the cancer research process. Clinical trials are done to find out if new cancer treatments are safe and effective or better than the standard treatment.

Many of today's standard treatments for cancer are based on earlier clinical trials. Patients who take part in a clinical trial may receive the standard treatment or be among the first to receive a new treatment.

Patients who take part in clinical trials also help improve the way cancer will be treated in the future. Even when clinical trials do not lead to effective new treatments, they often answer important questions and help move research forward.

Patients can enter clinical trials before, during, or after starting their cancer treatment.

Some clinical trials only include patients who have not yet received treatment. Other trials test treatments for patients whose cancer has not gotten better. There are also clinical trials that test new ways to stop cancer from recurring (coming back) or reduce the side effects of cancer treatment.

Clinical trials are taking place in many parts of the country.

Follow-up tests may be needed.

Some of the tests that were done to diagnose the cancer or to find out the stage of the cancer may be repeated. Some tests will be repeated in order to see how well the treatment is working. Decisions about whether to continue, change, or stop treatment may be based on the results of these tests. This is sometimes called re-staging.

Some of the tests will continue to be done from time to time after treatment has ended. The results of these tests can show if your condition has changed or if the cancer has recurred (come back). These tests are sometimes called follow-up tests or check-ups.

Section 32.2

Adult Hodgkin Lymphoma

Text in this section is excerpted from "Adult Hodgkin Lymphoma Treatment," National Cancer Institute at the National Institutes of Health (NIH), May 22, 2015.

General Information About Adult Hodgkin Lymphoma

Adult Hodgkin lymphoma is a disease in which malignant (cancer) cells form in the lymph system.

Adult Hodgkin lymphoma is a type of cancer that develops in the lymph system, part of the body's immune system.

The lymph system is made up of the following:

- Lymph: Colorless, watery fluid that travels through the lymph system and carries white blood cells called lymphocytes.

Lymphocytes protect the body against infections and the growth of tumors.

- Lymph vessels: A network of thin tubes that collect lymph from different parts of the body and return it to the bloodstream.

- Lymph nodes: Small, bean-shaped structures that filter lymph and store white blood cells that help fight infection and disease. Lymph nodes are located along the network of lymph vessels found throughout the body. Clusters of lymph nodes are found in the underarm, pelvis, neck, abdomen, and groin.

- Spleen: An organ that makes lymphocytes, filters the blood, stores blood cells, and destroys old blood cells. It is located on the left side of the abdomen near the stomach.

- Thymus: An organ in which lymphocytes grow and multiply. The thymus is in the chest behind the breast bone.

- Tonsils: Two small masses of lymph tissue at the back of the throat. The tonsils make lymphocytes.

- Bone marrow: The soft, spongy tissue in the center of large bones. Bone marrow makes white blood cells, red blood cells, and platelets.

Because lymph tissue is found throughout the body, Hodgkin lymphoma can begin in almost any part of the body and spread to almost any tissue or organ in the body.

Lymphomas are divided into two general types: Hodgkin lymphoma and non-Hodgkin lymphoma.

Hodgkin lymphoma can occur in both adults and children; however, treatment for adults may be different than treatment for children. Hodgkin lymphoma may also occur in patients who have acquired immunodeficiency syndrome (AIDS); these patients require special treatment.

Hodgkin lymphoma in pregnant women is the same as the disease in non-pregnant women of childbearing age. However, treatment is different for pregnant women.

There are two main types of Hodgkin lymphoma: classical and nodular lymphocyte-predominant.

Most Hodgkin lymphomas are the classical type. The classical type is broken down into the following four subtypes:

- Nodular sclerosing Hodgkin lymphoma.

- Mixed cellularity Hodgkin lymphoma.

- Lymphocyte depletion Hodgkin lymphoma.

- Lymphocyte-rich classical Hodgkin lymphoma.

Age, gender, and Epstein-Barr infection can affect the risk of adult Hodgkin lymphoma.

Anything that increases your risk of getting a disease is called a risk factor. Having a risk factor does not mean that you will get cancer; not having risk factors doesn't mean that you will not get cancer. Talk with your doctor if you think you may be at risk. Risk factors for adult Hodgkin lymphoma include the following:

- Being in young or late adulthood.

- Being male.

- Being infected with the Epstein-Barr virus.

- Having a first-degree relative (parent, brother, or sister) with Hodgkin lymphoma.

Pregnancy is not a risk factor for Hodgkin lymphoma.

Signs of adult Hodgkin lymphoma include swollen lymph nodes, fever, night sweats, and weight loss.

These and other signs and symptoms may be caused by adult Hodgkin lymphoma or by other conditions. Check with your doctor if any of the following do not go away:

- Painless, swollen lymph nodes in the neck, underarm, or groin.

- Fever for no known reason.

- Drenching night sweats.

- Weight loss for no known reason.

- Itchy skin.

- Feeling very tired.

Tests that examine the lymph nodes are used to detect (find) and diagnose adult Hodgkin lymphoma.

The following tests and procedures may be used:

- **Physical exam and history**: An exam of the body to check general signs of health, including checking for signs of disease, such as lumps or anything else that seems unusual. A history of the patient's past illnesses and treatments will also be taken.

- **Complete blood count (CBC)**: A procedure in which a sample of blood is drawn and checked for the following:

  - The number of red blood cells, white blood cells, and platelets.

  - The amount of hemoglobin (the protein that carries oxygen) in the red blood cells.

  - The portion of the sample made up of red blood cells.

- **Blood chemistry studies**: A procedure in which a blood sample is checked to measure the amounts of certain substances released into the blood by organs and tissues in the body. An unusual (higher or lower than normal) amount of a substance can be a sign of disease in the organ or tissue that makes it.

- **Sedimentation rate**: A procedure in which a sample of blood is drawn and checked for the rate at which the red blood cells settle to the bottom of the test tube.

- **Lymph node biopsy**: The removal of all or part of a lymph node. One of the following types of biopsies may be done:

  - **Excisional biopsy**: The removal of an entire lymph node.

  - **Incisional biopsy**: The removal of part of a lymph node.

  - **Core biopsy**: The removal of part of a lymph node using a wide needle.

A pathologist views the tissue under a microscope to look for cancer cells, especially Reed-Sternberg cells. Reed-Sternberg cells are common in classical Hodgkin lymphoma.

The following test may be done on tissue that was removed:

- **Immunophenotyping**: A laboratory test used to identify cells, based on the types of antigens or markers on the surface of the cell. This test is used to diagnose the specific type of lymphoma by comparing the cancer cells to normal cells of the immune system.

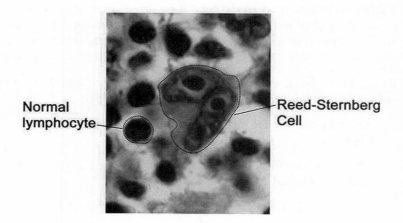

Fig 32.1 Reed-Sternberg cell. *Reed-Sternberg cells are large, abnormal lymphocytes that may contain more than one nucleus. These cells are found in Hodgkin lymphoma*

Certain factors affect prognosis (chance of recovery) and treatment options.

The prognosis (chance of recovery) and treatment options depend on the following:

- The patient's signs and symptoms.
- The stage of the cancer.
- The type of Hodgkin lymphoma.
- Blood test results.
- The patient's age, gender, and general health.
- Whether the cancer is recurrent or progressive.

For Hodgkin lymphoma during pregnancy, treatment options also depend on:

- The wishes of the patient.
- The age of the fetus.

Adult Hodgkin lymphoma can usually be cured if found and treated earl

Stages of Adult Hodgkin Lymphoma

After adult Hodgkin lymphoma has been diagnosed, tests are done to find out if cancer cells have spread within the lymph system or to other parts of the body.

The process used to find out if cancer has spread within the lymph system or to other parts of the body is called staging. The information gathered from the staging process determines the stage of the disease. It is important to know the stage in order to plan treatment. The following tests and procedures may be used in the staging process:

- **CT scan (CAT scan):** A procedure that makes a series of detailed pictures of areas inside the body, taken from different angles. The pictures are made by a computer linked to an x-ray machine. A dye may be injected into a vein or swallowed to help the organs or tissues show up more clearly. This procedure is also called computed tomography, computerized tomography, or computerized axial tomography. For adult Hodgkin lymphoma, CT scans of the neck, chest, abdomen, and pelvis are taken.

- **PET-CT scan:** A procedure that combines the pictures from a positron emission tomography (PET) scan and a computed tomography (CT) scan. The PET and CT scans are done at the same time on the same machine. The pictures from both scans are combined to make a more detailed picture than either test would make by itself. A PET scan is a procedure to find malignant tumor cells in the body. A small amount of radioactive glucose (sugar) is injected into a vein. The PET scanner rotates around the body and makes a picture of where glucose is being used in the body. Malignant tumor cells show up brighter in the picture because they are more active and take up more glucose than normal cells do.

- **Bone marrow aspiration and biopsy:** The removal of bone marrow, blood, and a small piece of bone by inserting a hollow needle into the hipbone or breastbone. A pathologist views the bone marrow, blood, and bone under a microscope to look for signs of cancer.

For pregnant women with Hodgkin lymphoma, staging tests that protect the fetus from the harms of radiation are used. These include:

- **MRI (magnetic resonance imaging):** A procedure that uses a magnet, radio waves, and a computer to make a series of

727

detailed pictures of areas inside the body. This procedure is also called nuclear magnetic resonance imaging (NMRI).

- **Ultrasound exam:** A procedure in which high-energy sound waves (ultrasound) are bounced off internal tissues or organs and make echoes. The echoes form a picture of body tissues called a sonogram.

There are three ways that cancer spreads in the body.

Cancer can spread through tissue, the lymph system, and the blood:

- Tissue. The cancer spreads from where it began by growing into nearby areas.
- Lymph system. The cancer spreads from where it began by getting into the lymph system. The cancer travels through the lymph vessels to other parts of the body.
- Blood. The cancer spreads from where it began by getting into the blood. The cancer travels through the blood vessels to other parts of the body.

Stages of adult Hodgkin lymphoma may include A, B, E, and S.

Adult Hodgkin lymphoma may be described as follows:

- A: The patient does not have B symptoms (fever, weight loss, or night sweats).
- B: The patient has B symptoms.
- E: Cancer is found in an organ or tissue that is not part of the lymph system but which may be next to an involved area of the lymph system.
- S: Cancer is found in the spleen.

The following stages are used for adult Hodgkin lymphoma:

Stage I

Stage I is divided into stage I and stage IE.

- Stage I: Cancer is found in one of the following places in the lymph system:

- One or more lymph nodes in one lymph node group.
- Waldeyer's ring.
- Thymus.
- Spleen.
- Stage IE: Cancer is found outside the lymph system in one organ or area.

Stage II

Stage II is divided into stage II and stage IIE.

- Stage II: Cancer is found in two or more lymph node groups either above or below the diaphragm (the thin muscle below the lungs that helps breathing and separates the chest from the abdomen).
- Stage IIE: Cancer is found in one or more lymph node groups either above or below the diaphragm and outside the lymph nodes in a nearby organ or area.

Stage III

Stage III is divided into stage III, stage IIIE, stage IIIS, and stage IIIE,S.

- Stage III: Cancer is found in lymph node groups above and below the diaphragm (the thin muscle below the lungs that helps breathing and separates the chest from the abdomen).
- Stage IIIE: Cancer is found in lymph node groups above and below the diaphragm and outside the lymph nodes in a nearby organ or area.
- Stage IIIS: Cancer is found in lymph node groups above and below the diaphragm, and in the spleen.
- Stage IIIE,S: Cancer is found in lymph node groups above and below the diaphragm, outside the lymph nodes in a nearby organ or area, and in the spleen.

Stage IV

In stage IV, the cancer:

- is found outside the lymph nodes throughout one or more organs, and may be in lymph nodes near those organs; or

- is found outside the lymph nodes in one organ and has spread to areas far away from that organ; or

- is found in the lung, liver, bone marrow, or cerebrospinal fluid (CSF). The cancer has not spread to the lung, liver, bone marrow, or CSF from nearby areas.

Adult Hodgkin lymphoma may be grouped for treatment as follows:

Early Favorable

Early favorable adult Hodgkin lymphoma is stage I or stage II, without risk factors.

Early Unfavorable

Early unfavorable adult Hodgkin lymphoma is stage I or stage II with **one or more** of the following risk factors:

- A tumor in the chest that is larger than 1/3 of the width of the chest or at least 10 centimeters.

- Cancer in an organ other than the lymph nodes.

- A high sedimentation rate (in a sample of blood, the red blood cells settle to the bottom of the test tube more quickly than normal).

- Three or more lymph nodes with cancer.

- Symptoms such as fever, weight loss, or night sweats.

Advanced Favorable

Advanced favorable adult Hodgkin lymphoma is stage III or stage IV with **three or fewer** of the following risk factors:

- Being male.

- Being aged 45 years or older.

- Having stage IV disease.

- Having a low blood albumin (protein) level (below 4).

- Having a low hemoglobin level (below 10.5).
- Having a high white blood cell count (15,000 or higher).
- Having a low lymphocyte count (below 600 or less than 8% of the white blood cell count).

Advanced Unfavorable

Advanced unfavorable Hodgkin lymphoma is stage III or stage IV with **four or more** of the following risk factors:

- Being male.
- Being aged 45 years or older.
- Having stage IV disease.
- Having a low blood albumin (protein) level (below 4).
- Having a low hemoglobin level (below 10.5).
- Having a high white blood cell count (15,000 or higher).
- Having a low lymphocyte count (below 600 or less than 8% of the white blood cell count).

Treatment Option Overview

There are different types of treatment for patients with adult Hodgkin lymphoma.

Different types of treatment are available for patients with adult Hodgkin lymphoma. Some treatments are standard (the currently used treatment), and some are being tested in clinical trials. A treatment clinical trial is a research study meant to help improve current treatments or obtain information on new treatments for patients with cancer. When clinical trials show that a new treatment is better than the standard treatment, the new treatment may become the standard treatment. Patients may want to think about taking part in a clinical trial. Some clinical trials are open only to patients who have not started treatment.

For pregnant women with Hodgkin lymphoma, treatment is carefully chosen to protect the fetus. Treatment decisions are based on the mother's wishes, the stage of the Hodgkin lymphoma, and the age of the fetus. The treatment plan may change as the signs and symptoms, cancer, and pregnancy change. Choosing the most appropriate cancer treatment is a decision that ideally involves the patient, family, and health care team.

Patients with Hodgkin lymphoma should have their treatment planned by a team of health care providers with expertise in treating lymphomas.

Treatment will be overseen by a medical oncologist, a doctor who specializes in treating cancer. The medical oncologist may refer you to other health care providers who have experience and expertise in treating adult Hodgkin lymphoma and who specialize in certain areas of medicine. These may include the following specialists:

- Neurosurgeon.

- Neurologist.

- Rehabilitation specialist.

- Radiation oncologist.

- Endocrinologist.

- Hematologist.

- Other oncology specialists.

Patients may develop late effects that appear months or years after their treatment for Hodgkin lymphoma.

Treatment with chemotherapy and/or radiation therapy for Hodgkin lymphoma may increase the risk of second cancers and other health problems for many months or years after treatment. These late effects depend on the type of treatment and the patient's age when treated, and may include:

- Acute myelogenous leukemia.
- Cancer of the breast, bone, cervix, gastrointestinal tract, head and neck, lung, soft tissue, and thyroid.
- Heart, lung, and thyroid disease.
- Avascular necrosis of bone (death of bone cells caused by lack of blood flow).
- Herpes zoster (shingles) or severe infection.
- Depression and fatigue.
- Infertility.
- Hypogonadism (low levels of testosterone and estrogen).

Regular follow-up by doctors who are expert in finding and treating late effects is important for the long-term health of patients treated for Hodgkin lymphoma.

Three types of standard treatment are used:

Chemotherapy

Chemotherapy is a cancer treatment that uses drugs to stop the growth of cancer cells, either by killing the cells or by stopping them from dividing. When chemotherapy is taken by mouth or injected into a vein or muscle, the drugs enter the bloodstream and can reach cancer cells throughout the body (systemic chemotherapy). When chemotherapy is placed directly into the cerebrospinal fluid, an organ, or a body cavity such as the abdomen, the drugs mainly affect cancer cells in those areas (regional chemotherapy). The way the chemotherapy is given depends on the type and stage of the cancer being treated. Combination chemotherapy is treatment with more than one anti-cancer drug.

When a pregnant woman is treated with chemotherapy for Hodgkin lymphoma, it isn't possible to protect the fetus from being exposed to the chemotherapy. Some chemotherapy regimens may cause birth defects if given in the first trimester. Vinblastine is an anticancer drug that has not been linked with birth defects when given in the second half of pregnancy.

Radiation therapy

Radiation therapy is a cancer treatment that uses high-energy x-rays or other types of radiation to kill cancer cells or keep them from growing. There are two types of radiation therapy. External radiation therapy uses a machine outside the body to send radiation toward the cancer. Internal radiation therapy uses a radioactive substance sealed in needles, seeds, wires, or catheters that are placed directly into or near the cancer. The way the radiation therapy is given depends on the type and stage of the cancer being treated.

For a pregnant woman with Hodgkin lymphoma, radiation therapy should be postponed until after delivery, if possible, to avoid any risk to the fetus. If immediate treatment is needed, the woman may decide to continue the pregnancy and receive radiation therapy. However, lead used to shield the fetus may not protect it from scattered radiation that could possibly cause cancer in the future.

Surgery

Laparotomy is a procedure in which an incision (cut) is made in the wall of the abdomen to check the inside of the abdomen for signs of disease. The size of the incision depends on the reason the laparotomy is being done. Sometimes organs are removed or tissue samples are taken and checked under a microscope for signs of disease. If cancer is found, the tissue or organ is removed during the laparotomy.

For pregnant patients with Hodgkin lymphoma, treatment options also include:

Watchful waiting

Watchful waiting is closely monitoring a patient's condition without giving any treatment unless signs or symptoms appear or change. Delivery may be induced when the fetus is 32 to 36 weeks old, so that the mother can begin treatment.

Steroid therapy

Steroids are hormones made naturally in the body by the adrenal glands and by reproductive organs. Some types of steroids are made in a laboratory. Certain steroid drugs have been found to help chemotherapy work better and help stop the growth of cancer cells. Steroids can also help the lungs of the fetus develop faster than normal. This is important when delivery is induced early.

New types of treatment are being tested in clinical trials.

Chemotherapy and radiation therapy with stem cell transplant

High-dose chemotherapy and radiation therapy with stem cell transplant is a way of giving high doses of chemotherapy and radiation therapy and replacing blood -forming cells destroyed by the cancer treatment. Stem cells (immature blood cells) are removed from the blood or bone marrow of the patient or a donor and are frozen and stored. After therapy is completed, the stored stem cells are thawed and given back to the patient through an infusion. These re-infused stem cells grow into (and restore) the body's blood cells. The use of lower-dose chemotherapy and radiation therapy with stem cell transplant is also being studied.

Monoclonal antibody therapy

Monoclonal antibody therapy is a cancer treatment that uses antibodies made in the laboratory, from a single type of immune system cell. These antibodies can identify substances on cancer cells or normal substances that may help cancer cells grow. The antibodies attach to the substances and kill the cancer cells, block their growth, or keep them from spreading. Monoclonal antibodies are given by infusion. They may be used alone or to carry drugs, toxins, or radioactive material directly to cancer cells.

Patients may want to think about taking part in a clinical trial.

For some patients, taking part in a clinical trial may be the best treatment choice. Clinical trials are part of the cancer research process. Clinical trials are done to find out if new cancer treatments are safe and effective or better than the standard treatment.

Many of today's standard treatments for cancer are based on earlier clinical trials. Patients who take part in a clinical trial may receive the standard treatment or be among the first to receive a new treatment.

Patients who take part in clinical trials also help improve the way cancer will be treated in the future. Even when clinical trials do not lead to effective new treatments, they often answer important questions and help move research forward.

Patients can enter clinical trials before, during, or after starting their cancer treatment.

Some clinical trials only include patients who have not yet received treatment. Other trials test treatments for patients whose cancer has not gotten better. There are also clinical trials that test new ways to stop cancer from recurring (coming back) or reduce the side effects of cancer treatment.

Clinical trials are taking place in many parts of the country.

Follow-up tests may be needed.

Some of the tests that were done to diagnose the cancer or to find out the stage of the cancer may be repeated. Some tests will be repeated in order to see how well the treatment is working. Decisions about whether to continue, change, or stop treatment may be based on the results of these tests. This is sometimes called re-staging.

Some of the tests will continue to be done from time to time after treatment has ended. The results of these tests can show if your condition has changed or if the cancer has recurred (come back). These tests are sometimes called follow-up tests or check-ups.

Section 32.3

Adult Non-Hodgkin Lymphoma

Text in this section is excerpted from "Adult Non Hodgkin Lymphoma Treatment," National Cancer Institute at the National Institutes of Health (NIH), April 25, 2014.

General Information About Adult Non-Hodgkin Lymphoma

Adult non-Hodgkin lymphoma is a disease in which malignant (cancer) cells form in the lymph system.

The lymph system is part of the immune system and is made up of the following:

- Lymph: Colorless, watery fluid that travels through the lymph system and carries white blood cells called lymphocytes. Lymphocytes protect the body against infections and the growth of tumors.

- Lymph vessels: A network of thin tubes that collect lymph from different parts of the body and return it to the bloodstream.

- Lymph nodes: Small, bean-shaped structures that filter lymph and store white blood cells that help fight infection and disease. Lymph nodes are located along the network of lymph vessels found throughout the body. Clusters of lymph nodes are found in the underarm, pelvis, neck, abdomen, and groin.

- Spleen: An organ that makes lymphocytes, filters the blood, stores blood cells, and destroys old blood cells. It is on the left side of the abdomen near the stomach.

- Thymus: An organ in which lymphocytes grow and multiply. The thymus is in the chest behind the breast bone.

- Tonsils: Two small masses of lymph tissue at the back of the throat. The tonsils make lymphocytes.

- Bone marrow: The soft, spongy tissue in the center of large bones. Bone marrow makes white blood cells, red blood cells, and platelets.

Because lymph tissue is found throughout the body, adult non-Hodgkin lymphoma can begin in almost any part of the body. Cancer can spread to the liver and many other organs and tissues.

Non-Hodgkin lymphoma in pregnant women is the same as the disease in non-pregnant women of childbearing age. However, treatment is different for pregnant women.

Non-Hodgkin lymphoma can occur in both adults and children. Treatment for children, however, is different than treatment for adults.

There are many different types of lymphoma.

Lymphomas are divided into two general types: Hodgkin lymphoma and non-Hodgkin lymphoma.

Waldenström macroglobulinemia is a type of non-Hodgkin lymphoma.

Waldenström macroglobulinemia begins in a type of white blood cell called B lymphocytes. Certain B lymphocytes multiply out of control and make large amounts of a protein called monoclonal immunoglobulin M (IgM) antibody. High levels of IgM in the blood cause the blood to thicken and leads to many of the symptoms of Waldenström macroglobulinemia. Waldenström macroglobulinemia is also called lymphoplasmacytic lymphoma.

Age, gender, and a weakened immune system can affect the risk of adult non-Hodgkin lymphoma.

Anything that increases your risk of getting a disease is called a risk factor. Having a risk factor does not mean that you will get cancer; not having risk factors doesn't mean that you will not get cancer. Talk with your doctor if you think you may be at risk. Risk factors for adult non-Hodgkin lymphoma include the following:

- Being older, male, or white.

- Having one of the following medical conditions:

  - An Inherited immune disorder (for example, hypogamma-globulinemia or Wiskott-Aldrich syndrome)

  - An autoimmune disease (for example, rheumatoid arthritis, psoriasis, or Sjögren syndrome).

  - HIV /AIDS.

  - Human T-lymphotrophic virus type I or Epstein-Barr virus.

  - A history of Helicobacter pylori infection.

- Taking immunosuppressant drugs after an organ transplant.

- Being exposed to certain pesticides.

- A diet high in meats and fat.

- Past treatment for Hodgkin lymphoma.

Signs and symptoms of adult non-Hodgkin lymphoma include fever, sweating, weight loss, and fatigue.

These and other signs and symptoms may be caused by adult non-Hodgkin lymphoma or by other conditions. Check with your doctor if you have any of the following:

- Painless swelling in the lymph nodes in the neck, underarm, groin, or stomach.

- Fever for no known reason.

- Drenching night sweats.

- Feeling very tired.

- Weight loss for no known reason.

- Skin rash or itchy skin.

- Pain in the chest, abdomen, or bones for no known reason.

Signs and symptoms of Waldenström macroglobulinemia depend on the part of the body affected. Most patients with Waldenström macroglobulinemia have no signs or symptoms. Check with your doctor if you have any of the following:

- Feeling very tired.

- Headache.

- Easy bruising or bleeding, such as nosebleeds or bleeding from the gums.

- Vision changes, such as blurred vision or blind spots.

- Dizziness.

- Pain, tingling, or numbness, especially in the hands, feet, fingers, or toes.

- Confusion.

- Pain or a feeling of fullness below the ribs on the left side.

- Painless lumps in the neck, underarm, stomach, or groin.

- Weight loss for no known reason.

Tests that examine the body and lymph system are used to help detect (find) and diagnose adult non-Hodgkin lymphoma.

The following tests and procedures may be used:

- **Physical exam and history:** An exam of the body to check general signs of health, including checking for signs of disease, such as lumps or anything else that seems unusual. A history of the patient's health habits and past illnesses and treatments will also be taken.

- **Blood and urine immunoglobulin studies:** A procedure in which a blood or urine sample is checked to measure the amounts of certain antibodies (immunoglobulins). In Waldenström macroglobulinemia, immunoglobulin M (IgM) and beta-2-microglobulin is measured. A higher- or lower-than-normal amount of these substances can be a sign of disease.

- **Blood viscosity test:** A procedure in which a blood sample is checked to see how "thick" the blood is. In Waldenström macroglobulinemia, when the amount of monoclonal immunoglobulin M (IgM) antibody in the blood becomes very high, the blood thickens and may cause signs or symptoms.

- **Flow cytometry:** A laboratory test that measures the number of cells in a sample, the percentage of live cells in a sample, and certain characteristics of cells, such as size, shape, and the presence of tumor markers on the cell surface. The cells are stained with a light-sensitive dye, placed in a fluid, and passed in a stream before a laser or other type of light. The measurements are based on how the light-sensitive dye reacts to the light. This test is used to diagnose Waldenström macroglobulinemia.

- **Bone marrow aspiration and biopsy:** The removal of bone marrow, blood, and a small piece of bone by inserting a needle into the hipbone or breastbone. A pathologist views the bone marrow, blood, and bone under a microscope to look for signs of cancer.

- **Lumbar puncture:** A procedure used to collect cerebrospinal fluid from the spinal column. This is done by placing a needle into the spinal column. This procedure is also called an LP or spinal tap. A pathologist views the cerebrospinal fluid under a microscope to look for signs of cancer.

- **Lymph node biopsy:** The removal of all or part of a lymph node. A pathologist views the tissue under a microscope to look for cancer cells. One of the following types of biopsies may be done:

  - **Excisional biopsy:** The removal of an entire lymph node.

  - **Incisional biopsy:** The removal of part of a lymph node.

  - **Core biopsy:** The removal of part of a lymph node using a wide needle.

  - **Fine-needle aspiration (FNA) biopsy:** The removal of tissue or fluid using a thin needle.

  - **Laparoscopy**: A surgical procedure to look at the organs inside the abdomen to check for signs of disease. Small incisions (cuts) are made in the wall of the abdomen and a laparoscope (a thin, lighted tube) is inserted into one of the incisions. Other instruments may be inserted through the same or other incisions to perform procedures such as removing organs or taking tissue samples to be checked under a microscope for signs of disease.

  - **Laparotomy**: A surgical procedure in which an incision (cut) is made in the wall of the abdomen to check the inside of the abdomen for signs of disease. The size of the incision depends on the reason the laparotomy is being done. Sometimes organs are removed or tissue samples are taken and checked under a microscope for signs of disease.

If cancer is found, the following tests may be done to study the cancer cells:

- **Immunohistochemistry**: A test that uses antibodies to check for certain antigens in a sample of tissue. The antibody is usually linked to a radioactive substance or a dye that causes the tissue to light up under a microscope. This type of test may be used to tell the difference between different types of cancer.

- **Cytogenetic analysis:** A laboratory test in which cells in a sample of tissue are viewed under a microscope to look for certain changes in the chromosomes.

- **Immunophenotyping:** A process used to identify cells, based on the types of antigens or markers on the surface of the cell. This process is used to diagnose specific types of leukemia and lymphoma by comparing the cancer cells to normal cells of the immune system.

Certain factors affect prognosis (chance of recovery) and treatment options.

The prognosis (chance of recovery) and treatment options depend on the following:

- The stage of the cancer.
- The type of non-Hodgkin lymphoma.
- The amount of lactate dehydrogenase (LDH) in the blood.
- The amount of beta-2-microglobulin in the blood (for Waldenström macroglobulinemia).
- The patient's age and general health.
- Whether the lymphoma has just been diagnosed or has recurred (come back).

For non-Hodgkin lymphoma during pregnancy, the treatment options also depend on:

- The wishes of the patient
- Which trimester of pregnancy the patient is in.

Some types of non-Hodgkin lymphoma spread more quickly than others do. Most non-Hodgkin lymphomas that occur during pregnancy are aggressive. Delaying treatment of aggressive lymphoma until after the baby is born may lessen the mother's chance of survival. Immediate treatment is often recommended, even during pregnancy.

Stages of Adult Non-Hodgkin Lymphoma

After adult non-Hodgkin lymphoma has been diagnosed, tests are done to find out if cancer cells have spread within the lymph system or to other parts of the body.

The process used to find out the type of cancer and if cancer cells have spread within the lymph system or to other parts of the body is called staging. The information gathered from the staging process determines the stage of the disease. It is important to know the stage of the disease in order to plan treatment. The following tests and procedures may be used in the staging process:

- **Complete blood count (CBC) with differential:** A procedure in which a sample of blood is drawn and checked for the following:

  - The number of red blood cells and platelets.

  - The number and type of white blood cells.

  - The amount of hemoglobin (the protein that carries oxygen) in the red blood cells.

  - The portion of the blood sample made up of red blood cells.

- **Blood chemistry studies**: A procedure in which a blood sample is checked to measure the amounts of certain substances released into the blood by organs and tissues in the body. An unusual (higher or lower than normal) amount of a substance can be a sign of disease in the organ or tissue that makes it.

- **CT scan (CAT scan):** A procedure that makes a series of detailed pictures of areas inside the body, such as the lung, lymph nodes, and liver, taken from different angles. The pictures are made by a computer linked to an x-ray machine. A dye may be injected into a vein or swallowed to help the organs or tissues show up more clearly. This procedure is also called computed tomography, computerized tomography, or computerized axial tomography.

- **PET scan (positron emission tomography scan):** A procedure to find malignant tumor cells in the body. A small amount of radioactive glucose (sugar) is injected into a vein. The PET scanner rotates around the body and makes a picture of where glucose is being used in the body. Malignant tumor cells show up brighter in the picture because they are more active and take up more glucose than normal cells do.

- **MRI (magnetic resonance imaging):** A procedure that uses a magnet, radio waves, and a computer to make a series of detailed pictures of areas inside the body. This procedure is also called nuclear magnetic resonance imaging (NMRI).

- **Bone marrow aspiration and biopsy:** The removal of bone marrow, blood, and a small piece of bone by inserting a needle into the hipbone or breast bone. A pathologist views the bone marrow, blood, and bone under a microscope to look for signs of cancer.

For pregnant women with non-Hodgkin lymphoma, staging tests that protect the fetus from the harms of radiation are used. These include MRI, bone marrow aspiration and biopsy, lumbar puncture, and ultrasound, which do not use radiation. An ultrasound exam is a procedure in which high-energy sound waves (ultrasound) are bounced off internal tissues or organs and make echoes. The echoes form a picture of body tissues called a sonogram.

There are three ways that cancer spreads in the body.

Cancer can spread through tissue, the lymph system, and the blood:

- Tissue. The cancer spreads from where it began by growing into nearby areas.
- Lymph system. The cancer spreads from where it began by getting into the lymph system. The cancer travels through the lymph vessels to other parts of the body.
- Blood. The cancer spreads from where it began by getting into the blood. The cancer travels through the blood vessels to other parts of the body.

Stages of adult non-Hodgkin lymphoma may include E and S.

Adult non-Hodgkin lymphoma may be described as follows:

- E: "E" stands for extranodal and means the cancer is found in an area or organ other than the lymph nodes or has spread to tissues beyond, but near, the major lymphatic areas.
- S: "S" stands for spleen and means the cancer is found in the spleen.

The following stages are used for adult non-Hodgkin lymphoma:

Stage I

Stage I adult non-Hodgkin lymphoma is divided into stage I and stage IE.

- Stage I: Cancer is found in one lymphatic area (lymph node group, tonsils and nearby tissue, thymus, or spleen).

- Stage IE: Cancer is found in one organ or area outside the lymph nodes.

Stage II

Stage II adult non-Hodgkin lymphoma is divided into stage II and stage IIE.

- Stage II: Cancer is found in two or more lymph node groups either above or below the diaphragm (the thin muscle below the lungs that helps breathing and separates the chest from the abdomen).

- Stage IIE: Cancer is found in one or more lymph node groups either above or below the diaphragm. Cancer is also found outside the lymph nodes in one organ or area on the same side of the diaphragm as the affected lymph nodes.

Stage III

Stage III adult non-Hodgkin lymphoma is divided into stage III, stage IIIE, stage IIIS, and stage IIIE+S.

- Stage III: Cancer is found in lymph node groups above and below the diaphragm (the thin muscle below the lungs that helps breathing and separates the chest from the abdomen).

- Stage IIIE: Cancer is found in lymph node groups above and below the diaphragm and outside the lymph nodes in a nearby organ or area.

- Stage IIIS: Cancer is found in lymph node groups above and below the diaphragm, and in the spleen.

- Stage IIIE+S: Cancer is found in lymph node groups above and below the diaphragm, outside the lymph nodes in a nearby organ or area, and in the spleen.

Stage IV

In stage IV adult non-Hodgkin lymphoma, the cancer:

- is found throughout one or more organs that are not part of a lymphatic area (lymph node group, tonsils and nearby tissue, thymus, or spleen), and may be in lymph nodes near those organs; or

- is found in one organ that is not part of a lymphatic area and has spread to organs or lymph nodes far away from that organ; or

- is found in the liver, bone marrow, cerebrospinal fluid (CSF), or lungs (other than cancer that has spread to the lungs from nearby areas).

Adult non-Hodgkin lymphomas are also described based on how fast they grow and where the affected lymph nodes are in the body.

Indolent or aggressive:

- Indolent lymphomas: These tend to grow and spread slowly and have few symptoms.

- Aggressive lymphomas: These grow and spread quickly and have severe symptoms. Lymphoblastic lymphoma, diffuse small non-cleaved cell lymphoma /Burkitt lymphoma, and mantle cell lymphoma are three types of aggressive adult non-Hodgkin lymphoma. Aggressive lymphomas are seen more often in patients who are HIV -positive (AIDS -related lymphoma).

Contiguous or noncontiguous:

- Contiguous lymphomas: Lymphomas in which the lymph nodes with cancer are next to each other.

- Noncontiguous lymphomas: Lymphomas in which the lymph nodes with cancer are not next to each other, but are on the same side of the diaphragm.

There is no standard staging system for Waldenström macroglobulinemia.

Treatment Options for Non-Hodgkin Lymphoma

Indolent, Stage I and Contiguous Stage II Adult Non-Hodgkin Lymphoma

Treatment of indolent, stage I and contiguous stage II adult non-Hodgkin lymphoma may include the following:

- Radiation therapy directed at the area where cancer is found.

- Watchful waiting.

- Chemotherapy with radiation therapy.

- Radiation therapy directed at the area where cancer is found and nearby lymph nodes.

- Monoclonal antibody therapy with or without chemotherapy.

- Treatments used for more advanced disease, in patients who can't be treated with radiation therapy.

Aggressive, Stage I and Contiguous Stage II Adult Non-Hodgkin Lymphoma

Treatment of aggressive, stage I and contiguous stage II adult non-Hodgkin lymphoma may include the following:

- Combination chemotherapy with or without radiation therapy to areas where cancer is found.

- A clinical trial of monoclonal antibody therapy and combination chemotherapy with steroids. Radiation therapy may also be given.

Indolent, Noncontiguous Stage II / III / IV Adult Non-Hodgkin Lymphoma

Treatment of indolent, noncontiguous stage II /III /IV adult non-Hodgkin lymphoma may include the following:

- Watchful waiting for patients who do not have symptoms.

- Chemotherapy with or without steroids.

- Combination chemotherapy with steroids.

- Monoclonal antibody therapy with or without chemotherapy.

- Radiolabeled monoclonal antibody therapy.

- Radiation therapy directed at the area where cancer is found and nearby lymph nodes, for patients who have stage II and stage III disease.

- A clinical trial of chemotherapy with or without total-body irradiation (radiation therapy to the entire body) or radiolabeled monoclonal antibody therapy, followed by autologous or allogeneic stem cell transplant.

- A clinical trial of chemotherapy with or without vaccine therapy.

Aggressive, Noncontiguous Stage II / III / IV Adult Non-Hodgkin Lymphoma

Treatment of aggressive, noncontiguous stage II /III /IV adult non-Hodgkin lymphoma may include the following:

- Combination chemotherapy with radiation therapy or monoclonal antibody therapy.

- Combination chemotherapy with CNS prophylaxis.

- A clinical trial of autologous or allogeneic stem cell transplant for patients who are likely to relapse.

Adult Lymphoblastic Lymphoma

Treatment of adult lymphoblastic lymphoma may include the following:

- Combination chemotherapy and CNS prophylaxis.

- A clinical trial of autologous or allogeneic stem cell transplant.

Diffuse Small Non-cleaved Cell / Burkitt Lymphoma

Treatment of adult diffuse small non-cleaved cell/Burkitt lymphoma may include the following:

- Combination chemotherapy and CNS prophylaxis.

- A clinical trial of combination chemotherapy.

- A clinical trial of autologous or allogeneic stem cell transplant.

Waldenström Macroglobulinemia

Treatment of Waldenström macroglobulinemia may include the following:

- Watchful waiting.

- Plasmapheresis and chemotherapy.

- Combinations of chemotherapy using one or more anticancer drugs and targeted therapy with amonoclonal antibody or a proteasome inhibitor.

- Biologic therapy with interferon.

- A clinical trial of stem cell transplant.

Recurrent Adult Non-Hodgkin Lymphoma

Indolent, Recurrent Adult Non-Hodgkin Lymphoma

Treatment of indolent, recurrent adult non-Hodgkin lymphoma may include the following:

- Chemotherapy with one or more drugs.

- Radiation therapy.

- Radiation therapy and/or chemotherapy as palliative therapy to relieve symptoms and improve quality of life.

- Monoclonal antibody therapy.

- A clinical trial of radiolabeled monoclonal antibody therapy.

- A clinical trial of monoclonal antibody therapy as palliative therapy to relieve symptoms and improve quality of life.

- A clinical trial of autologous or allogeneic stem cell transplant.

Treatment of indolent lymphoma that comes back as aggressive lymphoma may include the following:

- A clinical trial of autologous or allogeneic stem cell transplant.

- A clinical trial of combination chemotherapy followed by radiation therapy or stem cell transplant and radiation therapy.

- A clinical trial of monoclonal antibody therapy.

- A clinical trial of radiolabeled monoclonal antibody therapy.

Aggressive, Recurrent Adult Non-Hodgkin Lymphoma

Treatment of aggressive, recurrent adult non-Hodgkin lymphoma may include the following:

- Stem cell transplant.

- Monoclonal antibody therapy with or without combination chemotherapy followed by autologous stem cell transplant.

- Radiolabeled monoclonal antibody therapy.

- A clinical trial of autologous or allogeneic stem cell transplant.

- A clinical trial of combination chemotherapy followed by radiation therapy or stem cell transplant and radiation therapy.

Treatment of aggressive lymphoma that comes back as indolent lymphoma may include the following:

- Chemotherapy.

- Palliative therapy with low-dose radiation therapy to relieve symptoms and improve quality of life.

Non-Hodgkin Lymphoma During Pregnancy

Aggressive Non-Hodgkin Lymphoma During the First Trimester of Pregnancy

When aggressive non-Hodgkin lymphoma is diagnosed in the first trimester of pregnancy, medical oncologists may advise the patient to end her pregnancy so that treatment may begin. Treatment is usually chemotherapy with or without radiation therapy.

Aggressive Non-Hodgkin Lymphoma During the Second and Third Trimesters of Pregnancy

When possible, treatment should delayed until after an early delivery, so that the anticancer drugs or radiation therapy will not affect the fetus. However, sometimes the cancer will need to be treated right away to increase the mother's chance of survival.

Indolent Non-Hodgkin Lymphoma During Pregnancy

Women who have indolent (slow-growing) non-Hodgkin lymphoma can usually delay treatment with watchful waiting.

Chapter 33

Other Types of Hematological Cancer

Chapter Contents

Section 33.1

Chronic Myeloproliferative Neoplasms

Text in this section is excerpted from "Chronic Myelogenous
Leukemia Treatment," National Cancer Institute at the National
Institutes of Health (NIH), March 16, 2015.

General Information About Chronic Myeloproliferative Neoplasms

*Chronic myelogenous leukemia is a disease in which the
bone marrow makes too many white blood cells.*

Chronic myelogenous leukemia (also called CML or chronic granulocytic leukemia) is a slowly progressing blood and bone marrow disease that usually occurs during or after middle age, and rarely occurs in children.

*Leukemia may affect red blood cells, white blood cells, and
platelets.*

Normally, the bone marrow makes blood stem cells (immature cells) that become mature blood cells over time. A blood stem cell may become a myeloid stem cell or a lymphoid stem cell. A lymphoid stem cell becomes a white blood cell.

A myeloid stem cell becomes one of three types of mature blood cells:

- Red blood cells that carry oxygen and other substances to all tissues of the body.

- Platelets that form blood clots to stop bleeding.

- Granulocytes (white blood cells) that fight infection and disease.

In CML, too many blood stem cells become a type of white blood cell called granulocytes. These granulocytes are abnormal and do not become healthy white blood cells. They are also called leukemia cells. The leukemia cells can build up in the blood and bone marrow so there is less room for healthy white blood cells, red blood cells, and platelets. When this happens, infection, anemia, or easy bleeding may occur.

Signs and symptoms of chronic myelogenous leukemia include fever, night sweats, and tiredness.

These and other signs and symptoms may be caused by CML or by other conditions. Check with your doctor if you have any of the following:

- Feeling very tired.
- Weight loss for no known reason.
- Night sweats.
- Fever.
- Pain or a feeling of fullness below the ribs on the left side.

Sometimes CML does not cause any symptoms at all.

Most people with CML have a gene mutation (change) called the Philadelphia chromosome.

Every cell in the body contains DNA (genetic material) that determines how the cell looks and acts. DNA is contained inside chromosomes. In CML, part of the DNA from one chromosome moves to another chromosome. This change is called the "Philadelphia chromosome." It results in the bone marrow making an enzyme, called tyrosine kinase, that causes too many stem cells to become white blood cells (granulocytes or blasts).

The Philadelphia chromosome is not passed from parent to child.

Tests that examine the blood and bone marrow are used to detect (find) and diagnose chronic myelogenous leukemia.

The following tests and procedures may be used:

- **Physical exam and history:** An exam of the body to check general signs of health, including checking for signs of disease such as an enlarged spleen. A history of the patient's health habits and past illnesses and treatments will also be taken.

- **Complete blood count (CBC) with differential:** A procedure in which a sample of blood is drawn and checked for the following:

  - The number of red blood cells and platelets.

- The number and type of white blood cells.

- The amount of hemoglobin (the protein that carries oxygen) in the red blood cells.

- The portion of the blood sample made up of red blood cells.

- **Blood chemistry studies:** A procedure in which a blood sample is checked to measure the amounts of certain substances released into the blood by organs and tissues in the body. An unusual (higher or lower than normal) amount of a substance can be a sign of disease in the organ or tissue that makes it.

- **Bone marrow aspiration and biopsy:** The removal of bone marrow, blood, and a small piece of bone by inserting a needle into the hipbone or breastbone. A pathologist views the bone marrow, blood, and bone under a microscope to look for abnormal cells.

One of the following tests may be done on the samples of blood or bone marrow tissue that are removed:

- **Cytogenetic analysis:** A test in which cells in a sample of blood or bone marrow are viewed under a microscope to look for certain changes in the chromosomes, such as the Philadelphia chromosome.

- **FISH (fluorescence in situ hybridization):** A laboratory technique used to look at genes or chromosomes in cells and tissues. Pieces of DNA that contain a fluorescent dye are made in the laboratory and added to cells or tissues on a glass slide. When these pieces of DNA bind to specific genes or areas of chromosomes on the slide, they light up when viewed under a microscope with a special light.

- **Reverse transcription polymerase chain reaction test (RT–PCR):** A laboratory test in which cells in a sample of tissue are studied using chemicals to look for certain changes in the structure or function of genes.

Certain factors affect prognosis (chance of recovery) and treatment options.

The prognosis (chance of recovery) and treatment options depend on the following:

- The patient's age.
- The phase of CML.

- The amount of blasts in the blood or bone marrow.

- The size of the spleen at diagnosis.

- The patient's general health.

Stages of Chronic Myelogenous Leukemia

After chronic myelogenous leukemia has been diagnosed, tests are done to find out if the cancer has spread.

Staging is the process used to find out how far the cancer has spread. There is no standard staging system for chronic myelogenous leukemia (CML). Instead, the disease is classified by phase: chronic phase, accelerated phase, or blastic phase. It is important to know the phase in order to plan treatment. The information from tests and procedures done to detect (find) and diagnose chronic myelogenous leukemia is also used to plan treatment.

Chronic myelogenous leukemia has 3 phases.

As the amount of blast cells increases in the blood and bone marrow, there is less room for healthy white blood cells, red blood cells, and platelets. This may result in infections, anemia, and easy bleeding, as well as bone pain and pain or a feeling of fullness below the ribs on the left side. The number of blast cells in the blood and bone marrow and the severity of signs or symptoms determine the phase of the disease.

Chronic phase

In chronic phase CML, fewer than 10% of the cells in the blood and bone marrow are blast cells.

Accelerated phase

In accelerated phase CML, 10% to 19% of the cells in the blood and bone marrow are blast cells.

Blastic phase

In blastic phase CML, 20% or more of the cells in the blood or bone marrow are blast cells. When tiredness, fever, and an enlarged spleen occur during the blastic phase, it is called blast crisis.

Treatment Options for Chronic Myelogenous Leukemia

Chronic Phase Chronic Myelogenous Leukemia

Treatment of chronic phase chronic myelogenous leukemia may include the following:

- Targeted therapy with a tyrosine kinase inhibitor.
- High-dose chemotherapy with donor stem cell transplant.
- Chemotherapy.
- Splenectomy.
- A clinical trial of lower-dose chemotherapy with donor stem cell transplant.
- A clinical trial of a new treatment.

Accelerated Phase Chronic Myelogenous Leukemia

Treatment of accelerated phase chronic myelogenous leukemia may include the following:

- Donor stem cell transplant.
- Targeted therapy with a tyrosine kinase inhibitor.
- Tyrosine kinase inhibitor therapy followed by a donor stem cell transplant.
- Biologic therapy (interferon) with or without chemotherapy.
- High-dose chemotherapy.
- Chemotherapy.
- Transfusion therapy to replace red blood cells, platelets, and sometimes white blood cells, to relieve symptoms and improve quality of life.
- A clinical trial of a new treatment.

Blastic Phase Chronic Myelogenous Leukemia

Treatment of blastic phase chronic myelogenous leukemia may include the following:

- Targeted therapy with a tyrosine kinase inhibitor.
- Chemotherapy using one or more drugs.

- High-dose chemotherapy.

- Donor stem cell transplant.

- Chemotherapy as palliative therapy to relieve symptoms and improve quality of life.

- A clinical trial of a new treatment.

Relapsed Chronic Myelogenous Leukemia

Treatment of relapsed chronic myelogenous leukemia may include the following:

- Targeted therapy with a tyrosine kinase inhibitor.

- Donor stem cell transplant.

- Chemotherapy.

- Donor lymphocyte infusion.

- Biologic therapy (interferon).

- A clinical trial of new types or higher doses of targeted therapy or donor stem cell transplant.

Section 33.2

Langerhans Cell Histiocytosis

Text in this section is excerpted from "Langerhans Cell Histiocytosis
Treatment," National Cancer Institute at the National Institutes of
Health (NIH), May 22, 2015.

General Information About Langerhans Cell Histiocytosis

Langerhans cell histiocytosis is a type of cancer that can damage tissue or cause lesions to form in one or more places in the body.

Langerhans cell histiocytosis (LCH) is a rare cancer that begins in LCH cells (a type of dendritic cell which fights infection). Sometimes there are mutations (changes) in LCH cells as they form. These include mutations of the *BRAF* gene. These changes may make the LCH cells grow and multiply quickly. This causes LCH cells to build up in certain parts of the body, where they can damage tissue or form lesions.

LCH is not a disease of the Langerhans cells that normally occur in the skin.

LCH may occur at any age, but is most common in young children. Treatment of LCH in children is different from treatment of LCH in adults.

Family history or having a parent who was exposed to certain chemicals may increase the risk of LCH.

Anything that increases your risk of getting a disease is called a risk factor. Having a risk factor does not mean that you will get cancer; not having risk factors doesn't mean that you will not get cancer. Talk with your doctor if you think you may be at risk. Risk factors for LCH include the following:

- Having a parent who was exposed to certain chemicals such as benzene.

- Having a parent who was exposed to metal, granite, or wood dust in the workplace.

- A family history of cancer, including LCH.

- Having infections as a newborn.

- Having a personal history or family history of thyroid disease.

- Smoking, especially in young adults.

- Being Hispanic

The signs and symptoms of LCH depend on where it is in the body.

These and other signs and symptoms may be caused by LCH or by other conditions.

Check with your doctor if you or your child have any of the following:

Skin and nails

LCH in infants may affect the skin only. In some cases, skin-only LCH may get worse over weeks or months and become a form called high-risk multisystem LCH.

In infants, signs or symptoms of LCH that affects the skin may include:

- Flaking of the scalp that may look like "cradle cap".

- Raised, brown or purple skin rash anywhere on the body.

In children and adults, signs or symptoms of LCH that affects the skin and nails may include:

- Flaking of the scalp that may look like dandruff.

- Raised, red or brown, crusted rash in the groin area, abdomen, back, or chest, that may be itchy.

- Bumps or ulcers on the scalp.

- Ulcers behind the ears, under the breasts, or in the groin area.

- Fingernails that fall off or have discolored grooves that run the length of the nail.

Mouth

Signs or symptoms of LCH that affects the mouth may include:

- Swollen gums.
- Sores on the roof of the mouth, inside the cheeks, or on the tongue or lips.
- Teeth that become uneven.
- Tooth loss.

Bone

Signs or symptoms of LCH that affects the bone may include:

- Swelling or a lump over a bone, such as the skull, ribs, spine, thigh bone, upper arm bone, elbow, eye socket, or bones around the ear.
- Pain where there is swelling or a lump over a bone.

Children with LCH lesions in bones around the ears or eyes have a high risk for diabetes insipidus and other central nervous system disease.

Lymph nodes and thymus

Signs or symptoms of LCH that affects the lymph nodes or thymus may include:

- Swollen lymph nodes.
- Trouble breathing.
- Superior vena cava syndrome. This can cause coughing, trouble breathing, and swelling of the face, neck, and upper arms.

Endocrine system

Signs or symptoms of LCH that affects the pituitary gland may include:

- Diabetes insipidus. This can cause a strong thirst and frequent urination.
- Slow growth.
- Early or late puberty.
- Being very overweight.

Signs or symptoms of LCH that affects the thyroid may include:

- Swollen thyroid gland.
- Hypothyroidism. This can cause tiredness, lack of energy, being sensitive to cold, constipation, dry skin, thinning hair, memory problems, trouble concentrating, and depression. In infants, this can also cause a loss of appetite and choking on food. In children and teens, this can also cause behavior problems, weight gain, slow growth, and late puberty.
- Trouble breathing.

Central nervous system (CNS)

Signs or symptoms of LCH that affects the CNS (brain and spinal cord) may include:

- Loss of balance, uncoordinated body movements, and trouble walking.
- Trouble speaking.
- Trouble seeing.
- Headaches.
- Changes in behavior or personality.
- Memory problems.

These signs and symptoms may be caused by lesions in the CNS or by CNS neurodegenerative syndrome.

Liver and spleen

Signs or symptoms of LCH that affects the liver or spleen may include:

- Swelling in the abdomen caused by a buildup of extra fluid.
- Trouble breathing.
- Yellowing of the skin and whites of the eyes.
- Itching.
- Easy bruising or bleeding.
- Feeling very tired.

Lung

Signs or symptoms of LCH that affects the lung may include:

- Collapsed lung. This condition can cause chest pain or tightness, trouble breathing, feeling tired, and a bluish color to the skin.

- Trouble breathing, especially in adults who smoke.

- Dry cough.

- Chest pain.

Bone marrow

Signs or symptoms of LCH that affects the bone marrow may include:

- Easy bruising or bleeding.

- Fever.

- Frequent infections.

Tests that examine the organs and body systems where LCH may occur are used to detect (find) and diagnose LCH.

The following tests and procedures may be used to detect (find) and diagnose LCH or conditions caused by LCH:

- **Physical exam and history**: An exam of the body to check general signs of health, including checking for signs of disease, such as lumps or anything else that seems unusual. A history of the patient's health habits and past illnesses and treatments will also be taken.

- **Neurological exam:** A series of questions and tests to check the brain, spinal cord, and nerve function. The exam checks a person's mental status, coordination, and ability to walk normally, and how well the muscles, senses, and reflexes work. This may also be called a neuro exam or a neurologic exam.

- **Complete blood count (CBC) with differential:** A procedure in which a sample of blood is drawn and checked for the following:

  - The amount of hemoglobin (the protein that carries oxygen) in the red blood cells.

  - The portion of the blood sample made up of red blood cells.

- The number and type of white blood cells.

- The number of red blood cells and platelets.

- **Blood chemistry studies:** A procedure in which a blood sample is checked to measure the amounts of certain substances released into the body by organs and tissues in the body. An unusual (higher or lower than normal) amount of a substance can be a sign of disease in the organ or tissue that makes it.

- **Liver function test:** A blood test to measure the blood levels of certain substances released by the liver. A high or low level of these substances can be a sign of disease in the liver.

- **BRAF gene testing:** A laboratory test in which a sample of blood or tissue is tested for the *BRAF* gene.

- **Urinalysis:** A test to check the color of urine and its contents, such as sugar, protein, red blood cells, and white blood cells.

- **Water deprivation test:** A test to check how much urine is made and whether it becomes concentrated when little or no water is given. This test is used to diagnose diabetes insipidus, which may be caused by LCH.

- **Bone marrow aspiration and biopsy:** The removal of bone marrow and a small piece of bone by inserting a hollow needle into the hipbone. A pathologist views the bone marrow and bone under a microscope to look for signs of LCH.

The following tests may be done on the tissue that was removed:

- **Immunohistochemistry**: A test that uses antibodies to check for certain antigens in a sample of tissue. The antibody is usually linked to a radioactive substance or a dye that causes the tissue to light up under a microscope. This type of test may be used to tell the difference between different types of cancer.

- **Flow cytometry**: A laboratory test that measures the number of cells in a sample, how many cells are live, and the size of the cells. It also shows the shapes of the cells and whether there are tumor markers on the surface of the cells. The cells are stained with a light-sensitive dye, placed in a fluid, and passed in a stream before a laser or other type of light. The measurements are based on how the light-sensitive dye reacts to the light.

- **Bone scan**: A procedure to check if there are rapidly dividing cells in the bone. A very small amount of radioactive material is injected into a vein and travels through the bloodstream. The radioactive material collects in the bones with cancer and is detected by a scanner.

- **X-ray:** An x-ray of the organs and bones inside the body. An x-ray is a type of energy beam that can go through the body and onto film, making a picture of areas inside the body. Sometimes a skeletal survey is done. This is a procedure to x-ray all of the bones in the body.

- **CT scan (CAT scan):** A procedure that makes a series of detailed pictures of areas inside the body, taken from different angles. The pictures are made by a computer linked to an x-ray machine. A dye may be injected into a vein or swallowed to help the organs or tissues show up more clearly. This procedure is also called computed tomography, computerized tomography, or computerized axial tomography.

- **MRI (magnetic resonance imaging):** A procedure that uses a magnet, radio waves, and a computer to make a series of detailed pictures of areas inside the body. A substance called gadolinium may be injected into a vein. The gadolinium collects around the LCH cells so that they show up brighter in the picture. This procedure is also called nuclear magnetic resonance imaging (NMRI).

- **PET scan (positron emission tomography scan):** A procedure to find tumor cells in the body. A small amount of radioactive glucose (sugar) is injected into a vein. The PET scanner rotates around the body and makes a picture of where glucose is being used in the body. Tumor cells show up brighter in the picture because they are more active and take up more glucose than normal cells do.

- **Ultrasound exam:** A procedure in which high-energy sound waves (ultrasound) are bounced off internal tissues or organs and make echoes. The echoes form a picture of body tissues called a sonogram. The picture can be printed to be looked at later.

- **Bronchoscopy:** A procedure to look inside the trachea and large airways in the lung for abnormal areas. A bronchoscope is inserted through the nose or mouth into the trachea and lungs. A bronchoscope is a thin, tube-like instrument with a light and a lens for viewing. It may also have a tool to remove tissue samples, which are checked under a microscope for signs of cancer.

- **Endoscopy:** A procedure to look at organs and tissues inside the body to check for abnormal areas in the gastrointestinal tract or lungs. An endoscope is inserted through an incision (cut) in the skin or opening in the body, such as the mouth. An endoscope is a thin, tube-like instrument with a light and a lens for viewing. It may also have a tool to remove tissue or lymph node samples, which are checked under a microscope for signs of disease.

- **Biopsy:** The removal of cells or tissues so they can be viewed under a microscope by a pathologist to check for LCH cells. To diagnose LCH, a biopsy of bone lesions, skin, lymph nodes, or the liver may be done.

Certain factors affect prognosis (chance of recovery) and treatment options.

LCH in organs such as the skin, bones, lymph nodes, or pituitary gland usually gets better with treatment and is called "low- risk". LCH in the spleen, liver, or bone marrow is harder to treat and is called "high-risk".

The prognosis (chance of recovery) and treatment options depend on the following:

- How old the patient is when diagnosed with LCH.

- How many organs or body systems the cancer affects.

- Whether the cancer is found in the liver, spleen, bone marrow, or certain bones in the skull.

- How quickly the cancer responds to initial treatment.

- Whether the cancer has just been diagnosed or has come back (recurred).

In infants up to one year of age, LCH may go away without treatment.

Stages of LCH

There is no staging system for Langerhans cell histiocytosis (LCH).

The extent or spread of cancer is usually described as stages. There is no staging system for LCH.

Treatment of LCH is b ased on where LCH cells are found in the body and how many body systems are affected.

LCH is described as single-system disease or multisystem disease, depending on how many body systems are affected:

- **Single-system LCH:** LCH is found in one part of an organ or body system (unifocal) or in more than one part of that organ or body system (multifocal). Bone is the most common single place for LCH to be found.

- **Multisystem LCH:** LCH occurs in two or more organs or body systems or may be spread throughout the body. Multisystem LCH is less common than single-system LCH.

LCH may affect low-risk organs or high-risk organs:

- **Low-risk organs** include the skin, bone, lungs, lymph nodes, gastrointestinal tract, pituitary gland, and central nervous system (CNS).

- **High-risk organs** include the liver, spleen, and bone marrow.

Treatment Option Overview for LCH

There are different types of treatment for patients with Langerhans cell histiocytosis (LCH).

Different types of treatments are available for patients with LCH. Some treatments are standard (the currently used treatment), and some are being tested in clinical trials. A treatment clinical trial is a research study meant to help improve current treatments or obtain information on new treatments for patients with cancer. When clinical trials show that a new treatment is better than the standard treatment, the new treatment may become the standard treatment. Whenever possible, patients should take part in a clinical trial in order to receive new types of treatment for LCH. Some clinical trials are open only to patients who have not started treatment.

Clinical trials are taking place in many parts of the country.

Children with LCH should have their treatment planned by a team of health care providers who are experts in treating childhood cancer.

Treatment will be overseen by a pediatric oncologist, a doctor who specializes in treating children with cancer. The pediatric oncologist works with other pediatric healthcare providers who are experts in treating children with LCH and who specialize in certain areas of medicine. These may include the following specialists:

- Pediatrician.
- Primary care physician.
- Pediatric surgeon.
- Pediatric hematologist.
- Radiation oncologist.
- Neurologist.
- Endocrinologist.
- Pediatric nurse specialist.
- Rehabilitation specialist.
- Psychologist.
- Social worker.

Some cancer treatments cause side effects months or years after treatment for childhood cancer has ended.

Side effects from cancer treatment that begin during or after treatment and continue for months or years are called late effects. Late effects of cancer treatment may include the following:

- Slow growth and development.
- Hearing loss.
- Bone, tooth, liver, and lung problems.
- Changes in mood, feeling, learning, thinking, or memory.

- Second cancers, such as leukemia, retinoblastoma, Ewing sarcoma, brain or liver cancer.

Some late effects may be treated or controlled. It is important to talk with your child's doctors about the effects cancer treatment can have on your child.

Many patients with multisystem LCH have late effects caused by treatment or by the disease itself. These patients often have long-term health problems that affect their quality of life.

Nine types of standard treatment are used:

Chemotherapy

Chemotherapy is a cancer treatment that uses drugs to stop the growth of cancer cells, either by killing the cells or by stopping them from dividing. When chemotherapy is taken by mouth or injected into a vein or muscle, the drugs enter the bloodstream and can reach cancer cells throughout the body (systemic chemotherapy). When chemotherapy is placed directly onto the skin or into the cerebrospinal fluid, an organ, or a body cavity such as the abdomen, the drugs mainly affect cancer cells in those areas (regional chemotherapy).

Chemotherapy agents given by injection or by mouth are used to treat LCH. Chemotherapy agents include vinblastine, cytarabine, cladribine, and methotrexate. Nitrogen mustard is a drug that is put directly on the skin to treat small LCH lesions.

Surgery

Surgery may be used to remove LCH lesions and a small amount of nearby healthy tissue. Curettage is a type of surgery that uses a curette (a sharp, spoon-shaped tool) to scrape LCH cells from bone.

When there is severe liver or lung damage, the entire organ may be removed and replaced with a healthy liver or lung from a donor.

Radiation therapy

Radiation therapy is a cancer treatment that uses high-energy x-rays or other types of radiation to kill cancer cells or keep them from growing. External radiation therapy uses a machine outside the body to send radiation toward the cancer. In LCH, a special lamp may be used to send ultraviolet B (UVB) radiation toward LCH skin lesions.

Photodynamic therapy

Photodynamic therapy is a cancer treatment that uses a drug and a certain type of laser light to kill cancer cells. A drug that is not active until it is exposed to light is injected into a vein. The drug collects more in cancer cells than in normal cells. For LCH, laser light is aimed at the skin and the drug becomes active and kills the cancer cells. Photodynamic therapy causes little damage to healthy tissue. Patients who have photodynamic therapy should not spend too much time in the sun.

In one type of photodynamic therapy, called psoralen and ultraviolet A (PUVA) therapy, the patient receives a drug called psoralen and then ultraviolet A radiation is directed to the skin.

Biologic therapy

Biologic therapy is a treatment that uses the patient's immune system to fight cancer. Substances made by the body or made in a laboratory are used to boost, direct, or restore the body's natural defenses against cancer. This type of cancer treatment is also called biotherapy or immunotherapy.

Interferon is a type of biologic therapy used to treat LCH of the skin. Immunomodulators are also a type of biologic therapy. Thalidomide is an immunomodulator used to treat LCH.

Targeted therapy

Targeted therapy is a type of treatment that uses drugs or other substances to find and attack LCH cells without harming normal cells. Imatinib mesylate is a type of targeted therapy called a tyrosine kinase inhibitor. It stops blood stem cells from turning into dendritic cells that may become cancer cells. Other types of kinase inhibitors that affect cells with the *BRAF* gene, such as dabrafenib and vemurafenib, are being studied in clinical trials for LCH.

A family of genes, called ras genes, may cause cancer when they are mutated (changed). Ras genes make proteins that are involved in cell signaling pathways, cell growth, and cell death. Ras pathway inhibitors are a type of targeted therapy being studied in clinical trials. They block the actions of a mutated ras gene or its protein and may stop the growth of cancer.

Other drug therapy

Other drugs used to treat LCH include the following:

- Steroid therapy, such as prednisone, is used to treat LCH lesions.

- Bisphosphonate therapy (such as pamidronate, zoledronate, or alendronate) is used to treat LCH lesions of the bone and to lessen bone pain.

- Nonsteroidal anti-inflammatory drugs (NSAIDs) are drugs (such as aspirin and ibuprofen) that are commonly used to decrease fever, swelling, pain, and redness. Sometimes an NSAID called indomethacin is used to treat LCH.

- Retinoids, such as isotretinoin, are drugs related to vitamin A that can slow the growth of LCH cells in the skin. The retinoids are taken by mouth.

Stem cell transplant

Stem cell transplant is a method of giving chemotherapy and replacing blood-forming cells destroyed by the LCH treatment. Stem cells (immature blood cells) are removed from the blood or bone marrow of the patient or a donor and are frozen and stored. After the chemotherapy is completed, the stored stem cells are thawed and given back to the patient through an infusion. These re-infused stem cells grow into (and restore) the body's blood cells.

Observation

Observation is closely monitoring a patient's condition without giving any treatment until signs or symptoms appear or change.

Patients may want to think about taking part in a clinical trial.

For some patients, taking part in a clinical trial may be the best treatment choice. Clinical trials are part of the cancer research process. Clinical trials are done to find out if new cancer treatments are safe and effective or better than the standard treatment.

Many of today's standard treatments for cancer are based on earlier clinical trials. Patients who take part in a clinical trial may receive the standard treatment or be among the first to receive a new treatment.

Patients who take part in clinical trials also help improve the way cancer will be treated in the future. Even when clinical trials do not lead to effective new treatments, they often answer important questions and help move research forward.

Patients can enter clinical trials before, during, or after starting their treatment.

Some clinical trials only include patients who have not yet received treatment. Other trials test treatments for patients whose cancer has not gotten better. There are also clinical trials that test new ways to stop cancer from recurring (coming back) or reduce the side effects of cancer treatment.

Clinical trials are taking place in many parts of the country.

When treatment of LCH stops, new lesions may appear or old lesions may come back.

Many patients with LCH get better with treatment. However, when treatment stops, new lesions may appear or old lesions may come back. This is called reactivation (recurrence) and may occur within one year after stopping treatment. Patients with multisystem disease are more likely to have a reactivation. More common sites of reactivation are bone, ears, or skin. Diabetes insipidus also may develop. Less common sites of reactivation include lymph nodes, bone marrow, spleen, liver, or lung. Some patients may have more than one reactivation over a number of years.

Follow-up tests may be needed.

Some of the tests that were done to diagnose LCH may be repeated. This is to see how well the treatment is working and if there are any new lesions. These tests may include:

- Physical exam.
- Neurological exam.
- Ultrasound exam.
- MRI.
- CT scan.
- PET scan.

Other tests that may be needed include:

- **Brain stem auditory evoked response (BAER) test**: A test that measures the brain's response to clicking sounds or certain tones.

771

- **Pulmonary function test (PFT)**: A test to see how well the lungs are working. It measures how much air the lungs can hold and how quickly air moves into and out of the lungs. It also measures how much oxygen is used and how much carbon dioxide is given off during breathing. This is also called a lung function test.

- **Chest x-ray**: An x-ray of the organs and bones inside the chest. An x-ray is a type of energy beam that can go through the body and onto film, making a picture of areas inside the body.

- Decisions about whether to continue, change, or stop treatment may be based on the results of these tests.

- Some of the tests will continue to be done from time to time after treatment has ended. The results of these tests can show if your condition has changed or if the cancer has recurred (come back). These tests are sometimes called follow-up tests or check-ups.

Section 33.3

Plasma Cell Neoplasms

Text in this section is excerpted from "Plasma Cell Neoplasms (Including Multiple Myeloma) Treatment," National Cancer Institute at the National Institutes of Health (NIH), March 16, 2015.

General Information About Plasma Cell Neoplasms

Plasma cell neoplasms are diseases in which the body makes too many plasma cells.

Plasma cells develop from B lymphocytes (B cells), a type of white blood cell that is made in the bone marrow. Normally, when bacteria or viruses enter the body, some of the B cells will change into plasma cells. The plasma cells make antibodies to fight bacteria and viruses, to stop infection and disease.

Plasma cell neoplasms are diseases in which abnormal plasma cells or myeloma cells form tumors in the bones or soft tissues of the body.

The plasma cells also make an antibody protein, called M protein that is not needed by the body and does not help fight infection. These antibody proteins build up in the bone marrow and can cause the blood to thicken or can damage the kidneys.

Plasma cell neoplasms can be benign (not cancer) or malignant (cancer).

Monoclonal gammopathy of undetermined significance (MGUS) is not cancer but can become cancer. The following types of plasma cell neoplasms are cancer:

- Waldenström macroglobulinemia.

- Plasmacytoma.

- Multiple myeloma.

There are several types of plasma cell neoplasms.

Plasma cell neoplasms include the following:

Monoclonal gammopathy of undetermined significance (MGUS)

In this type of plasma cell neoplasm, less than 10% of the bone marrow is made up of abnormal plasma cells and there is no cancer. The abnormal plasma cells make M protein, which is sometimes found during a routine blood or urine test. In most patients, the amount of M protein stays the same and there are no signs, symptoms, or health problems. In some patients, MGUS may later become a more serious condition, such as amyloidosis. It can also become cancer, such as multiple myeloma, lymphoma, or chronic lymphocytic leukemia.

Plasmacytoma

In this type of plasma cell neoplasm, the abnormal plasma cells (myeloma cells) are in one place and form one tumor, called a plasmacytoma. Sometimes plasmacytoma can be cured. There are two types of plasmacytoma.

- In isolated plasmacytoma of bone, one plasma cell tumor is found in the bone, less than 10% of the bone marrow is made up of plasma cells, and there are no other signs of cancer. Plasmacytoma of the bone often becomes multiple myeloma.

- In extramedullary plasmacytoma, one plasma cell tumor is found in soft tissue but not in the bone or the bone marrow. Extramedullary plasmacytomas commonly form in tissues of the throat, tonsil, and paranasal sinuses.

Signs and symptoms depend on where the tumor is.

- In bone, the plasmacytoma may cause pain or broken bones.

- In soft tissue, the tumor may press on nearby areas and cause pain or other problems. For example, a plasmacytoma in the throat can make it hard to swallow.

Multiple myeloma

In multiple myeloma, abnormal plasma cells (myeloma cells) build up in the bone marrow and form tumors in many bones of the body. These tumors may keep the bone marrow from making enough healthy blood cells. Normally, the bone marrow makes stem cells (immature cells) that become three types of mature blood cells:

- Red blood cells that carry oxygen and other substances to all tissues of the body.

- White blood cells that fight infection and disease.

- Platelets that form blood clots to help prevent bleeding.

As the number of myeloma cells increases, fewer red blood cells, white blood cells, and platelets are made. The myeloma cells also damage and weaken the bone.

Sometimes multiple myeloma does not cause any signs or symptoms. It may be found when a blood or urine test is done for another condition. Signs and symptoms may be caused by multiple myeloma or other conditions. Check with your doctor if you have any of the following:

- Bone pain, especially in the back or ribs.

- Bones that break easily.

- Fever for no known reason or frequent infections.

- Easy bruising or bleeding.

- Trouble breathing.

- Weakness of the arms or legs.

- Feeling very tired.

A tumor can damage the bone and cause hypercalcemia (too much calcium in the blood). This can affect many organs in the body, including the kidneys, nerves, heart, muscles, and digestive tract, and cause serious health problems.

Hypercalcemia may cause the following signs and symptoms:

- Loss of appetite.
- Nausea or vomiting.
- Feeling thirsty.
- Frequent urination.
- Constipation.
- Feeling very tired.
- Muscle weakness.
- Restlessness.
- Confusion or trouble thinking.

Multiple myeloma and other plasma cell neoplasms may cause a condition called amyloidosis.

In rare cases, multiple myeloma can cause peripheral nerves (nerves that are not in the brain or spinal cord) and organs to fail. This may be caused by a condition called amyloidosis. Antibody proteins build up and stick together in peripheral nerves and organs, such as the kidney and heart. This can cause the nerves and organs to become stiff and unable to work the way they should.

Amyloidosis may cause the following signs and symptoms:

- Feeling very tired.
- Purple spots on the skin.
- Enlarged tongue.
- Diarrhea.
- Swelling caused by fluid in your body's tissues.
- Tingling or numbness in your legs and feet.

Age can affect the risk of plasma cell neoplasms.

Anything that increases your risk of getting a disease is called a risk factor. Having a risk factor does not mean that you will get cancer;

not having risk factors doesn't mean that you will not get cancer. Talk with your doctor if you think you may be at risk.

Plasma cell neoplasms are most common in people who are middle aged or older. For multiple myeloma and plasmacytoma, other risk factors include the following:

- Being black.

- Being male.

- Having a personal history of MGUS or plasmacytoma.

- Being exposed to radiation or certain chemicals.

Tests that examine the blood, bone marrow, and urine are used to detect (find) and diagnose multiple myeloma and other plasma cell neoplasms.

The following tests and procedures may be used:

- **Physical exam and history**: An exam of the body to check general signs of health, including checking for signs of disease, such as lumps or anything else that seems unusual. A history of the patient's health habits and past illnesses and treatments will also be taken.

- **Blood and urine immunoglobulin studies**: A procedure in which a blood or urine sample is checked to measure the amounts of certain antibodies (immunoglobulins). For multiple myeloma, beta-2-microglobulin, M protein, free light chains, and other proteins made by the myeloma cells are measured. A higher-than-normal amount of these substances can be a sign of disease.

- **Bone marrow aspiration and biopsy**: The removal of bone marrow, blood, and a small piece of bone by inserting a hollow needle into the hipbone or breastbone. A pathologist views the bone marrow, blood, and bone under a microscope to look for abnormal cells.

The following test may be done on the sample of tissue removed during the bone marrow aspiration and biopsy:

- **Cytogenetic analysis**: A test in which cells in a sample of bone marrow are viewed under a microscope to look for certain changes in the chromosomes. Other tests, such as fluorescence in situ hybridization (FISH), may also be done to look for certain changes in the chromosomes.

- **Skeletal bone survey:** In a skeletal bone survey, x-rays of all the bones in the body are taken. The x-rays are used to find areas where the bone is damaged. An x-ray is a type of energy beam that can go through the body and onto film, making a picture of areas inside the body.

- **Complete blood count (CBC) with differential:** A procedure in which a sample of blood is drawn and checked for the following:

  - The number of red blood cells and platelets.

  - The number and type of white blood cells.

  - The amount of hemoglobin (the protein that carries oxygen) in the red blood cells.

  - The portion of the blood sample made up of red blood cells.

- **Blood chemistry studies:** A procedure in which a blood sample is checked to measure the amounts of certain substances, such as calcium or albumin, released into the blood by organs and tissues in the body. An unusual (higher or lower than normal) amount of a substance can be a sign of disease in the organ or tissue that makes it.

- **Twenty-four-hour urine test:** A test in which urine is collected for 24 hours to measure the amounts of certain substances. An unusual (higher or lower than normal) amount of a substance can be a sign of disease in the organ or tissue that makes it. A higher than normal amount of protein may be a sign of multiple myeloma.

- **MRI (magnetic resonance imaging):** A procedure that uses a magnet, radio waves, and a computer to make a series of detailed pictures of areas inside the body. This procedure is also called nuclear magnetic resonance imaging (NMRI). An MRI may be used to find areas where the bone is damaged.

Certain factors affect prognosis (chance of recovery) and treatment options.

The prognosis (chance of recovery) depends on the following:

- The type of plasma cell neoplasm.

- The stage of the disease.

- Whether a certain immunoglobulin (antibody) is present.

- Whether there are certain genetic changes.

- Whether the kidney is damaged.

- Whether the cancer responds to initial treatment or recurs (comes back).

Treatment options depend on the following:

- The type of plasma cell neoplasm.

- The age and general health of the patient.

- Whether there are signs, symptoms, or health problems, such as kidney failure or infection, related to the disease.

- Whether the cancer responds to initial treatment or recurs (comes back).

Stages of Plasma Cell Neoplasms

There are no standard staging systems for monoclonal gammopathy of undetermined significance (MGUS), macroglobulinemia, and plasmacytoma.

After multiple myeloma has been diagnosed, tests are done to find out the amount of cancer in the body.

The process used to find out the amount of cancer in the body is called staging. It is important to know the stage in order to plan treatment. The following tests and procedures may be used in the staging process:

- **Skeletal bone survey:** In a skeletal bone survey, x-rays of all the bones in the body are taken. The x-rays are used to find areas where the bone is damaged. An x-ray is a type of energy beam that can go through the body and onto film, making a picture of areas inside the body.

- **MRI (magnetic resonance imaging):** A procedure that uses a magnet, radio waves, and a computer to make a series of detailed pictures of areas inside the body, such as the bone marrow. This procedure is also called nuclear magnetic resonance imaging (NMRI).

- **Bone densitometry:** A procedure that uses a special type of x-ray to measure bone density.

The stage of multiple myeloma is based on the levels of beta-2-microglobulin and albumin in the blood.

Beta-2-microglobulin and albumin are found in the blood. Beta-2-microglobulin is a protein found on plasma cells. Albumin makes up the biggest part of the blood plasma. It keeps fluid from leaking out of blood vessels. It also brings nutrients to tissues, and carries hormones, vitamins, drugs, and other substances, such as calcium, all through the body. In the blood of patients with multiple myeloma, the amount of beta-2-microglobulin is increased and the amount of albumin is decreased.

The following stages are used for multiple myeloma:

Stage I multiple myeloma

In stage I multiple myeloma, the blood levels are as follows:

- beta-2-microglobulin level is lower than 3.5 mg/L; and
- albumin level is 3.5 g/dL or higher.

Stage II multiple myeloma

In stage II multiple myeloma, the blood levels are as follows:

- beta-2-microglobulin level is lower than 3.5 mg/L and the albumin level is lower than 3.5 g/dL; or
- beta-2-microglobulin level is between 3.5 mg/L and 5.4 mg/L.

Stage III multiple myeloma

In stage III multiple myeloma, the blood level of beta-2-microglobulin is 5.5 mg/L or higher.

Treatment Options for Plasma Cell Neoplasms

Monoclonal Gammopathy of Undetermined Significance

Treatment of monoclonal gammopathy of undetermined significance (MGUS) is usually watchful waiting. Regular blood tests to check the level of M protein in the blood and physical exams to check for signs or symptoms of cancer will be done.

Isolated Plasmacytoma of Bone

Treatment of isolated plasmacytoma of bone is usually radiation therapy to the bone lesion.

Extramedullary Plasmacytoma

Treatment of extramedullary plasmacytoma may include the following:

- Radiation therapy to the tumor and nearby lymph nodes.
- Surgery, usually followed by radiation therapy.
- Watchful waiting after initial treatment, followed by radiation therapy, surgery, or chemotherapy if the tumor grows or causes signs or symptoms.

Multiple Myeloma

Patients without signs or symptoms may not need treatment. When signs or symptoms appear, the treatment of multiple myeloma may be done in phases:

- **Induction therapy:** This is the first phase of treatment. Its goal is to reduce the amount of disease, and may include one or more of the following:

  - Corticosteroid therapy.
  - Biologic therapy with thalidomide, lenalidomide, or pomalidomide therapy.
  - Targeted therapy with proteasome inhibitors (bortezomib or carfilzomib).
  - Chemotherapy.
  - A clinical trial of different combinations of treatment.

- **Consolidation chemotherapy:** This is the second phase of treatment. Treatment in the consolidation phase is to kill any remaining cancer cells. High-dose chemotherapy is followed by either:

  - one or two autologous stem cell transplants, in which the patient's stem cells from the blood or bone marrow are used; or
  - one allogeneic stem cell transplant, in which the patient receives stem cells from the blood or bone marrow of a donor.

- **Maintenance therapy**: After the initial treatment, maintenance therapy is often given to help keep the disease in remission for a longer time. Several types of treatment are being studied for this use, including the following:

  - Chemotherapy.

  - Biologic therapy with interferon.

  - Corticosteroid therapy.

  - Thalidomide or lenalidomide therapy.

  - Targeted therapy with a proteasome inhibitor (bortezomib).

Refractory Multiple Myeloma

Treatment of refractory multiple myeloma may include the following:

- Watchful waiting for patients whose disease is stable.

- A different treatment than treatment already given, for patients whose tumor kept growing during treatment.

Section 33.4

Myeloidysplastic Syndrome

Text in this section is excerpted from "Myelodysplastic Syndromes Treatment," National Cancer Institute at the National Institutes of Health (NIH), March 16, 2015.

General Information About Myelodysplastic Syndromes

A myelodysplastic syndrome is a type of cancer in which the bone marrow does not make enough healthy blood cells and there are abnormal (blast) cells in the blood and / or bone marrow.

In a healthy person, the bone marrow makes blood stem cells (immature cells) that become mature blood cells over time.

A blood stem cell may become a lymphoid stem cell or a myeloid stem cell. A lymphoid stem cell becomes a white blood cell. A myeloid stem cell becomes one of three types of mature blood cells:

- Red blood cells that carry oxygen and other substances to all tissues of the body.

- Platelets that form blood clots to stop bleeding.

- White blood cells that fight infection and disease.

In a patient with a myelodysplastic syndrome, the blood stem cells (immature cells) do not become healthy red blood cells, white blood cells, or platelets. These immature blood cells, called blasts, do not work the way they should and either die in the bone marrow or soon after they go into the blood. This leaves less room for healthy white blood cells, red blood cells, and platelets to form in the bone marrow. When there are fewer healthy blood cells, infection, anemia, or easy bleeding may occur.

The different types of myelodysplastic syndromes are diagnosed based on certain changes in the blood cells and bone marrow.

- **Refractory anemia**: There are too few red blood cells in the blood and the patient has anemia. The number of white blood cells and platelets is normal.

- **Refractory anemia with ring sideroblasts:** There are too few red blood cells in the blood and the patient has anemia. The red blood cells have too much iron inside the cell. The number of white blood cells and platelets is normal.

- **Refractory anemia with excess blasts:** There are too few red blood cells in the blood and the patient has anemia. Five percent to 19% of the cells in the bone marrow are blasts. There also may be changes to the white blood cells and platelets. Refractory anemia with excess blasts may progress to acute myeloid leukemia (AML).

- **Refractory cytopenia with multilineage dysplasia:** There are too few of at least two types of blood cells (red blood cells, platelets, or white blood cells). Less than 5% of the cells in the bone marrow are blasts and less than 1% of the cells in the blood are blasts. If red blood cells are affected, they may have extra iron. Refractory cytopenia may progress to acute myeloid leukemia (AML).

- **Refractory cytopenia with unilineage dysplasia:** There are too few of one type of blood cell (red blood cells, platelets, or white blood cells). There are changes in 10% or more of two other types of blood cells. Less than 5% of the cells in the bone marrow are blasts and less than 1% of the cells in the blood are blasts.

- **Unclassifiable myelodysplastic syndrome:** The numbers of blasts in the bone marrow and blood are normal, and the disease is not one of the other myelodysplastic syndromes.

- **Myelodysplastic syndrome associated with an isolated del(5q) chromosome abnormality:** There are too few red blood cells in the blood and the patient has anemia. Less than 5% of the cells in the bone marrow and blood are blasts. There is a specific change in the chromosome.

- **Chronic myelomonocytic leukemia (CMML)**

Age and past treatment with chemotherapy or radiation therapy affect the risk of a myelodysplastic syndrome.

Anything that increases your risk of getting a disease is called a risk factor. Having a risk factor does not mean that you will get a disease; not having risk factors doesn't mean that you will not get a disease. Talk with your doctor if you think you may be at risk. Risk factors for myelodysplastic syndromes include the following:

- Past treatment with chemotherapy or radiation therapy for cancer.

- Being exposed to certain chemicals, including tobacco smoke, pesticides, fertilizers, and solvents such as benzene.

- Being exposed to heavy metals, such as mercury or lead.

The cause of myelodysplastic syndromes in most patients is not known.

Signs and symptoms of a myelodysplastic syndrome include shortness of breath and feeling tired.

Myelodysplastic syndromes often do not cause early signs or symptoms. They may be found during a routine blood test. Signs and symptoms may be caused by myelodysplastic syndromes or by other conditions. Check with your doctor if you have any of the following:

- Shortness of breath.

- Weakness or feeling tired.

- Having skin that is paler than usual.

- Easy bruising or bleeding.

- Petechiae (flat, pinpoint spots under the skin caused by bleeding).

Tests that examine the blood and bone marrow are used to detect (find) and diagnose myelodysplastic syndromes.

The following tests and procedures may be used:

- **Physical exam and history:** An exam of the body to check general signs of health, including checking for signs of disease, such as lumps or anything else that seems unusual. A history of the patient's health habits and past illnesses and treatments will also be taken.

- **Complete blood count (CBC) with differential:** A procedure in which a sample of blood is drawn and checked for the following:

  - The number of red blood cells and platelets.

  - The number and type of white blood cells.

  - The amount of hemoglobin (the protein that carries oxygen) in the red blood cells.

  - The portion of the blood sample made up of red blood cells.

- **Peripheral blood smear:** A procedure in which a sample of blood is checked for changes in the number, type, shape, and size of blood cells and for too much iron in the red blood cells.

- **Cytogenetic analysis**: A test in which cells in a sample of blood or bone marrow are viewed under a microscope to look for certain changes in the chromosomes.

- **Blood chemistry studies:** A procedure in which a blood sample is checked to measure the amounts of certain substances, such as vitamin B12 and folate, released into the blood by organs and tissues in the body. An unusual (higher or lower than normal) amount of a substance can be a sign of disease in the organ or tissue that makes it.

- **Bone marrow aspiration and biopsy:** The removal of bone marrow, blood, and a small piece of bone by inserting a hollow needle into the hipbone or breastbone. A pathologist views the bone marrow, blood, and bone under a microscope to look for abnormal cells.

The following tests may be done on the sample of tissue that is removed:

- **Immunocytochemistry**: A test that uses antibodies to check for certain antigens in a sample of bone marrow. This type of test is used to tell the difference between myelodysplastic syndromes, leukemia, and other conditions.

- **Immunophenotyping**: A process used to identify cells, based on the types of antigens or markers on the surface of the cell. This process is used to diagnose specific types of leukemia and other blood disorders by comparing the cancer cells to normal cells of the immune system.

- **Flow cytometry:** A laboratory test that measures the number of cells in a sample, the percentage of live cells in a sample, and certain characteristics of cells, such as size, shape, and the presence of tumor markers on the cell surface. The cells are stained with a light-sensitive dye, placed in a fluid, and passed in a stream before a laser or other type of light. The measurements are based on how the light-sensitive dye reacts to the light.

- **FISH (fluorescence in situ hybridization):** A laboratory technique used to look at genes or chromosomes in cells and tissues. Pieces of DNA that contain a fluorescent dye are made in the laboratory and added to cells or tissues on a glass slide. When these pieces of DNA bind to specific genes or areas of chromosomes on the slide, they light up when viewed under a microscope with a special light.

Certain factors affect prognosis and treatment options.

The prognosis (chance of recovery) and treatment options depend on the following:

- The number of blast cells in the bone marrow.
- Whether one or more types of blood cells are affected.
- Whether the patient has signs or symptoms of anemia, bleeding, or infection.
- Whether the patient has a low or high risk of leukemia.
- Certain changes in the chromosomes.

- Whether the myelodysplastic syndrome occurred after chemotherapy or radiation therapy for cancer.

- The age and general health of the patient.

Treatment Option Overview

There are different types of treatment for patients with myelodysplastic syndromes.

Different types of treatment are available for patients with myelodysplastic syndromes. Some treatments are standard (the currently used treatment), and some are being tested in clinical trials. A treatment clinical trial is a research study meant to help improve current treatments or obtain information on new treatments for patients with cancer. When clinical trials show that a new treatment is better than the standard treatment, the new treatment may become the standard treatment. Patients may want to think about taking part in a clinical trial. Some clinical trials are open only to patients who have not started treatment.

Treatment for myelodysplastic syndromes includes supportive care, drug therapy, and stem cell transplantation.

Patients with a myelodysplastic syndrome who have symptoms caused by low blood counts are given supportive care to relieve symptoms and improve quality of life. Drug therapy may be used to slow progression of the disease. Certain patients can be cured with aggressive treatment with chemotherapy followed by stem cell transplant using stem cells from a donor.

Three types of standard treatment are used:

Supportive care

Supportive care is given to lessen the problems caused by the disease or its treatment. Supportive care may include the following:

- **Transfusion therapy**

   Transfusion therapy (blood transfusion) is a method of giving red blood cells, white blood cells, or platelets to replace blood cells destroyed by disease or treatment. A red blood cell transfusion is given when the red blood cell count is low and signs or symptoms of anemia, such as shortness of breath or feeling very tired, occur. A platelet transfusion is usually given when the patient is bleeding, is having a procedure that may cause bleeding, or when the platelet count is very low.

Patients who receive many blood cell transfusions may have tissue and organ damage caused by the buildup of extra iron. These patients may be treated with iron chelation therapy to remove the extra iron from the blood.

- **Erythropoiesis-stimulating agents**

  Erythropoiesis-stimulating agents (ESAs) may be given to increase the number of mature red blood cells made by the body and to lessen the effects of anemia. Sometimes granulocyte colony-stimulating factor (G-CSF) is given with ESAs to help the treatment work better.

Antibiotic therapy
Antibiotics may be given to fight infection.

Drug therapy

- **Lenalidomide**

  Patients with myelodysplastic syndrome associated with an isolated del (5q) chromosome abnormality who need frequent red blood cell transfusions may be treated with lenalidomide. Lenalidomide is used to lessen the need for red blood cell transfusions.

- **Immunosuppressive therapy**

  Antithymocyte globulin (ATG) works to suppress or weaken the immune system. It is used to lessen the need for red blood cell transfusions.

- **Azacitidine and decitabine**

  Azacitidine and decitabine are used to treat myelodysplastic syndromes by killing cells that are dividing rapidly. They also help genes that are involved in cell growth to work the way they should. Treatment with azacitidine and decitabine may slow the progression of myelodysplastic syndromes to acute myeloid leukemia.

- **Chemotherapy used in acute myeloid leukemia (AML)**

  Patients with a myelodysplastic syndrome and a high number of blasts in their bone marrow have a high risk of acute leukemia.

They may be treated with the same chemotherapy regimen used in patients with acute myeloid leukemia.

Chemotherapy with stem cell transplant

Stem cell transplant is a method of giving chemotherapy and replacing blood-forming cells destroyed by the treatment. Stem cells (immature blood cells) are removed from the blood or bone marrow of a donor and are frozen for storage. After the chemotherapy is completed, the stored stem cells are thawed and given back to the patient through an infusion. These re-infused stem cells grow into (and restore) the body's blood cells.

This treatment may not work as well in patients whose myelodysplastic syndrome was caused by past treatment for cancer.

Patients may want to think about taking part in a clinical trial.

For some patients, taking part in a clinical trial may be the best treatment choice. Clinical trials are part of the cancer research process. Clinical trials are done to find out if new cancer treatments are safe and effective or better than the standard treatment.

Many of today's standard treatments for cancer are based on earlier clinical trials. Patients who take part in a clinical trial may receive the standard treatment or be among the first to receive a new treatment.

Patients who take part in clinical trials also help improve the way cancer will be treated in the future. Even when clinical trials do not lead to effective new treatments, they often answer important questions and help move research forward.

Patients can enter clinical trials before, during, or after starting their treatment.

Some clinical trials only include patients who have not yet received treatment. Other trials test treatments for patients whose cancer has not gotten better. There are also clinical trials that test new ways to stop cancer from recurring (coming back) or reduce the side effects of cancer treatment.

Clinical trials are taking place in many parts of the country.

Follow-up tests may be needed.

Some of the tests that were done to diagnose the cancer or to find out the stage of the cancer may be repeated. Some tests will be repeated in order to see how well the treatment is working. Decisions about whether to continue, change, or stop treatment may be based on the results of these tests. This is sometimes called re-staging.

Some of the tests will continue to be done from time to time after treatment has ended. The results of these tests can show if your condition has changed or if the cancer has recurred (come back). These tests are sometimes called follow-up tests or check-ups.

Part Four

Cancer Detection and Diagnosis

Chapter 34

Cancer Staging

What is staging?

Staging describes the severity of a person's cancer based on the size and/or extent (reach) of the original (primary) tumor and whether or not cancer has spread in the body. Staging is important for several reasons:

- Staging helps the doctor plan the appropriate treatment.

- Cancer stage can be used in estimating a person's prognosis.

- Knowing the stage of cancer is important in identifying clinical trials that may be a suitable treatment option for a patient.

- Staging helps health care providers and researchers exchange information about patients; it also gives them a common terminology for evaluating the results of clinical trials and comparing the results of different trials.

Staging is based on knowledge of the way cancer progresses. Cancer cells grow and divide without control or order, and they do not die when they should. As a result, they often form a mass of tissue called a tumor. As a tumor grows, it can invade nearby tissues and organs. Cancer cells can also break away from a tumor and enter the bloodstream or the

---

Text in this chapter is excerpted from "Cancer Staging," National Cancer Institute at the National Institutes of Health (NIH), January 6, 2015.

lymphatic system. By moving through the bloodstream or lymphatic system, cancer cells can spread from the primary site to lymph nodes or to other organs, where they may form new tumors. The spread of cancer is called metastasis.

All cancers are staged when they are first diagnosed. This stage classification, which is typically assigned before treatment, is called the clinical stage. A cancer may be further staged after surgery or biopsy, when the extent of the cancer is better known. This stage designation (called the pathologic stage) combines the results of the clinical staging with the surgical results.

A cancer is always referred to by the stage it was given at diagnosis, even if it gets worse or spreads. New information about how a cancer changes over time simply gets added on to the original stage designation. The cancer stage designation doesn't change (even though the cancer itself might) because survival statistics and information on treatment by stage for specific cancer types are based on the original cancer stage at diagnosis.

What are the common elements of staging systems?

Staging systems for cancer have evolved over time. They continue to change as scientists learn more about cancer. Some staging systems cover many types of cancer; others focus on a particular type. The common elements considered in most staging systems are as follows:

- Site of the primary tumor and the cell type (e.g., adenocarcinoma, squamous cell carcinoma)

- Tumor size and/or extent (reach)

- Regional lymph node involvement (the spread of cancer to nearby lymph nodes)

- Number of tumors (the primary tumor and the presence of metastatic tumors, or metastases)

- Tumor grade (how closely the cancer cells and tissue resemble normal cells and tissue)

What is the TNM system?

The TNM system is one of the most widely used cancer staging systems. This system has been accepted by the Union for International Cancer Control (UICC) and the American Joint Committee on Cancer

(AJCC). Most medical facilities use the TNM system as their main method for cancer reporting.

The TNM system is based on the size and/or extent (reach) of the primary tumor (**T**), the amount of spread to nearby lymph nodes (**N**), and the presence of metastasis (**M**) or secondary tumors formed by the spread of cancer cells to other parts of the body. A number is added to each letter to indicate the size and/or extent of the primary tumor and the degree of cancer spread.

Primary Tumor (T)

TX: Primary tumor cannot be evaluated

T0: No evidence of primary tumor

Tis: Carcinoma in situ (CIS; abnormal cells are present but have not spread to neighboring tissue; although not cancer, CIS may become cancer and is sometimes called preinvasive cancer)

T1, T2, T3, T4: Size and/or extent of the primary tumor

Regional Lymph Nodes (N)

NX: Regional lymph nodes cannot be evaluated

N0: No regional lymph node involvement

N1, N2, N3: Degree of regional lymph node involvement (number and location of lymph nodes)

Distant Metastasis (M)

MX: Distant metastasis cannot be evaluated

M0: No distant metastasis

M1: Distant metastasis is present

For example, breast cancer classified as T3 N2 M0 refers to a large tumor that has spread outside the breast to nearby lymph nodes but not to other parts of the body. Prostate cancer T2 N0 M0 means that

Table 34.1. Cancer Stages

Stage	Definition
Stage 0	Carcinoma in situ
Stage I, Stage II, and Stage III	Higher numbers indicate more extensive disease: Larger tumor size and/or spread of the cancer beyond the organ in which it first developed to nearby lymph nodes and/or tissues or organs adjacent to the location of the primary tumor
Stage IV	The cancer has spread to distant tissues or organs

the tumor is located only in the prostate and has not spread to the lymph nodes or any other part of the body.

For many cancers, TNM combinations correspond to one of five stages. Criteria for stages differ for different types of cancer. For example, bladder cancer T3 N0 M0 is stage III, whereas colon cancer T3 N0 M0 is stage II.

Are all cancers staged with TNM classifications?

Most types of cancer have TNM designations, but some do not. For example, cancers of the brain and spinal cord are staged according to their cell type and grade. Different staging systems are also used for many cancers of the blood or bone marrow, such as lymphomas. The Ann Arbor staging classification is commonly used to stage lymphomas and has been adopted by both the AJCC and the UICC. However, other cancers of the blood or bone marrow, including most types of leukemia, do not have a clear-cut staging system. Another staging system, developed by the International Federation of Gynecology and Obstetrics (FIGO), is used to stage cancers of the cervix, uterus, ovary, vagina, and vulva. This system is also based on TNM information. Additionally, most childhood cancers are staged using either the TNM system or the staging criteria of the Children's Oncology Group (COG), which conducts pediatric clinical trials; however, other staging systems may be used for some childhood cancers.

Many cancer registries, such as those supported by NCI's Surveillance, Epidemiology, and End Results (SEER) Program, use "summary staging." This system is used for all types of cancer. It groups cancer cases into five main categories:

- In situ: Abnormal cells are present only in the layer of cells in which they developed

- Localized: Cancer is limited to the organ in which it began, without evidence of spread

- Regional: Cancer has spread beyond the primary site to nearby lymph nodes or tissues and organs

- Distant: Cancer has spread from the primary site to distant tissues or organs or to distant lymph nodes

- Unknown: There is not enough information to determine the stage

What types of tests are used to determine stage?

The types of tests used for staging depend on the type of cancer. Tests include the following:

- Physical exams are used to gather information about the cancer. The doctor examines the body by looking, feeling, and listening for anything unusual. The physical exam may show the location and size of the tumor(s) and the spread of the cancer to the lymph nodes and/or to other tissues and organs.

- Imaging studies produce pictures of areas inside the body. These studies are important tools in determining stage. Procedures such as x-rays, computed tomography (CT) scans, magnetic resonance imaging (MRI) scans, and positron emission tomography (PET) scans can show the location of the cancer, the size of the tumor, and whether the cancer has spread.

- Laboratory tests are studies of blood, urine, other fluids, and tissues taken from the body. For example, tests for liver function and tumor markers (substances sometimes found in increased amounts if cancer is present) can provide information about the cancer.

- Pathology reports may include information about the size of the tumor, the growth of the tumor into other tissues and organs, the type of cancer cells, and the grade of the tumor. A biopsy may be performed to provide information for the pathology report. Cytology reports also describe findings from the examination of cells in body fluids.

- Surgical reports tell what is found during surgery. These reports describe the size and appearance of the tumor and often include observations about lymph nodes and nearby organs.

What is restaging?

Doctors may reassess a person's cancer after their treatment has been completed to determine how the cancer responded to treatment. Such a reassessment, or restaging, may also be done when a cancer has recurred and may require more treatment. This reassessment involves the same tests that were done when the cancer was first diagnosed. After these tests, the doctor may assign a new stage to the cancer. The new stage will be preceded by an "r" to indicate that it reflects the restaging. The original stage at diagnosis does not change.

797

Chapter 35

Computed Tomography (CT) Scans and Cancer

What is computed tomography?

Computed tomography (CT) is an imaging procedure that uses special x-ray equipment to create detailed pictures, or scans, of areas inside the body. It is also called computerized tomography and computerized axial tomography (CAT).

The term tomography comes from the Greek words tomos (a cut, a slice, or a section) and graphein (to write or record). Each picture created during a CT procedure shows the organs, bones, and other tissues in a thin "slice" of the body. The entire series of pictures produced in CT is like a loaf of sliced bread—you can look at each slice individually (2-dimensional pictures), or you can look at the whole loaf (a 3-dimensional picture). Computer programs are used to create both types of pictures.

Most modern CT machines take continuous pictures in a helical (or spiral) fashion rather than taking a series of pictures of individual slices of the body, as the original CT machines did. Helical CT has several advantages over older CT techniques: it is faster, produces better 3-D pictures of areas inside the body, and may detect small

Text in this chapter is excerpted from "Computed Tomography (CT) Scans and Cancer," National Cancer Institute at the National Institutes of Health (NIH), July 16, 2013.

abnormalities better. The newest CT scanners, called multi slice CT or multi detector CT scanners, allow more slices to be imaged in a shorter period of time.

In addition to its use in cancer, CT is widely used to help diagnose circulatory (blood) system diseases and conditions, such as coronary artery disease (atherosclerosis), blood vessel aneurysms, and blood clots; spinal conditions; kidney and bladder stones; abscesses; inflammatory diseases, such as ulcerative colitis and sinusitis; and injuries to the head, skeletal system, and internal organs. CT can be a life-saving tool for diagnosing illness and injury in both children and adults.

What can a person expect during a CT procedure?

During a CT procedure, the person lies very still on a table, and the table passes slowly through the center of a large x-ray machine. With some types of CT scanners, the table stays still and the machine moves around the person. The person might hear whirring sounds during the procedure. At times during a CT procedure, the person may be asked to hold their breath to prevent blurring of the images.

Sometimes, CT involves the use of a contrast (imaging) agent, or "dye." The dye may be given by mouth, injected into a vein, given by enema, or given in all three ways before the procedure. The contrast dye highlights specific areas inside the body, resulting in clearer pictures. Iodine and barium are two dyes commonly used in CT.

In very rare cases, the contrast agents used in CT can cause allergic reactions. Some people experience mild itching or hives (small bumps on the skin). Symptoms of a more serious allergic reaction include shortness of breath and swelling of the throat or other parts of the body. People should tell the technologist immediately if they experience any of these symptoms, so they can be treated promptly. Very rarely, the contrast agents used in CT can also cause kidney problems in certain patients. These kidney problems usually do not have any symptoms, but they can be detected by running a simple test on a blood sample.

CT does not cause any pain. However, lying in one position during the procedure may be slightly uncomfortable. The length of a CT procedure depends on the size of the area being scanned, but it usually lasts only a few minutes to half an hour. For most people, the CT is performed on an outpatient basis at a hospital or a radiology center, without an overnight hospital stay.

Some people are concerned about experiencing claustrophobia during a CT procedure. However, most CT scanners surround only portions of the body, not the whole body. Therefore, people are not enclosed in a machine and are unlikely to feel claustrophobic.

Women should let their health care provider and the technologist know if there is any possibility that they are pregnant, because radiation from CT can harm a growing fetus.

How is CT used in cancer?

CT is used in cancer in many different ways:

- To detect abnormal growths

- To help diagnose the presence of a tumor

- To provide information about the stage of a cancer

- To determine exactly where to perform (i.e., guide) a biopsy procedure

- To guide certain local treatments, such as cryotherapy, radiofrequency ablation, and the implantation of radioactive seeds

- To help plan external-beam radiation therapy or surgery

- To determine whether a cancer is responding to treatment

- To detect recurrence of a tumor

How is CT used in cancer screening?

Studies have shown that CT can be effective in both colorectal cancer screening (including screening for large polyps) and lung cancer screening.

Colorectal cancer

CT colonography (also known as virtual colonoscopy) can be used to screen for both large colorectal polyps and colorectal tumors. CT colonography uses the same dose of radiation that is used in standard CT of the abdomen and pelvis, which is about 10 millisieverts (mSv). (By comparison, the estimated average annual dose received from natural sources of radiation is about 3 mSv.) As with standard (optical) colonoscopy, a thorough cleansing of the colon is performed before this test. During the examination, air or carbon dioxide gas is pumped into the colon to expand it for better viewing.

The National CT Colonography Trial, an NCI-sponsored clinical trial, found that the accuracy of CT colonography is similar to that of standard colonoscopy. CT colonography is less invasive than standard colonoscopy and has a lower risk of complications. However, if polyps or other abnormal growths are found on CT colonography, a standard colonoscopy is usually performed to remove them.

Whether CT colonography can help reduce the death rate from colorectal cancer is not yet known, and most insurance companies (and Medicare) do not currently reimburse the costs of this procedure. Also, because CT colonography can produce images of organs and tissues outside the colon, it is possible that non-colorectal abnormalities may be found. Some of these "extra-colonic" findings will be serious, but many will not be, leading to unnecessary additional tests and surgeries.

Lung cancer

The NCI-sponsored National Lung Screening Trial (NLST) showed that people aged 55 to 74 years with a history of heavy smoking are 20 percent less likely to die from lung cancer if they are screened with low-dose helical CT than if they are screened with standard chest x-rays. (Previous studies had shown that screening with standard chest x-rays does not reduce the death rate from lung cancer.) The estimated amount of radiation in a low-dose helical CT procedure is 1.5 mSv.

Despite the effectiveness of low-dose helical CT for lung cancer screening in heavy smokers, the NLST identified risks as well as benefits. For example, people screened with low-dose helical CT had a higher overall rate of false-positive results (that is, findings that appeared to be abnormal even though no cancer was present), a higher rate of false-positive results that led to an invasive procedure (such as bronchoscopy or biopsy), and a higher rate of serious complications from an invasive procedure than those screened with standard x-rays.

The benefits of helical CT in screening for lung cancer may vary, depending on how similar someone is to the people who participated in the NLST. The benefits may also be greater for those with a higher lung cancer risk, and the harms may be more pronounced for those who have more medical problems (like heart or other lung disease), which could increase problems arising from biopsies and other surgery.

People who think that they have an increased risk of lung cancer and are interested in screening with low-dose helical CT should discuss the appropriateness and the benefits and risks of lung cancer screening with their doctors. They should also be aware that, because the technique is fairly new, some insurance plans do not currently cover it.

What is total, or whole-body, CT?

Total, or whole-body, CT creates pictures of nearly every area of the body—from the chin to below the hips. This procedure, which is used routinely in patients who already have cancer, can also be used in people who do not have any symptoms of disease. However, whole-body CT has not been shown to be an effective screening method for healthy people. Most abnormal findings from this procedure do not indicate a serious health problem, but the tests that must be done to follow up and rule out a problem can be expensive, inconvenient, and uncomfortable. In addition, whole-body CT can expose people to relatively large amounts of ionizing radiation—about 12 mSv, or four times the estimated average annual dose received from natural sources of radiation. Most doctors recommend against whole-body CT for people without any signs or symptoms of disease.

What is combined PET/CT?

Combined PET/CT uses two imaging methods, CT and positron emission tomography (PET), in one procedure. CT is done first to create anatomic pictures of the organs and structures in the body, and then PET is done to create colored pictures that show chemical or other functional changes in tissues.

Different types of positron-emitting (radioactive) substances can be used in PET. Depending on the substance used, different kinds of chemical or functional changes can be imaged. The most common type of PET procedure uses an imaging agent called FDG (a radioactive form of the sugar glucose), which shows the metabolic activity of tissues. Because cancerous tumors are usually more metabolically active than normal tissues, they appear different from other tissues on a PET scan. Other PET imaging agents can provide information about the level of oxygen in a particular tissue, the formation of new blood vessels, the presence of bone growth, or whether tumor cells are actively dividing and growing.

Combining CT and PET may provide a more complete picture of a tumor's location and growth or spread than either test alone. The combined procedure may improve the ability to diagnose cancer, to determine how far a tumor has spread, to plan treatment, and to monitor response to treatment. Combined PET/CT may also reduce the number of additional imaging tests and other procedures a patient needs.

Is the radiation from CT harmful?

Some people may be concerned about the amount of radiation they receive during CT. CT imaging involves the use of x-rays, which are a form of ionizing radiation. Exposure to ionizing radiation is known to increase the risk of cancer. Standard x-ray procedures, such as routine chest x-rays and mammography, use relatively low levels of ionizing radiation. The radiation exposure from CT is higher than that from standard x-ray procedures, but the increase in cancer risk from one CT scan is still small. *Not* having the procedure can be much more risky than having it, especially if CT is being used to diagnose cancer or another serious condition in someone who has signs or symptoms of disease.

It is commonly thought that the extra risk of any one person developing a fatal cancer from a typical CT procedure is about 1 in 2,000. In contrast, the lifetime risk of dying from cancer in the U.S. population is about 1 in 5.

It is also important to note that everyone is exposed to some background level of naturally occurring ionizing radiation every day. The average person in the United States receives an estimated effective dose of about 3 millisieverts (mSv) per year from naturally occurring radioactive materials, such as radon and radiation from outer space. By comparison, the radiation exposure from one low-dose CT scan of the chest (1.5 mSv) is comparable to 6 months of natural background radiation, and a regular-dose CT scan of the chest (7 mSv) is comparable to 2 years of natural background radiation.

The widespread use of CT and other procedures that use ionizing radiation to create images of the body has raised concerns that even small increases in cancer risk could lead to large numbers of future cancers. People who have CT procedures as children may be at higher risk because children are more sensitive to radiation and have a longer life expectancy than adults. Women are at a somewhat higher risk than men of developing cancer after receiving the same radiation exposures at the same ages.

People considering CT should talk with their doctors about whether the procedure is necessary for them and about its risks and benefits. Some organizations recommend that people keep a record of the imaging examinations they have received in case their doctors don't have access to all of their health records. A sample form, called *My Medical*

Imaging History, was developed by the Radiological Society of North America, the American College of Radiology, and the U.S. Food and Drug Administration. It includes questions to ask the doctor before undergoing any x-ray exam or treatment procedure.

What are the risks of CT scans for children?

Radiation exposure from CT scans affects adults and children differently. Children are considerably more sensitive to radiation than adults because of their growing bodies and the rapid pace at which the cells in their bodies divide. In addition, children have a longer life expectancy than adults, providing a larger window of opportunity for radiation-related cancers to develop.

Individuals who have had multiple CT scans before the age of 15 were found to have an increased risk of developing leukemia, brain tumors, and other cancers in the decade following their first scan. However, the lifetime risk of cancer from a single CT scan was small—about one case of cancer for every 10,000 scans performed on children.

In talking with health care providers, three key questions that the parents can ask are: why is the test needed? Will the results change the treatment decisions? Is there an alternative test that doesn't involve radiation? If the test is clinically justified, then the parents can be reassured that the benefits will outweigh the small long-term risks.

What is being done to reduce the level of radiation exposure from CT?

In response to concerns about the increased risk of cancer associated with CT and other imaging procedures that use ionizing radiation, several organizations and government agencies have developed guidelines and recommendations regarding the appropriate use of these procedures.

- In 2010, the U.S. Food and Drug Administration (FDA) launched the Initiative to Reduce Unnecessary Radiation Exposure from Medical Imaging. This initiative focuses on the safe use of medical imaging devices, informed decision-making about when to use specific imaging procedures, and increasing patients' awareness of their radiation exposure. Key components of the initiative include avoiding repeat procedures, keeping doses as low as possible while maximizing image quality, and using imaging only when appropriate. The FDA also produced Reducing

Radiation from Medical X-rays, a guide for consumers that includes information about the risks of medical x-rays, steps consumers can take to reduce radiation risks, and a table that shows the radiation dose of some common medical x-ray exams.

- The NIH Clinical Center requires that radiation dose exposures from CT and other imaging procedures be included in the electronic medical records of patients treated at the center. In addition, all imaging equipment purchased by NIH must provide data on exposure in a form that can be tracked and reported electronically. This patient protection policy is being adopted by other hospitals and imaging facilities.

- NCI's website includes a guide for health care providers, Radiation Risks and Pediatric Computed Tomography (CT): A Guide for Health Care Providers. The guide addresses the value of CT as a diagnostic tool in children, unique considerations for radiation exposure in children, risks to children from radiation exposure, and measures to minimize exposure.

- The American College of Radiology (ACR) has developed the ACR Appropriateness Criteria®, evidence-based guidelines to help providers make appropriate imaging and treatment decisions for a number of clinical conditions.

- ACR has also established the Dose Index Registry, which collects anonymized information related to dose indices for all CT exams at participating facilities. Data from the registry can be used to compare radiology facilities and to establish national benchmarks.

- CT scanner manufacturers are developing newer cameras and detector systems that can provide higher quality images at much lower radiation doses.

What is NCI doing to improve CT imaging?

Researchers funded by NCI are studying ways to improve the use of CT in cancer screening, diagnosis, and treatment. NCI also conducts and sponsors clinical trials that are testing ways to improve CT or new uses of CT imaging technology. Some of these clinical trials are run by the American College of Radiology Imaging Network (ACRIN), a clinical trials cooperative group that is funded in part by NCI. ACRIN performed the National CT Colonography Trial, which tested the use of CT for colorectal cancer screening, and participated in the NLST, which tested the use of CT for lung cancer screening in high-risk individuals.

NCI's Cancer Imaging Program (CIP), part of the Division of Cancer Treatment and Diagnosis (DCTD), funds cancer-related basic, translational, and clinical research in imaging sciences and technology. CIP supports the development of novel imaging agents for CT and other types of imaging procedures to help doctors better locate cancer cells in the body.

Chapter 36

Mammograms

What is a mammogram?

A mammogram is an x-ray picture of the breast.

Mammograms can be used to check for breast cancer in women who have no signs or symptoms of the disease. This type of mammogram is called a screening mammogram. Screening mammograms usually involve two x-ray pictures, or images, of each breast. The x-ray images make it possible to detect tumors that cannot be felt. Screening mammograms can also find microcalcifications (tiny deposits of calcium) that sometimes indicate the presence of breast cancer.

Mammograms can also be used to check for breast cancer after a lump or other sign or symptom of the disease has been found. This type of mammogram is called a diagnostic mammogram. Besides a lump, signs of breast cancer can include breast pain, thickening of the skin of the breast, nipple discharge, or a change in breast size or shape; however, these signs may also be signs of benign conditions. A diagnostic mammogram can also be used to evaluate changes found during a screening mammogram or to view breast tissue when it is difficult to obtain a screening mammogram because of special circumstances, such as the presence of breast implants.

Text in this chapter is excerpted from "Mammograms," National Cancer Institute at the National Institutes of Health (NIH), March 25, 2014.

How are screening and diagnostic mammograms different?

Diagnostic mammography takes longer than screening mammography because more x-rays are needed to obtain views of the breast from several angles. The technician may magnify a suspicious area to produce a detailed picture that can help the doctor make an accurate diagnosis.

What are the benefits of screening mammograms?

Early detection of breast cancer with screening mammography means that treatment can be started earlier in the course of the disease, possibly before it has spread. Results from randomized clinical trials and other studies show that screening mammography can help reduce the number of deaths from breast cancer among women ages 40 to 74, especially for those over age 50. However, studies to date have not shown a benefit from regular screening mammography in women under age 40 or from baseline screening mammograms (mammograms used for comparison) taken before age 40.

What are some of the potential limitations of screening mammograms?

False-positive results. False-positive results occur when radiologists decide mammograms are abnormal but no cancer is actually present. All abnormal mammograms should be followed up with additional testing (diagnostic mammograms, ultrasound, and/or biopsy) to determine whether cancer is present.

False-positive results are more common for younger women, women who have had previous breast biopsies, women with a family history of breast cancer, and women who are taking estrogen (for example, menopausal hormone therapy).

False-positive mammogram results can lead to anxiety and other forms of psychological distress in affected women. The additional testing required to rule out cancer can also be costly and time consuming and can cause physical discomfort.

Overdiagnosis and overtreatment. Screening mammograms can find cancers and cases of ductal carcinoma in situ (DCIS, a noninvasive tumor in which abnormal cells that may become cancerous build up in the lining of breast ducts) that need to be treated. However, they can also find cancers and cases of DCIS that will never cause symptoms or threaten a woman's life, leading to "overdiagnosis" of breast cancer.

Treatment of these latter cancers and cases of DCIS is not needed and leads to "overtreatment." Overtreatment exposes women unnecessarily to the adverse effects associated with cancer therapy.

Because doctors often cannot distinguish cancers and cases of DCIS that need to be treated from those that do not, they are all treated.

False-negative results. False-negative results occur when mammograms appear normal even though breast cancer is present. Overall, screening mammograms miss about 20 percent of breast cancers that are present at the time of screening.

The main cause of false-negative results is high breast density. Breasts contain both dense tissue (i.e., glandular tissue and connective tissue, together known as fibro glandular tissue) and fatty tissue. Fatty tissue appears dark on a mammogram, whereas fibro glandular tissue appears as white areas. Because fibro glandular tissue and tumors have similar density, tumors can be harder to detect in women with denser breasts.

False-negative results occur more often among younger women than among older women because younger women are more likely to have dense breasts. As a woman ages, her breasts usually become more fatty, and false-negative results become less likely. False-negative results can lead to delays in treatment and a false sense of security for affected women.

Some of the cancers missed by screening mammograms can be detected by clinical breast exams (physical exams of the breast done by a health care provider).

Finding cancer early does not always reduce a woman's chance of dying from breast cancer. Even though mammograms can detect malignant tumors that cannot be felt, treating a small tumor does not always mean that the woman will not die from the cancer. A fast-growing or aggressive cancer may have already spread to other parts of the body before it is detected. Women with such tumors live a longer period of time knowing that they likely have a fatal disease.

In addition, screening mammograms may not help prolong the life of a woman who is suffering from other, more life-threatening health conditions.

Radiation exposure. Mammograms require very small doses of radiation. The risk of harm from this radiation exposure is extremely low, but repeated x-rays have the potential to cause cancer. The benefits of mammography, however, nearly always outweigh the potential harm from the radiation exposure. Nevertheless, women should talk with their health care providers about the need for each x-ray. In addition, they should always let their health care provider and the x-ray technician know if there is any possibility that they are pregnant, because radiation can harm a growing fetus.

Where can I find current recommendations for screening mammography?

Many organizations and professional societies, including the United States Preventive Services Task Force (which is convened by the Agency for Healthcare Research and Quality, a federal agency), have developed guidelines for mammography screening. All recommend that women should talk with their doctor about the benefits and harms of mammography, when to start screening, and how often to be screened.

Although NCI does not issue guidelines for cancer screening, it conducts and facilitates basic and translational research that informs standard clinical practice and medical decision making that other organizations may use to develop their guidelines.

What is the best method of detecting breast cancer as early as possible?

Getting a high-quality screening mammogram and having a clinical breast exam on a regular basis are the most effective ways to detect breast cancer early.

Checking one's own breasts for lumps or other unusual changes is called a breast self-exam, or BSE. This type of exam cannot replace regular screening mammograms or clinical breast exams. In clinical trials, BSE alone was not found to help reduce the number of deaths from breast cancer.

Although regular BSE is not specifically recommended for breast cancer screening, many women choose to examine their own breasts. Women who do so should remember that breast changes can occur because of pregnancy, aging, or menopause; during menstrual cycles; or when taking birth control pills or other hormones. It is normal for breasts to feel a little lumpy and uneven. Also, it is common for breasts to be swollen and tender right before or during a menstrual period. If a woman notices any unusual changes in her breasts, she should contact her health care provider.

What is the Breast Imaging Reporting and Database System (BI-RADS®)?

The American College of Radiology (ACR) has established a uniform way for radiologists to describe mammogram findings. The system, called BI-RADS, includes seven standardized categories, or levels. Each BI-RADS category has a follow-up plan associated with it to help radiologists and other physicians appropriately manage a patient's care.

How much does a mammogram cost?

For most women with private insurance, the cost of screening mammograms is covered without co-payments or deductibles, but women should contact their mammography facility or health insurance company for confirmation of the cost and coverage.

Medicare pays for annual screening mammograms for all female Medicare beneficiaries who are age 40 or older. Medicare will also pay for one baseline mammogram for female beneficiaries between

Table 36.1. Breast Imaging Reporting and Database System (BI-RADS)

Category	Assessment	Follow-up
0	Need additional imaging evaluation	Additional imaging needed before a category can be assigned
1	Negative	Continue regular screening mammograms (for women over age 40)
2	Benign (noncancerous) finding	Continue regular screening mammograms (for women over age 40)
3	Probably benign	Receive a 6-month follow-up mammogram
4	Suspicious abnormality	May require biopsy
5	Highly suggestive of malignancy (cancer)	Requires biopsy
6	Known biopsy-proven malignancy (cancer)	Biopsy confirms presence of cancer before treatment begins

the ages of 35 and 39. There is no deductible requirement for this benefit.

How can uninsured or low-income women obtain a free or low-cost screening mammogram?

Some state and local health programs and employers provide mammograms free or at low cost. For example, the Centers for Disease Control and Prevention (CDC) coordinates the National Breast and Cervical Cancer Early Detection Program. This program provides screening services, including clinical breast exams and mammograms, to low-income, uninsured women throughout the United States and in several U.S. territories.

Information about free or low-cost mammography screening programs is also available from NCI's Cancer Information Service at 1–800–4–CANCER (1–800–422–6237) and from local hospitals, health departments, women's centers, or other community groups.

Where can women get high-quality mammograms?

Women can get high-quality mammograms in breast clinics, hospital radiology departments, mobile vans, private radiology offices, and doctors' offices.

The Mammography Quality Standards Act (MQSA) is a Federal law that requires mammography facilities across the nation to meet uniform quality standards. Under the law, all mammography facilities must: 1) be accredited by an FDA-approved accreditation body; 2) be certified by the FDA, or an agency of a state that has been approved by the FDA, as meeting the standards; 3) undergo an annual MQSA inspection; and 4) prominently display the certificate issued by the agency.

Women can ask their doctors or staff at a local mammography facility about FDA certification before making an appointment. Women should look for the MQSA certificate at the mammography facility and check its expiration date. MQSA regulations also require that mammography facilities give patients an easy-to-read report of their mammogram results.

What should women with breast implants do about screening mammograms?

Women with breast implants should continue to have mammograms. (A woman who had an implant following a mastectomy should ask her doctor whether a mammogram of the reconstructed breast is necessary.) It is important to let the mammography facility know about breast implants when scheduling a mammogram. The technician and radiologist must be experienced in performing mammography on women who have breast implants. Implants can hide some breast tissue, making it more difficult for the radiologist to detect an abnormality on the mammogram. If the technician performing the procedure is aware that a woman has breast implants, steps can be taken to make sure that as much breast tissue as possible can be seen on the mammogram. A special technique called implant displacement views may be used.

What is digital mammography? How is it different from conventional (film) mammography?

Digital and conventional mammography both use x-rays to produce an image of the breast; however, in conventional mammography, the image is stored directly on film, whereas, in digital mammography, an electronic image of the breast is stored as a computer file. This digital information can be enhanced, magnified, or manipulated for further evaluation more easily than information stored on film.

Because digital mammography allows a radiologist to adjust, store, and retrieve digital images electronically, digital mammography may offer the following advantages over conventional mammography:

- Health care providers can share image files electronically, making long-distance consultations between radiologists and breast surgeons easier.

- Subtle differences between normal and abnormal tissues may be more easily noted.

- Fewer follow-up procedures may be needed.

- Fewer repeat images may be needed, reducing the exposure to radiation.

To date, there is no evidence that digital mammography helps to reduce a woman's risk of dying from breast cancer compared with film mammography. Results from a large NCI-sponsored clinical trial that compared digital mammography with film mammography found no difference between digital and film mammograms in detecting breast cancer in the general population of women in the trial; however, digital mammography appeared to be more accurate than conventional film

815

mammography in younger women with dense breasts. A subsequent analysis of women aged 40 through 79 who were undergoing screening in U.S. community-based imaging facilities also found that digital and film mammography had similar accuracy in most women. Digital screening had higher sensitivity in women with dense breasts.

Some health care providers recommend that women who have a very high risk of breast cancer, such as those with a known mutation in either the *BRCA1* or *BRCA2* gene or extremely dense breasts, have digital mammograms instead of conventional mammograms; however, no studies have shown that digital mammograms are superior to conventional mammograms in reducing the risk of death for these women.

Digital mammography can be done only in facilities that are certified to practice conventional mammography and have received FDA approval to offer digital mammography. The procedure for having a mammogram with a digital system is the same as with conventional mammography.

What is 3D mammography?

Three-dimensional (3D) mammography, also known as breast tomosynthesis, is a type of digital mammography in which x-ray machines are used to take pictures of thin slices of the breast from different angles and computer software is used to reconstruct an image. This process is similar to how a computed tomography (CT) scanner produces images of structures inside of the body. 3D mammography uses very low dose x-rays, but, because it is generally performed at the same time as standard two-dimensional (2D) digital mammography, the radiation dose is slightly higher than that of standard mammography. The accuracy of 3D mammography has not been compared with that of 2D mammography in randomized studies. Therefore, researchers do not know whether 3D mammography is better or worse than standard mammography at avoiding false-positive results and identifying early cancers.

Chapter 37

BRCA1 and BRCA2: Cancer Risk and Genetic Testing

What are BRCA1 and BRCA2?

BRCA1 and *BRCA2* are human genes that produce tumor suppressor proteins. These proteins help repair damaged DNA and, therefore, play a role in ensuring the stability of the cell's genetic material. When either of these genes is mutated, or altered, such that its protein product either is not made or does not function correctly, DNA damage may not be repaired properly. As a result, cells are more likely to develop additional genetic alterations that can lead to cancer.

Specific inherited mutations in *BRCA1* and *BRCA2* increase the risk of female breast and ovarian cancers, and they have been associated with increased risks of several additional types of cancer. Together, *BRCA1* and *BRCA2* mutations account for about 20 to 25 percent of hereditary breast cancers and about 5 to 10 percent of all breast cancers. In addition, mutations in *BRCA1* and *BRCA2* account for around 15 percent of ovarian cancers overall. Breast and ovarian cancers associated with *BRCA1* and *BRCA2* mutations tend to develop at younger ages than their nonhereditary counterparts.

Text in this chapter is excerpted from "*BRCA1* and *BRCA2*: Cancer Risk and Genetic Testing," National Cancer Institute at the National Institutes of Health (NIH), April 1, 2015.

A harmful *BRCA1* or *BRCA2* mutation can be inherited from a person's mother or father. Each child of a parent who carries a mutation in one of these genes has a 50 percent chance (or 1 chance in 2) of inheriting the mutation. The effects of mutations in *BRCA1* and *BRCA2* are seen even when a person's second copy of the gene is normal.

How much does having a BRCA1 or BRCA2 gene mutation increase a woman's risk of breast and ovarian cancer?

A woman's lifetime risk of developing breast and/or ovarian cancer is greatly increased if she inherits a harmful mutation in *BRCA1* or *BRCA2*.

- **Breast cancer:** About 12 percent of women in the general population will develop breast cancer sometime during their lives. By contrast, according to the most recent estimates, 55 to 65 percent of women who inherit a harmful *BRCA1* mutation and around 45 percent of women who inherit a harmful *BRCA2* mutation will develop breast cancer by age 70 years.

- **Ovarian cancer:** About 1.4 percent of women in the general population will develop ovarian cancer sometime during their lives. By contrast, according to the most recent estimates, 39 percent of women who inherit a harmful *BRCA1* mutation and 11 to 17 percent of women who inherit a harmful *BRCA2* mutation will develop ovarian cancer by age 70 years.

It is important to note that these estimated percentages of lifetime risk are different from those available previously; the estimates have changed as more information has become available, and they may change again with additional research. No long-term general population studies have directly compared cancer risk in women who have and do not have a harmful *BRCA1* or *BRCA2* mutation.

It is also important to note that other characteristics of a particular woman can make her cancer risk higher or lower than the average risks. These characteristics include her family history of breast, ovarian, and, possibly, other cancers; the specific mutation(s) she has inherited; and other risk factors, such as her reproductive history. However, at this time, based on current data, none of these other factors seems to be as strong as the effect of carrying a harmful *BRCA1* or *BRCA2* mutation.

What other cancers have been linked to mutations in BRCA1 and BRCA2?

Harmful mutations in *BRCA1* and *BRCA2* increase the risk of several cancers in addition to breast and ovarian cancer. *BRCA1* mutations may increase a woman's risk of developing fallopian tube cancer and peritoneal cancer. Men with *BRCA2* mutations, and to a lesser extent *BRCA1* mutations, are also at increased risk of breast cancer. Men with harmful *BRCA1* or *BRCA2* mutations have a higher risk of prostate cancer. Men and women with *BRCA1* or *BRCA2* mutations may be at increased risk of pancreatic cancer. Mutations in *BRCA2* (also known as *FANCD1*), if they are inherited from both parents, can cause a Fanconi anemia subtype (FA-D1), a syndrome that is associated with childhood solid tumors and development of acute myeloid leukemia. Likewise, mutations in *BRCA1* (also known as *FANCS*), if they are inherited from both parents, can cause another Fanconi anemia subtype.

Are mutations in BRCA1 and BRCA2 more common in certain racial/ethnic populations than others?

Yes. For example, people of Ashkenazi Jewish descent have a higher prevalence of harmful *BRCA1* and *BRCA2* mutations than people in the general U.S. population. Other ethnic and geographic populations around the world, such as the Norwegian, Dutch, and Icelandic peoples, also have a higher prevalence of specific harmful *BRCA1* and *BRCA2* mutations.

In addition, limited data indicate that the prevalence of specific harmful *BRCA1* and *BRCA2* mutations may vary among individual racial and ethnic groups in the United States, including African Americans, Hispanics, Asian Americans, and non-Hispanic whites.

Are genetic tests available to detect BRCA1 and BRCA2 mutations?

Yes. Several different tests are available, including tests that look for a known mutation in one of the genes (i.e., a mutation that has already been identified in another family member) and tests that check for all possible mutations in both genes. DNA (from a blood or saliva sample) is needed for mutation testing. The sample is sent to a laboratory for analysis. It usually takes about a month to get the test results.

Who should consider genetic testing for BRCA1 and BRCA2 mutations?

Because harmful *BRCA1* and *BRCA2* gene mutations are relatively rare in the general population, most experts agree that mutation testing of individuals who do not have cancer should be performed only when the person's individual or family history suggests the possible presence of a harmful mutation in *BRCA1* or *BRCA2*.

In December 2013, the United States Preventive Services Task Force recommended that women who have family members with breast, ovarian, fallopian tube, or peritoneal cancer be evaluated to see if they have a family history that is associated with an increased risk of a harmful mutation in one of these genes.

Several screening tools are now available to help health care providers with this evaluation. These tools assess family history factors that are associated with an increased likelihood of having a harmful mutation in *BRCA1* or *BRCA2*, including:

- Breast cancer diagnosed before age 50 years
- Cancer in both breasts in the same woman
- Both breast and ovarian cancers in either the same woman or the same family
- Multiple breast cancers
- Two or more primary types of *BRCA1*- or *BRCA2*-related cancers in a single family member
- Cases of male breast cancer
- Ashkenazi Jewish ethnicity

When an individual has a family history that is suggestive of the presence of a *BRCA1* or *BRCA2* mutation, it may be most informative to first test a family member who has cancer if that person is still alive and willing to be tested. If that person is found to have a harmful *BRCA1* or *BRCA2* mutation, then other family members may want to consider genetic counseling to learn more about their potential risks and whether genetic testing for mutations in *BRCA1* and *BRCA2* might be appropriate for them.

If it is not possible to confirm the presence of a harmful *BRCA1* or *BRCA2* mutation in a family member who has cancer, it is appropriate for both men and women who do not have cancer but have a family medical history that suggests the presence of such a mutation to have genetic counseling for possible testing.

Some individuals—for example, those who were adopted at birth—may not know their family history. In cases where a woman with an unknown family history has an early-onset breast cancer or ovarian cancer or a man with an unknown family history is diagnosed with breast cancer, it may be reasonable for that individual to consider genetic testing for a *BRCA1* or *BRCA2* mutation. Individuals with an unknown family history who do not have an early-onset cancer or male breast cancer are at very low risk of having a harmful *BRCA1* or *BRCA2* mutation and are unlikely to benefit from routine genetic testing.

Professional societies do not recommend that children, even those with a family history suggestive of a harmful *BRCA1* or *BRCA2* mutation, undergo genetic testing for *BRCA1* or *BRCA2*. This is because no risk-reduction strategies exist for children, and children's risks of developing a cancer type associated with a *BRCA1* or *BRCA2* mutation are extremely low. After children with a family history suggestive of a harmful *BRCA1* or *BRCA2* mutation become adults, however, they may want to obtain genetic counseling about whether or not to under-going genetic testing.

Should people considering genetic testing for BRCA1 and BRCA2 mutations talk with a genetic counselor?

Genetic counseling is generally recommended before and after any genetic test for an inherited cancer syndrome. This counseling should be performed by a health care professional who is experienced in cancer genetics. Genetic counseling usually covers many aspects of the testing process, including:

- A hereditary cancer risk assessment based on an individual's personal and family medical history
- Discussion of:
  - The appropriateness of genetic testing
  - The medical implications of a positive or a negative test result
  - The possibility that a test result might not be informative
  - The psychological risks and benefits of genetic test results
  - The risk of passing a mutation to children
- Explanation of the specific test(s) that might be used and the technical accuracy of the test(s)

How much does BRCA1 and BRCA2 mutation testing cost?

The Affordable Care Act considers genetic counseling and *BRCA1* and *BRCA2* mutation testing for individuals at high risk a covered preventive service. People considering *BRCA1* and *BRCA2* mutation testing may want to confirm their insurance coverage for genetic tests before having the test.

Some of the genetic testing companies that offer testing for *BRCA1* and *BRCA2* mutations may offer testing at no charge to patients who lack insurance and meet specific financial and medical criteria.

What does a positive BRCA1 or BRCA2 genetic test result mean?

BRCA1 and *BRCA2* gene mutation testing can give several possible results: a positive result, a negative result, or an ambiguous or uncertain result.

A positive test result indicates that a person has inherited a known harmful mutation in *BRCA1* or *BRCA2* and, therefore, has an increased risk of developing certain cancers. However, a positive test result cannot tell whether or when an individual will actually develop cancer. For example, some women who inherit a harmful *BRCA1* or *BRCA2* mutation will never develop breast or ovarian cancer.

A positive genetic test result may also have important health and social implications for family members, including future generations. Unlike most other medical tests, genetic tests can reveal information not only about the person being tested but also about that person's relatives:

- Both men and women who inherit a harmful *BRCA1* or *BRCA2* mutation, whether or not they develop cancer themselves, may pass the mutation on to their sons and daughters. Each child has a 50 percent chance of inheriting a parent's mutation.

- If a person learns that he or she has inherited a harmful *BRCA1* or *BRCA2* mutation, this will mean that each of his or her siblings has a 50 percent chance of having inherited the mutation as well.

What does a negative BRCA1 or BRCA2 test result mean?

A negative test result can be more difficult to understand than a positive result because what the result means depends in part on an individual's family history of cancer and whether a *BRCA1* or *BRCA2* mutation has been identified in a blood relative.

If a close (first- or second-degree) relative of the tested person is known to carry a harmful *BRCA1* or *BRCA2* mutation, a negative test result is clear: it means that person does not carry the harmful mutation that is responsible for the familial cancer, and thus cannot pass it on to their children. Such a test result is called a true negative. A person with such a test result is currently thought to have the same risk of cancer as someone in the general population.

If the tested person has a family history that suggests the possibility of having a harmful mutation in *BRCA1* or *BRCA2* but complete gene testing identifies no such mutation in the family, a negative result is less clear. The likelihood that genetic testing will miss a known harmful *BRCA1* or *BRCA2* mutation is very low, but it could happen. Moreover, scientists continue to discover new *BRCA1* and *BRCA2* mutations and have not yet identified all potentially harmful ones. Therefore, it is possible that a person in this scenario with a "negative" test result actually has an as-yet unknown harmful *BRCA1* or *BRCA2* mutation that has not been identified.

It is also possible for people to have a mutation in a gene other than *BRCA1* or *BRCA2* that increases their cancer risk but is not detectable by the test used. People considering genetic testing for *BRCA1* and *BRCA2* mutations may want to discuss these potential uncertainties with a genetic counselor before undergoing testing.

What does an ambiguous or uncertain BRCA1 or BRCA2 test result mean?

Sometimes, a genetic test finds a change in *BRCA1* or *BRCA2* that has not been previously associated with cancer. This type of test result may be described as "ambiguous" (often referred to as "a genetic variant of uncertain significance") because it isn't known whether this specific gene change affects a person's risk of developing cancer. One study found that 10 percent of women who underwent *BRCA1* and *BRCA2* mutation testing had this type of ambiguous result.

As more research is conducted and more people are tested for *BRCA1* and *BRCA2* mutations, scientists will learn more about these changes and cancer risk. Genetic counseling can help a person understand what an ambiguous change in *BRCA1* or *BRCA2* may mean in terms of cancer risk. Over time, additional studies of variants of uncertain significance may result in a specific mutation being re-classified as either harmful or clearly not harmful.

How can a person who has a positive test result manage their risk of cancer?

Several options are available for managing cancer risk in individuals who have a known harmful *BRCA1* or *BRCA2* mutation. These include enhanced screening, prophylactic (risk-reducing) surgery, and chemoprevention.

Enhanced Screening. Some women who test positive for *BRCA1* and *BRCA2* mutations may choose to start cancer screening at younger ages than the general population or to have more frequent screening. For example, some experts recommend that women who carry a harmful *BRCA1* or *BRCA2* mutation undergo clinical breast examinations beginning at age 25 to 35 years. And some expert groups recommend that women who carry such a mutation have a mammogram every year, beginning at age 25 to 35 years.

Enhanced screening may increase the chance of detecting breast cancer at an early stage, when it may have a better chance of being treated successfully. Women who have a positive test result should ask their health care provider about the possible harms of diagnostic tests that involve radiation (mammograms or x-rays).

Recent studies have shown that MRI may be more sensitive than mammography for women at high risk of breast cancer. However, mammography can also identify some breast cancers that are not identified by MRI, and MRI may be less specific (i.e., lead to more false-positive results) than mammography. Several organizations, such as the American Cancer Society and the National Comprehensive Cancer Network, now recommend annual screening with mammography and MRI for women who have a high risk of breast cancer.

No effective ovarian cancer screening methods currently exist. Some groups recommend transvaginal ultrasound, blood tests for the antigen CA-125, and clinical examinations for ovarian cancer screening in women with harmful *BRCA1* or *BRCA2* mutations, but none of these methods appears to detect ovarian tumors at an early enough stage to reduce the risk of dying from ovarian cancer. For a screening method to be considered effective, it must have demonstrated reduced mortality from the disease of interest. This standard has not yet been met for ovarian cancer screening.

The benefits of screening for breast and other cancers in men who carry harmful mutations in *BRCA1* or *BRCA2* is also not known, but some expert groups recommend that men who are known to carry a harmful mutation undergo regular mammography as well as testing for prostate cancer. The value of these screening strategies remains unproven at present.

Prophylactic (Risk-reducing) Surgery. Prophylactic surgery involves removing as much of the "at-risk" tissue as possible. Women may choose to have both breasts removed (bilateral prophylactic mastectomy) to reduce their risk of breast cancer. Surgery to remove a woman's ovaries and fallopian tubes (bilateral prophylactic salpingo-oophorectomy) can help reduce her risk of ovarian cancer. Removing the ovaries also reduces the risk of breast cancer in premenopausal women by eliminating a source of hormones that can fuel the growth of some types of breast cancer.

No evidence is available regarding the effectiveness of bilateral prophylactic mastectomy in reducing breast cancer risk in men with a harmful *BRCA1* or *BRCA2* mutation or a family history of breast cancer. Therefore, bilateral prophylactic mastectomy for men at high risk of breast cancer is considered an experimental procedure, and insurance companies will not normally cover it.

Prophylactic surgery does not completely guarantee that cancer will not develop because not all at-risk tissue can be removed by these procedures. Some women have developed breast cancer, ovarian cancer, or primary peritoneal carcinomatosis (a type of cancer similar to ovarian cancer) even after prophylactic surgery. Nevertheless, the mortality reduction associated with this surgery is substantial: Research demonstrates that women who underwent bilateral prophylactic salpingo-oophorectomy had a nearly 80 percent reduction in risk of dying from ovarian cancer, a 56 percent reduction in risk of dying from breast cancer, and a 77 percent reduction in risk of dying from any cause.

Emerging evidence suggests that the amount of protection that removing the ovaries and fallopian tubes provides against the development of breast and ovarian cancer may be similar for carriers of *BRCA1* and *BRCA2* mutations, in contrast to earlier studies.

Chemoprevention. Chemoprevention is the use of drugs, vitamins, or other agents to try to reduce the risk of, or delay the recurrence of, cancer. Although two chemopreventive drugs (tamoxifen and raloxifene) have been approved by the U.S. Food and Drug Administration (FDA) to reduce the risk of breast cancer in women at increased risk, the role of these drugs in women with harmful *BRCA1* or *BRCA2* mutations is not yet clear.

Data from three studies suggest that tamoxifen may be able to help lower the risk of breast cancer in *BRCA1* and *BRCA2* mutation carriers, including the risk of cancer in the opposite breast among women previously diagnosed with breast cancer. Studies have not examined the effectiveness of raloxifene in *BRCA1* and *BRCA2* mutation carriers specifically.

Oral contraceptives (birth control pills) are thought to reduce the risk of ovarian cancer by about 50 percent both in the general population and in women with harmful *BRCA1* or *BRCA2* mutations.

What are some of the benefits of genetic testing for breast and ovarian cancer risk?

There can be benefits to genetic testing, regardless of whether a person receives a positive or a negative result.

The potential benefits of a true negative result include a sense of relief regarding the future risk of cancer, learning that one's children are not at risk of inheriting the family's cancer susceptibility, and the possibility that special checkups, tests, or preventive surgeries may not be needed.

A positive test result may bring relief by resolving uncertainty regarding future cancer risk and may allow people to make informed decisions about their future, including taking steps to reduce their cancer risk. In addition, people who have a positive test result may choose to participate in medical research that could, in the long run, help reduce deaths from hereditary breast and ovarian cancer.

What are some of the possible harms of genetic testing for breast and ovarian cancer risk?

The direct medical harms of genetic testing are minimal, but knowledge of test results may have harmful effects on a person's emotions, social relationships, finances, and medical choices.

People who receive a positive test result may feel anxious, depressed, or angry. They may have difficulty making choices about whether to have preventive surgery or about which surgery to have.

People who receive a negative test result may experience "survivor guilt," caused by the knowledge that they likely do not have an increased risk of developing a disease that affects one or more loved ones.

Because genetic testing can reveal information about more than one family member, the emotions caused by test results can create tension within families. Test results can also affect personal life choices, such as decisions about career, marriage, and childbearing.

Violations of privacy and of the confidentiality of genetic test results are additional potential risks. However, the federal Health Insurance

Portability and Accountability Act and various state laws protect the privacy of a person's genetic information. Moreover, the federal Genetic Information Nondiscrimination Act, along with many state laws, prohibits discrimination based on genetic information in relation to health insurance and employment, although it does not cover life insurance, disability insurance, or long-term care insurance.

Finally, there is a small chance that test results may not be accurate, leading people to make decisions based on incorrect information. Although inaccurate results are unlikely, people with these concerns should address them during genetic counseling.

What are the implications of having a harmful BRCA1 or BRCA2 mutation for breast and ovarian cancer prognosis and treatment?

A number of studies have investigated possible differences between breast and ovarian cancers that are associated with harmful *BRCA1* or *BRCA2* mutations and cancers that are not associated with these mutations.

There is some evidence that, over the long term, women who carry these mutations are more likely to develop a second cancer in either the same (ipsilateral) breast or the opposite (contralateral) breast than women who do not carry these mutations. Thus, some women with a harmful *BRCA1* or *BRCA2* mutation who develop breast cancer in one breast opt for a bilateral mastectomy, even if they would otherwise be candidates for breast-conserving surgery. In fact, because of the increased risk of a second breast cancer among *BRCA1* and *BRCA2* mutation carriers, some doctors recommend that women with early-onset breast cancer and those whose family history is consistent with a mutation in one of these genes have genetic testing when breast cancer is diagnosed.

Breast cancers in women with a harmful *BRCA1* mutation are also more likely to be "triple-negative cancers," (i.e., the breast cancer cells do not have estrogen receptors, progesterone receptors, or large amounts of HER2/neu protein), which generally have poorer prognosis than other breast cancers.

Because the products of the *BRCA1* and *BRCA2* genes are involved in DNA repair, some investigators have suggested that cancer cells with a harmful mutation in either of these genes may be more sensitive to anticancer agents that act by damaging DNA, such as cisplatin. In preclinical studies, drugs called PARP inhibitors, which block the repair of DNA damage, have been found to arrest the growth of cancer cells that have *BRCA1* or *BRCA2* mutations. These drugs have also shown some activity in cancer patients who carry *BRCA1* or *BRCA2* mutations, and researchers are continuing to develop and test these drugs.

Do inherited mutations in other genes increase the risk of breast and/or ovarian tumors?

Yes. Although harmful mutations in *BRCA1* and *BRCA2* are responsible for the disease in nearly half of families with multiple cases of breast cancer and up to 90 percent of families with both breast and ovarian cancer, mutations in a number of other genes have been associated with increased risks of breast and/or ovarian cancers. These other genes include several that are associated with the inherited disorders Cowden syndrome, Peutz-Jeghers syndrome, Li-Fraumeni syndrome, and Fanconi anemia, which increase the risk of many cancer types.

Most mutations in these other genes are associated with smaller increases in breast cancer risk than are seen with mutations in *BRCA1* and *BRCA2*. However, researchers recently reported that inherited mutations in the *PALB2* gene are associated with a risk of breast cancer nearly as high as that associated with inherited *BRCA1* and *BRCA2* mutations. They estimated that 33 percent of women who inherit a harmful mutation in *PALB2* will develop breast cancer by age 70 years. The estimated risk of breast cancer associated with a harmful *PALB2* mutation is even higher for women who have a family history of breast cancer: 58 percent of those women will develop breast cancer by age 70 years.

PALB2, like *BRCA1* and *BRCA2*, is a tumor suppressor gene. The *PALB2* gene produces a protein that interacts with the proteins produced by the *BRCA1* and *BRCA2* genes to help repair breaks in DNA. Harmful mutations in *PALB2* (also known as *FANCN*) are associated with increased risks of ovarian, pancreatic, and prostate cancers in addition to an increased risk of breast cancer. Mutations in *PALB2*, when inherited from each parent, can cause a Fanconi anemia subtype, FA-N, that is associated with childhood solid tumors.

Although genetic testing for *PALB2* mutations is available, expert groups have not yet developed specific guidelines for who should be tested for, or the management of breast cancer risk in individuals with, *PALB2* mutations.

Chapter 38

Genetic Testing for Hereditary Cancer Syndromes

What is genetic testing?

Genetic testing looks for specific inherited changes (mutations) in a person's chromosomes, genes, or proteins. Genetic mutations can have harmful, beneficial, neutral (no effect), or uncertain effects on health. Mutations that are harmful may increase a person's chance, or risk, of developing a disease such as cancer. Overall, inherited mutations are thought to play a role in about 5 to 10 percent of all cancers.

Cancer can sometimes appear to "run in families" even if it is not caused by an inherited mutation. For example, a shared environment or lifestyle, such as tobacco use, can cause similar cancers to develop among family members. However, certain patterns—such as the types of cancer that develop, other non-cancer conditions that are seen, and the ages at which cancer typically develops—may suggest the presence of a hereditary cancer syndrome.

The genetic mutations that cause many of the known hereditary cancer syndromes have been identified, and genetic testing can confirm whether a condition is, indeed, the result of an inherited syndrome. Genetic testing is also done to determine whether family members

---

Text in this chapter is excerpted from "Genetic Testing for Hereditary Cancer Syndromes," National Cancer Institute at the National Institutes of Health (NIH), April 11, 2013.

without obvious illness have inherited the same mutation as a family member who is known to carry a cancer-associated mutation.

Inherited genetic mutations can increase a person's risk of developing cancer through a variety of mechanisms, depending on the function of the gene. Mutations in genes that control cell growth and the repair of damaged DNA are particularly likely to be associated with increased cancer risk.

Genetic testing of tumor samples can also be performed, but this Fact Sheet does not cover such testing.

Does someone who inherits a cancer-predisposing mutation always get cancer?

No. Even if a cancer-predisposing mutation is present in a family, it does not necessarily mean that everyone who inherits the mutation will develop cancer. Several factors influence the outcome in a given person with the mutation.

One factor is the pattern of inheritance of the cancer syndrome. To understand how hereditary cancer syndromes may be inherited, it is helpful to keep in mind that every person has two copies of most genes, with one copy inherited from each parent. Most mutations involved in hereditary cancer syndromes are inherited in one of two main patterns: autosomal dominant and autosomal recessive.

With autosomal dominant inheritance, a single altered copy of the gene is enough to increase a person's chances of developing cancer. In this case, the parent from whom the mutation was inherited may also show the effects of the gene mutation. The parent may also be referred to as a carrier.

With autosomal recessive inheritance, a person has an increased risk of cancer only if he or she inherits a mutant (altered) copy of the gene from each parent. The parents, who each carry one copy of the altered gene along with a normal (unaltered) copy, do not usually have an increased risk of cancer themselves. However, because they can pass the altered gene to their children, they are called carriers.

A third form of inheritance of cancer-predisposing mutations is X-linked recessive inheritance. Males have a single X chromosome, which they inherit from their mothers, and females have two X chromosomes (one from each parent). A female with a recessive cancer-predisposing mutation on one of her X chromosomes and a normal copy of the gene on her other X chromosome is a carrier but will not have an increased risk of cancer. Her sons, however, will have only the altered copy of the gene and will therefore have an increased risk of cancer.

Even when people have one copy of a dominant cancer-predisposing mutation, two copies of a recessive mutation, or, for males, one copy of an X-linked recessive mutation, they may not develop cancer. Some mutations are "incompletely penetrant," which means that only some people will show the effects of these mutations. Mutations can also "vary in their expressivity," which means that the severity of the symptoms may vary from person to person.

What genetic tests are available for cancer risk?

More than 50 hereditary cancer syndromes have been described. The majority of these are caused by highly penetrant mutations that are inherited in a dominant fashion. The list below includes some of the more common inherited cancer syndromes for which genetic testing is available, the gene(s) that are mutated in each syndrome, and the cancer types most often associated with these syndromes.

Hereditary breast cancer and ovarian cancer syndrome

- Genes: *BRCA1, BRCA2*
- Related cancer types: Female breast, ovarian, and other cancers, including prostate, pancreatic, and male breast cancer

Li-Fraumeni syndrome

- Gene: TP53
- Related cancer types: Breast cancer, soft tissue sarcoma, osteosarcoma (bone cancer), leukemia, brain tumors, adrenocortical carcinoma (cancer of the adrenal glands), and other cancers

Cowden syndrome (PTEN hamartoma tumor syndrome)

- Gene: PTEN
- Related cancer types: Breast, thyroid, endometrial (uterine lining), and other cancers

Lynch syndrome (hereditary nonpolyposis colorectal cancer)

- Genes: MSH2, MLH1, MSH6, PMS2, EPCAM
- Related cancer types: Colorectal, endometrial, ovarian, renal pelvis, pancreatic, small intestine, liver and biliary tract, stomach, brain, and breast cancers

Familial adenomatous polyposis

- Gene: APC

- Related cancer types: Colorectal cancer, multiple non-malignant colon polyps, and both non-cancerous (benign) and cancerous tumors in the small intestine, brain, stomach, bone, skin, and other tissues

Retinoblastoma

- Gene: RB1

- Related cancer types: Eye cancer (cancer of the retina), pineal-oma (cancer of the pineal gland), osteosarcoma, melanoma, and soft tissue sarcoma

Multiple endocrine neoplasia type 1 (Wermer syndrome)

- Gene: MEN1

- Related cancer types: Pancreatic endocrine tumors and (usually benign) parathyroid and pituitary gland tumors

Multiple endocrine neoplasia type 2

- Gene: RET

- Related cancer types: Medullary thyroid cancer and pheochro-mocytoma (benign adrenal gland tumor)

Von Hippel-Lindau syndrome

- Gene: VHL

- Related cancer types: Kidney cancer and multiple noncancerous tumors, including pheochromocytoma

Who should consider genetic testing for cancer risk?

Many experts recommend that genetic testing for cancer risk should be strongly considered when all three of the following criteria are met:

- The person being tested has a personal or family history that suggests an inherited cancer risk condition

- The test results can be adequately interpreted (that is, they can clearly tell whether a specific genetic change is present or absent)

- The results provide information that will help guide a person's future medical care

The features of a person's personal or family medical history that, particularly in combination, may suggest a hereditary cancer syndrome include:

- Cancer that was diagnosed at an unusually young age

- Several different types of cancer that have occurred independently in the same person

- Cancer that has developed in both organs in a set of paired organs, such as both kidneys or both breasts

- Several close blood relatives that have the same type of cancer (for example, a mother, daughter, and sisters with breast cancer)

- Unusual cases of a specific cancer type (for example, breast cancer in a man)

- The presence of birth defects, such as certain noncancerous (benign) skin growths or skeletal abnormalities, that are known to be associated with inherited cancer syndromes

- Being a member of a racial/ethnic group that is known to have an increased chance of having a certain hereditary cancer syndrome and having one or more of the above features as well

It is strongly recommended that a person who is considering genetic testing speak with a professional trained in genetics before deciding whether to be tested. These professionals can include doctors, genetic counselors, and other health care providers (such as nurses, psychologists, or social workers). Genetic counseling can help people consider the risks, benefits, and limitations of genetic testing in their particular situation. Sometimes the genetic professional finds that testing is not needed.

Genetic counseling includes a detailed review of the individual's personal and family medical history related to possible cancer risk. Counseling also includes discussions about such issues as:

- Whether genetic testing is appropriate, which specific test(s) might be used, and the technical accuracy of the test(s)

- The medical implications of a positive or a negative test result (see below)

- The possibility that a test result might not be informative—that is, that the information may not be useful in making health care decisions (see below)

- The psychological risks and benefits of learning one's genetic test results

- The risk of passing a genetic mutation (if one is present in a parent) to children

Learning about these issues is a key part of the informed consent process. Written informed consent is strongly recommended before a genetic test is ordered. People give their consent by signing a form saying that they have been told about, and understand, the purpose of the test, its medical implications, the risks and benefits of the test, possible alternatives to the test, and their privacy rights.

Unlike most other medical tests, genetic tests can reveal information not only about the person being tested but also about that person's relatives. The presence of a harmful genetic mutation in one family member makes it more likely that other blood relatives may also carry the same mutation. Family relationships can be affected when one member of a family discloses genetic test results that may have implications for other family members. Family members may have very different opinions about how useful it is to learn whether they do or do not have a disease-related genetic mutation. Health discussions may get complicated when some family members know their genetic status while other family members do not choose to know their test results. A conversation with genetics professionals may help family members better understand the complicated choices they may face.

How is genetic testing done?

Genetic tests are usually requested by a person's doctor or other health care provider. Although it may be possible to obtain some genetic tests without a health care provider's order, this approach is not recommended because it does not give the patient the valuable opportunity to discuss this complicated decision with a knowledgeable professional.

Testing is done on a small sample of body fluid or tissue—usually blood, but sometimes saliva, cells from inside the cheek, skin cells, or amniotic fluid (the fluid surrounding a developing fetus).

The sample is then sent to a laboratory that specializes in genetic testing. The laboratory returns the test results to the doctor or genetic counselor who requested the test. In some cases, the laboratory may send the results to the patient directly. It usually takes several weeks or longer to get the test results. Genetic counseling is recommended both before and after genetic testing to make sure that patients have accurate information about what a particular genetic test means for their health and care.

What do the results of genetic testing mean?

Genetic testing can have several possible results: positive, negative, true negative, uninformative negative, false negative, variant of unknown significance, or benign polymorphism. These results are described below.

A **"positive test result"** means that the laboratory found a specific genetic alteration (or mutation) that is associated with a hereditary cancer syndrome. A positive result may:

- Confirm the diagnosis of a hereditary cancer syndrome

- Indicate an increased risk of developing certain cancer(s) in the future

- Show that someone carries a particular genetic change that does not increase their own risk of cancer but that may increase the risk in their children if they also inherit an altered copy from their other parent (that is, if the child inherits two copies of the abnormal gene, one from their mother and one from their father).

- Suggest a need for further testing

- Provide important information that can help other family members make decisions about their own health care.

Also, people who have a positive test result that indicates that they have an increased risk of developing cancer in the future may be able to take steps to lower their risk of developing cancer or to find cancer earlier, including:

- Being checked at a younger age or more often for signs of cancer

- Reducing their cancer risk by taking medications or having surgery to remove "at-risk" tissue (These approaches to risk reduction are options for only a few inherited cancer syndromes.)

- Changing personal behaviors (like quitting smoking, getting more exercise, and eating a healthier diet) to reduce the risk of certain cancers.

A positive result on a prenatal genetic test for cancer risk may influence a decision about whether to continue a pregnancy. The results of pre-implantation testing (performed on embryos created by in vitro fertilization) can guide a doctor in deciding which embryo (or embryos) to implant in a woman's uterus.

Finally, in patients who have already been diagnosed with cancer, a positive result for a mutation associated with certain hereditary cancer syndromes can influence how the cancer is treated. For example, some hereditary cancer disorders interfere with the body's ability to repair damage that occurs to cellular DNA. If someone with one of these conditions receives a standard dose of radiation or chemotherapy to treat their cancer, they may experience severe, potentially life-threatening treatment side effects. Knowing about the genetic disorder before treatment begins allows doctors to modify the treatment and reduce the severity of the side effects.

A **"negative test result"** means that the laboratory did not find the specific alteration that the test was designed to detect. This result is most useful when working with a family in which the specific, disease-causing genetic alteration is already known to be present. In such a case, a negative result can show that the tested family member has not inherited the mutation that is present in their family and that this person therefore does not have the inherited cancer syndrome tested for, does not have an increased genetic risk of developing cancer, or is not a carrier of a mutation that increases cancer risk. Such a test result is called a **"true negative."** A true negative result does not mean that there is no cancer risk, but rather that the risk is probably the same as the cancer risk in the general population.

When a person has a strong family history of cancer but the family has not been found to have a known mutation associated with a hereditary cancer syndrome, a negative test result is classified as an **"uninformative negative"** (that is, does not provide useful information). It is not possible to tell whether someone has a harmful gene mutation that was not detected by the particular test used (a **"false negative"**) or whether the person truly has no cancer-predisposing genetic alterations in that gene. It is also possible for a person to have a mutation in a gene other than the gene that was tested.

If genetic testing shows a change that has not been previously associated with cancer in other people, the person's test result may report **"variant of unknown significance,"** or VUS. This result may be interpreted as "ambiguous" (uncertain), which is to say that the information does not help in making health care decisions.

If the test reveals a genetic change that is common in the general population among people without cancer, the change is called a **polymorphism.** Everyone has commonly occurring genetic variations (polymorphisms) that are not associated with any increased risk of disease.

Who can help people understand their test results?

A genetic counselor, doctor, or other health care professional trained in genetics can help an individual or family understand their test results. Such counseling may include discussing recommendations for preventive care and screening with the patient, referring the patient to support groups and other information resources, and providing emotional support to the person receiving the results.

In some cases, a genetic counselor or doctor may recommend that other family members consider being tested for specific gene changes that indicate an increased risk of cancer. The decision to test other family members is complicated. It requires a careful evaluation of family history and other factors as well as advice from a genetic counselor or other professional trained in genetics. In general, physicians rely on the family member who has been tested to share the genetic information with their relatives so that family members will know that a genetic condition has been identified in their family. Then, each family member will need to make their own decision regarding whether or not to be tested themselves.

Who has access to a person's genetic test results?

Medical test results are normally included in a person's medical records, particularly if a doctor or other health care provider has ordered the test or has been consulted about the test results. Therefore, people considering genetic testing must understand that their results may become known to other people or organizations that have legitimate, legal access to their medical records, such as their insurance company or employer, if their employer provides the patient's health insurance as a benefit.

However, legal protections are in place to prevent genetic discrimination, which would occur if insurance companies or employers were to treat people differently because they have a gene mutation that increases their risk of a disease such as cancer or because they have a strong family history of a disease such as cancer.

In 2008, the Genetic Information Non-discrimination Act (GINA) became federal law for all U.S. residents. GINA prohibits discrimination based on genetic information in determining health insurance eligibility or rates and suitability for employment. However, GINA does not cover members of the military, and it does not apply to life insurance, disability insurance, or long-term care insurance. Some states have additional genetic non-discrimination legislation that addresses the possibility of discrimination in those contexts.

In addition, because a person's genetic information is considered one kind of health information, it is covered by the Privacy Rule of the Health Information Portability and Accountability Act (HIPAA) of 1996. The Privacy Rule requires that health care providers and others with medical record access protect the privacy of health information, sets limits on the use and release of health records, and empowers people to control certain uses and sharing of their health-related information. Many states also have laws to protect patient privacy and limit the release of genetic and other health information.

What are at-home or direct-to-consumer genetic tests?

Some companies offer at-home genetic testing, also known as direct-to-consumer (DTC) genetic testing. People collect a tissue sample themselves and submit the sample through the mail. They learn about the test results online, by mail, or over the phone. DTC genetic testing is often done without a doctor's order or guidance from a doctor or genetic counselor before the test. Some states in the United States do not allow DTC genetic testing.

Whereas the genetic testing for cancer that is typically ordered by a doctor involves testing for rare major hereditary cancer syndromes, most DTC genetic testing for cancer risk involves the analysis of common inherited genetic variants, called single-nucleotide polymorphisms, that have been shown to be statistically associated with a particular type of cancer. Each individual variant is generally associated with only a minor increase in risk, and even when added together all the known variants for a particular cancer type account for only a small portion of a person's risk of that cancer. Although the identification and study of such variants is an active area of research, genetic tests based on these variants have not yet been found to help patients and their care providers make health care decisions and, therefore, they are not a part of recommended clinical practice.

Even when people have DTC genetic tests for known mutations in genes associated with hereditary cancer syndrome, there are potential risks and drawbacks to the use of DTC testing. In particular, without guidance about genetic test results from an informed, genetically knowledgeable health care provider, people may experience unneeded anxiety or false reassurance, or they may make important decisions about medical treatment or care based on incomplete information.

Also, although some people may view DTC genetic testing as a way to ensure the privacy of their genetic test results, companies that offer DTC genetic testing do not always tell the consumer the details of their privacy policies. In addition, if people consult their doctor or other health care provider about the test results obtained from a DTC testing vendor, the results may become part of the patient's medical record anyway. Also, companies that provide DTC testing may not be subject to current state and federal privacy laws and regulations. It is generally recommended that people considering DTC genetic testing make sure that they have chosen a reputable company.

The U.S. Federal Trade Commission (FTC) has a fact sheet about at-home genetic tests which offers advice for people who are considering such a test. As part of its mission, the FTC investigates complaints about false or misleading health claims in advertisements.

The American Society of Human Genetics, a membership organization of genetics professionals, has issued a statement about DTC genetic tests that recommends transparency in such testing, provider education about the testing, and the development of appropriate regulations to ensure test and laboratory quality.

How are genetic tests regulated?

U.S. laboratories that perform health-related testing, including genetic testing, are regulated under the Clinical Laboratory Improvement Amendments (CLIA) program. Laboratories that are certified under CLIA are required to meet federal standards for quality, accuracy, and reliability of tests. All laboratories that do genetic testing and share results must be CLIA certified. However, CLIA certification only indicates that appropriate laboratory quality control standards are being followed; it does not guarantee that a genetic test being done by a laboratory is medically useful.

The Centers for Medicare and Medicaid Services has more information about CLIA programs. The National Library of Medicine also has information about how genetic testing is regulated and how to judge the quality of a genetic test. This information is available in the Genetics Home Reference.

Chapter 39

Pap and HPV Testing

What causes cervical cancer?

Nearly all cases of cervical cancer are caused by infection with oncogenic, or high-risk, types of human papillomavirus, or HPV. There are about 12 high-risk HPV types. Infections with these sexually transmitted viruses also cause most anal cancers; many vaginal, vulvar, and penile cancers; and some oropharyngeal cancers.

Although HPV infection is very common, most infections will be suppressed by the immune system within 1 to 2 years without causing cancer. These transient infections may cause temporary changes in cervical cells. If a cervical infection with a high-risk HPV type persists, the cellular changes can eventually develop into more severe precancerous lesions. If precancerous lesions are not treated, they can progress to cancer. It can take 10 to 20 years or more for a persistent infection with a high-risk HPV type to develop into cancer.

What is cervical cancer screening?

Cervical cancer screening is an essential part of a woman's routine health care. It is a way to detect abnormal cervical cells, including precancerous cervical lesions, as well as early cervical cancers. Both precancerous lesions and early cervical cancers can be treated very

Text in this chapter is excerpted from "Pap and HPV Testing," National Cancer Institute at the National Institutes of Health (NIH), September 9, 2014.

successfully. Routine cervical screening has been shown to greatly reduce both the number of new cervical cancers diagnosed each year and deaths from the disease.

Cervical cancer screening includes two types of screening tests: cytology-based screening, known as the Pap test or Pap smear, and HPV testing. The main purpose of screening with the Pap test is to detect abnormal cells that may develop into cancer if left untreated. The Pap test can also find noncancerous conditions, such as infections and inflammation. It can also find cancer cells. In regularly screened populations, however, the Pap test identifies most abnormal cells before they become cancer.

HPV testing is used to look for the presence of high-risk HPV types in cervical cells. These tests can detect HPV infections that cause cell abnormalities, sometimes even before cell abnormalities are evident. Several different HPV tests have been approved for screening. Most tests detect the DNA of high-risk HPV, although one test detects the RNA of high-risk HPV. Some tests detect any high-risk HPV and do not identify the specific type or types that are present. Other tests specifically detect infection with HPV types 16 and 18, the two types that cause most HPV-associated cancers.

How is cervical cancer screening done?

Cervical cancer screening can be done in a medical office, a clinic, or a community health center. It is often done during a pelvic examination.

While a woman lies on an exam table, a health care professional inserts an instrument called a speculum into her vagina to widen it so that the upper portion of the vagina and the cervix can be seen. This procedure also allows the health care professional to take a sample of cervical cells. The cells are taken with a wooden or plastic scraper and/ or a cervical brush and are then prepared for Pap analysis in one of two ways. In a conventional Pap test, the specimen (or smear) is placed on a glass microscope slide and a fixative is added. In an automated liquid-based Pap cytology test, cervical cells collected with a brush or other instrument are placed in a vial of liquid preservative. The slide or vial is then sent to a laboratory for analysis.

In the United States, automated liquid-based Pap cytology testing has largely replaced conventional Pap tests. One advantage of liquid-based testing is that the same cell sample can also be tested for the presence of high-risk types of HPV, a process known as "Pap and HPV co-testing." In addition, liquid-based cytology appears to reduce the likelihood of an unsatisfactory specimen. However, conventional and liquid-based Pap tests appear to have a similar ability to detect cellular abnormalities.

When should a woman begin cervical cancer screening, and how often should she be screened?

Women should talk with their doctor about when to start screening and how often to be screened. In March 2012, updated screening guidelines were released by the United States Preventive Services Task Force and jointly by the American Cancer Society, the American Society for Colposcopy and Cervical Pathology, and the American Society for Clinical Pathology. These guidelines recommend that women have their first Pap test at age 21. Although previous guidelines recommended that women have their first Pap test 3 years after they start having sexual intercourse, waiting until age 21 is now recommended because adolescents have a very low risk of cervical cancer and a high likelihood that cervical cell abnormalities will go away on their own.

According to the updated guidelines, women ages 21 through 29 should be screened with a Pap test every 3 years. Women ages 30 through 65 can then be screened every 5 years with Pap and HPV co-testing or every 3 years with a Pap test alone.

The guidelines also note that women with certain risk factors may need to have more frequent screening or to continue screening beyond age 65. These risk factors include being infected with the human immunodeficiency virus (HIV), being immunosuppressed, having been exposed to diethylstilbestrol before birth, and having been treated for a precancerous cervical lesion or cervical cancer.

Women who have had a hysterectomy (surgery to remove the uterus and cervix) do not need to have cervical screening, unless the hysterectomy was done to treat a precancerous cervical lesion or cervical cancer.

What are the benefits of Pap and HPV co-testing?

For women age 30 and older, Pap and HPV co-testing is less likely to miss an abnormality (i.e., has a lower false-negative rate) than Pap testing alone. Therefore, a woman with a negative HPV test and normal Pap test has very little risk of a serious abnormality developing over the next several years. In fact, researchers have found that, when Pap and HPV co-testing is used, lengthening the screening interval to 5 years still allows abnormalities to be detected in time to treat them

843

while also reducing the detection of HPV infections that would have gone away on their own.

Adding HPV testing to Pap testing may also improve the detection of glandular cell abnormalities, including adenocarcinoma of the cervix (cancer of the glandular cells of the cervix). Glandular cells are mucus-producing cells found in the endocervical canal (the opening in the center of the cervix) or in the lining of the uterus. Glandular cell abnormalities and adenocarcinoma of the cervix are much less common than squamous cell abnormalities and squamous cell carcinoma. There is some evidence that Pap testing is not as good at detecting adenocarcinoma and glandular cell abnormalities as it is at detecting squamous cell abnormalities and cancers.

Can HPV testing be used alone for cervical cancer screening?

On April 24, 2014, the Food and Drug Administration (FDA) approved the use of one HPV DNA test (cobas HPV test, Roche Molecular Systems, Inc.) as a first-line primary screening test for use alone for women age 25 and older. This test detects each of HPV types 16 and 18 and gives pooled results for 12 additional high-risk HPV types.

The new approval was based on long-term findings from the ATHENA trial, a clinical trial that included more than 47,000 women. The results showed that the HPV test used in the study performed better than the Pap test at identifying women at risk of developing severe cervical cell abnormalities.

The greater assurance against future cervical cancer risk with HPV testing has also been demonstrated by a cohort study of more than a million women, which found that, after 3 years, women who tested negative on the HPV test had an extremely low risk of developing cervical cancer—about half the already low risk of women who tested negative on the Pap test.

First-line HPV testing has not yet been incorporated into the current professional cervical cancer screening guidelines. Professional societies are developing interim guidance documents, and some medical practices might incorporate primary HPV screening.

How are the results of cervical cancer screening tests reported?

A doctor may simply describe Pap test results to a patient as "normal" or "abnormal." Likewise, HPV test results can either be "positive," meaning that a patient's cervical cells are infected with high-risk HPV, or "negative," indicating that high-risk HPV types were not found. A woman may want to ask her doctor for specific information about her Pap and HPV test results and what these results mean.

Most laboratories in the United States use a standard set of terms, called the Bethesda System, to report Pap test results. Under the Bethesda System, samples that have no cell abnormalities are reported as "negative for intraepithelial lesion or malignancy." A negative Pap test report may also note certain benign (non-neoplastic) findings, such as common infections or inflammation. Pap test results also indicate whether the specimen was satisfactory or unsatisfactory for examination.

The Bethesda System considers abnormalities of squamous cells and glandular cells separately. Squamous cell abnormalities are divided into the following categories, ranging from the mildest to the most severe.

Atypical squamous cells (ASC) are the most common abnormal finding in Pap tests. The Bethesda System divides this category into two groups, ASC-US and ASC-H.

- **ASC-US:** atypical squamous cells of undetermined significance. The squamous cells do not appear completely normal, but doctors are uncertain about what the cell changes mean. The changes may be related to an HPV infection, but they can also be caused by other factors.

- **ASC-H:** atypical squamous cells, cannot exclude a high-grade squamous intraepithelial lesion. The cells do not appear normal, but doctors are uncertain about what the cell changes mean. ASC-H lesions may be at higher risk of being precancerous compared with ASC-US lesions.

Low-grade squamous intraepithelial lesions (LSILs) are considered mild abnormalities caused by HPV infection. Low-grade means that there are early changes in the size and shape of cells. Intraepithelial refers to the layer of cells that forms the surface of the cervix. When cells from the abnormal area are removed and examined under a microscope (in a procedure called a biopsy), LSILs are usually found to have mild cell changes that may be classified as mild dysplasia or as cervical intraepithelial neoplasia, grade 1 (CIN-1).

High-grade squamous intraepithelial lesions (HSILs) are more severe abnormalities that have a higher likelihood of progressing to cancer if left untreated. High-grade means that there are more evident changes in the size and shape of the abnormal (precancerous) cells and that the cells look very different from normal cells. When examined under a microscope, the cells from HSILs are often found to have more extensive changes that may be classified as moderate or severe dysplasia or as CIN-2, CIN-2/3, or CIN-3 (in order of increasing severity). Microscopic examination of HSILs may also reveal carcinoma in situ (CIS), which is commonly included in the CIN-3 category.

Squamous cell carcinoma is cervical cancer. The abnormal squamous cells have invaded more deeply into the cervix or into other tissues or organs. In a well-screened population, such as that in the United States, a finding of cancer during cervical screening is extremely rare.

Glandular cell abnormalities describe abnormal changes that occur in the glandular tissues of the cervix. These abnormalities are divided into the following categories:

Atypical glandular cells (AGC), meaning the glandular cells do not appear normal, but doctors are uncertain about what the cell changes mean.

Endocervical adenocarcinoma in situ (AIS), meaning that severely abnormal cells are found but have not spread beyond the glandular tissue of the cervix.

Adenocarcinoma includes not only cancer of the endocervical canal itself but also, in some cases, endometrial, extrauterine, and other cancers.

What follow-up tests are done if cervical cancer screening results are abnormal?

For a woman receiving Pap and HPV co-testing:

If a woman is found to have a **normal Pap test result with a positive HPV test** that detects the group of high-risk HPV types, the doctor will usually have her return in a year for repeat screening to see if the HPV infection persists and whether any cell changes have developed that need further follow-up testing. Alternatively, the woman may have another HPV test that looks specifically for HPV-16 and HPV-18, the two HPV types that cause most cervical cancers.

If either of these two HPV types is present, a woman will usually have follow-up testing with colposcopy. Colposcopy is the use of an instrument much like a microscope (called a colposcope) to examine the vagina and the cervix. During a colposcopy, the doctor inserts a speculum into the vagina to widen it and may apply a dilute vinegar solution to the cervix, which causes abnormal areas to turn white. The doctor then uses the colposcope (which remains outside the body) to observe the cervix. When a doctor performs colposcopy, he or she will usually remove cells or tissues from the abnormal area for examination under a microscope, a procedure called a biopsy.

If a woman is found to have an **abnormal Pap test result with a negative (normal) HPV test,** the follow-up tests will depend on the Pap test result. If the Pap test result is ASC-US, the doctor will usually have the woman return in 3 to 5 years for a repeat screen. If the Pap test result is LSIL, the doctor may recommend colposcopy or might have the woman return in a year for repeat screening.

If a woman is found to have an **abnormal Pap test result with a positive HPV test** that detects any high-risk HPV type, the doctor will usually have the woman receive follow-up testing with colposcopy.

For a woman receiving Pap testing alone:

If a woman who is receiving Pap testing alone is found to have an **ASC-US Pap test result,** her doctor may have the sample tested for high-risk HPV types or may repeat the Pap test to determine whether further follow-up is needed. Many times, ASC-US cell changes in the cervix go away without treatment, especially if there is no evidence of infection with high-risk HPV. Doctors may prescribe estrogen cream for women with ASC-US who are near or past menopause. Because ASC-US cell changes can be caused by low hormone levels, applying an estrogen cream to the cervix for a few weeks can usually help to clarify their cause.

Follow-up testing for **all other abnormal Pap results** will typically involve a colposcopy.

For a woman receiving HPV-alone testing:

If a woman who is having HPV-alone testing **tests positive for HPV types 16 or 18,** she should, according to guidance from the FDA, have a colposcopy. A women who tests negative for types 16 and 18 but is positive for one of the 12 other high-risk HPV types should have a Pap test to determine whether a colposcopy is needed.

How are cervical abnormalities treated?

If biopsy analysis of cells from the affected area of the cervix shows that the cells have CIN-2 or more severe abnormalities, further treatment is probably needed depending on a woman's age, pregnancy status, and future fertility concerns. Without treatment, these cells may turn into cancer. Treatment options include the following:

- LEEP (loop electrosurgical excision procedure), in which an electrical current that is passed through a thin wire loop acts as a knife to remove tissue

- Cryotherapy, in which abnormal tissue is destroyed by freezing it

- Laser therapy, the use of a narrow beam of intense light to destroy or remove abnormal cells

- Conization, the removal of a cone-shaped piece of tissue using a knife, a laser, or the LEEP technique.

The screening guidelines call for women who have been treated for CIN-2 or more severe abnormalities to continue screening for at least 20 years, even if they are over 65.

Do women who have been vaccinated against HPV still need to be screened for cervical cancer?

Yes. Because current HPV vaccines do not protect against all HPV types that cause cervical cancer, it is important for vaccinated women to continue to undergo routine cervical cancer screening.

What are the limitations of cervical cancer screening?

Although cervical cancer screening tests are highly effective, they are not completely accurate. Sometimes a patient can be told that she has abnormal cells when the cells are actually normal (a false-positive result), or she can be told that her cells are normal when in fact there is an abnormality that was not detected (a false-negative result).

Cervical cancer screening has another limitation, caused by the nature of HPV infections. Because most HPV infections are transient and produce only temporary changes in cervical cells, overly frequent cervical screening could detect HPV infections or cervical cell changes that would never cause cancer. Treating abnormalities that would have gone away on their own can cause needless psychological stress. In addition, follow-up tests and treatments can be uncomfortable, and some treatments that remove cervical tissue, such as LEEP and conization, have the potential to weaken the cervix and may affect fertility or slightly increase the rate of premature delivery, depending on how much tissue is removed.

The screening intervals in the 2012 guidelines are intended to minimize the harms caused by treating abnormalities that would never progress to cancer while also limiting false-negative results that would delay the diagnosis and treatment of a precancerous condition or cancer. With these intervals, if an HPV infection or abnormal cells are missed at one screen, chances are good that abnormal cells will be detected at the next screening exam, when they can still be treated successfully.

Chapter 40

Prostate-Specific Antigen (PSA) Test

What is the PSA test?

Prostate-specific antigen, or PSA, is a protein produced by cells of the prostate gland. The PSA test measures the level of PSA in a man's blood. For this test, a blood sample is sent to a laboratory for analysis. The results are usually reported as nanograms of PSA per milliliter (ng/mL) of blood.

The blood level of PSA is often elevated in men with prostate cancer, and the PSA test was originally approved by the FDA in 1986 to monitor the progression of prostate cancer in men who had already been diagnosed with the disease. In 1994, the FDA approved the use of the PSA test in conjunction with a digital rectal exam (DRE) to test asymptomatic men for prostate cancer. Men who report prostate symptoms often undergo PSA testing (along with a DRE) to help doctors determine the nature of the problem.

In addition to prostate cancer, a number of benign (not cancerous) conditions can cause a man's PSA level to rise. The most frequent benign prostate conditions that cause an elevation in PSA level are prostatitis (inflammation of the prostate) and benign prostatic hyperplasia (BPH)

Text in this chapter is excerpted from "Prostate-Specific Antigen (PSA) Test," National Cancer Institute at the National Institutes of Health (NIH), July 24, 2012.

(enlargement of the prostate). There is no evidence that prostatitis or BPH leads to prostate cancer, but it is possible for a man to have one or both of these conditions and to develop prostate cancer as well.

Is the PSA test recommended for prostate cancer screening?

Until recently, many doctors and professional organizations encouraged yearly PSA screening for men beginning at age 50. Some organizations recommended that men who are at higher risk of prostate cancer, including African American men and men whose father or brother had prostate cancer, begin screening at age 40 or 45. However, as more has been learned about both the benefits and harms of prostate cancer screening, a number of organizations have begun to caution against routine population screening. Although some organizations continue to recommend PSA screening, there is widespread agreement that any man who is considering getting tested should first be informed in detail about the potential harms and benefits.

Currently, Medicare provides coverage for an annual PSA test for all Medicare-eligible men age 50 and older. Many private insurers cover PSA screening as well.

What is a normal PSA test result?

There is no specific normal or abnormal level of PSA in the blood. In the past, most doctors considered PSA levels of 4.0 ng/mL and lower as normal. Therefore, if a man had a PSA level above 4.0 ng/mL, doctors would often recommend a prostate biopsy to determine whether prostate cancer was present.

However, more recent studies have shown that some men with PSA levels below 4.0 ng/mL have prostate cancer and that many men with higher levels do not have prostate cancer. In addition, various factors can cause a man's PSA level to fluctuate. For example, a man's PSA level often rises if he has prostatitis or a urinary tract infection. Prostate biopsies and prostate surgery also increase PSA level. Conversely, some drugs—including finasteride and dutasteride, which are used to treat BPH—lower a man's PSA level. PSA level may also vary somewhat across testing laboratories.

Another complicating factor is that studies to establish the normal range of PSA levels have been conducted primarily in populations of white men. Although expert opinions vary, there is no clear consensus regarding the optimal PSA threshold for recommending a prostate biopsy for men of any racial or ethnic group.

In general, however, the higher a man's PSA level, the more likely it is that he has prostate cancer. Moreover, continuous rise in a man's PSA level over time may also be a sign of prostate cancer.

What if a screening test shows an elevated PSA level?

If a man who has no symptoms of prostate cancer chooses to undergo prostate cancer screening and is found to have an elevated PSA level, the doctor may recommend another PSA test to confirm the original finding. If the PSA level is still high, the doctor may recommend that the man continue with PSA tests and DREs at regular intervals to watch for any changes over time.

If a man's PSA level continues to rise or if a suspicious lump is detected during a DRE, the doctor may recommend additional tests to determine the nature of the problem. A urine test may be recommended to check for a urinary tract infection. The doctor may also recommend imaging tests, such as a transrectal ultrasound, x-rays, or cystoscopy.

If prostate cancer is suspected, the doctor will recommend a prostate biopsy. During this procedure, multiple samples of prostate tissue are collected by inserting hollow needles into the prostate and then withdrawing them. Most often, the needles are inserted through the wall of the rectum (transrectal biopsy); however, the needles may also be inserted through the skin between the scrotum and the anus (transperineal biopsy). A pathologist then examines the collected tissue under a microscope. The doctor may use ultrasound to view the prostate during the biopsy, but ultrasound cannot be used alone to diagnose prostate cancer.

What are some of the limitations and potential harms of the PSA test for prostate cancer screening?

Detecting prostate cancer early may not reduce the chance of dying from prostate cancer. When used in screening, the PSA test can help detect small tumors that do not cause symptoms. Finding a small tumor, however, may not necessarily reduce a man's chance of dying from prostate cancer. Some tumors found through PSA testing grow so slowly that they are unlikely to threaten a man's life. Detecting tumors that are not life threatening is called "overdiagnosis," and treating these tumors is called "overtreatment."

Overtreatment exposes men unnecessarily to the potential complications and harmful side effects of treatments for early prostate cancer, including surgery and radiation therapy. The side effects of these treatments include urinary incontinence (inability to control urine flow), problems with bowel function, erectile dysfunction (loss of erections, or having erections that are inadequate for sexual intercourse), and infection.

In addition, finding cancer early may not help a man who has a fast-growing or aggressive tumor that may have spread to other parts of the body before being detected.

The PSA test may give false-positive or false-negative results. A false-positive test result occurs when a man's PSA level is elevated but no cancer is actually present. A false-positive test result may create anxiety for a man and his family and lead to additional medical procedures, such as a prostate biopsy, that can be harmful. Possible side effects of biopsies include serious infections, pain, and bleeding.

Most men with an elevated PSA level turn out not to have prostate cancer; only about 25 percent of men who have a prostate biopsy due to an elevated PSA level actually have prostate cancer.

A false-negative test result occurs when a man's PSA level is low even though he actually has prostate cancer. False-negative test results may give a man, his family, and his doctor false assurance that he does not have cancer, when he may in fact have a cancer that requires treatment.

What research has been done to study prostate cancer screening?

Several randomized trials of prostate cancer screening have been carried out. One of the largest is the Prostate, Lung, Colorectal, and Ovarian (PLCO) Cancer Screening Trial, which NCI conducted to determine whether certain screening tests can help reduce the numbers of deaths from several common cancers. In the prostate portion of the trial, the PSA test and DRE were evaluated for their ability to decrease a man's chances of dying from prostate cancer.

The PLCO investigators found that men who underwent annual prostate cancer screening had a higher incidence of prostate cancer than men in the control group but the same rate of deaths from the disease. Overall, the results suggest that many men were treated for prostate cancers that would not have been detected in their lifetime without screening. Consequently, these men were exposed unnecessarily to the potential harms of treatment.

A second large trial, the European Randomized Study of Screening for Prostate Cancer (ERSPC), compared prostate cancer deaths in men randomly assigned to PSA-based screening or no screening. As in the PLCO, men in ERSPC who were screened for prostate cancer had a higher incidence of the disease than control men. In contrast to the PLCO, however, men who were screened had a lower rate of death from prostate cancer.

The United States Preventive Services Task Force has analyzed the data from the PLCO, ERSPC, and other trials and estimated that, for every 1,000 men ages 55 to 69 years who are screened every 1 to 4 years for a decade:

- 0 to 1 death from prostate cancer would be avoided.

- 100 to 120 men would have a false-positive test result that leads to a biopsy, and about one-third of the men who get a biopsy would experience at least moderately bothersome symptoms from the biopsy.

- 110 men would be diagnosed with prostate cancer. About 50 of these men would have a complication from treatment, including erectile dysfunction in 29 men, urinary incontinence in 18 men, serious cardiovascular events in 2 men, deep vein thrombosis or pulmonary embolism in 1 man, and death due to the treatment in less than 1 man.

How is the PSA test used in men who have been treated for prostate cancer?

The PSA test is used to monitor patients who have a history of prostate cancer to see if their cancer has recurred (come back). If a man's PSA level begins to rise after prostate cancer treatment, it may be the first sign of a recurrence. Such a "biochemical relapse" typically appears months or years before other clinical signs and symptoms of prostate cancer recurrence.

However, a single elevated PSA measurement in a patient who has a history of prostate cancer does not always mean that the cancer has come back. A man who has been treated for prostate cancer should discuss an elevated PSA level with his doctor. The doctor may recommend repeating the PSA test or performing other tests to check for evidence of a recurrence. The doctor may look for a trend of rising PSA level over time rather than a single elevated PSA level.

What does an increase in PSA level mean for a man who has been treated for prostate cancer?

If a man's PSA level rises after prostate cancer treatment, his doctor will consider a number of factors before recommending further treatment. Additional treatment based on a single PSA test is not recommended. Instead, a rising trend in PSA level over time in combination with other findings, such as an abnormal result on imaging tests, may lead a man's doctor to recommend further treatment.

How are researchers trying to improve the PSA test?

Scientists are investigating ways to improve the PSA test to give doctors the ability to better distinguish cancerous from benign conditions and slow-growing cancers from fast-growing, potentially lethal cancers. Some of the methods being studied include:

- **Free versus total PSA.** The amount of PSA in the blood that is "free" (not bound to other proteins) divided by the total amount of PSA (free plus bound). Some evidence suggests that a lower proportion of free PSA may be associated with more aggressive cancer.

- **PSA density of the transition zone.** The blood level of PSA divided by the volume of the transition zone of the prostate. The transition zone is the interior part of the prostate that surrounds the urethra. Some evidence suggests that this measure may be more accurate at detecting prostate cancer than the standard PSA test.

- **Age-specific PSA reference ranges.** Because a man's PSA level tends to increase with age, it has been suggested that the use of age-specific PSA reference ranges may increase the accuracy of PSA tests. However, age-specific reference ranges have not been generally favored because their use may delay the detection of prostate cancer in many men.

- **PSA velocity and PSA doubling time.** PSA velocity is the rate of change in a man's PSA level over time, expressed as ng/mL per year. PSA doubling time is the period of time over which a man's PSA level doubles. Some evidence suggests that the rate of increase in a man's PSA level may be helpful in predicting whether he has prostate cancer.

- **Pro-PSA.** Pro-PSA refers to several different inactive precursors of PSA. There is some evidence that pro-PSA is more strongly associated with prostate cancer than with BPH. One recently approved test combines measurement of a form of pro-PSA called [-2]proPSA with measurements of PSA and free PSA. The resulting "prostate health index" can be used to help a man with a PSA level of between 4 and 10 ng/mL decide whether he should have a biopsy.

Chapter 41

Sentinel Lymph Node Biopsy

What are lymph nodes?

Lymph nodes are small round organs that are part of the body's lymphatic system. They are found widely throughout the body and are connected to one another by lymph vessels. Groups of lymph nodes are located in the neck, underarms, chest, abdomen, and groin. A clear fluid called lymph flows through lymph vessels and lymph nodes.

Lymph originates from a fluid, known as interstitial fluid that has diffused, or "leaked," out of small blood vessels called capillaries. This fluid contains many substances, including blood plasma, proteins, glucose, and oxygen. It bathes most of the body's cells, providing them with the oxygen and nutrients they need for growth and survival. Interstitial fluid also picks up waste products from cells as well as other materials, such as bacteria and viruses, to help remove them from the body's tissues. Interstitial fluid eventually collects in lymph vessels, where it becomes known as lymph. Lymph flows through the body's lymph vessels to reach two large ducts at the base of the neck, where it is emptied into the bloodstream.

Lymph nodes are important parts of the body's immune system. They contain B lymphocytes, T lymphocytes, and other types of immune system cells. These cells monitor lymph for the presence of "foreign" substances, such as bacteria and viruses. If a foreign substance is

Text in this chapter is excerpted from "Sentinel Lymph Node Biopsy," National Cancer Institute at the National Institutes of Health (NIH), August 11, 2011.

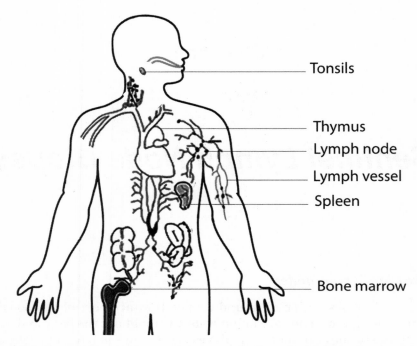

Tonsils

Thymus
Lymph node
Lymph vessel
Spleen

Bone marrow

Figure 41.1. *Anatomy of the lymphatic system, showing the lymph vessels and lymph organs, including lymph nodes, tonsils, thymus, spleen, and bone marrow.*

detected, some of the cells will become activated and an immune response will be triggered.

Lymph nodes are also important in helping to determine whether cancer cells have developed the ability to spread to other parts of the body. Many types of cancer spread through the lymphatic system, and one of the earliest sites of spread for these cancers is nearby lymph nodes.

What is a sentinel lymph node?

A sentinel lymph node is defined as the first lymph node to which cancer cells are most likely to spread from a primary tumor. Sometimes, there can be more than one sentinel lymph node.

What is a sentinel lymph node biopsy?

A sentinel lymph node biopsy (SLNB) is a procedure in which the sentinel lymph node is identified, removed, and examined to determine whether cancer cells are present.

A negative SLNB result suggests that cancer has not developed the ability to spread to nearby lymph nodes or other organs. A positive SLNB result indicates that cancer is present in the sentinel lymph node and may be present in other nearby lymph nodes (called regional lymph nodes) and, possibly, other organs. This information can help a doctor determine the stage of the cancer (extent of the disease within the body) and develop an appropriate treatment plan.

What happens during an SLNB?

A surgeon injects a radioactive substance, a blue dye, or both near the tumor to locate the position of the sentinel lymph node. The surgeon then uses a device that detects radioactivity to find the sentinel node or looks for lymph nodes that are stained with the blue dye. Once the sentinel lymph node is located, the surgeon makes a small incision (about 1/2 inch) in the overlying skin and removes the node.

The sentinel node is then checked for the presence of cancer cells by a pathologist. If cancer is found, the surgeon may remove additional lymph nodes, either during the same biopsy procedure or during a follow-up surgical procedure. SLNBs may be done on an outpatient basis or may require a short stay in the hospital.

SLNB is usually done at the same time the primary tumor is removed. However, the procedure can also be done either before or after removal of the tumor.

What are the benefits of SLNB?

In addition to helping doctors stage cancers and estimate the risk that tumor cells have developed the ability to spread to other parts of the body, SLNB may help some patients avoid more extensive lymph node surgery. Removing additional nearby lymph nodes to look for cancer cells may not be necessary if the sentinel node is negative for cancer. All lymph node surgery can have adverse effects, and some of these effects may be reduced or avoided if fewer lymph nodes are removed. The potential adverse effects of lymph node surgery include the following:

- Lymphedema, or tissue swelling. During SLNB or more extensive lymph node surgery, lymph vessels leading to and from the sentinel node or group of nodes are cut, thereby disrupting the normal flow of lymph through the affected area. This disruption may lead to an abnormal buildup of lymph fluid. In addition to swelling, patients with lymphedema may experience pain or discomfort in the affected area, and the overlying skin may become thickened or hard. In the case of extensive lymph node surgery in an armpit or groin, the swelling may affect an entire arm or leg. In addition, there is an increased risk of infection in the affected area or limb. Very rarely, chronic lymphedema due to extensive lymph node removal may cause a cancer of the lymphatic vessels called lymphangiosarcoma.

- Seroma, or the buildup of lymph fluid at the site of the surgery.
- Numbness, tingling, or pain at the site of the surgery.
- Difficulty moving the affected body part.

Is SLNB associated with other harms?

SLNB, like other surgical procedures, can cause short-term pain, swelling, and bruising at the surgical site and increase the risk of infection. In addition, some patients may have skin or allergic reactions to the blue dye used in SLNB. Another potential harm is a false-negative biopsy result—that is, cancer cells are not seen in the sentinel lymph node although they are present and may have already spread to other regional lymph nodes or other parts of the body. A false-negative biopsy result gives the patient and the doctor a false sense of security about the extent of cancer in the patient's body.

Is SLNB used to help stage all types of cancer?

No. SLNB is most commonly used to help stage breast cancer and melanoma. However, it is being studied with other cancer types, including colorectal cancer, gastric cancer, esophageal cancer, head and neck cancer, thyroid cancer, and non-small cell lung cancer.

What has research shown about the use of SLNB in breast cancer?

Breast cancer cells are most likely to spread first to lymph nodes located in the axilla, or armpit area, next to the affected breast. However, in breast cancers close to the center of the chest (near the breastbone), cancer cells may spread first to lymph nodes inside the chest (under the breastbone) before they can be detected in the axilla.

The number of lymph nodes in the axilla varies from person to person but usually ranges from 20 to 40. Historically, removal of these lymph nodes (in an operation called axillary lymph node dissection, or ALND) was done for two reasons: to help stage breast cancer and to help prevent a regional recurrence of the disease. (Regional recurrence of breast cancer occurs when breast cancer cells that have migrated to nearby lymph nodes give rise to a new tumor.)

Because removing multiple lymph nodes at the same time has been associated with adverse effects, the possibility that SLNB alone might be sufficient for staging breast cancer in women who have no clinical signs of axillary lymph node metastasis, such as swollen or "matted" (clumped or stuck together) nodes, was investigated.

In a phase III trial involving 5,611 women with breast cancer and no clinical signs of axillary metastasis, researchers from the National Surgical Adjuvant Breast and Bowel Project, which is a National Cancer Institute (NCI) clinical trials cooperative group, randomly assigned participants to receive SLNB alone or SLNB plus ALND. The women in the two groups whose sentinel lymph node(s) were negative for cancer (a total of 3,989 women) were then followed for an average of 8 years. Most of the women (87.5 percent) had a lumpectomy, and the rest had a mastectomy. Nearly 88 percent of the women also received adjuvant systemic therapy (chemotherapy, hormonal, or both), and 82 percent had external-beam radiation therapy to the affected breast.

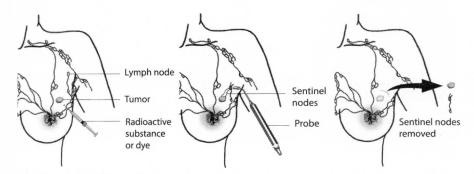

Figure 41.2. *Sentinel lymph node biopsy of the breast.*

A radioactive substance and/or blue dye is injected near the tumor (first panel). The injected material is located visually and/or with a device that detects radioactivity (middle panel). The sentinel node(s) (the first lymph node(s) to take up the material) is (are) removed and checked for cancer cells (last panel). Sentinel lymph node biopsy can be done before or after the tumor is removed.

The researchers found no differences in overall survival and disease-free survival between the two groups of women. Based on these results, it was concluded that ALND might not be necessary for women with clinically negative axillary lymph nodes and a negative SLNB whose breast cancer is treated with surgery, adjuvant systemic therapy, and external-beam radiation therapy.

Subsequently, the American College of Surgeons Oncology Group, which is another NCI clinical trials cooperative group, reported findings from an additional phase III clinical trial, this one testing whether women with a positive sentinel lymph node but no clinical evidence of axillary lymph node metastasis could be safely treated with tumor removal and no further lymph node surgery other than the SLNB. In this trial, 891 women were randomly assigned to SLNB only or ALND after SLNB. All of the women were treated with lumpectomy. More than 95 percent of them also received adjuvant systemic therapy (chemotherapy, hormone therapy, or both), and about 90 percent received external-beam radiation therapy to the affected breast.

When the results of this trial were reported, the patients had been followed for a median of 6.3 years. The two groups of women had similar 5-year overall survival (92.5 percent in the SLNB-only group versus 91.8 percent in the SLNB plus ALND group) and 5-year disease-free survival (83.9 percent in the SLNB-only group and 82.2 percent in the SLNB plus ALND group). The researchers concluded that SLNB alone is safe and does not affect the survival of women who have sentinel lymph node metastasis but no clinical signs of other lymph node involvement and whose breast cancer is treated with surgery, systemic therapy, and external-beam radiation therapy. The excellent outcome in this trial for women treated with SLNB without ALND is likely due, at least in part, to the ability of local radiation therapy and modern systemic treatments to effectively treat breast cancer cells that may have spread to other axillary lymph nodes besides the sentinel node or to other parts of the body.

What has research shown about the use of SLNB in melanoma?

Researchers have investigated whether patients with melanoma whose sentinel lymph node is negative for cancer and who have no clinical signs of other lymph node involvement can also be spared more extensive lymph node surgery at the time of primary tumor removal. A meta-analysis of 71 studies that involved data from 25,240 patients suggests that the answer to this question is "yes." This meta-analysis

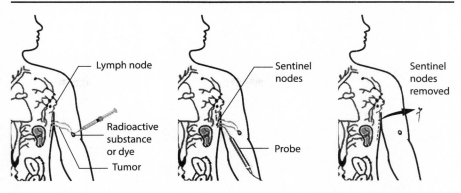

Figure 41.3. *Sentinel lymph node biopsy in a patient with melanoma.*

A radioactive substance and/or blue dye is injected near the tumor (first panel). The injected material is located visually and/or with a device that detects radioactivity (middle panel). The sentinel node(s) (the first lymph node(s) to take up the material) is (are) removed and checked for cancer cells (last panel). Sentinel lymph node biopsy can be done before or after the tumor is removed.

found that the risk of regional lymph node recurrence in patients with a negative SLNB was 5 percent or less.

Another question posed by researchers is whether SLNB plus the removal of the remaining regional lymph nodes (called completion lymph node dissection, or CLND) if the sentinel lymph node is positive for cancer has a therapeutic benefit for melanoma patients in terms of disease-free survival and melanoma-specific survival (length of time until death from melanoma). To address this question, NCI, the National Institutes of Health, and the John Wayne Cancer Institute are sponsoring a large phase III clinical trial called the Multicenter Selective Lymphadenectomy Trial II, or MSLT-II. In this trial, more than 1,900 patients with positive sentinel lymph nodes but no clinical evidence of other lymph node involvement are being randomly assigned to immediate CLND or regular ultrasound examination of the remaining regional lymph nodes and CLND if signs of additional lymph node metastasis appear. The patients in this trial will be followed for 10 years.

Chapter 42

Tests to Detect Colorectal Cancer and Polyps

What is colorectal cancer?

Colorectal cancer is a disease in which abnormal cells in the colon or rectum divide uncontrollably, ultimately forming a malignant tumor. (The colon and rectum are parts of the body's digestive system, which takes up nutrients from food and water and stores solid waste until it passes out of the body.)

Most colorectal cancers begin as a polyp, a growth in the tissue that lines the inner surface of the colon or rectum. Polyps may be flat, or they may be raised. Raised polyps may grow on the inner surface of the colon or rectum like mushrooms without a stalk (sessile polyps), or they may grow like a mushroom with a stalk (pedunculated polyps). Polyps are common in people older than 50 years of age, and most are not cancers. However, a certain type of polyp known as an adenoma may have a higher risk of becoming a cancer.

Colorectal cancer is the third most common type of non-skin cancer in both men (after prostate cancer and lung cancer) and women (after breast cancer and lung cancer). It is the second leading cause of cancer death in the United States after lung cancer. The rates of new

Text in this chapter is excerpted from "Tests to Detect Colorectal Cancer and Polyps," National Cancer Institute at the National Institutes of Health (NIH), November 12, 2014.

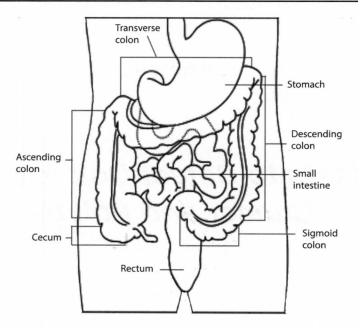

Figure 42.1. *Parts of the colon.*

Drawing of the front of the abdomen that shows the four sections of the colon: the ascending colon, the transverse colon, the descending colon, and the sigmoid colon. Also shown are the small intestine, the cecum, and the rectum. The cecum, colon, rectum, and anal canal make up the large intestine. The cecum, ascending colon, and transverse colon make up the upper, or proximal, colon; the descending colon and sigmoid colon make up the lower, or distal, colon.

colorectal cancer cases and deaths among adults aged 50 years or older are decreasing in this country. However, the incidence is increasing among younger adults. It is estimated that a total of 136,830 people in the United States would be diagnosed with colorectal cancer and 50,310 people would die from it in 2014.

Although the major risk factors for colorectal cancer are a family history and older age, several other factors have been associated with increased risk, including excessive alcohol use, obesity, being physically inactive, cigarette smoking, and, possibly, diet.

In addition, people with a history of inflammatory bowel disease (such as ulcerative colitis or Crohn disease) have a higher risk of colorectal cancer than people without such conditions. And people who have a family history of colorectal cancer or certain inherited conditions (such as Lynch syndrome and familial adenomatous polyposis) also have an increased risk of colorectal cancer.

Several screening tests have been developed to help doctors find colorectal cancer early, when it may be more treatable. Some tests that detect adenomas and polyps can actually prevent the development of cancer because these tests allow growths that might otherwise become cancer to be detected and removed. That is, colorectal cancer screening may be a form of cancer prevention, not just early detection.

What methods are used to screen people for colorectal cancer?

Expert medical groups, including the U.S. Preventive Services Task Force, strongly recommend screening for colorectal cancer. Although minor details of the recommendations may vary, these groups generally recommend that people at average risk of colorectal cancer get screened at regular intervals with high-sensitivity fecal occult blood tests (FOBT), sigmoidoscopy, or colonoscopy beginning at age 50. People at increased risk because of a family history of colorectal cancer or polyps or because they have inflammatory bowel disease or certain inherited conditions may be advised to start screening before age 50 and/or have more frequent screening.

- **High-sensitivity fecal occult blood tests (FOBT):** Both polyps and colorectal cancers can bleed, and FOBT checks for tiny amounts of blood in feces (stool) that cannot be seen. (Blood in stool may also indicate the presence of conditions that are not cancer, such as hemorrhoids.) Currently, two types of FOBT are approved by the Food and Drug Administration (FDA) to screen for colorectal cancer: guaiac FOBT (gFOBT) and the fecal immunochemical (or immunohistochemical) test (FIT, also known as iFOBT). With both types of FOBT, stool samples are collected by the patient using a kit, and the samples are returned to the doctor.

  - Guaiac FOBT uses a chemical to detect heme, a component of the blood protein hemoglobin. Because the guaiac FOBT can also detect heme in some foods (e.g., red meat), people have to avoid certain foods before having this test.

  - FIT uses antibodies to detect human hemoglobin specifically. Dietary restrictions are typically not required for FIT.

  Studies have shown that guaiac FOBT, when performed every 1 to 2 years in people aged 50 to 80 years, can help reduce the number of deaths due to colorectal cancer by 15 to 33 percent.

If FOBT is the only type of colorectal cancer screening test performed, The U.S. Preventive Services Task Force recommends yearly testing.

- **Sigmoidoscopy:** In this test, the rectum and sigmoid colon are examined using a sigmoidoscope, a flexible lighted tube with a lens for viewing and a tool for removing tissue. This instrument is inserted through the anus into the rectum and sigmoid colon as air (or carbon dioxide) is pumped into the colon to expand it so the doctor can see the colon lining more clearly. During sigmoidoscopy, abnormal growths in the rectum and sigmoid colon can be removed for analysis (biopsied). The lower colon must be cleared of stool before sigmoidoscopy, but the preparation is less involved than that required for colonoscopy. People are usually not sedated for this test.

  Studies have shown that people who have regular screening with sigmoidoscopy after age 50 years have a 60 to 70 percent lower risk of death due to cancer of the rectum and lower colon than people who do not have screening. One randomized controlled clinical trial found that even just one sigmoidoscopy screening between 55 and 64 years of age can substantially reduce colorectal cancer incidence and mortality. The U.S. Preventive Services Task Force recommends sigmoidoscopy every 5 years along with FOBT every 3 years for people at average risk who have had negative test results.

- **Standard (or optical) colonoscopy:** In this test, the rectum and entire colon are examined using a colonoscope, a flexible lighted tube with a lens for viewing and a tool for removing tissue. Like the shorter sigmoidoscope, the colonoscope is inserted through the anus into the rectum and the colon as air (or carbon dioxide) is pumped into the colon to expand it so the doctor can see the colon lining more clearly. During colonoscopy, any abnormal growths in the colon and the rectum can be removed, including growths in the upper parts of the colon that are not reached by sigmoidoscopy. A thorough cleansing of the entire colon is necessary before this test. Most patients receive some form of sedation during the test.

  Studies suggest that colonoscopy reduces deaths from colorectal cancer by about 60 to 70 percent. Additional studies are currently being done to better evaluate how effective colonoscopy screening methods are (8). The U.S. Preventive Services Task

Force recommends colonoscopy every 10 years for people at average risk as long as their test results are negative (2).

- **Other methods:** Although most expert groups generally recommend high-sensitivity FOBT, sigmoidoscopy, and colonoscopy as standard colorectal cancer screening tests, several other types of tests exist.

Cologuard®. This test detects tiny amounts of blood in stool (with an immunochemical test similar to FIT) as well as nine DNA biomarkers in three genes that have been found in colorectal cancer and precancerous advanced adenomas. The DNA comes from cells from the lining of the colon and rectum that collect in stool as it passes through the large intestine and rectum. As with both types of FOBT, the stool sample for the Cologuard test is collected by the patient using a kit; the sample is mailed to a laboratory for testing. A computer program analyzes the results of the two tests (blood and DNA biomarkers) and provides a finding of negative or positive. People who have a positive finding with this test are advised to undergo a colonoscopy.

In one study of people who were at average risk for developing colon cancer and had no symptoms of colon problems, this test detected more cancers and adenomas than the FIT test (that is, it was more sensitive). However, the Cologuard test also was more likely to identify an abnormality when none was actually present (that is, it had more false-positive results).

In August 2014, the FDA approved the Cologuard test. At the same time, in a pilot program known as parallel review, the Centers for Medicare & Medicaid Services proposed national coverage for this test. This test is still being evaluated to see where it fits in screening guidelines. To date, it has not been incorporated into clinical practice guidelines or recommended by the U.S. Preventive Services Task Force as a method to screen for colorectal cancer. The Task Force is currently updating its guideline and is examining recent evidence on the Cologuard test.

Virtual colonoscopy. This screening method, also called computed tomographic [CT] colonography), uses special x-ray equipment (a CT scanner) is to produce a series of pictures of the colon and the rectum from outside the body. A computer then assembles these pictures into detailed images that can show polyps and other abnormalities. Virtual colonoscopy is less invasive than standard colonoscopy and does not require sedation. As with standard colonoscopy, a thorough cleansing of the colon is necessary before this test, and air (or carbon dioxide) is pumped into the colon to expand it for better viewing of the colon's lining. The accuracy of virtual colonoscopy is similar to that of standard colonoscopy, and virtual colonoscopy has a lower risk of complications. However, if polyps or other abnormal growths are found during a virtual colonoscopy, a standard colonoscopy is usually performed to remove them.

Whether virtual colonoscopy can help reduce deaths from colorectal cancer is not yet known, and Medicare and some insurance companies currently do not pay for the costs of this procedure. Studies are ongoing to compare virtual colonoscopy with other screening methods.

Double-contrast barium enema. This test, also called DCBE, is another method of visualizing the colon from outside the body. In DCBE, a series of x-ray images of the entire colon and rectum is taken after the patient is given an enema with a barium solution. The barium helps to outline the colon and the rectum on the images. DCBE is rarely used for screening because it is less sensitive than colonoscopy for detecting small polyps and cancers. However, it may be used for people who cannot undergo standard colonoscopy—for example, because they are at particular risk for complications.

Single-specimen guaiac FOBT done in a doctor's office. Doctors sometimes perform a single-specimen guaiac FOBT on a stool sample collected during a digital rectal examination done as part of a routine physical examination. However, this approach has not been shown to be an effective way to screen for colorectal cancer.

How can people and their health care providers decide which colorectal cancer screening test(s) to use?

People should talk with their health care provider about when to begin screening for colorectal cancer, what test(s) to have, the advantages and disadvantages of each test, how often to undergo colorectal cancer screening, and when to stop.

The decision about which test to have usually takes into account several factors, including:

- The person's age, medical history, family history, and general health
- The potential harms of the test
- The preparation required for the test
- Whether sedation may be needed for the test
- The follow-up care needed after the test
- The convenience of the test
- The cost of the test and the availability of insurance coverage

The commonly used colorectal cancer screening tests all have advantages and disadvantages:

Fecal Occult Blood Test (guaiac FOBT or fecal immunochemical test [FIT])

Advantages:

- No cleansing of the colon is necessary.
- No dietary restrictions are needed before FIT.
- Samples can be collected at home.
- Cost is low compared with other colorectal cancer screening tests.
- There is no risk of damage to the lining of the colon.
- No sedation is needed.

Disadvantages:

- The test does not detect some polyps and cancers.
- False-positive test results (i.e., the test suggests an abnormality when none is present) are possible.
- Dietary restrictions are needed before guaiac FOBT.
- Additional procedures, such as colonoscopy, may be needed if the test result shows blood in the stool.

Sigmoidoscopy

Advantages:

- For most patients, discomfort is minimal, and complications are rare.

- The doctor can perform a biopsy or polypectomy (removal of a polyp or adenoma) during the test, if necessary.

- Less extensive cleansing of the colon is necessary for this test than for a colonoscopy.

- Sedation is often not required.

Disadvantages:

- Abnormal growths in the upper part of the colon will be missed because the test allows the doctor to view only the rectum and the lower part of the colon.

- Bowel cleansing is needed before the test.

- Medication and diet changes may be needed before the test.

- There is a very small risk of bleeding or of tearing or perforation of the lining of the colon.

- Additional procedures, such as colonoscopy, may be needed if the test finds an abnormality.

- The availability of sigmoidoscopy has decreased substantially in the United States in recent years.

Standard Colonoscopy

Advantages:

- This test is one of the most sensitive currently available.

- It allows the doctor to view the rectum and the entire colon.

- The doctor can perform a biopsy or polypectomy during the test if necessary.

Disadvantages:

- Even though this test is highly sensitive, it still may not detect all small polyps, non-polypoid lesions, or cancers.

- A thorough cleansing of the colon is required before the test.

- Diet changes are needed before the test, and medications may need to be adjusted.

- Some form of sedation is almost always used. As a result, the patient must have someone accompany them to the procedure and drive them home afterward, and they may not be able to work the day of the procedure.

- There is a small risk of bleeding or of tearing or perforation of the lining of the colon; this risk increases with age, the presence of other health problems, and when polyps are removed.

Does health insurance pay for colorectal cancer screening?

The Affordable Care Act requires coverage of colorectal cancer screening tests by health plans that started on or after September 23, 2010. (For health plans that started before September 23, 2010, the rules about insurance coverage are covered by state laws, which vary, and by other federal laws.) People should check with their health insurance provider to determine their colorectal cancer screening coverage. Medicare covers several colorectal cancer screening tests for its beneficiaries.

What happens if a colorectal cancer screening test finds an abnormality?

If a screening test finds an abnormality, additional tests may be recommended. These tests may include x-rays of the gastrointestinal tract, a sigmoidoscopy, or, most often, a colonoscopy if it has not already been done. If a polyp or tumor is found during a sigmoidoscopy, a biopsy or polypectomy may be performed during the test, and a colonoscopy may be recommended. If a polyp or tumor is found during a standard colonoscopy, a biopsy or polypectomy may be performed during the test to determine whether cancer is present. If a polyp or tumor is detected during virtual colonoscopy, the patient will be referred for a standard colonoscopy.

What new tests are being developed for colorectal cancer screening?

Colorectal polyps and tumors can release cells and DNA into the bloodstream as well as into stool. Researchers are studying whether the presence of an altered gene called SEPT9 in blood can be used to screen for early-stage colorectal cancer and advanced adenomas. In clinical studies, a biomarker test that detects altered SEPT9 DNA in blood (Epi proColon®) was no less sensitive than FIT, but it was less specific. In March 2014, the FDA recommended premarket approval, a process of scientific and regulatory review to evaluate safety and effectiveness, for this test.

New approaches to visualize the colon that avoid the need for thorough cleansing of the colon that is currently required for virtual colonoscopy are being studied and refined. One approach is "fecal tagging" with a contrast agent that is ingested over several days before the procedure. This technique allows fecal material in the colon to be differentiated from colon tissue; computer software can be used to electronically remove the tagged fecal material from images.

Chapter 43

Tumor Grade

What is tumor grade?

Tumor grade is the description of a tumor based on how abnormal the tumor cells and the tumor tissue look under a microscope. It is an indicator of how quickly a tumor is likely to grow and spread. If the cells of the tumor and the organization of the tumor's tissue are close to those of normal cells and tissue, the tumor is called "well-differentiated." These tumors tend to grow and spread at a slower rate than tumors that are "undifferentiated" or "poorly differentiated," which have abnormal-looking cells and may lack normal tissue structures. Based on these and other differences in microscopic appearance, doctors assign a numerical "grade" to most cancers. The factors used to determine tumor grade can vary between different types of cancer.

Tumor grade is not the same as the stage of a cancer. Cancer stage refers to the size and/or extent (reach) of the original (primary) tumor and whether or not cancer cells have spread in the body. Cancer stage is based on factors such as the location of the primary tumor, tumor size, regional lymph node involvement (the spread of cancer to nearby lymph nodes), and the number of tumors present.

Text in this chapter is excerpted from "Tumor Grade," National Cancer Institute at the National Institutes of Health (NIH), May 3, 2013.

How is tumor grade determined?

If a tumor is suspected to be malignant, a doctor removes all or part of it during a procedure called a biopsy. A pathologist (a doctor who identifies diseases by studying cells and tissues under a microscope) then examines the biopsied tissue to determine whether the tumor is benign or malignant. The pathologist also determines the tumor's grade and identifies other characteristics of the tumor.

How are tumor grades classified?

Grading systems differ depending on the type of cancer. In general, tumors are graded as 1, 2, 3, or 4, depending on the amount of abnormality. In Grade 1 tumors, the tumor cells and the organization of the tumor tissue appear close to normal. These tumors tend to grow and spread slowly. In contrast, the cells and tissue of Grade 3 and Grade 4 tumors do not look like normal cells and tissue. Grade 3 and Grade 4 tumors tend to grow rapidly and spread faster than tumors with a lower grade.

If a grading system for a tumor type is not specified, the following system is generally used:

- GX: Grade cannot be assessed (undetermined grade)
- G1: Well differentiated (low grade)
- G2: Moderately differentiated (intermediate grade)
- G3: Poorly differentiated (high grade)
- G4: Undifferentiated (high grade)

What are some of the cancer type-specific grading systems?

Breast and prostate cancers are the most common types of cancer that have their own grading systems.

Breast cancer. Doctors most often use the Nottingham grading system (also called the Elston-Ellis modification of the Scarff-Bloom-Richardson grading system) for breast cancer. This system grades breast tumors based on the following features:

- Tubule formation: how much of the tumor tissue has normal breast (milk) duct structures
- Nuclear grade: an evaluation of the size and shape of the nucleus in the tumor cells

- Mitotic rate: how many dividing cells are present, which is a measure of how fast the tumor cells are growing and dividing

Each of the categories gets a score between 1 and 3; a score of "1" means the cells and tumor tissue look the most like normal cells and tissue, and a score of "3" means the cells and tissue look the most abnormal. The scores for the three categories are then added, yielding a total score of 3 to 9. Three grades are possible:

- Total score = 3–5: G1 (Low grade or well differentiated)
- Total score = 6–7: G2 (Intermediate grade or moderately differentiated)
- Total score = 8–9: G3 (High grade or poorly differentiated)

Prostate cancer. The Gleason scoring system is used to grade prostate cancer. The Gleason score is based on biopsy samples taken from the prostate. The pathologist checks the samples to see how similar the tumor tissue looks to normal prostate tissue. Both a primary and a secondary pattern of tissue organization are identified. The primary pattern represents the most common tissue pattern seen in the tumor, and the secondary pattern represents the next most common pattern. Each pattern is given a grade from 1 to 5, with 1 looking the most like normal prostate tissue and 5 looking the most abnormal. The two grades are then added to give a Gleason score. The American Joint Committee on Cancer recommends grouping Gleason scores into the following categories:

- Gleason X: Gleason score cannot be determined
- Gleason 2–6: The tumor tissue is well differentiated
- Gleason 7: The tumor tissue is moderately differentiated
- Gleason 8–10: The tumor tissue is poorly differentiated or undifferentiated

How does tumor grade affect a patient's treatment options?

Doctors use tumor grade and other factors, such as cancer stage and a patient's age and general health, to develop a treatment plan and to determine a patient's prognosis (the likely outcome or course of a disease; the chance of recovery or recurrence). Generally, a lower grade indicates a better prognosis. A higher-grade cancer may grow and spread more quickly and may require immediate or more aggressive treatment.

The importance of tumor grade in planning treatment and determining a patient's prognosis is greater for certain types of cancer, such as soft tissue sarcoma, primary brain tumors, and breast and prostate cancer.

Patients should talk with their doctor for more information about tumor grade and how it relates to their treatment and prognosis.

Chapter 44

Tumor Markers

What are tumor markers?

Tumor markers are substances that are produced by cancer or by other cells of the body in response to cancer or certain benign (noncancerous) conditions. Most tumor markers are made by normal cells as well as by cancer cells; however, they are produced at much higher levels in cancerous conditions. These substances can be found in the blood, urine, stool, tumor tissue, or other tissues or bodily fluids of some patients with cancer. Most tumor markers are proteins. However, more recently, patterns of gene expression and changes to DNA have also begun to be used as tumor markers. Markers of the latter type are assessed in tumor tissue specifically.

Thus far, more than 20 different tumor markers have been characterized and are in clinical use. Some are associated with only one type of cancer, whereas others are associated with two or more cancer types. There is no "universal" tumor marker that can detect any type of cancer.

There are some limitations to the use of tumor markers. Sometimes, noncancerous conditions can cause the levels of certain tumor markers to increase. In addition, not everyone with a particular type of cancer will have a higher level of a tumor marker associated with that cancer. Moreover, tumor markers have not been identified for every type of cancer.

Text in this chapter is excerpted from "Tumor Markers," National Cancer Institute at the National Institutes of Health (NIH), December 7, 2011.

881

How are tumor markers used in cancer care?

Tumor markers are used to help detect, diagnose, and manage some types of cancer. Although an elevated level of a tumor marker may suggest the presence of cancer, this alone is not enough to diagnose cancer. Therefore, measurements of tumor markers are usually combined with other tests, such as biopsies, to diagnose cancer.

Tumor marker levels may be measured before treatment to help doctors plan the appropriate therapy. In some types of cancer, the level of a tumor marker reflects the stage (extent) of the disease and/or the patient's prognosis (likely outcome or course of disease).

Tumor markers may also be measured periodically during cancer therapy. A decrease in the level of a tumor marker or a return to the marker's normal level may indicate that the cancer is responding to treatment, whereas no change or an increase may indicate that the cancer is not responding.

Tumor markers may also be measured after treatment has ended to check for recurrence (the return of cancer).

How are tumor markers measured?

A doctor takes a sample of tumor tissue or bodily fluid and sends it to a laboratory, where various methods are used to measure the level of the tumor marker.

If the tumor marker is being used to determine whether treatment is working or whether there is a recurrence, the marker's level will be measured in multiple samples taken over time. Usually these "serial measurements," which show whether the level of a marker is increasing, staying the same, or decreasing, are more meaningful than a single measurement.

Does NCI have guidelines for the use of tumor markers?

NCI does not have such guidelines. However, some national and international organizations do have guidelines for the use of tumor markers for some types of cancer:

- The American Society of Clinical Oncology (ASCO) has published clinical practice guidelines on a variety of topics, including tumor markers for breast cancer, gastrointestinal cancers, and testicular cancer and extragonadal germ cell tumors in males. These guidelines, called What to Know: ASCO's Guidelines, are available on the ASCO website.

- The National Academy of Clinical Biochemistry publishes laboratory medicine practice guidelines, including Use of Tumor Markers in Clinical Practice: Quality Requirements, which focuses on the appropriate use of tumor markers for specific cancers.

What tumor markers are currently being used, and for which cancer types?

A number of tumor markers are currently being used for a wide range of cancer types. Although most of these can be tested in laboratories that meet standards set by the Clinical Laboratory Improvement Amendments, some cannot be and may therefore be considered experimental. Tumor markers that are currently in common use are listed below.

ALK gene rearrangements

- Cancer types: Non-small cell lung cancer and anaplastic large cell lymphoma
- Tissue analyzed: Tumor
- How used: To help determine treatment and prognosis

Alpha-fetoprotein (AFP)

- Cancer types: Liver cancer and germ cell tumors
- Tissue analyzed: Blood
- How used: To help diagnose liver cancer and follow response to treatment; to assess stage, prognosis, and response to treatment of germ cell tumors

Beta-2-microglobulin (B2M)

- Cancer types: Multiple myeloma, chronic lymphocytic leukemia, and some lymphomas
- Tissue analyzed: Blood, urine, or cerebrospinal fluid
- How used: To determine prognosis and follow response to treatment

Beta-human chorionic gonadotropin (Beta-hCG)

- Cancer types: Choriocarcinoma and testicular cancer
- Tissue analyzed: Urine or blood
- How used: To assess stage, prognosis, and response to treatment

BCR-ABL fusion gene

- Cancer type: Chronic myeloid leukemia
- Tissue analyzed: Blood and/or bone marrow
- How used: To confirm diagnosis and monitor disease status

BRAF mutation V600E

- Cancer types: Cutaneous melanoma and colorectal cancer
- Tissue analyzed: Tumor
- How used: To predict response to targeted therapies

CA15-3/CA27.29

- Cancer type: Breast cancer
- Tissue analyzed: Blood
- How used: To assess whether treatment is working or disease has recurred

CA19-9

- Cancer types: Pancreatic cancer, gallbladder cancer, bile duct cancer, and gastric cancer
- Tissue analyzed: Blood
- How used: To assess whether treatment is working

CA-125

- Cancer type: Ovarian cancer
- Tissue analyzed: Blood
- How used: To help in diagnosis, assessment of response to treatment, and evaluation of recurrence

Calcitonin

- Cancer type: Medullary thyroid cancer
- Tissue analyzed: Blood
- How used: To aid in diagnosis, check whether treatment is working, and assess recurrence

Carcinoembryonic antigen (CEA)

- Cancer types: Colorectal cancer and breast cancer
- Tissue analyzed: Blood
- How used: To check whether colorectal cancer has spread; to look for breast cancer recurrence and assess response to treatment

CD20

- Cancer type: Non-Hodgkin lymphoma
- Tissue analyzed: Blood
- How used: To determine whether treatment with a targeted therapy is appropriate

Chromogranin A (CgA)

- Cancer type: Neuroendocrine tumors
- Tissue analyzed: Blood
- How used: To help in diagnosis, assessment of treatment response, and evaluation of recurrence

Chromosomes 3, 7, 17, and 9p21

- Cancer type: Bladder cancer
- Tissue analyzed: Urine
- How used: To help in monitoring for tumor recurrence

Cytokeratin fragments 21-1

- Cancer type: Lung cancer
- Tissue analyzed: Blood
- How used: To help in monitoring for recurrence

EGFR mutation analysis

- Cancer type: Non-small cell lung cancer
- Tissue analyzed: Tumor
- How used: To help determine treatment and prognosis

Estrogen receptor (ER)/progesterone receptor (PR)

- Cancer type: Breast cancer
- Tissue analyzed: Tumor
- How used: To determine whether treatment with hormonal therapy (such as tamoxifen) is appropriate

Fibrin/fibrinogen

- Cancer type: Bladder cancer
- Tissue analyzed: Urine
- How used: To monitor progression and response to treatment

HE4

- Cancer type: Ovarian cancer
- Tissue analyzed: Blood
- How used: To assess disease progression and monitor for recurrence

HER2/neu

- Cancer types: Breast cancer, gastric cancer, and esophageal cancer
- Tissue analyzed: Tumor
- How used: To determine whether treatment with trastuzumab is appropriate

Immunoglobulins

- Cancer types: Multiple myeloma and Waldenström macroglobulinemia
- Tissue analyzed: Blood and urine
- How used: To help diagnose disease, assess response to treatment, and look for recurrence

KIT

- Cancer types: Gastrointestinal stromal tumor and mucosal melanoma

- Tissue analyzed: Tumor
- How used: To help in diagnosing and determining treatment

KRAS mutation analysis

- Cancer types: Colorectal cancer and non-small cell lung cancer
- Tissue analyzed: Tumor
- How used: To determine whether treatment with a particular type of targeted therapy is appropriate

Lactate dehydrogenase

- Cancer type: Germ cell tumors
- Tissue analyzed: Blood
- How used: To assess stage, prognosis, and response to treatment

Nuclear matrix protein 22

- Cancer type: Bladder cancer
- Tissue analyzed: Urine
- How used: To monitor response to treatment

Prostate-specific antigen (PSA)

- Cancer type: Prostate cancer
- Tissue analyzed: Blood
- How used: To help in diagnosis, assess response to treatment, and look for recurrence

Thyroglobulin

- Cancer type: Thyroid cancer
- Tissue analyzed: Tumor
- How used: To evaluate response to treatment and look for recurrence

Urokinase plasminogen activator (uPA) and plasminogen activator inhibitor (PAI-1)

- Cancer type: Breast cancer
- Tissue analyzed: Tumor

- How used: To determine aggressiveness of cancer and guide treatment

5-Protein signature (Oval)

- Cancer type: Ovarian cancer
- Tissue analyzed: Blood
- How used: To pre-operatively assess pelvic mass for suspected ovarian cancer

21-Gene signature (Oncotype DX)

- Cancer type: Breast cancer
- Tissue analyzed: Tumor
- How used: To evaluate risk of recurrence

70-Gene signature (Mammaprint)

- Cancer type: Breast cancer
- Tissue analyzed: Tumor
- How used: To evaluate risk of recurrence

Can tumor markers be used in cancer screening?

Because tumor markers can be used to assess the response of a tumor to treatment and for prognosis, researchers have hoped that they might also be useful in screening tests that aim to detect cancer early, before there are any symptoms. For a screening test to be useful, it should have very high sensitivity (ability to correctly identify people who have the disease) and specificity (ability to correctly identify people who do *not* have the disease). If a test is highly sensitive, it will identify most people with the disease—that is, it will result in very few false-negative results. If a test is highly specific, only a small number of people will test positive for the disease who do not have it—in other words, it will result in very few false-positive results.

Although tumor markers are extremely useful in determining whether a tumor is responding to treatment or assessing whether it has recurred, no tumor marker identified to date is sufficiently sensitive or specific to be used on its own to screen for cancer.

For example, the prostate-specific antigen (PSA) test, which measures the level of PSA in the blood, is often used to screen men for prostate cancer. However, an increased PSA level can be caused by benign prostate conditions as well as by prostate cancer, and most men with an elevated PSA level do not have prostate cancer. Initial results from two large randomized controlled trials, the NCI-conducted Prostate, Lung, Colorectal, and Ovarian Cancer Screening Trial, or PLCO, and the European Randomized Study of Screening for Prostate Cancer, showed that PSA testing at best leads to only a small reduction in the number of prostate cancer deaths. Moreover, it is not clear whether the benefits of PSA screening outweigh the harms of follow-up diagnostic tests and treatments for cancers that in many cases would never have threatened a man's life.

Similarly, results from the PLCO trial showed that CA-125, a tumor marker that is sometimes elevated in the blood of women with ovarian cancer but can also be elevated in women with benign conditions, is not sufficiently sensitive or specific to be used together with transvaginal ultrasound to screen for ovarian cancer in women at average risk of the disease. An analysis of 28 potential markers for ovarian cancer in blood from women who later went on to develop ovarian cancer found that none of these markers performed even as well as CA-125 at detecting the disease in women at average risk.

What kind of research is under way to develop more accurate tumor markers?

Cancer researchers are turning to proteomics (the study of protein structure, function, and patterns of expression) in hopes of developing new biomarkers that can be used to identify disease in its early stages, to predict the effectiveness of treatment, or to predict the chance of cancer recurrence after treatment has ended.

Scientists are also evaluating patterns of gene expression for their ability to help determine a patient's prognosis or response to therapy. For example, the NCI-sponsored TAILORx trial assigned women with lymph node-negative, hormone receptor–positive breast cancer who have undergone surgery to different treatments based on their recurrence scores in the Oncotype DX test. One of the goals of the trial is to determine whether women whose score indicates that they have an intermediate risk of recurrence will benefit from the addition of chemotherapy to hormonal therapy or whether such women can safely avoid chemotherapy. The trial has accrued its required number of subjects and these subjects will be followed for several years before results are available.

NCI's Early Detection Research Network is developing and testing a number of genomic- and proteomic-based biomarkers.

The Program for the Assessment of Clinical Cancer Tests (PACCT), an initiative of the Cancer Diagnosis Program of NCI's Division of Cancer Diagnosis and Treatment, has been developed to ensure that development of the next generation of laboratory tests is efficient and effective. The PACCT strategy group, which includes scientists from academia, industry, and NCI, is developing criteria for assessing which markers are ready for further development. PACCT also aims to improve access to human specimens, make standardized reagents and control materials, and support validation studies. A new program, the Clinical Assay Development Program, allows NCI to assist in the development of promising assays that may predict which treatment may be better or that will help indicate a particular cancer's aggressiveness.

Chapter 45

Understanding Laboratory Tests

What are laboratory tests?

A laboratory test is a procedure in which a sample of blood, urine, other bodily fluid, or tissue is examined to get information about a person's health. Some laboratory tests provide precise and reliable information about specific health problems. Other tests provide more general information that helps doctors identify or rule out possible health problems. Doctors often use other types of tests, such as imaging tests, in addition to laboratory tests to learn more about a person's health.

How are laboratory tests used in cancer medicine?

Laboratory tests are used in cancer medicine in many ways:

- To screen for cancer or precancerous conditions before a person has any symptoms of disease

- To help diagnose cancer

Text in this chapter is excerpted from "Understanding Laboratory Tests," National Cancer Institute at the National Institutes of Health (NIH), December 11, 2013.

- To provide information about the stage of a cancer (that is, its severity); for malignant tumors, this includes the size and/or extent (reach) of the original (primary) tumor and whether or not the tumor has spread (metastasized) to other parts of the body

- To plan treatment

- To monitor a patient's general health during treatment and to check for potential side effects of the treatment

- To determine whether a cancer is responding to treatment

- To find out whether a cancer has recurred (come back)

Which laboratory tests are used in cancer medicine?

Categories of some common laboratory tests used in cancer medicine are listed below in alphabetical order.

- **Blood chemistry test**

  What it measures: The amounts of certain substances that are released into the blood by the organs and tissues of the body, such as metabolites, electrolytes, fats, and proteins, including enzymes. Blood chemistry tests usually include tests for blood urea nitrogen (BUN) and creatinine.

  How it is used: Diagnosis and monitoring of patients during and after treatment. High or low levels of some substances can be signs of disease or side effects of treatment.

- **Cancer gene mutation testing**

  What it measures: The presence or absence of specific inherited mutations in genes that are known to play a role in cancer development. Examples include tests to look for *BRCA1* and *BRCA2* gene mutations, which play a role in development of breast, ovarian, and other cancers.

  How it is used: Assessment of cancer risk

- **Complete blood count (CBC)**

  What it measures: Numbers of the different types of blood cells, including red blood cells, white blood cells, and platelets, in a sample of blood. This test also measures the amount of hemoglobin (the protein that carries oxygen) in the blood, the percentage of the total blood volume that is taken up by red blood cells (hematocrit), the size of the red blood cells, and the amount of hemoglobin in red blood cells.

How it is used: Diagnosis, particularly in leukemias, and monitoring during and after treatment

- **Cytogenetic analysis**

  What it measures: Changes in the number and/or structure of chromosomes in a patient's white blood cells or bone marrow cells

  How it is used: Diagnosis, deciding on appropriate treatment

- **Immunophenotyping**

  What it measures: Identifies cells based on the types of antigens present on the cell surface

  How it is used: Diagnosis, staging, and monitoring of cancers of the blood system and other hematologic disorders, including leukemias, lymphomas, myelodysplastic syndromes, and myeloproliferative disorders. It is most often done on blood or bone marrow samples, but it may also be done on other bodily fluids or biopsy tissue samples.

- **Sputum cytology (also called sputum culture)**

  What it measures: The presence of abnormal cells in sputum (mucus and other matter brought up from the lungs by coughing)

  How it is used: Diagnosis of lung cancer

- **Tumor marker tests**

  What they measure: Some measure the presence, levels, or activity of specific proteins or genes in tissue, blood, or other bodily fluids that may be signs of cancer or certain benign (noncancerous) conditions. A tumor that has a greater than normal level of a tumor marker may respond to treatment with a drug that targets that marker. For example, cancer cells that have high levels of the HER2/neu gene or protein may respond to treatment with a drug that targets the HER2/neu protein.

  Some tumor marker tests analyze DNA to look for specific gene mutations that may be present in cancers but not normal tissues. Examples include EGFR gene mutation analysis to help

893

determine treatment and assess prognosis in non-small cell lung cancer and *BRAF* gene mutation analysis to predict response to targeted therapies in melanoma and colorectal cancer.

Still other tumor marker tests, called multi-gene tests (or multi-parameter gene expression tests), analyze the expression of a specific group of genes in tumor samples. These tests are used for prognosis and treatment planning. For example, the 21-gene signature can help patients with lymph node–negative, estrogen receptor–positive breast cancer decide if there may be benefit to treating with chemotherapy in addition to hormone therapy, or not.

How they are used: Diagnosis, deciding on appropriate treatment, assessing response to treatment, and monitoring for cancer recurrence

- **Urinalysis**

  What it measures: The color of urine and its contents, such as sugar, protein, red blood cells, and white blood cells.

  How it is used: Detection and diagnosis of kidney cancer and urothelial cancers

- **Urine cytology**

  What it measures: The presence of abnormal cells shed from the urinary tract into urine to detect disease.

  How it is used: Detection and diagnosis of bladder cancer and other urothelial cancers, monitoring patients for cancer recurrence

How do I interpret my test results?

With some laboratory tests, the results obtained for healthy people can vary somewhat from person to person. Factors that can cause person-to-person variation in laboratory test results include a person's age, sex, race, medical history, and general health. In fact, the results obtained from a single person given the same test on different days can also vary. For these tests, therefore, the results are considered normal if they fall between certain lower and upper limits or values. This range of normal values is known as the "normal range," the "reference range," and the "reference interval." When healthy people take such tests, it is expected that their results will fall within the normal range 95 percent of the time. (Five percent of the time, the results from healthy people will fall outside the normal range and will be marked as "abnormal.") Reference ranges are based on test results from large numbers of people who have been tested in the past.

Some test results can be affected by certain foods and medications. For this reason, people may be asked to not eat or drink for several hours before a laboratory test or to delay taking medications until after the test.

For many tests, it is possible for someone with cancer to have results that fall within the normal range. Likewise, it is possible for someone who doesn't have cancer to have test results that fall outside the normal range. This is one reason that many laboratory tests alone cannot provide a definitive diagnosis of cancer or other diseases.

In general, laboratory test results must be interpreted in the context of the overall health of the patient and are considered along with the results of other examinations, tests, and procedures. A doctor who is familiar with a patient's medical history and current situation is the best person to explain test results and what they mean.

What if a laboratory test result is unclear or inconclusive?

If a test result is unclear or inconclusive, the doctor will likely repeat the test to be certain of the result and may order additional tests. The doctor may also compare the latest test result to previous results, if available, to get a better idea of what is normal for that person.

What are some questions to ask the doctor about laboratory tests?

It can be helpful to take a list of questions to the doctor's office. Questions about a laboratory test might include:

- What will this test measure?
- Why is this test being ordered?
- Does this test have any risks or side effects?
- How should I prepare for the test?
- When will the test results be available?
- How will the results be given (a letter, a phone call, online)?
- Will this test need to be done more than once?

How reliable are laboratory tests and their results?

The results of laboratory tests affect many of the decisions a doctor makes about a person's health care, including whether additional tests are necessary, developing a treatment plan, or monitoring a person's response to treatment. It is very important, therefore, that the laboratory tests themselves are trustworthy and that the laboratory that performs the tests meets rigorous state and federal regulatory standards.

The Food and Drug Administration (FDA) regulates the development and marketing of all laboratory tests that use test kits and equipment that are commercially manufactured in the United States. After the FDA approves a laboratory test, other federal and state agencies make sure that the test materials and equipment meet strict standards while they are being manufactured and then used in a medical or clinical laboratory.

All laboratory testing that is performed on humans in the United States (except testing done in clinical trials and other types of human research) is regulated through the Clinical Laboratory Improvement Amendments (CLIA), which were passed by Congress in 1988. The CLIA laboratory certification program is administered by the Centers for Medicare & Medicaid Services (CMS) in conjunction with the FDA and the Centers for Disease Control and Prevention. CLIA ensures that laboratory staff are appropriately trained and supervised and that testing laboratories have quality control programs in place so that test results are accurate and reliable.

To enroll in the CLIA program, laboratories must complete a certification process that is based on the level of complexity of tests that the laboratory will perform. The more complicated the test, the more demanding the requirements for certification. Laboratories must demonstrate that they can perform tests as accurately and as precisely as the manufacturer did to gain FDA approval of the test. Laboratories must also evaluate the tests regularly to make sure that they continue to meet the manufacturer's specifications. Laboratories undergo regular unannounced on-site inspections to ensure they are following the requirements outlined in CLIA to receive and maintain certification.

Some states have additional requirements that are equal to or more stringent than those outlined in CLIA. CMS has determined that Washington and New York have state licensure programs that are exempt from CLIA program requirements. Therefore, licensing authorities in Washington and New York have primary responsibility for oversight of their state's laboratory practices.

What new laboratory tests for cancer medicine are on the horizon?

Tests that measure the number of cancer cells in a sample of blood (circulating tumors cells) or examine the DNA of such cells are of great interest in cancer medicine because research suggests that levels of these cells might be useful for evaluating response to treatment and detecting cancer recurrence. One circulating tumor cell test has been approved by the Food and Drug Administration (FDA) to monitor patients with breast, colorectal, or prostate cancer. However, such tests are still being studied in clinical trials and are not routinely used in clinical practice.

Tests that determine the sequences of a large number of genes at one time using next generation DNA sequencing methods are being developed to provide gene mutation profiles of solid tumors (e.g., lung cancer). Some of these tests are being used to help choose the best treatment, but none are FDA approved.

Part Five

Cancer Treatment

Chapter 46

Chemotherapy

Chapter Contents

Text in this chapter is excerpted from "Chemotherapy and You," National Cancer Institute at the National Institutes of Health (NIH), June 2011.

Section 46.1

Questions and Answers about Chemotherapy

What is chemotherapy?

Chemotherapy (also called chemo) is a type of cancer treatment that uses drugs to destroy cancer cells.

How does chemotherapy work?

Chemotherapy works by stopping or slowing the growth of cancer cells, which grow and divide quickly. But it can also harm healthy cells that divide quickly, such as those that line your mouth and intestines or cause your hair to grow. Damage to healthy cells may cause side effects. Often, side effects get better or go away after chemotherapy is over.

What does chemotherapy do?

Depending on your type of cancer and how advanced it is, chemotherapy can:

- **Cure cancer**—when chemotherapy destroys cancer cells to the point that your doctor can no longer detect them in your body and they will not grow back.

- **Control cancer**—when chemotherapy keeps cancer from spreading, slows its growth, or destroys cancer cells that have spread to other parts of your body.

- **Ease cancer symptoms (also called palliative care)**—when chemotherapy shrinks tumors that are causing pain or pressure.

How is chemotherapy used?

Sometimes, chemotherapy is used as the only cancer treatment. But more often, you will get chemotherapy along with surgery, **radiation therapy**, or **biological therapy**. Chemotherapy can:

- Make a tumor smaller before surgery or radiation therapy. This is called **neo-adjuvant chemotherapy**.

- Destroy cancer cells that may remain after surgery or radiation therapy. This is called **adjuvant chemotherapy**.

- Help radiation therapy and biological therapy work better.

- Destroy cancer cells that have come back (**recurrent** cancer) or spread to other parts of your body (**metastatic** cancer).

How does my doctor decide which chemotherapy drugs to use?

This choice depends on:

- The type of cancer you have. Some types of chemotherapy drugs are used for many types of cancer. Other drugs are used for just one or two types of cancer.

- Whether you have had chemotherapy before.

- Whether you have other health problems, such as diabetes or heart disease.

Where do I go for chemotherapy?

You may receive chemotherapy during a hospital stay, at home, or in a doctor's office, clinic, or outpatient unit in a hospital (which means you do not have to stay overnight). No matter where you go for chemotherapy, your doctor and nurse will watch for side effects and make any needed drug changes.

How often will I receive chemotherapy?

Treatment schedules for chemotherapy vary widely. How often and how long you get chemotherapy depends on:

- Your type of cancer and how advanced it is

- The goals of treatment (whether chemotherapy is used to cure your cancer, control its growth, or ease the symptoms)

- The type of chemotherapy

- How your body reacts to chemotherapy

You may receive chemotherapy in cycles. A cycle is a period of chemotherapy treatment followed by a period of rest. For instance, you might receive 1 week of chemotherapy followed by 3 weeks of rest.

These 4 weeks make up one cycle. The rest period gives your body a chance to build new healthy cells.

Can I miss a dose of chemotherapy?

It is not good to skip a chemotherapy treatment. But sometimes your doctor or nurse may change your chemotherapy schedule. This can be due to side affects you are having. If this happens, your doctor or nurse will explain what to do and when to start treatment again.

How is chemotherapy given?

Chemotherapy may be given in many ways.

- Injection. The chemotherapy is given by a shot in a muscle in your arm, thigh, or hip, or right under the skin in the fatty part of your arm, leg, or belly.

- Intra-arterial (IA). The chemotherapy goes directly into the artery that is feeding the cancer.

- Intraperitoneal (IP). The chemotherapy goes directly into the peritoneal cavity (the area that contains organs such as your intestines, stomach, liver, and ovaries).

- Intravenous (IV). The chemotherapy goes directly into a vein.

- Topical. The chemotherapy comes in a cream that you rub onto your skin.

- Oral. The chemotherapy comes in pills, capsules, or liquids that you swallow.

How will I feel during chemotherapy?

Chemotherapy affects people in different ways. How you feel depends on how healthy you are before treatment, your type of cancer, how advanced it is, the kind of chemotherapy you are getting, and the dose. Doctors and nurses cannot know for certain how you will feel during chemotherapy. Some people do not feel well right after chemotherapy. The most common side effect is fatigue, feeling exhausted and worn out. You can prepare for fatigue by:

- Asking someone to drive you to and from chemotherapy
- Planning time to rest on the day of and day after chemotherapy

- Getting help with meals and childcare the day of and at least 1 day after chemotherapy.

There are many ways you can help manage chemotherapy side effects.

Editor's Note: For more information, see Section 46.4. Side Effects and Ways to Manage them.

Can I work during chemotherapy?

Many people can work during chemotherapy, as long as they match their schedule to how they feel. Whether or not you can work may depend on what kind of work you do. If your job allows, you may want to see if you can work part-time or work from home on days you do not feel well.

Many employers are required by law to change your work schedule to meet your needs during cancer treatment. Talk with your employer about ways to adjust your work during chemotherapy. You can learn more about these laws by talking with a social worker.

Can I take over-the-counter and prescription drugs while I get chemotherapy?

This depends on the type of chemotherapy you get and the other types of drugs you plan to take. Take only drugs that are approved by your doctor or nurse. Tell your doctor or nurse about all the over-the-counter and prescription drugs you take, including laxatives, allergy medicines, cold medicines, pain relievers, aspirin, and ibuprofen. One way to let your doctor or nurse know about these drugs is by bringing in all your pill bottles. Your doctor or nurse needs to know:

- The name of each drug
- The reason you take it
- How much you take
- How often you take it

Can I take vitamins, minerals, dietary supplements, or herbs while I get chemotherapy?

Some of these products can change how chemotherapy works. For this reason, it is important to tell your doctor or nurse about all the vitamins, minerals, dietary supplements, and herbs that you take before you start chemotherapy. During chemotherapy, talk with your doctor before you take any of these products.

How will I know if my chemotherapy is working?

Your doctor will give you physical exams and medical tests (such as blood tests and x-rays). He or she will also ask you how you feel.

You cannot tell if chemotherapy is working based on its side effects. Some people think that severe side effects mean that chemotherapy is working well, or that no side effects mean that chemotherapy is not working. The truth is that side effects have nothing to do with how well chemotherapy is fighting your cancer.

How much does chemotherapy cost?

It is hard to say how much chemotherapy will cost. It depends on:

- The types and doses of chemotherapy used
- How long and how often chemotherapy is given
- Whether you get chemotherapy at home, in a clinic or office, or during a hospital stay
- The part of the country where you live

Does my health insurance pay for chemotherapy?

- Talk with your health insurance company about what costs it will pay for. Questions to ask include:
- What will my insurance pay for?
- Do I need to call my insurance company before each treatment for it to be covered? Or, does my doctor's office need to call?
- What do I have to pay for?
- Can I see any doctor I want or do I need to choose from a list of preferred providers?
- Do I need a written referral to see a specialist?
- Is there a co-pay (money I have to pay) each time I have an appointment?

- Is there a deductible (certain amount I need to pay) before my insurance pays?

- Where should I get my prescription drugs?

- Does my insurance pay for all my tests and treatments, whether I am an inpatient or outpatient?

How can I best work with my insurance plan?

- Read your insurance policy before treatment starts to find out what your plan will and will not pay for.

- Keep records of all your treatment costs and insurance claims.

- Send your insurance company all the paperwork it asks for. This may include receipts from doctors' visits, prescriptions, and lab work. Be sure to also keep copies for your own records.

- As needed, ask for help with the insurance paperwork. You can ask a friend, family member, social worker, or local group such as a senior center.

- If your insurance does not pay for something you think it should, find out why the plan refused to pay. Then talk with your doctor or nurse about what to do next. He or she may suggest ways to appeal the decision or other actions to take.

What are clinical trials and are they an option for me?

Cancer clinical trials (also called cancer treatment studies or research studies) test new treatments for people with cancer. These can be studies of new types of chemotherapy, other types of treatment, or new ways to combine treatments. The goal of all these clinical trials is to find better ways to help people with cancer. Your doctor or nurse may suggest you take part in a clinical trial. You can also suggest the idea. Before you agree to be in a clinical trial, learn about:

- **Benefits**. All clinical trials offer quality cancer care. Ask how this clinical trial could help you or others. For instance, you may be one of the first people to get a new treatment or drug.

- **Risks**. New treatments are not always better or even as good as **standard treatments**. And even if this new treatment is good, it may not work well for you.

907

- **Payment**. Your insurance company may or may not pay for treatment that is part of a clinical trial. Before you agree to be in a trial, check with your insurance company to make sure it will pay for this treatment.

Section 46.2

Tips for Meeting with Your Doctor or Nurse

- Make a list of your questions before each appointment. Some people keep a "running list" and write down new questions as they think of them. Make sure to have space on this list to write down the answers from your doctor or nurse.

- Bring a family member or trusted friend to your medical visits. This person can help you understand what the doctor or nurse says and talk with you about it after the visit is over.

- Ask all your questions. There is no such thing as a stupid question. If you do not understand an answer, keep asking until you do.

- Take notes. You can write them down or use a tape recorder. Later, you can review your notes and remember what was said.

- Ask for printed information about your type of cancer and chemotherapy.

- Let your doctor or nurse know how much information you want to know, when you want to learn it, and when you have learned enough. Some people want to learn everything they can about cancer and its treatment. Others only want a little information. The choice is yours.

- Find out how to contact your doctor or nurse in an emergency. This includes who to call and where to go.

Questions to Ask

About My Cancer
- What kind of cancer do I have?

- What is the stage of my cancer?

About Chemotherapy

- Why do I need chemotherapy?
- What is the goal of this chemotherapy?
- What are the benefits of chemotherapy?
- What are the risks of chemotherapy?

About My Treatment

- Are there other ways to treat my type of cancer?
- What is the standard care for my type of cancer?
- Are there any clinical trials for my type of cancer?
- How many cycles of chemotherapy will I get? How long is each treatment? How long between treatments?
- What types of chemotherapy will I get?
- How will these drugs be given?
- Where do I go for this treatment?
- How long does each treatment last?
- Should someone drive me to and from treatments?

About Side Effects

- What side effects can I expect right away?
- What side effects can I expect later?
- How serious are these side effects?
- How long will these side effects last?
- Will all the side effects go away when treatment is over?
- What can I do to manage or ease these side effects?
- What can my doctor or nurse do to manage or ease side effects?
- When should I call my doctor or nurse about these side effects?

Section 46.3

Your Feelings During Chemotherapy

At some point during chemotherapy, you may feel:

- Frustrated

- Helpless

- Lonely

- Anxious

- Depressed

- Afraid

- Angry

It is normal to have a wide range of feelings while going through chemotherapy. After all, living with cancer and getting treatment can be stressful. You may also feel fatigue, which can make it harder to cope with your feelings.

How can I cope with my feelings during chemotherapy?

- **Relax**. Find some quiet time and think of yourself in a favorite place. Breathe slowly or listen to soothing music. This may help you feel calmer and less stressed.

- **Exercise**. Many people find that light exercise helps them feel better. There are many ways for you to exercise, such as walking, riding a bike, and doing yoga. Talk with your doctor or nurse about ways you can exercise.

- **Talk with others**. Talk about your feelings with someone you trust. Choose someone who can focus on you, such as a close friend, family member, chaplain, nurse, or social worker. You may also find it helpful to talk with someone else who is getting chemotherapy.

- **Join a support group**. Cancer support groups provide support for people with cancer. These groups allow you to meet others with the same problems. You will have a chance to talk about your feelings and listen to other people talk about theirs. You can find out how others cope with cancer, chemotherapy, and side effects. Your doctor, nurse, or social worker may know about support groups near where you live. Some support groups also meet online (over the Internet), which can be helpful if you cannot travel. Talk to your doctor or nurse about things that worry or upset you. You may want to ask about seeing a counselor. Your doctor may also suggest that you take medication if you find it very hard to cope with your feelings.

Section 46.4

Side Effects and Ways to Manage Them

What are side effects?

Side effects are problems caused by cancer treatment. Some common side effects from chemotherapy are fatigue, **nausea, vomiting**, decreased **blood cell counts**, hair loss, mouth sores, and pain.

What causes side effects?

Chemotherapy is designed to kill fast-growing cancer cells. But it can also affect healthy cells that grow quickly. These include cells that line your mouth and intestines, cells in your **bone marrow** that make blood cells, and cells that make your hair grow. Chemotherapy causes side effects when it harms these healthy cells.

Will I get side effects from chemotherapy?

You may have a lot of side effects, some, or none at all. This depends on the type and amount of chemotherapy you get and how your body reacts. Before you start chemotherapy, talk with your doctor or nurse about which side effects to expect.

How long do side effects last?

How long side effects last depends on your health and the kind of chemotherapy you get. Most side effects go away after chemotherapy is over. But sometimes it can take months or even years for them to go away. Sometimes, chemotherapy causes long-term side effects that do not go away. These may include damage to your heart, lungs, nerves, kidneys, or reproductive organs. Some types of chemotherapy may cause a second cancer years later. Ask your doctor or nurse about your chance of having long-term side effects.

What can be done about side effects?

Doctors have many ways to prevent or treat chemotherapy side effects and help you heal after each treatment session. Talk with your doctor or nurse about which ones to expect and what to do about them. Make sure to let your doctor or nurse know about any changes you notice—they may be signs of a side effect.

Side Effects at a Glance

Anemia

What it is and why it occurs?

Red blood cells carry oxygen throughout your body. **Anemia** is when you have too few red blood cells to carry the oxygen your body needs. Your heart works harder when your body does not get enough oxygen. This can make it feel like your heart is pounding or beating very fast. Anemia can also make you feel short of breath, weak, dizzy, faint, or very tired. Some types of chemotherapy cause anemia because they make it harder for bone marrow to produce new red blood cells.

Ways to manage

- **Get plenty of rest.** Try to sleep at least 8 hours each night. You might also want to take 1 to 2 short naps (1 hour or less) during the day.

- **Limit your activities.** This means doing only the activities that are most important to you. For example, you might go to work but not clean the house. Or you might order takeout food instead of cooking dinner.

- **Accept help.** When your family or friends offer to help, let them. They can help care for your children, pick up groceries, run errands, drive you to doctor's visits, or do other chores you feel too tired to do.

- **Eat a well-balanced diet.** Choose a diet that contains all the calories and protein your body needs. Calories will help keep your weight up, and extra protein can help repair tissues that have been harmed by cancer treatment. Talk to your doctor, nurse, or dietitian about the diet that is right for you.

- **Stand up slowly.** You may feel dizzy if you stand up too fast. When you get up from lying down, sit for a minute before you stand.

Your doctor or nurse will check your blood cell count throughout your chemotherapy. You may need a blood transfusion if your red blood cell count falls too low. Your doctor may also prescribe a medicine to boost (speed up) the growth of red blood cells or suggest that you take iron or other vitamins.

Appetite Changes

What they are and why they occur

Chemotherapy can cause appetite changes. You may lose your appetite because of nausea (feeling like you are going to throw up), mouth and throat problems that make it painful to eat, or drugs that cause you to lose your taste for food. The changes can also come from feeling depressed or tired. Appetite loss may last for a day, a few weeks, or even months.

It is important to eat well, even when you have no appetite. This means eating and drinking foods that have plenty of protein, vitamins, and calories. Eating well helps your body fight infection and repair tissues that are damaged by chemotherapy. Not eating well can lead to weight loss, weakness, and fatigue.

Some cancer treatments cause weight gain or an increase in your appetite. Be sure to ask your doctor, nurse, or dietitian what types of appetite changes you might expect and how to manage them.

Ways to manage

- **Eat 5 to 6 small meals or snacks each day instead of 3 big meals.** Choose foods and drinks that are high in calories and protein.

- **Set a daily schedule for eating your meals and snacks.** Eat when it is time to eat, rather than when you feel hungry. You may not feel hungry while you are on chemotherapy, but you still need to eat.

- **Drink milkshakes, smoothies, juice, or soup if you do not feel like eating solid foods.** Liquids like these can help provide the protein, vitamins, and calories your body needs.

- **Use plastic forks and spoons. Some types of chemo give you a metal taste in your mouth.** Eating with plastic can help decrease the metal taste. Cooking in glass pots and pans can also help.

- **Increase your appetite by doing something active.** For instance, you might have more of an appetite if you take a short walk before lunch. Also, be careful not to decrease your appetite by drinking too much liquid before or during meals.

- **Change your routine.** This may mean eating in a different place, such as the dining room rather than the kitchen. It can also mean eating with other people instead of eating alone. If you eat alone, you may want to listen to the radio or watch TV. You may also want to vary your diet by trying new foods and recipes.

- **Talk with your doctor, nurse, or dietitian.** He or she may want you to take extra vitamins or nutrition supplements (such as high protein drinks). If you cannot eat for a long time and are losing weight, you may need to take drugs that increase your appetite or receive nutrition through an IV or feeding tube.

Bleeding

What it is and why it occurs

Platelets are cells that make your blood clot when you bleed. Chemotherapy can lower the number of platelets because it affects your bone marrow's ability to make them. A low platelet count is called

thrombocytopenia. This condition may cause bruises (even when you have not been hit or have not bumped into anything), bleeding from your nose or in your mouth, or a rash of tiny, red dots.

Ways to manage

Do:

- Brush your teeth with a very soft toothbrush
- Soften the bristles of your toothbrush by running hot water over them before you brush
- Blow your nose gently
- Be careful when using scissors, knives, or other sharp objects
- Use an electric shaver instead of a razor
- Apply gentle but firm pressure to any cuts you get until the bleeding stops
- Wear shoes all the time, even inside the house or hospital

Do not:

- Use dental floss or toothpicks
- Play sports or do other activities during which you could get hurt. Use tampons, enemas, suppositories, or rectal thermometers
- Wear clothes with tight collars, wrists, or waistbands

Check with your doctor or nurse before:

- Drinking beer, wine, or other types of alcohol
- Having sex
- Taking vitamins, herbs, minerals, dietary supplements, aspirin, or other over-the counter medicines. Some of these products can change how chemotherapy works

Let your doctor know if you are constipated.

He or she may prescribe a stool softener to prevent straining and rectal bleeding when you go to the bathroom.

Your doctor or nurse will check your platelet count often.

You may need medication, a platelet transfusion, or a delay in your chemotherapy treatment if your platelet count is too low.

Call your doctor or nurse if you have any of these symptoms:

- Bruises, especially if you did not bump into anything
- Small, red spots on your skin
- Red- or pink-colored urine
- Black or bloody bowel movements
- Bleeding from your gums or nose
- Heavy bleeding during your menstrual period or for a prolonged period
- Vaginal bleeding not caused by your period
- Headaches or changes in your vision
- A warm or hot feeling in your arm or leg
- Feeling very sleepy or confused

Constipation

What it is and why it occurs

Constipation is when bowel movements become less frequent and stools are hard, dry, and difficult to pass. You may have painful bowel movements and feel bloated or nauseous. You may belch, pass a lot of gas, and have stomach cramps or pressure in the rectum.

Drugs such as chemotherapy and pain medicine can cause constipation. It can also happen when people are not active and spend a lot of time sitting or lying down. Constipation can also be due to eating foods that are low in fiber or not drinking enough fluids.

Ways to manage

- **Keep a record of your bowel movements.** Show this record to your doctor or nurse and talk about what is normal for you. This makes it easier to figure out whether you have constipation.

- **Drink at least 8 cups of water or other fluids each day.** Many people find that drinking warm or hot fluids, such as coffee and tea, helps with constipation. Fruit juices, such as prune juice, may also be helpful.

- **Be active every day. You can be active by walking, riding a bike, or doing yoga.** If you cannot walk, ask about exercises that you can do in a chair or bed. Talk with your doctor or nurse about ways you can be more active.

- **Ask your doctor, nurse, or dietitian about foods that are high in fiber.** Eating high-fiber foods and drinking lots of fluids can help soften your stools. Good sources of fiber include whole-grain breads and cereals, dried beans and peas, raw vegetables, fresh and dried fruit, nuts, seeds, and popcorn.

- **Let your doctor or nurse know if you have not had a bowel movement in 2 days.** Your doctor may suggest a fiber supplement, laxative, stool softener, or enema. Do not use these treatments without first checking with your doctor or nurse.

Diarrhea

What it is and why it occurs

Diarrhea is frequent bowel movements that may be soft, loose, or watery. Chemotherapy can cause diarrhea because it harms healthy cells that line your large and small intestines. It may also speed up your bowels. Diarrhea can also be caused by infections or drugs used to treat constipation.

Ways to manage

- **Eat 5 or 6 small meals and snacks each day instead of 3 large meals.**

- **Ask your doctor or nurse about foods that are high in salts such as sodium and potassium.** Your body can lose these salts when you have diarrhea, and it is important to replace them. Foods that are high in sodium or potassium include bananas, oranges, peach and apricot nectar, and boiled or mashed potatoes.

- **Drink 8 to 12 cups of clear liquids each day.** These include water, clear broth, ginger ale, or sports drinks such as Gatorade® or Propel®. Drink slowly, and choose drinks that are at room temperature. Let carbonated drinks lose their fizz before you drink them. Add extra water if drinks make you thirsty or nauseous (feeling like you are going to throw up).

- **Eat low-fiber foods.** Foods that are high in fiber can make diarrhea worse. Low-fiber foods include bananas, white rice, white toast, and plain or vanilla yogurt. See page 56 for other low-fiber foods.

- **Let your doctor or nurse know if your diarrhea lasts for more than 24 hours or if you have pain and cramping along with diarrhea.** Your doctor may prescribe a medicine to control the diarrhea. You may also need IV fluids to replace the water and nutrients you lost. Do not take any medicine for diarrhea without first asking your doctor or nurse.

- **Be gentle when you wipe yourself after a bowel movement.** Instead of toilet paper, use a baby wipe or squirt of water from a spray bottle to clean yourself after bowel movements. Let your doctor or nurse know if your rectal area is sore or bleeds or if you have hemorrhoids.

- **Ask your doctor if you should try a clear liquid diet.** This can give your bowels time to rest. Most people stay on this type of diet for 5 days or less.

Stay away from:

- Drinks that are very hot or very cold

- Beer, wine, and other types of alcohol

- Milk or milk products, such as ice cream, milkshakes, sour cream, and cheese

- Spicy foods, such as hot sauce, salsa, chili, and curry dishes

- Greasy and fried foods, such as french fries and hamburgers

- Foods or drinks with caffeine, such as regular coffee, black tea, cola, and chocolate

- Foods or drinks that cause gas, such as cooked dried beans, cabbage, broccoli, and soy milk and other soy products

- Foods that are high in fiber, such as cooked dried beans, raw fruits and vegetables, nuts, and whole-wheat breads and cereal

Fatigue

What it is and why it occurs

Fatigue from chemotherapy can range from a mild to extreme feeling of being tired. Many people describe fatigue as feeling weak, weary, worn out, heavy, or slow. Resting does not always help.

Many people say they feel fatigue during chemotherapy and even for weeks or months after treatment is over. Fatigue can be caused by the type of chemotherapy, the effort of making frequent visits to the doctor, or feelings such as stress, anxiety, and depression. If you receive radiation therapy along with chemotherapy, your fatigue may be more severe. Fatigue can also be caused by:

- Anemia

- Pain

- Medications

- Appetite changes

- Trouble sleeping

- Lack of activity

- Trouble breathing

- Infection

- Doing too much at one time

- Other medical problems

Fatigue can happen all at once or little by little. People feel fatigue in different ways. You may feel more or less fatigue than someone else who gets the same type of chemotherapy.

Ways to manage

- **Relax.** You might want to try meditation, prayer, yoga, guided imagery, visualization, or other ways to relax and decrease stress.

- **Eat and drink well.** Often, this means 5 to 6 small meals and snacks rather than 3 large meals. Keep foods around that are easy to fix, such as canned soups, frozen meals, yogurt, and cottage cheese. Drink plenty of fluids each day—about 8 cups of water or juice.

- **Plan time to rest.** You may feel better when you rest or take a short nap during the day. Many people say that it helps to rest for just 10 to 15 minutes rather than nap for a long time. If you nap, try to sleep for less than 1 hour. Keeping naps short will help you sleep better at night.

- **Be active.** Research shows that exercise can ease fatigue and help you sleep better at night. Try going for a 15-minute walk, doing yoga, or riding an exercise bike. Plan to be active when you have the most energy. Talk with your doctor or nurse about ways you can be active while getting chemotherapy.

- **Try not to do too much.** With fatigue, you may not have enough energy to do all the things you want to do. Choose the activities you want to do and let someone else help with the others. Try quiet activities, such as reading, knitting, or learning a new language on tape.

- **Sleep at least 8 hours each night.** This may be more sleep than you needed before chemotherapy. You are likely to sleep better at night when you are active during the day. You may also find it helpful to relax before going to bed. For instance, you might read a book, work on a jigsaw puzzle, listen to music, or do other quiet hobbies.

- **Plan a work schedule that works for you.** Fatigue may affect the amount of energy you have for your job. You may feel well enough to work your full schedule. Or you may need to work less—maybe just a few hours a day or a few days each week. If your job allows, you may want to talk with your boss about ways to work from home. Or you may want to go on medical leave (stop working for a while) while getting chemotherapy.

- **Let others help.** Ask family members and friends to help when you feel fatigue. Perhaps they can help with household chores or drive you to and from doctor's visits. They might also help by shopping for food and cooking meals for you to eat now or freeze for later.

- **Learn from others who have cancer.** People who have cancer can help by sharing ways that they manage fatigue. One way to meet others is by joining a support group—either in person or online. Talk with your doctor or nurse to learn more.

- **Keep a diary of how you feel each day.** This will help you plan how to best use your time. Share your diary with your nurse.

Let your doctor or nurse know if you notice changes in your energy level, whether you have lots of energy or are very tired.

- **Talk with your doctor or nurse.** Your doctor may prescribe medication that can help decrease fatigue, give you a sense of well-being, and increase your appetite. He or she may also suggest treatment if your fatigue is from anemia.

Hair Loss

What it is and why it occurs

Hair loss (also called **alopecia**) is when some or all of your hair falls out. This can happen anywhere on your body: your head, face, arms, legs, underarms, or the pubic area between your legs. Many people are upset by the loss of their hair and find it the most difficult part of chemotherapy.

Some types of chemotherapy damage the cells that cause hair growth. Hair loss often starts 2 to 3 weeks after chemotherapy begins. Your scalp may hurt at first. Then you may lose your hair, either a little at a time or in clumps. It takes about 1 week for all your hair to fall out. Almost always, your hair will grow back 2 to 3 months after chemotherapy is over. You may notice that your hair starts growing back even while you are getting chemotherapy.

Your hair will be very fine when it starts growing back. Also, your new hair may not look or feel the same as it did before. For instance, your hair may be thin instead of thick, curly instead of straight, and darker or lighter in color.

Ways to manage

Before hair loss:

- **Talk with your doctor or nurse.** He or she will know if you are likely to have hair loss.

- **Cut your hair short or shave your head.** You might feel more in control of hair loss if you first cut your hair or shave your head. This often makes hair loss easier to manage. If you shave your head, use an electric shaver instead of a razor.

- **The best time to choose your wig is before chemotherapy starts.** This way, you can match the wig to the color and style of your hair. You might also take it to your hair dresser who can

921

style the wig to look like your own hair. Make sure to choose a wig that feels comfortable and does not hurt your scalp.

- **Ask if your insurance company will pay for a wig.** If it will not, you can deduct the cost of your wig as a medical expense on your income tax. Some groups also have free "wig banks." Your doctor, nurse, or social worker will know if there is a wig bank near you.

- **Be gentle when you wash your hair.** Use a mild shampoo, such as a baby shampoo. Dry your hair by patting (not rubbing) it with a soft towel.

- **Do not use items that can hurt your scalp.** These include:
  - Straightening or curling irons
  - Brush rollers or curlers
  - Electric hair dryers
  - Hair bands and clips
  - Hairsprays
  - Hair dyes
  - Products to perm or relax your hair

After hair loss:

- **Protect your scalp.** Your scalp may hurt during and after hair loss. Protect it by wearing a hat, turban, or scarf when you are outside. Try to avoid places that are very hot or very cold. This includes tanning beds and outside in the sun or cold air. And always apply sunscreen or sunblock to protect your scalp.

- **Stay warm.** You may feel colder once you lose your hair. Wear a hat, turban, scarf, or wig to help you stay warm.

- **Sleep on a satin pillow case.** Satin creates less friction than cotton when you sleep on it. Therefore, you may find satin pillow cases more comfortable.

- **Talk about your feelings.** Many people feel angry, depressed, or embarrassed about hair loss. If you are very worried or upset, you might want to talk about these feelings with a doctor, nurse, family member, close friend, or someone who has had hair loss caused by cancer treatment.

Infection

What it is and why it occurs

Some types of chemotherapy make it harder for your bone marrow to produce new white blood cells. **White blood cells** help your body fight infection. Therefore, it is important to avoid infections, since chemotherapy decreases the number of your white blood cells.

There are many types of white blood cells. One type is called **neutrophil**. When your neutrophil count is low, it is called **neutropenia**. Your doctor or nurse may do blood tests to find out whether you have neutropenia.

It is important to watch for signs of infection when you have neutropenia. Check for fever at least once a day, or as often as your doctor or nurse tells you to. You may find it best to use a digital thermometer. Call your doctor or nurse if your temperature is 100.5°F or higher.

Ways to manage

- **Your doctor or nurse will check your white blood cell count throughout your treatment.** If chemotherapy is likely to make your white blood cell count very low, you may get medicine to raise your white blood cell count and lower your risk of infection.

- **Wash your hands often with soap and water.** Be sure to wash your hands before cooking and eating, and after you use the bathroom, blow your nose, cough, sneeze, or touch animals. Carry hand sanitizer for times when you are not near soap and water.

- **Use sanitizing wipes to clean surfaces and items that you touch.** This includes public telephones, ATM machines, doorknobs, and other common items.

- **Be gentle and thorough when you wipe yourself after a bowel movement.** Instead of toilet paper, use a baby wipe or squirt of water from a spray bottle to clean yourself. Let your doctor or nurse know if your rectal area is sore or bleeds or if you have hemorrhoids.

- **Stay away from people who are sick.** This includes people with colds, flu, measles, or chicken pox. You also need to stay away from children who just had a "live virus" vaccine for chicken pox or polio. Call your doctor, nurse, or local health department if you have any questions.

923

- **Stay away from crowds.** Try not to be around a lot of people. For instance, plan to go shopping or to the movies when the stores and theaters are less crowded.

- **Be careful not to cut or nick yourself.** Do not cut or tear your nail cuticles. Use an electric shaver instead of a razor. And be extra careful when using scissors, needles, or knives.

- **Watch for signs of infection around your catheter.** Signs include drainage, redness, swelling, or soreness. Let your doctor or nurse know about any changes you notice near your catheter.

- **Maintain good mouth care.** Brush your teeth after meals and before you go to bed. Use a very soft toothbrush. You can make the bristles even softer by running hot water over them just before you brush. Use a mouth rinse that does not contain alcohol. Check with your doctor or nurse before going to the dentist.

- **Take good care of your skin.** Do not squeeze or scratch pimples. Use lotion to soften and heal dry, cracked skin. Dry yourself after a bath or shower by gently patting (not rubbing) your skin.

- **Clean cuts right away.** Use warm water, soap, and an antiseptic to clean your cuts. Do this every day until your cut has a scab over it.

- **Be careful around animals.** Do not clean your cat's litter box, pick up dog waste, or clean bird cages or fish tanks. Be sure to wash your hands after touching pets and other animals.

- **Do not get a flu shot or other type of vaccine without first asking your doctor or nurse.** Some vaccines contain a live virus, which you should not be exposed to.

- **Keep hot foods hot and cold foods cold.** Do not leave leftovers sitting out. Put them in the refrigerator as soon as you are done eating. Wash raw vegetables and fruits well before eating them.

- **Do not eat raw or undercooked fish, seafood, meat, chicken, or eggs.** These may have bacteria that can cause infection.

- **Do not have food or drinks that are moldy, spoiled, or past the freshness date.**

Call your doctor right away (even on the weekend or in the middle of the night) if you think you have an infection. Be sure you know how to reach your doctor after office hours and on weekends. Call if you have a fever of 100.5°F or higher, or when you have chills or sweats. Do not take aspirin, acetaminophen (such as Tylenol®), ibuprofen products, or any other drugs that reduce fever without first talking with your doctor or nurse. Other signs of infection include:

- Redness
- Swelling
- Rash
- Chills
- Cough
- Earache
- Headache
- Stiff neck
- Bloody or cloudy urine
- Painful or frequent need to urinate
- Sinus pain or pressure

Infertility

What it is and why it occurs

Some types of chemotherapy can cause **infertility**. For a woman, this means that you may not be able to get pregnant. For a man, this means you may not be able to get a woman pregnant.

In women, chemotherapy may damage the ovaries. This damage can lower the number of healthy eggs in the ovaries. It can also lower the **hormones** produced by them. The drop in hormones can lead to early menopause. Early menopause and fewer healthy eggs can cause infertility.

In men, chemotherapy may damage sperm cells, which grow and divide quickly. Infertility may occur because chemotherapy can lower the number of sperm, make sperm less able to move, or cause other types of damage.

Whether or not you become infertile depends on the type of chemotherapy you get, your age, and whether you have other health problems. Infertility can last the rest of your life.

Ways to manage

For WOMEN, talk with your doctor or nurse about:

- **Whether you want to have children.** Before you start chemotherapy, let your doctor or nurse know if you might want to get pregnant in the future. He or she may talk with you about ways to preserve your eggs to use after treatment ends or refer you to a fertility specialist.

- **Birth control.** It is very important that you do not get pregnant while getting chemotherapy. These drugs can hurt the fetus, especially in the first 3 months of pregnancy. If you have not yet gone through menopause, talk with your doctor or nurse about birth control and ways to keep from getting pregnant.

- **Pregnancy.** If you still have menstrual periods, your doctor or nurse may ask you to have a pregnancy test before you start chemotherapy. If you are pregnant, your doctor or nurse will talk with you about other treatment options.

For MEN, talk with your doctor or nurse about:

- **Whether you want to have children.** Before you start chemotherapy, let your doctor or nurse know if you might want to father children in the future. He or she may talk with you about ways to preserve your sperm to use in the future or refer you to a fertility specialist.

- **Birth control.** It is very important that your spouse or partner does not get pregnant while you are getting chemotherapy. Chemotherapy can damage your sperm and cause birth defects.

Mouth and Throat Changes

What they are and why they occur

Some types of chemotherapy harm fast-growing cells, such as those that line your mouth, throat, and lips. This can affect your teeth, gums, the lining of your mouth, and the glands that make saliva. Most mouth problems go away a few days after chemotherapy is over.

Mouth and throat problems may include:

- Dry mouth (having little or no saliva)
- Changes in taste and smell (such as when food tastes like metal or chalk, has no taste, or does not taste or smell like it used to)
- Infections of your gums, teeth, or tongue
- Increased sensitivity to hot or cold foods
- Mouth sores
- Trouble eating when your mouth gets very sore

Ways to manage

- **Visit a dentist at least 2 weeks before starting chemotherapy.** It is important to have your mouth as healthy as possible. This means getting all your dental work done before chemotherapy starts. If you cannot go to the dentist before chemotherapy starts, ask your doctor or nurse when it is safe to go. Be sure to tell your dentist that you have cancer and about your treatment plan.

- **Check your mouth and tongue every day.** This way, you can see or feel problems (such as mouth sores, white spots, or infections) as soon as they start. Inform your doctor or nurse about these problems right away.

- **Keep your mouth moist.** You can keep your mouth moist by sipping water throughout the day, sucking on ice chips or sugar free hard candy, or chewing sugar-free gum. Ask your doctor or nurse about saliva substitutes if your mouth is always dry.

- **Clean your mouth, teeth, gums, and tongue.**
  - Brush your teeth, gums, and tongue after each meal and at bedtime.
  - Use an extra-soft toothbrush. You can make the bristles even softer by rinsing your toothbrush in hot water before you brush.
  - If brushing is painful, try cleaning your teeth with cotton swabs or Toothettes®.
  - Use a fluoride toothpaste or special fluoride gel that your dentist prescribes.

927

- Do not use mouthwash that has alcohol. Instead, rinse your mouth 3 to 4 times a day with a solution of 1/4 teaspoon baking soda and 1/8 teaspoon salt in 1 cup of warm water. Follow this with a plain water rinse.

- Gently floss your teeth every day. If your gums bleed or hurt, avoid those areas but floss your other teeth. Ask your doctor or nurse about flossing if your platelet count is low.

- If you wear dentures, make sure they fit well and keep them clean. Also, limit the length of time that you wear them.

- Be careful what you eat when your mouth is sore.

  - Choose foods that are moist, soft, and easy to chew or swallow. These include cooked cereals, mashed potatoes, and scrambled eggs.

  - Use a blender to puree cooked foods so that they are easier to eat. To help avoid infection, be sure to wash all blender parts before and after using them. If possible, it is best to wash them in a dishwasher.

  - Take small bites of food, chew slowly, and sip liquids while you eat.

  - Soften food with gravy, sauces, broth, yogurt, or other liquids.

  - Eat foods that are cool or at room temperature. You may find that warm and hot foods hurt your mouth or throat.

  - Suck on ice chips or popsicles. These can relieve mouth pain.

  - Ask your dietitian for ideas of foods that are easy to eat. For ideas of soft foods that are easy on a sore mouth.

Call your doctor, nurse, or dentist if your mouth hurts a lot. Your doctor or dentist may prescribe medicine for pain or to keep your mouth moist. Make sure to give your dentist the phone number of your doctor and nurse.

- **Stay away from** things that can hurt, scrape, or burn your mouth, such as:

  - Sharp or crunchy foods, such as crackers and potato or corn chips

  - Spicy foods, such as hot sauce, curry dishes, salsa, and chili

- Citrus fruits or juices such as orange, lemon, and grapefruit

- Food and drinks that have a lot of sugar, such as candy or soda

- Beer, wine, and other types of alcohol

- Toothpicks or other sharp objects

- Tobacco products, including cigarettes, pipes, cigars, and chewing tobacco

Nausea and Vomiting

What they are and why they occur

Some types of chemotherapy can cause nausea, vomiting, or both. Nausea is when you feel sick to your stomach, like you are going to throw up. Vomiting is when you throw up. You may also have **dry heaves,** which is when your body tries to vomit even though your stomach is empty.

Nausea and vomiting can occur while you are getting chemotherapy, right after, or many hours or days later. You will most likely feel better on the days you do not get chemotherapy.

New drugs can help prevent nausea and vomiting. These are called **antiemetic** or **antinausea** drugs. You may need to take these drugs 1 hour before each chemotherapy treatment and for a few days after. How long you take them after chemotherapy will depend on the type of chemotherapy you are getting and how you react to it. If one anti-nausea drug does not work well for you, your doctor can prescribe a different one. You may need to take more than one type of drug to help with nausea. **Acupuncture** may also help. Talk with your doctor or nurse about treatments to control nausea and vomiting caused by chemotherapy.

Ways to manage

- **Prevent nausea.** One way to prevent vomiting is to prevent nausea. Try having bland, easy-to-digest foods and drinks that do not upset your stomach. These include plain crackers, toast, and gelatin.

- **Plan when it's best for you to eat and drink.** Some people feel better when they eat a light meal or snack before

929

chemotherapy. Others feel better when they have chemotherapy on an empty stomach (nothing to eat or drink for 2 to 3 hours before treatment). After treatment, wait at least 1 hour before you eat or drink.

- **Eat small meals and snacks.** Instead of 3 large meals each day, you might feel better if you eat 5 or 6 small meals and snacks. Do not drink a lot before or during meals. Also, do not lie down right after you eat.

- **Have foods and drinks that are warm or cool (not hot or cold).** Give hot foods and drinks time to cool down, or make them colder by adding ice. You can warm up cold foods by taking them out of the refrigerator 1 hour before you eat or warming them slightly in a microwave. Drink cola or ginger ale that is warm and has lost its fizz.

- **Stay away from foods and drinks with strong smells.** These include coffee, fish, onions, garlic, and foods that are cooking.

- **Try small bites of popsicles or fruit ices.** You may also find sucking on ice chips helpful.

- **Suck on sugar-free mints or tart candies.** But do not use tart candies if you have mouth or throat sores.

- **Relax before treatment.** You may feel less nausea if you relax before each chemotherapy treatment. Meditate, do deep breathing exercises, or imagine scenes or experiences that make you feel peaceful. You can also do quiet hobbies such as reading, listening to music, or knitting.

- **When you feel like vomiting, breathe deeply and slowly or get fresh air.** You might also distract yourself by chatting with friends or family, listening to music, or watching a movie or TV.

- **Talk with your doctor or nurse.** Your doctor can give you drugs to help prevent nausea during and after chemotherapy. Be sure to take these drugs as ordered and let your doctor or nurse know if they do not work. You might also ask your doctor or nurse about acupuncture, which can help relieve nausea and vomiting caused by cancer treatment.

Tell your doctor or nurse if you vomit for more than 1 day or right after you drink.

Nervous System Changes

What they are and why they occur

Chemotherapy can cause damage to your nervous system. Many nervous system problems get better within a year of when you finish chemotherapy, but some may last the rest of your life. Symptoms may include:

- Tingling, burning, weakness, or numbness in your hands or feet
- Feeling colder than normal
- Pain when walking
- Weak, sore, tired, or achy muscles
- Being clumsy and losing your balance
- Trouble picking up objects or buttoning your clothes
- Shaking or trembling
- Hearing loss
- Stomach pain, such as constipation or heartburn
- Fatigue
- Confusion and memory problems
- Dizziness
- Depression

Ways to Manage

- **Let your doctor or nurse know right away if you notice any nervous system changes.** It is important to treat these problems as soon as possible.

- **Be careful when handling knives, scissors, and other sharp or dangerous objects.**

- **Avoid falling.** Walk slowly, hold onto handrails when using the stairs, and put no-slip bath mats in your bathtub or shower. Make sure there are no area rugs or cords to trip over.

- **Always wear sneakers, tennis shoes, or other footwear with rubber soles.**

- **Check the temperature of your bath water with a thermometer.** This will keep you from getting burned by water that is too hot.

- **Be extra careful to avoid burning or cutting yourself while cooking.**

- **Wear gloves when working in the garden, cooking, or washing dishes.**

- **Rest when you need to.**

- **Steady yourself when you walk by using a cane or other device.**

- **Talk to your doctor or nurse if you notice memory problems, feel confused, or are depressed.**

- **Ask your doctor for pain medicine if you need it.**

Pain

What it is and why it occurs

Some types of chemotherapy cause painful side effects. These include burning, numbness, and tingling or shooting pains in your hands and feet. Mouth sores, headaches, muscle pains, and stomach pains can also occur.

Pain can be caused by the cancer itself or by chemotherapy. Doctors and nurses have ways to decrease or relieve your pain.

Ways to manage

- **Talk about your pain with a doctor, nurse, or pharmacist. Be specific and describe:**

  - Where you feel pain. Is it in one part of your body or all over?

  - What the pain feels like. Is it sharp, dull, or throbbing? Does it come and go, or is it steady?

  - How strong the pain is. Describe it on a scale of 0 to 10.

  - How long the pain lasts. Does it last for a few minutes, an hour, or longer?

  - What makes the pain better or worse. For instance, does an ice pack help? Or does the pain get worse if you move a certain way?

  - Which medicines you take for pain. Do they help? How long do they last? How much do you take? How often?

- **Let your family and friends know about your pain.** They need to know about your pain so they can help you. If you are very tired or in a lot of pain, they can call your doctor or nurse for you. Knowing about your pain can also help them understand why you may be acting differently.

- **Practice pain control**
  - Take your pain medicine on a regular schedule (by the clock) even when you are not in pain. This is very important when you have pain most of the time.
  - Do not skip doses of your pain medicine. Pain is harder to control and manage if you wait until you are in a lot of pain before taking medicine.
  - Try deep breathing, yoga, or other ways to relax. This can help reduce muscle tension, anxiety, and pain.

- **Ask to meet with a pain or palliative care specialist.** This can be an oncologist, anesthesiologist, neurologist, neurosurgeon, nurse, or pharmacist who will talk with you about ways to control your pain.

- **Let your doctor, nurse, or pain specialist know if your pain changes.** Your pain can change over the course of your treatment. When this happens, your pain medications may need to be changed.

Sexual Changes

What they are and why they occur

Some types of chemotherapy can cause sexual changes. These changes are different for women and men.

In women, chemotherapy may damage the ovaries, which can cause changes in hormone levels. Hormone changes can lead to problems like vaginal dryness and early menopause.

In men, chemotherapy can cause changes in hormone levels, decreased blood supply to the penis, or damage to the nerves that control the penis, all of which can lead to impotence.

Whether or not you have sexual changes during chemotherapy depends on if you have had these problems before, the type of chemotherapy you are getting, your age, and whether you have any other illnesses. Some problems, such as loss of interest in sex, are likely to improve once chemotherapy is over.

Problems for WOMEN include:

- Symptoms of menopause (for women not yet in menopause). These symptoms include:
  - Hot flashes
  - Vaginal dryness
  - Feeling irritable
  - Irregular or no menstrual periods
- Bladder or vaginal infections
- Vaginal discharge or itching
- Being too tired to have sex or not being interested in having sex
- Feeling too worried, stressed, or depressed to have sex

Problems for MEN include:

- Not being able to reach climax
- Impotence (not being able to get or keep an erection)
- Being too tired to have sex or not being interested in having sex
- Feeling too worried, stressed, or depressed to have sex

Ways to manage for WOMEN:

- **Talk with your doctor or nurse about:**
  - **Sex.** Ask your doctor or nurse if it is okay for you to have sex during chemotherapy. Most women can have sex, but it is a good idea to ask.
  - **Birth control.** It is very important that you not get pregnant while having chemotherapy. Chemotherapy may hurt the fetus, especially in the first 3 months of pregnancy. If you have not yet gone through menopause, talk with your doctor or nurse about birth control and ways to keep from getting pregnant.
  - **Medications.** Talk with your doctor, nurse, or pharmacist about medications that help with sexual problems. These include products to relieve vaginal dryness or a vaginal cream or suppository to reduce the chance of infection.

- **Wear cotton underwear (cotton underpants and panty-hose with cotton linings).**

- **Do not wear tight pants or shorts.**

- **Use a water-based vaginal lubricant (such as K-Y Jelly® or Astroglide®) when you have sex.**

- **If sex is still painful because of dryness, ask your doctor or nurse about medications to help restore moisture in your vagina.**

- **Cope with hot flashes by:**

  - **Dressing in layers,** with an extra sweater or jacket that you can take off.

  - **Being active.** This includes walking, riding a bike, or other types of exercise.

  - **Reducing stress.** Try yoga, meditation, or other ways to relax.

For MEN:

- **Talk with your doctor or nurse about:**

  - **Sex.** Ask your doctor or nurse if it is okay for you to have sex during chemotherapy. Most men can have sex, but it is a good idea to ask. Also, ask if you should use a condom when you have sex, since traces of chemotherapy may be in your semen.

  - **Birth control.** It is very important that your spouse or partner not get pregnant while you are getting chemother-apy. Chemotherapy can damage your sperm and cause birth defects.

For men AND women:

- **Be open and honest with your spouse or partner.** Talk about your feelings and concerns.

- **Explore new ways to show love.** You and your spouse or partner may want to show your love for each other in new ways while you go through chemotherapy. For instance, if you are having sex less often, you may want to hug and cuddle more, bathe together, give each other massages, or try other activities that make you feel close to each other.

935

- **Talk with a doctor, nurse, social worker, or counselor.** If you and your spouse or partner are concerned about sexual problems, you may want to talk with someone who can help. This can be a psychiatrist, psychologist, social worker, marriage counselor, sex therapist, or clergy member.

Skin and Nail Changes

What they are and why they occur

Some types of chemotherapy can damage the fast-growing cells in your skin and nails. While these changes may be painful and annoying, most are minor and do not require treatment. Many of them will get better once you have finished chemotherapy. However, major skin changes need to be treated right away because they can cause lifelong damage.

Minor skin changes may include:

- **Itching, dryness, redness, rashes, and peeling**

- **Darker veins.** Your veins may look darker when you get chemotherapy through an IV.

- **Sensitivity to the sun** (when you burn very quickly). This can happen even to people who have very dark skin color.

- **Nail problems.** This is when your nails become dark, turn yellow, or become brittle and cracked. Sometimes your nails will loosen and fall off, but new nails will grow back in.

Major skin changes can be caused by:

- **Radiation recall.** Some chemotherapy causes skin in the area where you had radiation therapy to turn red (ranging from very light to bright red). Your skin may blister, peel, or be very painful.

- **Chemotherapy leaking from your IV.** You need to let your doctor or nurse know right away if you have burning or pain when you get IV chemotherapy.

- **Allergic reactions to chemotherapy.** Some skin changes mean that you are allergic to the chemotherapy. Let your doctor or nurse know right away if you have sudden and severe itching, rashes, or hives, along with wheezing or other trouble breathing.

Ways to manage

- **Itching, dryness, redness, rashes, and peeling**
  - Apply cornstarch, as you would dusting powder.
  - Take quick showers or sponge baths instead of long, hot baths.
  - Pat (do not rub) yourself dry after bathing.
  - Wash with a mild, moisturizing soap.
  - Put on cream or lotion while your skin is still damp after washing. Tell your doctor or nurse if this does not help.
  - Do not use perfume, cologne, or aftershave lotion that has alcohol.
  - Take a colloidal oatmeal bath (special powder you add to bath water) when your whole body itches.

- **Acne**
  - Keep your face clean and dry.
  - Ask your doctor or nurse if you can use medicated creams or soaps and which ones to use.

- **Sensitivity to the sun**
  - Avoid direct sunlight. This means not being in the sun from 10 a.m. until 4 p.m. It is the time when the sun is strongest.
  - Use sunscreen lotion with an SPF (skin protection factor) of 15 or higher. Or use ointments that block the sun's rays, such as those with zinc oxide.
  - Keep your lips moist with a lip balm that has an SPF of 15 or higher.
  - Wear light-colored pants, long-sleeve cotton shirts, and hats with wide brims.
  - Do not use tanning beds.

- **Nail problems**
  - Wear gloves when washing dishes, working in the garden, or cleaning the house.
  - Use products to make your nails stronger. (Stop using these products if they hurt your nails or skin.)

- Let your doctor or nurse know if your cuticles are red and painful.

- **Radiation recall**

  - Protect the area of your skin that received radiation therapy from the sun.

  - Do not use tanning beds.

  - Place a cool, wet cloth where your skin hurts.

  - Wear clothes that are made of cotton or other soft fabrics. This includes your underwear (bras, underpants, and t-shirts).

  - Let your doctor or nurse know if you think you have radiation recall.

Urinary, Kidney, and Bladder Changes

What they are and why they occur

Some types of chemotherapy damage cells in the kidneys and bladder. Problems may include:

- Burning or pain when you begin to urinate or after you empty your bladder

- Frequent, more urgent need to urinate

- Not being able to urinate

- Not able to control the flow of urine from the bladder (incontinence)

- Blood in the urine

- Fever

- Chills

- Urine that is orange, red, green, or dark yellow or has a strong medicine odor

Some kidney and bladder problems will go away after you finish chemotherapy. Other problems can last for the rest of your life.

Ways to manage

- **Your doctor or nurse will take urine and blood samples to check how well your bladder and kidneys are working.**

- **Drink plenty of fluids.** Fluids will help flush the chemotherapy out of your bladder and kidneys.

- **Limit drinks that contain caffeine** (such as black tea, coffee, and some cola products).

- **Talk with your doctor or nurse if you have any of the problems listed above.**

Other Side Effects

Flu-like symptoms

Some types of chemotherapy can make you feel like you have the flu. This is more likely to happen if you get chemotherapy along with biological therapy.

Flu-like symptoms may include:

- Muscle and joint aches
- Headache
- Fatigue
- Nausea
- Fever
- Chills
- Appetite loss

These symptoms may last from 1 to 3 days. An infection or the cancer itself can also cause them. Let your doctor or nurse know if you have any of these symptoms.

Fluid retention

Fluid retention is a buildup of fluid caused by chemotherapy, hormone changes caused by treatment, or your cancer. It can cause your face, hands, feet, or stomach to feel swollen and puffy. Sometimes fluid builds up around your lungs and heart, causing coughing, shortness of breath, or an irregular heartbeat. Fluid can also build up in the lower part of your belly, which can cause bloating.

You and your doctor or nurse can help manage fluid retention by:

- Weighing yourself at the same time each day, using the same scale. Let your doctor or nurse know if you gain weight quickly.

- Avoiding table salt or salty foods.

- Limiting the liquids you drink.

- If you retain a lot of fluid, your doctor may prescribe medicine to get rid of the extra fluid.

Eye changes

- **Trouble wearing contact lenses.** Some types of chemotherapy can bother your eyes and make wearing contact lenses painful. Ask your doctor or nurse if you can wear contact lenses while getting chemotherapy.

- **Blurry vision.** Some types of chemotherapy can clog your tear ducts, which can cause blurry vision.

- **Watery eyes.** Sometimes, chemotherapy can seep out in your tears, which can cause your eyes to water more than usual.

If your vision gets blurry or your eyes water more than usual, tell your doctor or nurse.

Section 46.5

Foods to Help with Side Effects

Clear Liquids

This list may help if you have:

- Diarrhea
- Urinary, kidney, or bladder changes

Table 46.1. Clear Liquids

Types	Examples
Soups	Bouillon Clear, fat-free broth Consommé
Drinks	Clear apple juice Clear carbonated beverages Fruit-flavored drinks Fruit juice, such as cranberry or grape Fruit punch Sports drinks Water Weak tea with no caffeine
Sweets	Fruit ices made without fruit pieces or milk Gelatin Honey Jelly Popsicles

Liquid Foods

This list may help if you:

- Do not feel like eating solid foods
- Have urinary, kidney, or bladder changes

Table 46.2. Liquid Foods

Types	Examples
Soups	Bouillon
	Broth Clear
	Cheese soup
	Soup that has been strained or put through a blender
	Soup with pureed potatoes
	Tomato soup
Drinks	Carbonate beverages
	Coffee
	Eggnog (pasteurized and alcohol free)
	Fruit drinks
	Fruit juices
	Fruit punch
	Milk (all types)
	Milkshakes
	Smoothies
	Sports drinks
	Tea
	Tomato juice
	Vegetable juice
	Water
Fats	Butter
	Cream
	Margarine
	Oil
	Sour cream
Sweets	Custard (soft or baked)
	Frozen yogurt
	Fruit purees that are watered down
	Gelatin
	Honey
	Ice cream with no chunks (such as nuts or cookie pieces)
	Ice milk
	Jelly
	Pudding
	Syrup
	Yogurt (plain or vanilla)
Replacement and Supplement	Instant breakfast drinks
	Liquid meal replacements

Foods and Drinks That Are High in Calories or Protein

This list may help if you do not feel like eating.

Table 46.3. Foods and Drinks That Are High in Calories or Protein

Types	Examples
Soups	Cream soups Soups with lentils, dried peas, or beans (such as pinto, black, red, or kidney)
Drinks	Instant breakfast drinks Milkshakes Smoothies Whole milk
Main meals and other foods	Beef Butter, margarine, or oil added to your food Cheese Chicken Cooked dried peas and beans (such as pinto, black, red, or kidney) Cottage cheese Cream cheese Croissants Deviled ham Eggs Fish Nuts, Seeds, and wheat germ Peanut butter Sour cream
Sweets	Custards (soft or baked) Frozen yogurt Ice cream Muffins Pudding Yogurt (plain or vanilla)
Replacement and Supplement	Liquid meal replacements Powdered milk added to foods such as pudding, milkshakes, and scrambled eggs

High-Fiber Foods

This list may help if you have constipation.

Table 46.4. High-Fiber Foods

Types	Examples
Main Meals and Other Foods	Bran muffins Bran or whole-grain cereals Brown or wild rice Cooked dried peas and beans (such as pinto, black, red, or kidney) Whole-wheat bread Whole-wheat pastas
Fruits and Vegetables	Dried fruit, such as apricots, dates, prunes, and raisins Fresh fruit, such as apples, blueberries, and grapes Raw or cooked vegetables, such as broccoli, corn, green beans, peas, and spinach
Snacks	Granola Nuts Popcorn Seeds, such as sunflower Trail mix

Low-Fiber Foods

This list may help if you have diarrhea.

Table 46.5. Low-Fiber Foods

Types	Examples
Main Meals and Other Foods	Chicken or turkey (skinless) Cooked refined cereals Cottage cheese Eggs Fish Noodles Potatoes (baked or mashed without the skin) White bread White rice

Types	Examples
Fruits and Vegetables	Asparagus Bananas Canned fruit, such as peaches, pears, and applesauce Clear fruit juice Vegetable juice
Snacks	Angel food cake Gelatin Saltine crackers Sherbet or sorbet Yogurt (plain or vanilla)

Foods That Are Easy on a Sore Mouth

This list may help if your mouth or throat are sore.

Table 46.6. Foods That Are Easy on a Sore Mouth

Types	Examples
Main Meals and Other Foods	Baby food Cooked refined cereals Cottage cheese Eggs (soft boiled or scrambled) Macaroni and cheese Mashed potatoes Pureed cooked foods Soups
Sweets	Custards Fruit (pureed or baby food) Gelatin Ice cream Milkshakes Puddings Smoothies Soft fruits (bananas and applesauce) Yogurt (plain or vanilla)

Foods and Drinks That Are Easy on the Stomach

This list may help if you have nausea and vomiting.

Table 46.7. Foods and Drinks That Are Easy on the Stomach

Types	Examples
Soups	Clear broth, such as chicken, vegetable, or beef
Drinks	Clear carbonated beverages that have lost their fizz Cranberry or grape juice Fruit-flavored drinks Fruit punch Sports drinks Tea Water
Main meals and other foods	Chicken (broiled or baked without its skin) Cream of rice Instant oatmeal Noodles Potatoes (boiled without skins) Pretzels Saltine crackers White rice White toast
Sweets	Angel food cake Canned fruit, such as applesauce, peaches, and pears Gelatin Popsicles Sherbet or sorbet Yogurt (plain or vanilla)

Chapter 47

Radiation Therapy

Chapter Contents

Text in this chapter is excerpted from "Radiation Therapy and You," National
Cancer Institute at the National Institutes of Health (NIH), May 2012.

Section 47.1

Questions and Answers About Radiation Therapy

What is radiation therapy?

Radiation therapy (also called **radiotherapy**) is a cancer treatment that uses high doses of radiation to kill cancer cells and stop them from spreading. At low doses, radiation is used as an x-ray to see inside your body and take pictures, such as x-rays of your teeth or broken bones. Radiation used in cancer treatment works in much the same way, except that it is given at higher doses.

How is radiation therapy given?

Radiation therapy can be **external beam** (when a machine outside your body aims radiation at cancer cells) or **internal** (when radiation is put inside your body, in or near the cancer cells). Sometimes people get both forms of radiation therapy.

Who gets radiation therapy?

Many people with cancer need radiation therapy. In fact, more than half (about 60 percent) of people with cancer get radiation therapy. Sometimes, radiation therapy is the only kind of cancer treatment people need.

What does radiation therapy do to cancer cells?

Given in high doses, radiation kills or slows the growth of cancer cells. Radiation therapy is used to:

- **Treat cancer.** Radiation can be used to cure, stop, or slow the growth of cancer.

- **Reduce symptoms.** When a cure is not possible, radiation may be used to shrink cancer tumors in order to reduce pressure.

Radiation therapy used in this way can treat problems such as pain, or it can prevent problems such as blindness or loss of bowel and bladder control.

How long does radiation therapy take to work?

Radiation therapy does not kill cancer cells right away. It takes days or weeks of treatment before cancer cells start to die. Then, cancer cells keep dying for weeks or months after radiation therapy ends.

What does radiation therapy do to healthy cells?

Radiation not only kills or slows the growth of cancer cells, it can also affect nearby healthy cells. The healthy cells almost always recover after treatment is over. But sometimes people may have side effects that do not get better or are severe. Doctors try to protect healthy cells during treatment by:

- **Using as low a dose of radiation as possible.** The radiation dose is balanced between being high enough to kill cancer cells yet low enough to limit damage to healthy cells.

- **Spreading out treatment over time.** You may get radiation therapy once a day for several weeks or in smaller doses twice a day. Spreading out the radiation dose allows normal cells to recover while cancer cells die.

- **Aiming radiation at a precise part of your body.** New techniques, such as **IMRT** and **3-D conformal radiation therapy,** allow your doctor to aim higher doses of radiation at your cancer while reducing the radiation to nearby healthy tissue.

- **Using medicines.** Some drugs can help protect certain parts of your body, such as the salivary glands that make saliva (spit).

Does radiation therapy hurt?

No, radiation therapy does not hurt while it is being given. But the side effects that people may get from radiation therapy can cause pain or discomfort. This chapter has a lot of information about ways that you, your doctor, and your nurse can help manage side effects.

Is radiation therapy used with other types of cancer treatment?

Yes, radiation therapy is often used with other cancer treatments. Here are some examples:

- **Radiation therapy and surgery.** Radiation may be given before, during, or after surgery. Doctors may use radiation to shrink the size of the cancer before surgery, or they may use radiation after surgery to kill any cancer cells that remain. Sometimes, radiation therapy is given during surgery so that it goes straight to the cancer without passing through the skin. This is called intraoperative radiation.

- **Radiation therapy and chemotherapy.** Radiation may be given before, during, or after chemotherapy. Before or during chemotherapy, radiation therapy can shrink the cancer so that chemotherapy works better. Sometimes, chemotherapy is given to help radiation therapy work better. After chemotherapy, radiation therapy can be used to kill any cancer cells that remain.

Who is on my radiation therapy team?

Many people help with your radiation treatment and care. This group of health care providers is often called the "radiation therapy team." They work together to provide care that is just right for you. Your radiation therapy team can include:

- **Radiation oncologist.** This is a doctor who specializes in using radiation therapy to treat cancer. He or she prescribes how much radiation you will receive, plans how your treatment will be given, closely follows you during your course of treatment, and prescribes care you may need to help with side effects. He or she works closely with the other doctors, nurses, and health care providers on your team. After you are finished with radiation therapy, your radiation oncologist will see you for follow-up visits. During these visits, this doctor will check for late side effects and assess how well the radiation has worked.

- **Nurse practitioner.** This is a nurse with advanced training. He or she can take your medical history, do physical exams, order tests, manage side effects, and closely watch your response to treatment. After you are finished with radiation therapy, your nurse practitioner may see you for follow-up visits to check for late side effects and assess how well the radiation has worked.

- **Radiation nurse.** This person provides nursing care during radiation therapy, working with all the members of your radiation therapy team. He or she will talk with you about your radiation treatment and help you manage side effects.

- **Radiation therapist.** This person works with you during each radiation therapy session. He or she positions you for treatment and runs the machines to make sure you get the dose of radiation prescribed by your radiation oncologist.

- **Other health care providers.** Your team may also include a dietitian, physical therapist, social worker, and others.

- **You.** You are also part of the radiation therapy team. Your role is to:

  - Arrive on time for all radiation therapy sessions
  - Ask questions and talk about your concerns
  - Let someone on your radiation therapy team know when you have side effects
  - Tell your doctor or nurse if you are in pain
  - Follow the advice of your doctors and nurses about how to care for yourself at home, such as:
    - Taking care of your skin
    - Drinking liquids
    - Eating foods that they suggest
    - Keeping your weight the same

Is radiation therapy expensive?

Yes, radiation therapy costs a lot of money. It uses complex machines and involves the services of many health care providers. The exact cost of your radiation therapy depends on the cost of health care where you live, what kind of radiation therapy you get, and how many treatments you need.

Talk with your health insurance company about what services it will pay for. Most insurance plans pay for radiation therapy for their members. To learn more, talk with the business office where you get treatment.

Should I follow a special diet while I am getting radiation therapy?

Your body uses a lot of energy to heal during radiation therapy. It is important that you eat enough calories and protein to keep your weight the same during this time. Ask your doctor or nurse if you need a special diet while you are getting radiation therapy. You might also find it helpful to speak with a dietitian.

Can I go to work during radiation therapy?

Some people are able to work full-time during radiation therapy. Others can only work part-time or not at all. How much you are able to work depends on how you feel. Ask your doctor or nurse what you may expect based on the treatment you are getting.

You are likely to feel well enough to work when you start radiation therapy. As time goes on, do not be surprised if you are more tired, have less energy, or feel weak. Once you have finished your treatment, it may take a few weeks or many months for you to feel better.

You may get to a point during your radiation therapy when you feel too sick to work. Talk with your employer to find out if you can go on medical leave. Make sure that your health insurance will pay for treatment when you are on medical leave.

What happens when radiation therapy is over?

Once you have finished radiation therapy, you will need **follow-up care** for the rest of your life. Follow-up care refers to checkups with your radiation oncologist or nurse practitioner after your course of radiation therapy is over. During these checkups, your doctor or nurse will see how well the radiation therapy worked, check for other signs of cancer, look for late side effects, and talk with you about your treatment and care. Your doctor or nurse will:

- **Examine you and review how you have been feeling.** Your doctor or nurse practitioner can prescribe medicine or suggest other ways to treat any side effects you may have.

- **Order lab and imaging tests.** These may include blood tests, x-rays, or CT, MRI, or PET scans.

- **Discuss treatment.** Your doctor or nurse practitioner may suggest that you have more treatment, such as extra radiation treatments, chemotherapy, or both.

- **Answer your questions and respond to your concerns.** It may be helpful to write down your questions ahead of time and bring them with you.

After radiation therapy is over, what symptoms should I look for?

You have gone through a lot with cancer and radiation therapy. Now you may be even more aware of your body and how you feel each day. Pay attention to changes in your body and let your doctor or nurse know if you have:

- A pain that does not go away

- New lumps, bumps, swellings, rashes, bruises, or bleeding

- Appetite changes, nausea, vomiting, diarrhea, or constipation

- Weight loss that you cannot explain

- A fever, cough, or hoarseness that does not go away

- Any other symptoms that worry you

Section 47.2

External Beam Radiation Therapy

What is external beam radiation therapy?

External beam radiation therapy comes from a machine that aims radiation at your cancer. The machine is large and may be noisy. It does not touch you, but rotates around you, sending radiation to your body from many directions.

External beam radiation therapy is a **local treatment**, meaning that the radiation is aimed only at a specific part of your body. For example, if you have lung cancer, you will get radiation to your chest only and not the rest of your body.

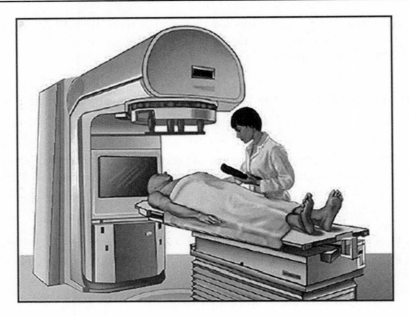

Figure 47.1. *External Beam Radiation Therapy*

External beam radiation therapy comes from a machine that aims radiation at your cancer.

How often will I get external beam radiation therapy?

Most people get external beam radiation therapy once a day, 5 days a week, Monday through Friday. Treatment lasts for 2 to 10 weeks, depending on the type of cancer you have and the goal of your treatment. The time between your first and last radiation therapy sessions is called a course of treatment.

Radiation is sometimes given in smaller doses twice a day (**hyper fractionated radiation therapy**). Your doctor may prescribe this type of treatment if he or she feels that it will work better. Although side effects may be more severe, there may be fewer late side effects. Doctors are doing research to see which types of cancer are best treated this way.

Where do I go for external beam radiation therapy?

Most of the time, you will get external beam radiation therapy as an outpatient. This means that you will have treatment at a clinic or radiation therapy center and will not have to stay in the hospital.

What happens before my first external beam radiation treatment?

You will have a 1- to 2-hour meeting with your doctor or nurse before you begin radiation therapy. At this time, you will have a physical exam, talk about your medical history, and maybe have imaging tests. Your doctor or nurse will discuss external beam radiation therapy, its benefits and side effects, and ways you can care for yourself during and after treatment. You can then choose whether to have external beam radiation therapy.

If you agree to have external beam radiation therapy, you will be scheduled for a treatment planning session called a **simulation**. At this time:

- A radiation oncologist and radiation therapist will define your treatment area (also called a **treatment port** or **treatment field**). This refers to the places in your body that will get radiation. You will be asked to lie very still while x-rays or scans are taken to define the treatment area.

- The radiation therapist will then put small marks (tattoos or dots of colored ink) on your skin to mark the treatment area. You will need these marks throughout the course of radiation therapy. The radiation therapist will use them each day to make sure you are in the correct position. Tattoos are about the size of a freckle and will remain on your skin for the rest of your life. Ink markings will fade over time. Be careful not to remove them and make sure to tell the radiation therapist if they fade or lose color.

- You may need a body mold. This is a plastic or plaster form that helps keep you from moving during treatment. It also helps make sure that you are in the exact same position each day of treatment.

- If you are getting radiation to the head, you may need a mask. The mask has air holes, and holes can be cut for your eyes, nose, and mouth. It attaches to the table where you will lie to receive your treatments. The mask helps keep your head from moving so that you are in the exact same position for each treatment.

If the body mold or mask makes you feel anxious, look for ways to relax during treatment.

What should I wear when I get external beam radiation therapy?

Wear clothes that are comfortable and made of soft fabric, such as cotton. Choose clothes that are easy to take off, since you may need to change into a hospital gown or show the area that is being treated. Do not wear clothes that are tight, such as close-fitting collars or waistbands, near your treatment area. Also, do not wear jewelry, BAND-AIDS®, powder, lotion, or deodorant in or near your treatment area, and do not use deodorant soap before your treatment.

What happens during treatment sessions?

- You may be asked to change into a hospital gown or robe.

- You will go to a treatment room where you will receive radiation.

- Depending on where your cancer is, you will either sit in a chair or lie down on a treatment table. The radiation therapist will use your body mold and skin marks to help you get into position.

- You may see colored lights pointed at your skin marks. These lights are harmless and help the therapist position you for treatment each day.

- You will need to stay very still so the radiation goes to the exact same place each time. You can breathe as you always do and do not have to hold your breath.

The radiation therapist will leave the room just before your treatment begins. He or she will go to a nearby room to control the radiation machine and watch you on a TV screen or through a window. You are not alone, even though it may feel that way. The radiation therapist can see you on the screen or through the window. He or she can hear and talk with you through a speaker in your treatment room. Make sure to tell the therapist if you feel sick or are uncomfortable. He or she can stop the radiation machine at any time. You cannot feel, hear, see, or smell radiation.

Your entire visit may last from 30 minutes to 1 hour. Most of that time is spent setting you in the correct position. You will get radiation for only 1 to 5 minutes. If you are getting IMRT, your treatment may last longer. Your visit may also take longer if your treatment team needs to take and review x-rays.

Will external beam radiation therapy make me radioactive?

No, external beam radiation therapy does not make people radioactive. You may safely be around other people, even babies and young children.

How can I relax during my treatment sessions?

- Bring something to read or do while in the waiting room.

- Ask if you can listen to music or books on tape.

- Meditate, breathe deeply, use imagery, or find other ways to relax.

Section 47.3

Internal Radiation Therapy

What is internal radiation therapy?

Internal radiation therapy is a form of treatment where a source of radiation is put inside your body. One form of internal radiation therapy is called **brachytherapy**. In brachytherapy, the radiation source is a solid in the form of seeds, ribbons, or capsules, which are placed in your body in or near the cancer cells. This allows treatment with a high dose of radiation to a smaller part of your body. Internal radiation can also be in a liquid form. You receive liquid radiation by drinking it, by swallowing a pill, or through an IV. Liquid radiation travels throughout your body, seeking out and killing cancer cells.

Brachytherapy may be used with people who have cancers of the head, neck, breast, uterus, cervix, prostate, gall bladder, esophagus, eye, and lung. Liquid forms of internal radiation are most often used with people who have thyroid cancer or non-Hodgkin's lymphoma. You may also get internal radiation along with other types of treatment, including external beam radiation, chemotherapy, or surgery.

What happens before my first internal radiation treatment?

You will have a 1- to 2-hour meeting with your doctor or nurse before you begin internal radiation therapy. At this time, you will have a physical exam, talk about your medical history, and maybe have imaging tests. Your doctor will discuss the type of internal radiation therapy that is best for you, its benefits and side effects, and ways you can care for yourself during and after treatment. You can then choose whether to have internal radiation therapy.

How is brachytherapy put in place?

Most brachytherapy is put in place through a **catheter**, which is a small, stretchy tube. Sometimes, it is put in place through a larger device called an **applicator**. When you decide to have brachytherapy, your doctor will place the catheter or applicator into the part of your body that will be treated.

What happens when the catheter or applicator is put in place?

You will most likely be in the hospital when your catheter or applicator is put in place. Here is what to expect:

- You will either be put to sleep or the area where the catheter or applicator goes will be numbed. This will help prevent pain when it is put in.

- Your doctor will place the catheter or applicator in your body.

- If you are awake, you may be asked to lie very still while the catheter or applicator is put in place. If you feel any discomfort, tell your doctor or nurse so he or she can give you medicine to help manage the pain.

What happens after the catheter or applicator is placed in my body?

Once your treatment plan is complete, radiation will be placed inside the catheter or applicator. The radiation source may be kept in place for a few minutes, many days, or the rest of your life. How long the radiation is in place depends on which type of brachytherapy you get, your type of cancer, where the cancer is in your body, your health, and other cancer treatments you have had.

What are the types of brachytherapy?

There are three types of brachytherapy:

- **Low-dose rate (LDR) implants.** In this type of brachytherapy, radiation stays in place for 1 to 7 days. You are likely to be in the hospital during this time. Once your treatment is finished, your doctor will remove the radiation sources and your catheter or applicator.

- **High-dose rate (HDR) implants.** In this type of brachytherapy, the radiation source is in place for 10 to 20 minutes at a time and then taken out. You may have treatment twice a day for 2 to 5 days or once a week for 2 to 5 weeks. The schedule depends on your type of cancer. During the course of treatment, your catheter or applicator may stay in place, or it may be put in place before each treatment. You may be in the hospital during this time, or you may make daily trips to the hospital to have the radiation source put in place. Like LDR implants, your doctor will remove your catheter or applicator once you have finished treatment.

- **Permanent implants.** After the radiation source is put in place, the catheter is removed. The implants always stay in your body, while the radiation gets weaker each day. You may need to limit your time around other people when the radiation is first put in place. Be extra careful not to spend time with children or pregnant women. As time goes by, almost all the radiation will go away, even though the implant stays in your body.

What happens while the radiation is in place?

- Your body will give off radiation once the radiation source is in place. With brachytherapy, your body fluids (urine, sweat, and saliva) will not give off radiation. With liquid radiation, your body fluids will give off radiation for a while.

- Your doctor or nurse will talk with you about safety measures that you need to take.

- If the radiation you receive is a very high dose, safety measures may include:

  - Staying in a private hospital room to protect others from radiation coming from your body.

959

- Being treated quickly by nurses and other hospital staff. They will provide all the care you need, but they may stand at a distance and talk with you from the doorway to your room.
- Your visitors will also need to follow safety measures, which may include:
  - Not being allowed to visit when the radiation is first put in
  - Needing to check with the hospital staff before they go to your room
  - Keeping visits short (30 minutes or less each day). The length of visits depends on the type of radiation being used and the part of your body being treated.
  - Standing by the doorway rather than going into your hospital room
  - Not having visits from children younger than 18 and pregnant women

You may also need to follow safety measures once you leave the hospital, such as not spending much time with other people. Your doctor or nurse will talk with you about the safety measures you should follow when you go home.

What happens when the catheter is taken out after treatment with LDR or HDR implants?

- You will get medicine for pain before the catheter or applicator is removed.
- The area where the catheter or applicator was might be tender for a few months.
- There is no radiation in your body after the catheter or applicator is removed. It is safe for people to be near you— even young children and pregnant women.
- For 1 to 2 weeks, you may need to limit activities that take a lot of effort. Ask your doctor what kinds of activities are safe for you.

Section 47.4

Your Feelings During Radiation Therapy

At some point during radiation therapy, you may feel:

- Anxious

- Depressed

- Afraid

- Angry

- Frustrated

- Helpless

- Alone

It is normal to have these kinds of feelings. Living with cancer and going through treatment is stressful. You may also feel **fatigue**, which can make it harder to cope with these feelings.

How can I cope with my feelings during radiation therapy?

There are many things you can do to cope with your feelings during treatment. Here are some things that have worked for other people:

- **Relax and meditate.** You might try thinking of yourself in a favorite place, breathing slowly while paying attention to each breath, or listening to soothing music. These kinds of activities can help you feel calmer and less stressed.

- **Exercise.** Many people find that light exercise (such as walking, biking, yoga, or water aerobics) helps them feel better. Talk with your doctor or nurse about types of exercise that you can do.

- **Talk with others.** Talk about your feelings with someone you trust. You may choose a close friend, family member, chaplain,

961

nurse, social worker, or psychologist. You may also find it helpful to talk to someone else who is going through radiation therapy.

- **Join a support group.** Cancer support groups are meetings for people with cancer. These groups allow you to meet others facing the same problems. You will have a chance to talk about your feelings and listen to other people talk about theirs. You can learn how others cope with cancer, radiation therapy, and side effects. Your doctor, nurse, or social worker can tell you about support groups near where you live. Some support groups also meet over the Internet, which can be helpful if you cannot travel or find a meeting in your area.

- **Talk to your doctor or nurse about things that worry or upset you.** You may want to ask about seeing a counselor. Your doctor may also suggest that you take medicine if you find it very hard to cope with these feelings.

Section 47.5

Radiation Therapy Side Effects

Side effects are problems that can happen as a result of treatment. They may happen with radiation therapy because the high doses of radiation used to kill cancer cells can also damage healthy cells in the treatment area. Side effects are different for each person. Some people have many side effects; others have hardly any. Side effects may be more severe if you also receive chemotherapy before, during, or after your radiation therapy.

Talk to your radiation therapy team about your chances of having side effects. The team will watch you closely and ask if you notice any problems. If you do have side effects or other problems, your doctor or nurse will talk with you about ways to manage them.

Common Side Effects

Many people who get radiation therapy have skin changes and some fatigue. Other side effects depend on the part of your body being treated.

Skin changes may include dryness, itching, peeling, or blistering. These changes occur because radiation therapy damages healthy skin cells in the treatment area. You will need to take special care of your skin during radiation therapy.

Fatigue is often described as feeling worn out or exhausted. There are many ways to manage fatigue.

Depending on the part of your body being treated, you may also have:

- Diarrhea
- Hair loss in treatment area
- Mouth problems
- Nausea and vomiting
- Sexual changes
- Swelling
- Trouble swallowing
- Urinary and bladder changes

Most of these side effects go away within 2 months after radiation therapy is finished.

Late side effects may first occur 6 or more months after radiation therapy is over. They vary by the part of your body that was treated and the dose of radiation you received. Late side effects may include **infertility**, joint problems, lymphedema, mouth problems, and secondary cancer. Everyone is different, so talk to your doctor or nurse about whether you might have late side effects and what signs to look for.

Radiation Therapy Side Effects At-A-Glance

Radiation therapy side effects depend on the part of your body being treated. Find the part of your body being treated in the column on the left, then read across the row to see the side effects. A checkmark means that you may get this side effect. Ask your doctor or nurse about your chances of getting each side effect.

Table 47.1. Side effects of Radiation Therapy

	Diarrhea	Fatigue	Hair Loss (on the part of the body being treated)	Mouth Changes	Nausea and Vomiting	Sexual and Fertility Changes	Skin Changes	Throat Changes	Urinary and Bladder Changes	Other Side Effects
Brain		✓	✓		✓		✓			Headache Blurry vision
Breast		✓	✓				✓			Tenderness Swelling
Chest		✓	✓				✓	✓		Cough Shortness of breath
Head and Neck		✓	✓	✓			✓	✓		Earaches Taste changes
Pelvic Area	✓	✓	✓		✓	✓	✓		✓	
Rectum	✓	✓	✓			✓	✓		✓	
Stomach and Abdomen	✓	✓	✓		✓		✓		✓	

Find the part of your body being treated in the column on the left. Read across the row. A checkmark means you may get the side effect listed.

964

Radiation Therapy Side Effects and Ways to Manage Them

Diarrhea

What it is

Diarrhea is frequent bowel movements which may be soft, formed, loose, or watery. Diarrhea can occur at any time during radiation therapy.

Why it occurs

Radiation therapy to the pelvis, stomach, and abdomen can cause diarrhea. People get diarrhea because radiation harms the healthy cells in the large and small bowels. These areas are very sensitive to the amount of radiation needed to treat cancer.

Ways to manage

When you have diarrhea:

- **Drink 8 to 12 cups of clear liquid per day.**

  If you drink liquids that are high in sugar (such as fruit juice, sweet iced tea, Kool-Aid®, or Hi-C®) ask your nurse or dietitian if you should mix them with water.

- **Eat many small meals and snacks.** For instance, eat 5 or 6 small meals and snacks rather than 3 large meals.

- **Eat foods that are easy on the stomach (which means foods that are low in fiber, fat, and lactose).** If your diarrhea is severe, your doctor or nurse may suggest the BRAT diet, which stands for bananas, rice, applesauce, and toast.

- **Take care of your rectal area.** Instead of toilet paper, use a baby wipe or squirt of water from a spray bottle to clean yourself after bowel movements. Also, ask your nurse about taking sitz baths, which is a warm-water bath taken in a sitting position that covers only the hips and buttocks. Be sure to tell your doctor or nurse if your rectal area gets sore.

- **Stay away from:**
  - Milk and dairy foods, such as ice cream, sour cream, and cheese

- Spicy foods, such as hot sauce, salsa, chili, and curry dishes

- Foods or drinks with caffeine, such as regular coffee, black tea, soda, and chocolate

- Foods or drinks that cause gas, such as cooked dried beans, cabbage, broccoli, soy milk, and other soy products

- Foods that are high in fiber, such as raw fruits and vegetables, cooked dried beans, and whole wheat breads and cereals

- Fried or greasy foods

- Food from fast food restaurants

- **Talk to your doctor or nurse.** Tell them if you are having diarrhea. He or she will suggest ways to manage it. He or she may also suggest taking medicine, such as Imodium®.

Fatigue

What it is

Fatigue from radiation therapy can range from a mild to an extreme feeling of being tired. Many people describe fatigue as feeling weak, weary, worn out, heavy, or slow.

Why it occurs

Fatigue can happen for many reasons. These include:

- Anemia

- Anxiety

- Depression

- Infection

- Lack of activity

- Medicines

Fatigue can also come from the effort of going to radiation therapy each day or from stress. Most of the time, you will not know why you feel fatigue.

How long it lasts

When you first feel fatigue depends on a few factors, which include your age, health, level of activity, and how you felt before radiation therapy started.

Fatigue can last from 6 weeks to 12 months after your last radiation therapy session. Some people may always feel fatigue and, even after radiation therapy is over, will not have as much energy as they did before.

Ways to manage

- **Try to sleep at least 8 hours each night.** This may be more sleep than you needed before radiation therapy. One way to sleep better at night is to be active during the day. For example, you could go for walks, do yoga, or ride a bike. Another way to sleep better at night is to relax before going to bed. You might read a book, work on a jigsaw puzzle, listen to music, or do other calming hobbies.

- **Plan time to rest.** You may need to nap during the day. Many people say that it helps to rest for just 10 to 15 minutes. If you do nap, try to sleep for less than 1 hour at a time.

- **Try not to do too much.** With fatigue, you may not have enough energy to do all the things you want to do. Stay active, but choose the activities that are most important to you. For example, you might go to work but not do housework, or watch your children's sports events but not go out to dinner.

- **Exercise.** Most people feel better when they get some exercise each day. Go for a 15- to 30-minute walk or do stretches or yoga. Talk with your doctor or nurse about how much exercise you can do while having radiation therapy.

- **Plan a work schedule that is right for you.** Fatigue may affect the amount of energy you have for your job. You may feel well enough to work your full schedule, or you may need to work less—maybe just a few hours a day or a few days each week. You may want to talk with your boss about ways to work from home so you do not have to commute. And you may want to think about going on medical leave while you have radiation therapy.

- **Plan a radiation therapy schedule that makes sense for you.** You may want to schedule your radiation therapy around

967

your work or family schedule. For example, you might want to have radiation therapy in the morning so you can go to work in the afternoon.

- **Let others help you at home.** Check with your insurance company to see whether it covers home care services. You can also ask family members and friends to help when you feel fatigue. Home care staff, family members, and friends can assist with household chores, running errands, or driving you to and from radiation therapy visits. They might also help by cooking meals for you to eat now or freeze for later.

- **Learn from others who have cancer.** People who have cancer can help each other by sharing ways to manage fatigue. One way to meet other people with cancer is by joining a support group—either in person or online. Talk with your doctor or nurse to learn more about support groups.

- **Talk with your doctor or nurse.** If you have trouble dealing with fatigue, your doctor may prescribe medicine (called psychostimulants) that can help decrease fatigue, give you a sense of well-being, and increase your appetite. Your doctor may also suggest treatments if you have anemia, depression, or are not able to sleep at night.

Hair Loss

What it is

Hair loss (also called **alopecia**) is when some or all of your hair falls out.

Why it occurs

Radiation therapy can cause hair loss because it damages cells that grow quickly, such as those in your hair roots.

Hair loss from radiation therapy only happens on the part of your body being treated. This is not the same as hair loss from chemotherapy, which happens all over your body. For instance, you may lose some or all of the hair on your head when you get radiation to your brain. But if you get radiation to your hip, you may lose pubic hair (between your legs) but not the hair on your head.

How long it lasts

You may start losing hair in your treatment area 2 to 3 weeks after your first radiation therapy session. It takes about a week for all the hair in your treatment area to fall out. Your hair may grow back 3 to 6 months after treatment is over. Sometimes, though, the dose of radiation is so high that your hair never grows back.

Once your hair starts to grow back, it may not look or feel the way it did before. Your hair may be thinner, or curly instead of straight. Or it may be darker or lighter in color than it was before.

Ways to manage hair loss on your head

Before hair loss:

- **Decide whether to cut your hair or shave your head.** You may feel more in control of hair loss when you plan ahead. Use an electric razor to prevent nicking yourself if you decide to shave your head.

- **If you plan to buy a wig, do so while you still have hair.** The best time to select your wig is before radiation therapy begins or soon after it starts. This way, the wig will match the color and style of your own hair. Some people take their wig to their hair stylist. You will want to have your wig fitted once you have lost your hair. Make sure to choose a wig that feels comfortable and does not hurt your scalp.

- **Check with your health insurance company to see whether it will pay for your wig.** If it does not, you can deduct the cost of your wig as a medical expense on your income taxes. Some groups also sponsor free wig banks. Ask your doctor, nurse, or social worker if he or she can refer you to a free wig bank in your area.

- **Be gentle when you wash your hair.** Use a mild shampoo, such as a baby shampoo. Dry your hair by patting (not rubbing) it with a soft towel.

- **Do not use curling irons, electric hair dryers, curlers, hair bands, clips, or hair sprays.** These can hurt your scalp or cause early hair loss.

- **Do not use products that are harsh on your hair.** These include hair colors, perms, gels, mousse, oil, grease, or pomade.

969

After hair loss:

- **Protect your scalp.** Your scalp may feel tender after hair loss. Cover your head with a hat, turban, or scarf when you are outside. Try not to be in places where the temperature is very cold or very hot. This means staying away from the direct sun, sun lamps, and very cold air.

- **Stay warm.** Your hair helps keep you warm, so you may feel colder once you lose it. You can stay warmer by wearing a hat, turban, scarf, or wig.

Mouth Changes

What they are

Radiation therapy to the head or neck can cause problems such as:

- Mouth sores (little cuts or ulcers in your mouth)
- Dry mouth (also called **xerostomia**) and throat
- Loss of taste
- Tooth decay
- Changes in taste (such as a metallic taste when you eat meat)
- Infections of your gums, teeth, or tongue
- Jaw stiffness and bone changes
- Thick, rope-like saliva

Why they occur

Radiation therapy kills cancer cells and can also damage healthy cells such as those in the glands that make saliva and the soft, moist lining of your mouth.

How long they last

Some problems, like mouth sores, may go away after treatment ends. Others, such as taste changes, may last for months or even years. Some problems, like dry mouth, may never go away.

Ways to manage

- If you are getting radiation therapy to your head or neck, **visit a dentist at least 2 weeks before treatment starts.** At this time, your dentist will examine your teeth and mouth and do any needed dental work to make sure your mouth is as healthy as possible before radiation therapy. If you cannot get to the dentist before treatment starts, ask your doctor if you should schedule a visit soon after treatment begins.

- **Check your mouth every day.** This way, you can see or feel problems as soon as they start. Problems can include mouth sores, white patches, or infection.

- **Keep your mouth moist.** You can do this by:
  - Sipping water often during the day
  - Sucking on ice chips
  - Chewing sugar-free gum or sucking on sugar-free hard candy
  - Using a saliva substitute to help moisten your mouth
  - Asking your doctor to prescribe medicine that helps increase saliva

- **Clean your mouth, teeth, gums, and tongue.**
  - Brush your teeth, gums, and tongue after every meal and at bedtime.
  - Use an extra-soft toothbrush. You can make the bristles softer by running warm water over them just before you brush.
  - Use a fluoride toothpaste.
  - Use a special fluoride gel that your dentist can prescribe.
  - Do not use mouthwashes that contain alcohol.
  - Gently floss your teeth every day. If your gums bleed or hurt, avoid those areas but floss your other teeth.
  - Rinse your mouth every 1 to 2 hours with a solution of 1/4 teaspoon baking soda and 1/8 teaspoon salt mixed in 1 cup of warm water.
  - If you have dentures, make sure they fit well and limit how long you wear them each day. If you lose weight, your dentist may need to adjust them.
  - Keep your dentures clean by soaking or brushing them each day.

971

- **Be careful what you eat when your mouth is sore.**
  - Choose foods that are easy to chew and swallow.
  - Take small bites, chew slowly, and sip liquids with your meals.
  - Eat moist, soft foods such as cooked cereals, mashed potatoes, and scrambled eggs.
  - Wet and soften food with gravy, sauce, broth, yogurt, or other liquids.
  - Eat foods that are warm or at room temperature.
- **Stay away from things that can hurt, scrape, or burn your mouth, such as:**
  - Sharp, crunchy foods such as potato or corn chips
  - Hot foods
  - Spicy foods such as hot sauce, curry dishes, salsa, and chili
  - Fruits and juices that are high in acid such as tomatoes, oranges, lemons, and grapefruits
  - Toothpicks or other sharp objects
  - All tobacco products, including cigarettes, pipes, cigars, and chewing tobacco
  - Drinks that contain alcohol
- **Stay away from foods and drinks that are high in sugar.** Foods and drinks that have a lot sugar (such as regular soda, gum, and candy) can cause tooth decay.
- **Exercise your jaw muscles.** Open and close your mouth 20 times as far as you can without causing pain. Do this exercise 3 times a day, even if your jaw isn't stiff.
- **Medicine.** Ask your doctor or nurse about medicines that can protect your saliva glands and the moist tissues that line your mouth.
- **Call your doctor or nurse when your mouth hurts.** There are medicines and other products, such as mouth gels, that can help control mouth pain.
- **You will need to take extra good care of your mouth for the rest of your life.** Ask your dentist how often you will need

dental check-ups and how best to take care of your teeth and mouth after radiation therapy is over.

Nausea and Vomiting

What they are

Radiation therapy can cause nausea, vomiting, or both. Nausea is when you feel sick to your stomach and feel like you are going to throw up. Vomiting is when you throw up food and fluids. You may also have **dry heaves**, which happen when your body tries to vomit even though your stomach is empty. Radiation Therapy Side Effects and Ways to Manage Them Radiation to the shaded area may cause nausea and vomiting.

Why they occur

Nausea and vomiting can occur after radiation therapy to the stomach, small intestine, colon, or parts of the brain. Your risk for nausea and vomiting depends on how much radiation you are getting, how much of your body is in the treatment area, and whether you are also having chemotherapy.

How long they last

Nausea and vomiting may occur 30 minutes to many hours after your radiation therapy session ends. You are likely to feel better on days that you do not have radiation therapy.

Ways to manage

- **Prevent nausea.** The best way to keep from vomiting is to prevent nausea. One way to do this is by having bland, easy-to-digest foods and drinks that do not upset your stomach. These include toast, gelatin, and apple juice.

- **Try to relax before treatment.** You may feel less nausea if you relax before each radiation therapy treatment. You can do this by spending time doing activities you enjoy, such as reading a book, listening to music, or other hobbies.

- **Plan when to eat and drink.** Some people feel better when they eat before radiation therapy; others do not. Learn the best time

973

for you to eat and drink. For example, you might want a snack of crackers and apple juice 1 to 2 hours before radiation therapy. Or, you might feel better if you have treatment on an empty stomach, which means not eating 2 to 3 hours before treatment.

- **Eat small meals and snacks.** Instead of eating 3 large meals each day, you may want to eat 5 or 6 small meals and snacks. Make sure to eat slowly and do not rush.

- **Have foods and drinks that are warm or cool (not hot or cold).** Before eating or drinking, let hot food and drinks cool down and cold food and drinks warm up.

- **Talk with your doctor or nurse.** He or she may suggest a special diet of foods to eat or prescribe medicine to help prevent nausea, which you can take 1 hour before each radiation therapy session. You might also ask your doctor or nurse about acupuncture, which may help relieve nausea and vomiting caused by cancer treatment.

Sexual and Fertility Changes

What they are

Radiation therapy sometimes causes sexual changes, which can include hormone changes and loss of interest in or ability to have sex. It can also affect fertility during and after radiation therapy. For a woman, this means that she might not be able to get pregnant and have a baby. For a man, this means that he might not be able to get a woman pregnant. Sexual and fertility changes differ for men and women.

Problems for women include:

- Pain or discomfort when having sex

- Vaginal itching, burning, dryness, or atrophy (when the muscles in the vagina become weak and the walls of the vagina become thin)

- **Vaginal stenosis**, when the vagina becomes less elastic, narrows, and gets shorter

- Symptoms of menopause for women not yet in menopause. These include hot flashes, vaginal dryness, and not having your period

- Not being able to get pregnant after radiation therapy is over

Problems for men include:

- **Impotence** (also called **erectile dysfunction** or ED), which means not being able to have or keep an erection

- Not being able to get a woman pregnant after radiation therapy is over due to fewer or less effective sperm

Why they occur

Sexual and fertility changes can happen when people get radiation therapy to the pelvic area. For women, this includes radiation to the vagina, uterus, or ovaries. For men, this includes radiation to the testicles or prostate. Many sexual side effects are caused by scar tissue from radiation therapy. Other problems, such as fatigue, pain, anxiety, or depression, can affect your interest in having sex.

How long they last

After radiation therapy is over, most people want to have sex as much as they did before treatment. Many sexual side effects go away after treatment ends. But you may have problems with hormone changes and fertility for the rest of your life. If you are able to get pregnant or father a child after you have finished radiation therapy, it should not affect the health of the baby.

Ways to manage

For both men and women, it is important to be open and honest with your spouse or partner about your feelings, concerns, and how you prefer to be intimate while you are getting radiation therapy.

For women, here are some issues to discuss with your doctor or nurse:

- **Fertility.** Before radiation therapy starts, let your doctor or nurse know if you think you might want to get pregnant after your treatment ends. He or she can talk with you about ways to preserve your fertility, such as preserving your eggs to use in the future.

- **Sexual problems.** You may or may not have sexual problems. Your doctor or nurse can tell you about side effects, you can expect and suggest ways for coping with them.

- **Birth control.** It is very important that you do not get pregnant while having radiation therapy. Radiation therapy can hurt the fetus at all stages of pregnancy. If you have not yet gone through menopause, talk with your doctor or nurse about birth control and ways to keep from getting pregnant.

- **Pregnancy.** Make sure to tell your doctor or nurse if you are already pregnant.

- **Stretching your vagina.** Vaginal stenosis is a common problem for women who have radiation therapy to the pelvis. This can make it painful to have sex. You can help by stretching your vagina using a dilator (a device that gently stretches the tissues of the vagina). Ask your doctor or nurse where to find a dilator and how to use it.

- **Lubrication.** Use a special lotion for your vagina (such as Replens®) once a day to keep it moist. When you have sex, use a water- or mineral oil-based lubricant (such as K-Y Jelly® or Astroglide®).

- **Sex.** Ask your doctor or nurse whether it is okay for you to have sex during radiation therapy. Most women can have sex, but it is a good idea to ask and be sure. If sex is painful due to vaginal dryness, you can use a water- or mineral oil-based lubricant.

For men, here are some issues to discuss with your doctor or nurse:

- **Fertility.** Before you start radiation therapy, let your doctor or nurse know if you think you might want to father children in the future. He or she may talk with you about ways to preserve your fertility before treatment starts, such as banking your sperm. Your sperm will need to be collected before you begin radiation therapy.

- **Impotence.** Your doctor or nurse can let you know whether you are likely to become impotent and how long it might last. Your doctor can prescribe medicine or other treatments that may help.

- **Sex.** Ask if it is okay for you to have sex during radiation therapy. Most men can have sex, but it is a good idea to ask and be sure.

Skin Changes

What they are

Radiation therapy can cause skin changes in your treatment area. Here are some common skin changes:

- **Redness.** Your skin in the treatment area may look as if you have a mild to severe sunburn or tan. This can occur on any part of your body where you are getting radiation.

- **Pruritus.** The skin in your treatment area may itch so much that you always feel like scratching. This causes problems because scratching too much can lead to **skin breakdown** and infection.

- **Dry and peeling skin.** This is when the skin in your treatment area gets very dry—much drier than normal. In fact, your skin may be so dry that it peels like it does after a sunburn.

- **Moist reaction.** Radiation kills skin cells in your treatment area, causing your skin to peel off faster than it can grow back. When this happens, you can get sores or ulcers. The skin in your treatment area can also become wet, sore, or infected. This is more common where you have skin folds, such as your buttocks, behind your ears, under your breasts. It may also occur where your skin is very thin, such as your neck.

- **Swollen skin.** The skin in your treatment area may be swollen and puffy.

Why they occur

Radiation therapy causes skin cells to break down and die. When people get radiation almost every day, their skin cells do not have enough time to grow back between treatments. Skin changes can happen on any part of the body that gets radiation.

How long they last

Skin changes may start a few weeks after you begin radiation therapy. Many of these changes often go away a few weeks after treatment is over. But even after radiation therapy ends, you may still have skin changes. Your treated skin may always look darker and blotchy.

It may feel very dry or thicker than before. And you may always burn quickly and be sensitive to the sun. You will always be at risk for skin cancer in the treatment area. Be sure to avoid tanning beds and protect yourself from the sun by wearing a hat, long sleeves, long pants, and sunscreen with an SPF of 30 or higher.

Ways to manage

- **Skin care.** Take extra good care of your skin during radiation therapy. Be gentle and do not rub, scrub, or scratch in the treatment area. Also, use creams that your doctor prescribes.

- **Do not put anything on your skin that is very hot or cold.** This means not using heating pads, ice packs, or other hot or cold items on the treatment area. It also means washing with lukewarm water.

- **Be gentle when you shower or take a bath.** You can take a lukewarm shower every day. If you prefer to take a lukewarm bath, do so only every other day and soak for less than 30 minutes. Whether you take a shower or bath, make sure to use a mild soap that does not have fragrance or deodorant in it. Dry yourself with a soft towel by patting, not rubbing, your skin. Be careful not to wash off the ink markings that you need for radiation therapy.

- **Use only those lotions and skin products that your doctor or nurse suggests.** If you are using a prescribed cream for a skin problem or acne, you must tell your doctor or nurse before you begin radiation treatment. Check with your doctor or nurse before using any of the following skin products:
  - Bubble bath
  - Cornstarch
  - Cream
  - Deodorant
  - Hair removers
  - Makeup
  - Oil
  - Ointment
  - Perfume

- Powder

- Soap

- Sunscreen

- **Cool, humid places.** Your skin may feel much better when you are in cool, humid places. You can make rooms more humid by putting a bowl of water on the radiator or using a humidifier. If you use a humidifier, be sure to follow the directions about cleaning it to prevent bacteria.

- **Soft fabrics.** Wear clothes and use bed sheets that are soft, such as those made from cotton.

- **Do not wear clothes that are tight and do not breathe,** such as girdles and pantyhose.

- **Protect your skin from the sun every day.** The sun can burn you even on cloudy days or when you are outside for just a few minutes. Do not go to the beach or sun bathe. Wear a broad brimmed hat, long-sleeved shirt, and long pants when you are outside. Talk with your doctor or nurse about sunscreen lotions. He or she may suggest that you use a sunscreen with an SPF of 30 or higher. You will need to protect your skin from the sun even after radiation therapy is over, since you will have an increased risk of skin cancer for the rest of your life.

- **Do not use tanning beds.** Tanning beds expose you to the same harmful effects as the sun.

- **Adhesive tape.** Do not put bandages, BAND-AIDS®, or other types of sticky tape on your skin in the treatment area. Talk with your doctor or nurse about ways to bandage without tape.

- **Shaving.** Ask your doctor or nurse if you can shave the treated area. If you can shave, use an electric razor and do not use pre-shave lotion.

- **Rectal area.** If you have radiation therapy to the rectal area, you are likely to have skin problems. These problems are often worse after a bowel movement. Clean yourself with a baby wipe or squirt of water from a spray bottle. Also ask your nurse about sitz baths (a warm-water bath taken in a sitting position that covers only the hips and buttocks.)

- **Talk with your doctor or nurse.** Some skin changes can be very serious. Your treatment team will check for skin changes each time you have radiation therapy. Make sure to report any skin changes that you notice.

- **Medicine.** Medicines can help with some skin changes. They include lotions for dry or itchy skin, antibiotics to treat infection, and other drugs to reduce swelling or itching.

Throat Changes

What they are

Radiation therapy to the neck or chest can cause the lining of your throat to become inflamed and sore. This is called **esophagitis**. You may feel as if you have a lump in your throat or burning in your chest or throat. You may also have trouble swallowing.

Why they occur

Radiation therapy to the neck or chest can cause throat changes because it not only kills cancer cells, but can also damage the healthy cells that line your throat. Your risk for throat changes depends on how much radiation you are getting, whether you are also having chemotherapy, and whether you use tobacco and alcohol while you are getting radiation therapy.

How long they last

You may notice throat changes 2 to 3 weeks after starting radiation. You will most likely feel better 4 to 6 weeks after radiation therapy has finished.

Ways to manage

- **Be careful what you eat when your throat is sore.**
  - Choose foods that are easy to swallow.
  - Cut, blend, or shred foods to make them easier to eat.
  - Eat moist, soft foods such as cooked cereals, mashed potatoes, and scrambled eggs.
  - Wet and soften food with gravy, sauce, broth, yogurt, or other liquids.
  - Drink cool drinks.

- Sip drinks through a straw.

- Eat foods that are cool or at room temperature.

- **Eat small meals and snacks.** It may be easier to eat a small amount of food at one time. Instead of eating 3 large meals each day, you may want to eat 5 or 6 small meals and snacks.

- **Choose foods and drinks that are high in calories and protein.** When it hurts to swallow, you may eat less and lose weight. It is important to keep your weight the same during radiation therapy. Having foods and drinks that are high in calories and protein can help you.

- **Sit upright and bend your head slightly forward when you are eating or drinking.** Remain sitting or standing upright for at least 30 minutes after eating.

- **Don't have things that can burn or scrape your throat, such as:**

  - Hot foods and drinks

  - Spicy foods

  - Foods and juices that are high in acid, such as tomatoes and oranges

  - Sharp, crunchy foods such as potato or corn chips

  - All tobacco products, such as cigarettes, pipes, cigars, and chewing tobacco

  - Drinks that contain alcohol

- **Talk with a dietitian.** He or she can help make sure you eat enough to maintain your weight. This may include choosing foods that are high in calories and protein and foods that are easy to swallow.

- **Talk with your doctor or nurse.** Let your doctor or nurse know if you notice throat changes, such as trouble swallowing, feeling as if you are choking, or coughing while eating or drinking. Also, let him or her know if you have pain or lose any weight. Your doctor can prescribe medicines that may help relieve your symptoms, such as antacids, gels that coat your throat, and pain killers.

Urinary and Bladder Changes

What they are

Radiation therapy can cause urinary and bladder problems, which can include:

- Burning or pain when you begin to **urinate** or after you empty your bladder
- Trouble starting to urinate
- Trouble emptying your bladder
- Frequent, urgent need to urinate
- Cystitis, a swelling (**inflammation**) in your urinary tract
- **Incontinence**, when you cannot control the flow of urine from your bladder, especially when coughing or sneezing
- Frequent need to get up during sleep to urinate
- Blood in your urine
- Bladder spasms, which are like painful muscle cramps

Why they occur

Urinary and bladder problems may occur when people get radiation therapy to the prostate or bladder. Radiation therapy can harm the healthy cells of the bladder wall and urinary tract, which can cause inflammation, ulcers, and infection.

How long they last

Urinary and bladder problems often start 3 to 5 weeks after radiation therapy begins. Most problems go away 2 to 8 weeks after treatment is over.

Ways to manage

- **Drink a lot of fluids.** This means 6 to 8 cups of fluids each day. Drink enough fluids so that your urine is clear to light yellow in color.
- **Avoid coffee, black tea, alcohol, spices, and all tobacco products.**

- **Talk with your doctor or nurse if you think you have urinary or bladder problems.** He or she may ask for a urine sample to make sure that you do not have an infection.

- **Talk to your doctor or nurse if you have incontinence.** He or she may refer you to a physical therapist who will assess your problem. The therapist can give you exercises to improve bladder control.

- **Medicine.** Your doctor may prescribe antibiotics if your problems are caused by an infection. Other medicines can help you urinate, reduce burning or pain, and ease bladder spasms.

Questions to Ask Your Doctor or Nurse

Here are some questions you might want to ask your doctor or nurse. You may want to write down their answers so you can review them again later.

- What kind of radiation therapy will I get?

- How can radiation therapy help?

- How many weeks will my course of radiation therapy last?

- What kinds of side effects should I expect during my course of radiation therapy?

- Will these side effects go away after radiation therapy is over?

- What kind of late side effects should I expect after radiation therapy is over?

- What can I do to manage these side effects?

- What will you do to manage these side effects?

- How can I learn more about radiation therapy?

- Which sections should I read in this book?

Section 47.6

Lists of Foods and Liquids

Clear Liquids

This list may help if you have diarrhea.

Table 47.2. Clear Liquids

Types of Liquids	Includes...
Soups	Bouillon Clear, fat-free broth Consommé Strained vegetable broth
Drinks	Apple juice Clear carbonated beverages Cranberry or grape juice Fruit-flavored drinks Fruit punch Sports drinks Tea Water
Types of Liquids	Includes...
Sweets	Fruit ices without fruit pieces Fruit ices without milk Honey Jelly Plain gelatin dessert Popsicles

Foods and Drinks that are High in Calories or Protein

This list may help if you need ideas for keeping your weight the same.

Table 47.3. Foods and Drinks that are High in Calories or Protein

Types of Food and Drinks	Includes...
Soups	Cream soups
Drinks	Instant breakfast shakes Milkshakes Whole milk (instead of low-fat or skim)
Main Meals and Other Foods	Beans, legumes, Butter, margarine, or oil Cheese Chicken, fish, or beef Cottage cheese Cream cheese on crackers or celery Deviled ham Eggs, such as scrambled or deviled eggs Muffins, Nuts, seeds, wheat germ Peanut butter
Desserts and Other Sweets	Custards Frozen yogurt Ice cream Puddings Yogurt
Replacement and Other Supplements	Powdered milk added to foods (pudding, milkshakes, or scrambled eggs) High-protein supplements, such as Ensure® and Carnation® Instant Breakfast®

Foods and Drinks that are Easy on the Stomach

This list may help if you have diarrhea or nausea and vomiting.

Table 47.4. Foods and Drinks that are Easy on the Stomach

Types of Food and Drinks	Includes...
Soups	Clear broth, such as chicken or beef
Drinks	Clear carbonated beverages Cranberry or grape juice Fruit-flavored drinks Fruit punch Sports drinks Tea Water
Main Meals and Snacks	Boiled potatoes Chicken, broiled or baked without the skin Crackers Cream of wheat Noodles Oatmeal Pretzels Rice Toast
Sweets	Angel food cake Canned peaches Gelatin Sherbet Yogurt

Chapter 48

Biological Therapy

What is biological therapy?

Biological therapy involves the use of living organisms, substances derived from living organisms, or laboratory-produced versions of such substances to treat disease. Some biological therapies for cancer use vaccines or bacteria to stimulate the body's immune system to act against cancer cells. These types of biological therapy, which are sometimes referred to collectively as "immunotherapy" or "biological response modifier therapy," do not target cancer cells directly. Other biological therapies, such as antibodies or segments of genetic material (RNA or DNA), do target cancer cells directly. Biological therapies that interfere with specific molecules involved in tumor growth and progression are also referred to as targeted therapies.

For patients with cancer, biological therapies may be used to treat the cancer itself or the side effects of other cancer treatments. Although many forms of biological therapy have been approved by the U.S. Food and Drug Administration (FDA), others remain experimental and are available to cancer patients principally through participation in clinical trials (research studies involving people).

Text in this chapter is excerpted from "Biological Therapies for Cancer," National Cancer Institute at the National Institutes of Health (NIH), June 12, 2013

What is the immune system and what role does it have in biological therapy for cancer?

The immune system is a complex network of organs, tissues, and specialized cells. It recognizes and destroys foreign invaders, such as bacteria or viruses, as well as some damaged, diseased, or abnormal cells in the body, including cancer cells. An immune response is triggered when the immune system encounters a substance, called an antigen, it recognizes as "foreign."

White blood cells are the primary players in immune system responses. Some white blood cells, including macrophages and natural killer cells, patrol the body, seeking out foreign invaders and diseased, damaged, or dead cells. These white blood cells provide a general—or nonspecific—level of immune protection.

Other white blood cells, including cytotoxic T cells and B cells, act against specific targets. Cytotoxic T cells release chemicals that can directly destroy microbes or abnormal cells. B cells make antibodies that latch onto foreign intruders or abnormal cells and tag them for destruction by another component of the immune system. Still other white blood cells, including dendritic cells, play supporting roles to ensure that cytotoxic T cells and B cells do their jobs effectively.

It is generally believed that the immune system's natural capacity to detect and destroy abnormal cells prevents the development of many cancers. Nevertheless, some cancer cells are able to evade detection by using one or more strategies. For example, cancer cells can undergo genetic changes that lead to the loss of cancer-associated antigens, making them less "visible" to the immune system. They may also use several different mechanisms to suppress immune responses or to avoid being killed by cytotoxic T cells.

The goal of immunotherapy for cancer is to overcome these barriers to an effective anticancer immune response. These biological therapies restore or increase the activities of specific immune-system components or counteract immunosuppressive signals produced by cancer cells.

What are monoclonal antibodies, and how are they used in cancer treatment?

Monoclonal antibodies, or MAbs, are laboratory-produced antibodies that bind to specific antigens expressed by cancer cells, such as a protein that is present on the surface of cancer cells but is absent from (or expressed at lower levels by) normal cells.

To create MAbs, researchers inject mice with an antigen from human cancer cells. They then harvest the antibody-producing cells from the mice and individually fuse them with a myeloma cell (cancerous B cell) to produce a fusion cell known as a hybridoma. Each hybridoma then divides to produce identical daughter cells or clones—hence the term "monoclonal"—and antibodies secreted by different clones are tested to identify the antibodies that bind most strongly to the antigen. Large quantities of antibodies can be produced by these immortal hybridoma cells. Because mouse antibodies can themselves elicit an immune response in humans, which would reduce their effectiveness, mouse antibodies are often "humanized" by replacing as much of the mouse portion of the antibody as possible with human portions. This is done through genetic engineering.

Some MAbs stimulate an immune response that destroys cancer cells. Similar to the antibodies produced naturally by B cells, these MAbs "coat" the cancer cell surface, triggering its destruction by the immune system. FDA-approved MAbs of this type include rituximab, which targets the CD20 antigen found on non-Hodgkin lymphoma cells, and alemtuzumab, which targets the CD52 antigen found on B-cell chronic lymphocytic leukemia (CLL) cells. Rituximab may also trigger cell death (apoptosis) directly.

Another group of MAbs stimulates an anticancer immune response by binding to receptors on the surface of immune cells and inhibiting signals that prevent immune cells from attacking the body's own tissues, including cancer cells. One such MAb, ipilimumab, has been approved by the FDA for treatment of metastatic melanoma, and others are being investigated in clinical studies.

Other MAbs interfere with the action of proteins that are necessary for tumor growth. For example, bevacizumab targets vascular endothelial growth factor (VEGF), a protein secreted by tumor cells and other cells in the tumor's microenvironment that promotes the development of tumor blood vessels. When bound to bevacizumab, VEGF cannot interact with its cellular receptor, preventing the signaling that leads to the growth of new blood vessels.

Similarly, cetuximab and panitumumab target the epidermal growth factor receptor (EGFR), and trastuzumab targets the human epidermal growth factor receptor 2 (HER-2). MAbs that bind to cell surface growth factor receptors prevent the targeted receptors from sending their normal growth-promoting signals. They may also trigger apoptosis and activate the immune system to destroy tumor cells.

Another group of cancer therapeutic MAbs are the immunoconjugates. These MAbs, which are sometimes called immunotoxins or antibody-drug conjugates, consist of an antibody attached to a cell-killing substance, such as a plant or bacterial toxin, a chemotherapy drug, or a radioactive molecule. The antibody latches onto its specific antigen on the surface of a cancer cell, and the cell-killing substance is taken up by the cell. FDA-approved conjugated MAbs that work this way include 90Y-ibritumomab tiuxetan, which targets the CD20 antigen to deliver radioactive yttrium-90 to B-cell non-Hodgkin lymphoma cells, and ado-trastuzumab emtansine, which targets the HER-2 molecule to deliver the drug DM1, which inhibits cell proliferation, to HER-2 expressing metastatic breast cancer cells.

What are cytokines, and how are they used in cancer treatment?

Cytokines are signaling proteins that are produced by white blood cells. They help mediate and regulate immune responses, inflammation, and hematopoiesis (new blood cell formation). Two types of cytokines are used to treat patients with cancer: interferons (INFs) and interleukins (ILs). A third type, called hematopoietic growth factors, is used to counteract some of the side effects of certain chemotherapy regimens.

Researchers have found that one type of INF, INF-alfa, can enhance a patient's immune response to cancer cells by activating certain white blood cells, such as natural killer cells and dendritic cells. INF-alfa may also inhibit the growth of cancer cells or promote their death. INF-alfa has been approved for the treatment of melanoma, Kaposi sarcoma, and several hematologic cancers.

Like INFs, ILs play important roles in the body's normal immune response and in the immune system's ability to respond to cancer. Researchers have identified more than a dozen distinct ILs, including IL-2, which is also called T-cell growth factor. IL-2 is naturally produced by activated T cells. It increases the proliferation of white blood cells, including cytotoxic T cells and natural killer cells, leading to an enhanced anticancer immune response. IL-2 also facilitates the production of antibodies by B cells to further target cancer cells. Aldesleukin, IL-2 that is made in a laboratory, has been approved for the treatment of metastatic kidney cancer and metastatic melanoma. Researchers are currently investigating whether combining aldesleukin treatment with other types of biological therapies may enhance its anticancer effects.

Hematopoietic growth factors are a special class of naturally occurring cytokines. All blood cells arise from hematopoietic stem cells in the bone marrow. Because chemotherapy drugs target proliferating cells, including normal blood stem cells, chemotherapy depletes these stem cells and the blood cells that they produce. Loss of red blood cells, which transport oxygen and nutrients throughout the body, can cause anemia. A decrease in platelets, which are responsible for blood clotting, often leads to abnormal bleeding. Finally, lower white blood cell counts leave chemotherapy patients vulnerable to infections.

Several growth factors that promote the growth of these various blood cell populations have been approved for clinical use. Erythropoietin stimulates red blood cell formation, and IL-11 increases platelet production. Granulocyte-macrophage colony-stimulating factor (GM-CSF) and granulocyte colony-stimulating factor (G-CSF) both increase the number of white blood cells, reducing the risk of infections. Treatment with these factors allows patients to continue chemotherapy regimens that might otherwise be stopped temporarily or modified to reduce the drug doses because of low blood cell numbers.

G-CSF and GM-CSF can also enhance the immune system's specific anticancer responses by increasing the number of cancer-fighting T cells. Thus, GM-CSF and G-CSF are used in combination with other biological therapies to strengthen anticancer immune responses.

What are cancer treatment vaccines?

Cancer treatment vaccines are designed to treat cancers that have already developed rather than to prevent them in the first place. Cancer treatment vaccines contain cancer-associated antigens to enhance the immune system's response to a patient's tumor cells. The cancer-associated antigens can be proteins or another type of molecule found on the surface of or inside cancer cells that can stimulate B cells or killer T cells to attack them.

Some vaccines that are under development target antigens that are found on or in many types of cancer cells. These types of cancer vaccines are being tested in clinical trials in patients with a variety of cancers, including prostate, colorectal, lung, breast, and thyroid cancers. Other cancer vaccines target antigens that are unique to a specific cancer type. Still other vaccines are designed against an antigen specific to one patient's tumor and need to be customized for each patient. The one cancer treatment vaccine that has received FDA approval, sipuleucel-T, is this type of vaccine.

Because of the limited toxicity seen with cancer vaccines, they are also being tested in clinical trials in combination with other forms of therapy, such as hormonal therapy, chemotherapy, radiation, and targeted therapies.

What is bacillus Calmette-Guérin therapy?

Bacillus Calmette-Guérin (BCG) was the first biological therapy to be approved by the FDA. It is a weakened form of a live tuberculosis bacterium that does not cause disease in humans. It was first used medically as a vaccine against tuberculosis. When inserted directly into the bladder with a catheter, BCG stimulates a general immune response that is directed not only against the foreign bacterium itself but also against bladder cancer cells. How and why BCG exerts this anticancer effect is not well understood, but the efficacy of the treatment is well documented. Approximately 70 percent of patients with early-stage bladder cancer experience a remission after BCG therapy.

BCG is also being studied in the treatment of other types of cancer.

What is oncolytic virus therapy?

Oncolytic virus therapy is an experimental form of biological therapy that involves the direct destruction of cancer cells. Oncolytic viruses infect both cancer and normal cells, but they have little effect on normal cells. In contrast, they readily replicate, or reproduce, inside cancer cells and ultimately cause the cancer cells to die. Some viruses, such as reovirus, Newcastle disease virus, and mumps virus, are naturally oncolytic, whereas others, including measles virus, adenovirus, and vaccinia virus, can be adapted or modified to replicate efficiently only in cancer cells. In addition, oncolytic viruses can be genetically engineered to preferentially infect and replicate in cancer cells that produce a specific cancer-associated antigen, such as EGFR or HER-2.

One of the challenges in using oncolytic viruses is that they may themselves be destroyed by the patient's immune system before they have a chance to attack the cancer. Researchers have developed several strategies to overcome this challenge, such as administering a combination of immune-suppressing chemotherapy drugs like cyclophosphamide along with the virus or "cloaking" the virus within a protective envelope. But an immune reaction in the patient may actually have xbenefits: although it may hamper oncolytic virus therapy at the time of viral delivery, it may enhance cancer cell destruction after the virus has infected the tumor cells.

No oncolytic virus has been approved for use in the United States, although H101, a modified form of adenovirus, was approved in China in 2006 for the treatment of patients with head and neck cancer. Several oncolytic viruses are currently being tested in clinical trials. Researchers are also investigating whether oncolytic viruses can be combined with other types of cancer therapies or can be used to sensitize patients' tumors to additional therapy.

What is gene therapy?

Still an experimental form of treatment, gene therapy attempts to introduce genetic material (DNA or RNA) into living cells. Gene therapy is being studied in clinical trials for many types of cancer.

In general, genetic material cannot be inserted directly into a person's cells. Instead, it is delivered to the cells using a carrier, or "vector." The vectors most commonly used in gene therapy are viruses, because they have the unique ability to recognize certain cells and insert genetic material into them. Scientists alter these viruses to make them more safe for humans (e.g., by inactivating genes that enable them to reproduce or cause disease) and/or to improve their ability to recognize and enter the target cell. A variety of liposomes (fatty particles) and nanoparticles are also being used as gene therapy vectors, and scientists are investigating methods of targeting these vectors to specific cell types.

Researchers are studying several methods for treating cancer with gene therapy. Some approaches target cancer cells, to destroy them or prevent their growth. Others target healthy cells to enhance their ability to fight cancer. In some cases, researchers remove cells from the patient, treat the cells with the vector in the laboratory, and return the cells to the patient. In others, the vector is given directly to the patient. Some gene therapy approaches being studied are described below.

- Replacing an altered tumor suppressor gene that produces a nonfunctional protein (or no protein) with a normal version of the gene. Because tumor suppressor genes (e.g., *TP53*) play a role in preventing cancer, restoring the normal function of these genes may inhibit cancer growth or promote cancer regression.

- Introducing genetic material to block the expression of an oncogene whose product promotes tumor growth. Short RNA or DNA molecules with sequences complementary to the gene's messenger RNA (mRNA) can be packaged into vectors or given to cells directly. These short molecules, called oligonucleotides, can bind

993

to the target mRNA, preventing its translation into protein or even causing its degradation.

- Improving a patient's immune response to cancer. In one approach, gene therapy is used to introduce cytokine-producing genes into cancer cells to stimulate the immune response to the tumor.

- Inserting genes into cancer cells to make them more sensitive to chemotherapy, radiation therapy, or other treatments

- Inserting genes into healthy blood-forming stem cells to make them more resistant to the side effects of cancer treatments, such as high doses of anticancer drugs

- Introducing "suicide genes" into a patient's cancer cells. A suicide gene is a gene whose product is able to activate a "pro-drug" (an inactive form of a toxic drug), causing the toxic drug to be produced only in cancer cells in patients given the pro-drug. Normal cells, which do not express the suicide genes, are not affected by the pro-drug.

- Inserting genes to prevent cancer cells from developing new blood vessels (angiogenesis)

Proposed gene therapy clinical trials, or protocols, must be approved by at least two review boards at the researchers' institution before they can be conducted. Gene therapy protocols must also be approved by the FDA, which regulates all gene therapy products. In addition, gene therapy trials that are funded by the National Institutes of Health must be registered with the NIH Recombinant DNA Advisory Committee.

What is adoptive T-cell transfer therapy?

Adoptive cell transfer is an experimental anticancer therapy that attempts to enhance the natural cancer-fighting ability of a patient's T cells. In one form of this therapy, researchers first harvest cytotoxic T cells that have invaded a patient's tumor. They then identify the cells with the greatest antitumor activity and grow large populations of those cells in a laboratory. The patients are then treated to deplete their immune cells, and the laboratory-grown T cells are infused into the patients.

In another, more recently developed form of this therapy, which is also a kind of gene therapy, researchers isolate T cells from a small sample of the patient's blood. They genetically modify the cells by inserting the gene for a receptor that recognizes an antigen specific to the patient's cancer cells and grow large numbers of these modified cells in culture. The genetically modified cells are then infused into patients whose immune cells have been depleted. The receptor expressed by the modified T cells allows these cells to attach to antigens on the surface of the tumor cells, which activates the T cells to attack and kill the tumor cells.

Adoptive T-cell transfer was first studied for the treatment of metastatic melanoma because melanomas often cause a substantial immune response, with many tumor-invading cytotoxic T cells. Adoptive cell transfer with genetically modified T cells is also being investigated as a treatment for other solid tumors, as well as for hematologic cancers.

What are the side effects of biological therapies?

The side effects associated with various biological therapies can differ by treatment type. However, pain, swelling, soreness, redness, itchiness, and rash at the site of infusion or injection are fairly common with these treatments.

Less common but more serious side effects tend to be more specific to one or a few types of biological therapy. For example, therapies intended to prompt an immune response against cancer can cause an array of flu-like symptoms, including fever, chills, weakness, dizziness, nausea or vomiting, muscle or joint aches, fatigue, headache, occasional breathing difficulties, and lowered or heightened blood pressure. Biological therapies that provoke an immune system response also pose a risk of severe or even fatal hypersensitivity (allergic) reactions.

Potential serious side effects of specific biological therapies are as follows:

MAbs

- Flu-like symptoms
- Severe allergic reaction
- Lowered blood counts
- Changes in blood chemistry
- Organ damage (usually to heart, lungs, kidneys, liver or brain)

Cytokines (interferons, interleukins, hematopoietic growth factors)

- Flu-like symptoms
- Severe allergic reaction

- Lowered blood counts
- Changes in blood chemistry
- Organ damage (usually to heart, lungs, kidneys, liver or brain)

Treatment vaccines

- Flu-like symptoms
- Severe allergic reaction

BCG

- Flu-like symptoms
- Severe allergic reaction
- Urinary side effects
  - Pain or burning sensation during urination
  - Increased urgency or frequency of urination
  - Blood in the urine

Oncolytic viruses

- Flu-like symptoms
- Tumor lysis syndrome: severe, sometimes life-threatening alterations in blood chemistry following the release of materials formerly contained within cancer cells into the bloodstream

Gene therapy

- Flu-like symptoms
- Secondary cancer: techniques that insert DNA into a host cell chromosome can cause cancer to develop if the insertion inhibits expression of a tumor suppressor gene or activates an oncogene; researchers are working to minimize this possibility
- Mistaken introduction of a gene into healthy cells, including reproductive cells
- Overexpression of the introduced gene may harm healthy tissues
- Virus vector transmission to other individuals or into the environment

Chapter 49

Targeted Cancer Therapies

What are targeted cancer therapies?

Targeted cancer therapies are drugs or other substances that block the growth and spread of cancer by interfering with specific molecules ("molecular targets") that are involved in the growth, progression, and spread of cancer. Targeted cancer therapies are sometimes called "molecularly targeted drugs," "molecularly targeted therapies," "precision medicines," or similar names.

Targeted therapies differ from standard chemotherapy in several ways:

- Targeted therapies act on specific molecular targets that are associated with cancer, whereas most standard chemotherapies act on all rapidly dividing normal and cancerous cells.

- Targeted therapies are deliberately chosen or designed to interact with their target, whereas many standard chemotherapies were identified because they kill cells.

- Targeted therapies are often cytostatic (that is, they block tumor cell proliferation), whereas standard chemotherapy agents are cytotoxic (that is, they kill tumor cells).

Targeted therapies are currently the focus of much anticancer drug development. They are a cornerstone of precision medicine, a form of

Text in this chapter is excerpted from "Targeted Cancer Therapies," National Cancer Institute at the National Institutes of Health (NIH), April 25, 2014 medicine that uses information about a person's genes and proteins to prevent, diagnose, and treat disease.

Many targeted cancer therapies have been approved by the Food and Drug Administration (FDA) to treat specific types of cancer. Others are being studied in clinical trials (research studies with people), and many more are in preclinical testing (research studies with animals).

How are targets for targeted cancer therapies identified?

The development of targeted therapies requires the identification of good targets—that is, targets that play a key role in cancer cell growth and survival. (It is for this reason that targeted therapies are sometimes referred to as the product of "rational" drug design.)

One approach to identify potential targets is to compare the amounts of individual proteins in cancer cells with those in normal cells. Proteins that are present in cancer cells but not normal cells or that are more abundant in cancer cells would be potential targets, especially if they are known to be involved in cell growth or survival. An example of such a differentially expressed target is the human epidermal growth factor receptor 2 protein (HER-2). HER-2 is expressed at high levels on the surface of some cancer cells. Several targeted therapies are directed against HER-2, including trastuzumab (Herceptin®), which is approved to treat certain breast and stomach cancers that overexpress HER-2.

Another approach to identify potential targets is to determine whether cancer cells produce mutant (altered) proteins that drive cancer progression. For example, the cell growth signaling protein BRAF is present in an altered form (known as BRAF V600E) in many melanomas. Vemurafenib (Zelboraf®) targets this mutant form of the BRAF protein and is approved to treat patients with inoperable or metastatic melanoma that contains this altered BRAF protein.

Researchers also look for abnormalities in chromosomes that are present in cancer cells but not in normal cells. Sometimes these chromosome abnormalities result in the creation of a fusion gene (a gene that incorporates parts of two different genes) whose product, called a fusion protein, may drive cancer development. Such fusion proteins are potential targets for targeted cancer therapies. For example, imatinib mesylate (Gleevec®) targets the BCR-ABL fusion protein, which is made from pieces of two genes that get joined together in some leukemia cells and promotes the growth of leukemic cells.

How are targeted therapies developed?

Once a candidate target has been identified, the next step is to develop a therapy that affects the target in a way that interferes with its ability to promote cancer cell growth or survival. For example, a targeted therapy could reduce the activity of the target or prevent it from binding to a receptor that it normally activates, among other possible mechanisms.

Most targeted therapies are either small molecules or monoclonal antibodies. Small-molecule compounds are typically developed for targets that are located inside the cell because such agents are able to enter cells relatively easily. Monoclonal antibodies are relatively large and generally cannot enter cells, so they are used only for targets that are outside cells or on the cell surface.

Candidate small molecules are usually identified in what are known as "high-throughput screens," in which the effects of thousands of test compounds on a specific target protein are examined. Compounds that affect the target (sometimes called "lead compounds") are then chemically modified to produce numerous closely related versions of the lead compound. These related compounds are then tested to determine which are most effective and have the fewest effects on nontarget molecules.

Monoclonal antibodies are developed by injecting animals (usually mice) with purified target proteins, causing the animals to make many different types of antibodies against the target. These antibodies are then tested to find the ones that bind best to the target without binding to nontarget proteins.

Before monoclonal antibodies are used in humans, they are "humanized" by replacing as much of the mouse antibody molecule as possible with corresponding portions of human antibodies. Humanizing is necessary to prevent the human immune system from recognizing the monoclonal antibody as "foreign" and destroying it before it has a chance to bind to its target protein. Humanization is not an issue for small-molecule compounds because they are not typically recognized by the body as foreign.

What types of targeted therapies are available?

Many different targeted therapies have been approved for use in cancer treatment. These therapies include hormone therapies, signal transduction inhibitors, gene expression modulator, apoptosis inducer, angiogenesis inhibitor, immunotherapies, and toxin delivery molecules.

- **Hormone therapies** slow or stop the growth of hormone-sensitive tumors, which require certain hormones to grow. Hormone therapies act by preventing the body from producing the hormones or by interfering with the action of the hormones. Hormone therapies have been approved for both breast cancer and prostate cancer.

- **Signal transduction inhibitors** block the activities of molecules that participate in signal transduction, the process by which a cell responds to signals from its environment. During this process, once a cell has received a specific signal, the signal is relayed within the cell through a series of biochemical reactions that ultimately produce the appropriate response(s). In some cancers, the malignant cells are stimulated to divide continuously without being prompted to do so by external growth factors. Signal transduction inhibitors interfere with this inappropriate signaling.

- **Gene expression modulators** modify the function of proteins that play a role in controlling gene expression.

- **Apoptosis inducers** cause cancer cells to undergo a process of controlled cell death called apoptosis. Apoptosis is one method the body uses to get rid of unneeded or abnormal cells, but cancer cells have strategies to avoid apoptosis. Apoptosis inducers can get around these strategies to cause the death of cancer cells.

- **Angiogenesis inhibitors** block the growth of new blood vessels to tumors (a process called tumor angiogenesis). A blood supply is necessary for tumors to grow beyond a certain size because blood provides the oxygen and nutrients that tumors need for continued growth. Treatments that interfere with angiogenesis may block tumor growth. Some targeted therapies that inhibit angiogenesis interfere with the action of vascular endothelial growth factor (VEGF), a substance that stimulates new blood vessel formation. Other angiogenesis inhibitors target other molecules that stimulate new blood vessel growth.

- **Immunotherapies** trigger the immune system to destroy cancer cells. Some immunotherapies are monoclonal antibodies that recognize specific molecules on the surface of cancer cells. Binding of the monoclonal antibody to the target molecule results in the immune destruction of cells that express that target molecule. Other monoclonal antibodies bind to certain immune cells to help these cells better kill cancer cells.

- **Monoclonal antibodies that deliver toxic molecules** can cause the death of cancer cells specifically. Once the antibody has bound to its target cell, the toxic molecule that is linked to the antibody—such as a radioactive substance or a poisonous chemical—is taken up by the cell, ultimately killing that cell. The toxin will not affect cells that lack the target for the antibody—i.e., the vast majority of cells in the body.

Cancer vaccines and gene therapy are sometimes considered targeted therapies because they interfere with the growth of specific cancer cells.

How is it determined whether a patient is a candidate for targeted therapy?

For some types of cancer, most patients with that cancer will have an appropriate target for a particular targeted therapy and, thus, will be candidates to be treated with that therapy. CML is an example: most patients have the *BCR-ABL* fusion gene. For other cancer types, however, a patient's tumor tissue must be tested to determine whether or not an appropriate target is present. The use of a targeted therapy may be restricted to patients whose tumor has a specific gene mutation that codes for the target; patients who do not have the mutation would not be candidates because the therapy would have nothing to target.

Sometimes, a patient is a candidate for a targeted therapy only if he or she meets specific criteria (for example, their cancer did not respond to other therapies, has spread, or is inoperable). These criteria are set by the FDA when it approves a specific targeted therapy.

What are the limitations of targeted cancer therapies?

Targeted therapies do have some limitations. One is that cancer cells can become resistant to them. Resistance can occur in two ways: the target itself changes through mutation so that the targeted therapy no longer interacts well with it, and/or the tumor finds a new pathway to achieve tumor growth that does not depend on the target.

For this reason, targeted therapies may work best in combination. For example, a recent study found that using two therapies that target different parts of the cell signaling pathway that is altered in melanoma by the BRAF V600E mutation slowed the development of resistance and disease progression to a greater extent than using just one targeted therapy.

Another approach is to use a targeted therapy in combination with one or more traditional chemotherapy drugs. For example, the targeted therapy trastuzumab (Herceptin®) has been used in combination with docetaxel, a traditional chemotherapy drug, to treat women with metastatic breast cancer that overexpresses the protein HER2/neu.

Another limitation of targeted therapy at present is that drugs for some identified targets are difficult to develop because of the target's structure and/or the way its function is regulated in the cell. One example is Ras, a signaling protein that is mutated in as many as one-quarter of all cancers (and in the majority of certain cancer types, such as pancreatic cancer). To date, it has not been possible to develop inhibitors of Ras signaling with existing drug development technologies. However, promising new approaches are offering hope that this limitation can soon be overcome.

What are the side effects of targeted cancer therapies?

Scientists had expected that targeted cancer therapies would be less toxic than traditional chemotherapy drugs because cancer cells are more dependent on the targets than are normal cells. However, targeted cancer therapies can have substantial side effects.

The most common side effects seen with targeted therapies are diarrhea and liver problems, such as hepatitis and elevated liver enzymes. Other side effects seen with targeted therapies include:

- Skin problems (acneiform rash, dry skin, nail changes, hair depigmentation)

- Problems with blood clotting and wound healing

- High blood pressure

- Gastrointestinal perforation (a rare side effect of some targeted therapies)

Certain side effects of some targeted therapies have been linked to better patient outcomes. For example, patients who develop acneiform rash (skin eruptions that resemble acne) while being treated with the signal transduction inhibitors erlotinib (Tarceva®) or gefitinib (Iressa®), both of which target the epidermal growth factor receptor, have tended to respond better to these drugs than patients who do not develop the rash. Similarly, patients who develop high blood pressure while being treated with the angiogenesis inhibitor bevacizumab generally have had better outcomes.

The few targeted therapies that are approved for use in children can have different side effects in children than in adults, including immunosuppression and impaired sperm production.

What targeted therapies have been approved for specific types of cancer?

The FDA has approved targeted therapies for the treatment of some patients with the following types of cancer (some targeted therapies have been approved to treat more than one type of cancer):

Adenocarcinoma of the stomach or gastroesophageal junction: Trastuzumab (Herceptin®), ramucirumab (Cyramza™)

Basal cell carcinoma: Vismodegib (Erivedge™)

Brain cancer: Bevacizumab (Avastin®), everolimus (Afinitor®)

Breast cancer: Everolimus (Afinitor®), tamoxifen, toremifene (Fareston®), Trastuzumab (Herceptin®), fulvestrant (Faslodex®), anastrozole (Arimidex®), exemestane (Aromasin®), lapatinib (Tykerb®), letrozole (Femara®), pertuzumab (Perjeta™), ado-trastuzumab emtansine (Kadcyla™), palbociclib (Ibrance®)

Cervical cancer: Bevacizumab (Avastin®)

Colorectal cancer: Cetuximab (Erbitux®), panitumumab (Vectibix®), bevacizumab (Avastin®),ziv-aflibercept (Zaltrap®), regorafenib (Stivarga®)

Dermatofibrosarcoma protuberans: Imatinib mesylate (Gleevec®)

Endocrine/neuroendocrine tumors: Lanreotide acetate (Somatuline® Depot)

Head and neck cancer: Cetuximab (Erbitux®)

Gastrointestinal stromal tumor: Imatinib mesylate (Gleevec®), sunitinib (Sutent®), regorafenib (Stivarga®)

Giant cell tumor of the bone: Denosumab (Xgeva®)

Kaposi sarcoma: Alitretinoin (Panretin®)

Kidney cancer: Bevacizumab (Avastin®), sorafenib (Nexavar®), sunitinib (Sutent®), pazopanib (Votrient®), temsirolimus (Torisel®), everolimus (Afinitor®), axitinib (Inlyta®)

Leukemia: Tretinoin (Vesanoid®), imatinib mesylate (Gleevec®), dasatinib (Sprycel®), nilotinib (Tasigna®), bosutinib (Bosulif®), rituximab (Rituxan®), alemtuzumab (Campath®), ofatumumab (Arzerra®), obinutuzumab (Gazyva™), ibrutinib (Imbruvica™), idelalisib (Zydelig®), blinatumomab (Blincyto™)

Liver cancer: Sorafenib (Nexavar®)

Lung cancer: Bevacizumab (Avastin®), crizotinib (Xalkori®), erlotinib (Tarceva®), gefitinib (Iressa®), afatinib dimaleate (Gilotrif®), ceritinib (LDK378/Zykadia), ramucirumab (Cyramza™)

Lymphoma: Ibritumomab tiuxetan (Zevalin®), denileukin diftitox (Ontak®), brentuximab vedotin (Adcetris®), rituximab (Rituxan®), vorinostat (Zolinza®), romidepsin (Istodax®), bexarotene (Targretin®), bortezomib (Velcade®), pralatrexate (Folotyn®), lenaliomide (Revlimid®), ibrutinib (Imbruvica™), siltuximab (Sylvant™), idelalisib (Zydelig®), belinostat (Beleodaq™)

Melanoma: Ipilimumab (Yervoy®), vemurafenib (Zelboraf®), trametinib (Mekinist®), dabrafenib (Tafinlar®), pembrolizumab (Keytruda®), nivolumab (Opdivo®)

Multiple myeloma: Bortezomib (Velcade®), carfilzomib (Kyprolis®), lenaliomide (Revlimid®),pomalidomide (Pomalyst®)

Myelodysplastic/myeloproliferative disorders: Imatinib mesylate (Gleevec®), ruxolitinib phosphate (Jakafi™)

Ovarian epithelial/fallopian tube/primary peritoneal cancers: Bevacizumab (Avastin®),olaparib (Lynparza™)

Pancreatic cancer: Erlotinib (Tarceva®), everolimus (Afinitor®), sunitinib (Sutent®)

Prostate cancer: Cabazitaxel (Jevtana®), enzalutamide (Xtandi®), abiraterone acetate (Zytiga®), radium 223 chloride (Xofigo®)

Soft tissue sarcoma: Pazopanib (Votrient®)

Systemic mastocytosis: Imatinib mesylate (Gleevec®)

Thyroid cancer: Cabozantinib (Cometriq™), vandetanib (Caprelsa®), sorafenib (Nexavar®)

Chapter 50

Hyperthermia in Cancer Treatment

What is hyperthermia?

Hyperthermia (also called thermal therapy or thermotherapy) is a type of cancer treatment in which body tissue is exposed to high temperatures (up to 113°F). Research has shown that high temperatures can damage and kill cancer cells, usually with minimal injury to normal tissues. By killing cancer cells and damaging proteins and structures within cells, hyperthermia may shrink tumors.

Hyperthermia is under study in clinical trials (research studies with people) and is not widely available.

How is hyperthermia used to treat cancer?

Hyperthermia is almost always used with other forms of cancer therapy, such as radiation therapy and chemotherapy. Hyperthermia may make some cancer cells more sensitive to radiation or harm other cancer cells that radiation cannot damage. When hyperthermia and radiation therapy are combined, they are often given within an hour of each other. Hyperthermia can also enhance the effects of certain anticancer drugs.

Text in this chapter is excerpted from "Hyperthermia in Cancer Treatment," National Cancer Institute at the National Institutes of Health (NIH), August 31, 2011.

Numerous clinical trials have studied hyperthermia in combination with radiation therapy and/or chemotherapy. These studies have focused on the treatment of many types of cancer, including sarcoma, melanoma, and cancers of the head and neck, brain, lung, esophagus, breast, bladder, rectum, liver, appendix, cervix, and peritoneal lining (mesothelioma). Many of these studies, but not all, have shown a significant reduction in tumor size when hyperthermia is combined with other treatments. However, not all of these studies have shown increased survival in patients receiving the combined treatments.

What are the different methods of hyperthermia?

Several methods of hyperthermia are currently under study, including local, regional, and whole-body hyperthermia.

- In **local hyperthermia**, heat is applied to a small area, such as a tumor, using various techniques that deliver energy to heat the tumor. Different types of energy may be used to apply heat, including microwave, radiofrequency, and ultrasound. Depending on the tumor location, there are several approaches to local hyperthermia:
    - **External** approaches are used to treat tumors that are in or just below the skin. External applicators are positioned around or near the appropriate region, and energy is focused on the tumor to raise its temperature.
    - **Intraluminal or endocavitary** methods may be used to treat tumors within or near body cavities, such as the esophagus or rectum. Probes are placed inside the cavity and inserted into the tumor to deliver energy and heat the area directly.
    - **Interstitial** techniques are used to treat tumors deep within the body, such as brain tumors. This technique allows the tumor to be heated to higher temperatures than external techniques. Under anesthesia, probes or needles are inserted into the tumor. Imaging techniques, such as ultrasound, may be used to make sure the probe is properly positioned within the tumor. The heat source is then inserted into the probe. Radiofrequency (RFA) is a type of interstitial hyperthermia that uses radio waves to heat and kill cancer cells.
- In **regional hyperthermia**, various approaches may be used to heat large areas of tissue, such as a body cavity, organ, or limb.

- **Deep tissue** approaches may be used to treat cancers within the body, such as cervical or bladder cancer. External applicators are positioned around the body cavity or organ to be treated, and microwave or radiofrequency energy is focused on the area to raise its temperature.

- **Regional perfusion** techniques can be used to treat cancers in the arms and legs, such as melanoma, or cancer in some organs, such as the liver or lung. In this procedure, some of the patient's blood is removed, heated, and then pumped (perfused) back into the limb or organ. Anticancer drugs are commonly given during this treatment.

- **Continuous hyperthermic peritoneal perfusion (CHPP)** is a technique used to treat cancers within the peritoneal cavity (the space within the abdomen that contains the intestines, stomach, and liver), including primary peritoneal mesothelioma and stomach cancer. During surgery, heated anticancer drugs flow from a warming device through the peritoneal cavity. The peritoneal cavity temperature reaches 106–108°F.

- **Whole-body hyperthermia** is used to treat metastatic cancer that has spread throughout the body. This can be accomplished by several techniques that raise the body temperature to 107–108°F, including the use of thermal chambers (similar to large incubators) or hot water blankets.

The effectiveness of hyperthermia treatment is related to the temperature achieved during the treatment, as well as the length of treatment and cell and tissue characteristics. To ensure that the desired temperature is reached, but not exceeded, the temperature of the tumor and surrounding tissue is monitored throughout hyperthermia treatment. Using local anesthesia, the doctor inserts small needles or tubes with tiny thermometers into the treatment area to monitor the temperature. Imaging techniques, such as CT (computed tomography), may be used to make sure the probes are properly positioned.

Does hyperthermia have any complications or side effects?

Most normal tissues are not damaged during hyperthermia if the temperature remains under 111°F. However, due to regional differences in tissue characteristics, higher temperatures may occur in various spots. This can result in burns, blisters, discomfort, or pain.

Perfusion techniques can cause tissue swelling, blood clots, bleeding, and other damage to the normal tissues in the perfused area; however, most of these side effects are temporary. Whole-body hyperthermia can cause more serious side effects, including cardiac and vascular disorders, but these effects are uncommon. Diarrhea, nausea, and vomiting are commonly observed after whole-body hyperthermia.

What does the future hold for hyperthermia?

A number of challenges must be overcome before hyperthermia can be considered a standard treatment for cancer. Many clinical trials are being conducted to evaluate the effectiveness of hyperthermia. Some trials continue to research hyperthermia in combination with other therapies for the treatment of different cancers. Other studies focus on improving hyperthermia techniques.

Chapter 51

Lasers in Cancer Treatment

What is laser light?

The term "laser" stands for light amplification by stimulated emission of radiation. Ordinary light, such as that from a light bulb, has many wavelengths and spreads in all directions. Laser light, on the other hand, has a specific wavelength. It is focused in a narrow beam and creates a very high-intensity light. This powerful beam of light may be used to cut through steel or to shape diamonds. Because lasers can focus very accurately on tiny areas, they can also be used for very precise surgical work or for cutting through tissue (in place of a scalpel).

What is laser therapy, and how is it used in cancer treatment?

Laser therapy uses high-intensity light to treat cancer and other illnesses. Lasers can be used to shrink or destroy tumors or precancerous growths. Lasers are most commonly used to treat superficial cancers (cancers on the surface of the body or the lining of internal organs) such as basal cell skin cancer and the very early stages of some cancers, such as cervical, penile, vaginal, vulvar, and non-small cell lung cancer.

Text in this chapter is excerpted from "Lasers in Cancer Treatment," National Cancer Institute at the National Institutes of Health (NIH), September 13, 2011.

Lasers also may be used to relieve certain symptoms of cancer, such as bleeding or obstruction. For example, lasers can be used to shrink or destroy a tumor that is blocking a patient's trachea (windpipe) or esophagus. Lasers also can be used to remove colon polyps or tumors that are blocking the colon or stomach.

Laser therapy can be used alone, but most often it is combined with other treatments, such as surgery, chemotherapy, or radiation therapy. In addition, lasers can seal nerve endings to reduce pain after surgery and seal lymph vessels to reduce swelling and limit the spread of tumor cells.

How is laser therapy given to the patient?

Laser therapy is often given through a flexible endoscope (a thin, lighted tube used to look at tissues inside the body). The endoscope is fitted with optical fibers (thin fibers that transmit light). It is inserted through an opening in the body, such as the mouth, nose, anus, or vagina. Laser light is then precisely aimed to cut or destroy a tumor.

Laser-induced interstitial thermotherapy (LITT), or interstitial laser photo coagulation, also uses lasers to treat some cancers. LITT is similar to a cancer treatment called hyperthermia, which uses heat to shrink tumors by damaging or killing cancer cells. During LITT, an optical fiber is inserted into a tumor. Laser light at the tip of the fiber raises the temperature of the tumor cells and damages or destroys them. LITT is sometimes used to shrink tumors in the liver.

Photodynamic therapy (PDT) is another type of cancer treatment that uses lasers. In PDT, a certain drug, called a photosensitizer or photosensitizing agent, is injected into a patient and absorbed by cells all over the patient's body. After a couple of days, the agent is found mostly in cancer cells. Laser light is then used to activate the agent and destroy cancer cells. Because the photosensitizer makes the skin and eyes sensitive to light afterwards, patients are advised to avoid direct sunlight and bright indoor light during that time.

What types of lasers are used in cancer treatment?

Three types of lasers are used to treat cancer: carbon dioxide (CO_2) lasers, argon lasers, and neodymium: yttrium-aluminum-garnet (Nd:YAG) lasers. Each of these can shrink or destroy tumors and can be used with endoscopes.

CO_2 and argon lasers can cut the skin's surface without going into deeper layers. Thus, they can be used to remove superficial cancers, such as skin cancer. In contrast, the Nd:YAG laser is more commonly applied through an endoscope to treat internal organs, such as the uterus, esophagus, and colon.

Nd:YAG laser light can also travel through optical fibers into specific areas of the body during LITT. Argon lasers are often used to activate the drugs used in PDT.

What are the advantages of laser therapy?

Lasers are more precise than standard surgical tools (scalpels), so they do less damage to normal tissues. As a result, patients usually have less pain, bleeding, swelling, and scarring. With laser therapy, operations are usually shorter. In fact, laser therapy can often be done on an outpatient basis. It takes less time for patients to heal after laser surgery, and they are less likely to get infections. Patients should consult with their health care provider about whether laser therapy is appropriate for them.

What are the disadvantages of laser therapy?

Laser therapy also has several limitations. Surgeons must have specialized training before they can do laser therapy, and strict safety precautions must be followed. Laser therapy is expensive and requires bulky equipment. In addition, the effects of laser therapy may not last long, so doctors may have to repeat the treatment for a patient to get the full benefit.

Chapter 52

Photodynamic Therapy for Cancer

What is photodynamic therapy?

Photodynamic therapy (PDT) is a treatment that uses a drug, called a photosensitizer or photosensitizing agent, and a particular type of light. When photosensitizers are exposed to a specific wavelength of light, they produce a form of oxygen that kills nearby cells.

Each photosensitizer is activated by light of a specific wavelength. This wavelength determines how far the light can travel into the body. Thus, doctors use specific photosensitizers and wavelengths of light to treat different areas of the body with PDT.

How is PDT used to treat cancer?

In the first step of PDT for cancer treatment, a photosensitizing agent is injected in to the bloodstream. The agent is absorbed by cells all over the body but stays in cancer cells longer than it does in normal cells. Approximately 24 to 72 hours after injection, when most of the agent has left normal cells but remains in cancer cells, the tumor is exposed to light. The photosensitizer in the tumor absorbs the light

Text in this chapter is excerpted from "Photodynamic Therapy for Cancer," National Cancer Institute at the National Institutes of Health (NIH), September 6, 2011.

and produces an active form of oxygen that destroys nearby cancer cells.

In addition to directly killing cancer cells, PDT appears to shrink or destroy tumors in two other ways. The photosensitizer can damage blood vessels in the tumor, thereby preventing the cancer from receiving necessary nutrients. PDT also may activate the immune system to attack the tumor cells.

The light used for PDT can come from a laser or other sources. Laser light can be directed through fiber optic cables (thin fibers that transmit light) to deliver light to areas inside the body. For example, a fiber optic cable can be inserted through an endoscope (a thin, lighted tube used to look at tissues inside the body) into the lungs or esophagus to treat cancer in these organs. Other light sources include light-emitting diodes (LEDs), which may be used for surface tumors, such as skin cancer.

PDT is usually performed as an outpatient procedure. PDT may also be repeated and may be used with other therapies, such as surgery, radiation, or chemotherapy.

Extracorporeal photopheresis (ECP) is a type of PDT in which a machine is used to collect the patient's blood cells, treat them outside the body with a photosensitizing agent, expose them to light, and then return them to the patient. The U.S. Food and Drug Administration (FDA) has approved ECP to help lessen the severity of skin symptoms of cutaneous T-cell lymphoma that has not responded to other therapies. Studies are under way to determine if ECP may have some application for other blood cancers, and also to help reduce rejection after transplants.

What types of cancer are currently treated with PDT?

To date, the FDA has approved the photosensitizing agent called porfimer sodium, or Photofrin®, for use in PDT to treat or relieve the symptoms of esophageal cancer and non-small cell lung cancer. Porfimer sodium is approved to relieve symptoms of esophageal cancer when the cancer obstructs the esophagus or when the cancer cannot be satisfactorily treated with laser therapy alone. Porfimer sodium is used to treat non-small cell lung cancer in patients for whom the usual treatments are not appropriate, and to relieve symptoms in patients with non-small cell lung cancer that obstructs the airways. In 2003, the FDA approved porfimer sodium for the treatment of precancerous lesions in patients with Barrett esophagus, a condition that can lead to esophageal cancer.

What are the limitations of PDT?

The light needed to activate most photosensitizers cannot pass through more than about one-third of an inch of tissue (1 centimeter). For this reason, PDT is usually used to treat tumors on or just under the skin or on the lining of internal organs or cavities. PDT is also less effective in treating large tumors, because the light cannot pass far into these tumors. PDT is a local treatment and generally cannot be used to treat cancer that has spread (metastasized).

Does PDT have any complications or side effects?

Porfimer sodium makes the skin and eyes sensitive to light for approximately 6 weeks after treatment. Thus, patients are advised to avoid direct sunlight and bright indoor light for at least 6 weeks.

Photosensitizers tend to build up in tumors and the activating light is focused on the tumor. As a result, damage to healthy tissue is minimal. However, PDT can cause burns, swelling, pain, and scarring in nearby healthy tissue. Other side effects of PDT are related to the area that is treated. They can include coughing, trouble swallowing, stomach pain, painful breathing, or shortness of breath; these side effects are usually temporary.

Chapter 53

Cancer Vaccines

What are vaccines?

Vaccines are medicines that boost the immune system's natural ability to protect the body against "foreign invaders," mainly infectious agents that may cause disease.

The immune system is a complex network of organs, tissues, and specialized cells that act collectively to defend the body. When an infectious microbe invades the body, the immune system recognizes it as foreign, destroys it, and "remembers" it to prevent another infection should the microbe invade the body again in the future. Vaccines take advantage of this response.

Traditional vaccines usually contain harmless versions of microbes—killed or weakened microbes, or parts of microbes—that do not cause disease but are able to stimulate an immune response against the microbes. When the immune system encounters these substances through vaccination, it responds to them, eliminates them from the body, and develops a memory of them. This vaccine-induced memory enables the immune system to act quickly to protect the body if it becomes infected by the same microbes in the future.

The immune system's role in defending against disease-causing microbes has long been recognized. Scientists have also discovered that the immune system can protect the body against threats posed by certain damaged, diseased, or abnormal cells, including cancer cells.

Text in this section is excerpted from "Cancer Vaccines," National Cancer Institute at the National Institutes of Health (NIH), November 15, 2011.

How do vaccines stimulate the immune system?

White blood cells, or leukocytes, play the main role in immune responses. These cells carry out the many tasks required to protect the body against disease-causing microbes and abnormal cells.

Some types of leukocytes patrol the circulation, seeking foreign invaders and diseased, damaged, or dead cells. These white blood cells provide a general—or nonspecific—level of immune protection.

Other types of leukocytes, known as lymphocytes, provide targeted protection against specific threats, whether from a specific microbe or a diseased or abnormal cell. The most important groups of lymphocytes responsible for carrying out immune responses against such threats are B cells and cytotoxic (cell-killing) T cells.

B cells make antibodies, which are large secreted proteins that bind to, inactivate, and help destroy foreign invaders or abnormal cells. Most preventive vaccines, including those aimed at hepatitis B virus (HBV) and human papillomavirus (HPV), stimulate the production of antibodies that bind to specific, targeted microbes and block their ability to cause infection. Cytotoxic T cells, which are also known as killer T cells, kill infected or abnormal cells by releasing toxic chemicals or by prompting the cells to self-destruct (a process known as apoptosis).

Other types of lymphocytes and leukocytes play supporting roles to ensure that B cells and killer T cells do their jobs effectively. These supporting cells include helper T cells and dendritic cells, which help activate killer T cells and enable them to recognize specific threats.

Cancer treatment vaccines are designed to work by activating B cells and killer T cells and directing them to recognize and act against specific types of cancer. They do this by introducing one or more molecules known as antigens into the body, usually by injection. An antigen is a substance that stimulates a specific immune response. An antigen can be a protein or another type of molecule found on the surface of or inside a cell.

Microbes are recognized by the immune system as a potential threat that should be destroyed because they carry foreign or "non-self" antigens. In contrast, normal cells in the body have antigens that identify them as "self." Self-antigens tell the immune system that normal cells are not a threat and should be ignored.

Cancer cells can carry both self-antigens and cancer-associated antigens. The cancer-associated antigens mark the cancer cells as abnormal, or foreign, and can cause B cells and killer T cells to mount an attack against them.

Cancer cells may also make much larger amounts of certain self-antigens than normal cells. Because of their high abundance, these self-antigens may be viewed by the immune system as being foreign and, therefore, may trigger an immune response against the cancer cells.

What are cancer vaccines?

Cancer vaccines are medicines that belong to a class of substances known as biological response modifiers. Biological response modifiers work by stimulating or restoring the immune system's ability to fight infections and disease. There are two broad types of cancer vaccines:

- **Preventive (or prophylactic) vaccines**, which are intended to prevent cancer from developing in healthy people; and

- **Treatment (or therapeutic) vaccines**, which are intended to treat an existing cancer by strengthening the body's natural defenses against the cancer.

Two types of cancer preventive vaccines are available in the United States, and one cancer treatment vaccine has recently become available.

How do cancer preventive vaccines work?

Cancer preventive vaccines target infectious agents that cause or contribute to the development of cancer. They are similar to traditional vaccines, which help prevent infectious diseases, such as measles or polio, by protecting the body against infection. Both cancer preventive vaccines and traditional vaccines are based on antigens that are carried by infectious agents and that are relatively easy for the immune system to recognize as foreign.

What cancer preventive vaccines are approved in the United States?

The U.S. Food and Drug Administration (FDA) has approved two vaccines, Gardasil® and Cervarix®, that protect against infection by the two types of HPV—types 16 and 18—that cause approximately 70 percent of all cases of cervical cancer worldwide. At least 17 other types of HPV are responsible for the remaining 30 percent of cervical cancer cases. HPV types 16 and/or 18 also cause some vaginal, vulvar, anal, penile, and oropharyngeal cancers.

In addition, Gardasil protects against infection by two additional HPV types, 6 and 11, which are responsible for about 90 percent of all cases of genital warts in males and females but do not cause cervical cancer.

Gardasil, manufactured by Merck & Company, is based on HPV antigens that are proteins. These proteins are used in the laboratory to make four different types of "virus-like particles," or VLPs, that correspond to HPV types 6, 11, 16, and 18. The four types of VLPs are then combined to make the vaccine. Because Gardasil targets four HPV types, it is called a quadrivalent vaccine. In contrast with traditional vaccines, which are often composed of weakened whole microbes, VLPs are not infectious. However, the VLPs in Gardasil are still able to stimulate the production of antibodies against HPV types 6, 11, 16, and 18.

Cervarix, manufactured by GlaxoSmithKline, is a bivalent vaccine. It is composed of VLPs made with proteins from HPV types 16 and 18. In addition, there is some initial evidence that Cervarix provides partial protection against a few additional HPV types that can cause cancer. However, more studies will be needed to understand the magnitude and impact of this effect.

Gardasil is approved for use in females to prevent cervical cancer and some vulvar and vaginal cancers caused by HPV types 16 and 18, and for use in males and females to prevent anal cancer and precancerous anal lesions caused by these HPV types. Gardasil is also approved for use in males and females to prevent genital warts caused by HPV types 6 and 11. The vaccine is approved for these uses in females and males ages 9 to 26. Cervarix is approved for use in females ages 9 to 25 to prevent cervical cancer caused by HPV types 16 and 18.

The FDA has also approved a cancer preventive vaccine that protects against HBV infection. Chronic HBV infection can lead to liver cancer. The original HBV vaccine was approved in 1981, making it the first cancer preventive vaccine to be successfully developed and marketed. Today, most children in the United States are vaccinated against HBV shortly after birth.

Have other microbes been associated with cancer?

Many scientists believe that microbes cause or contribute to between 15 percent and 25 percent of all cancers diagnosed worldwide each year, with the percentage being lower in developed than developing countries

The International Agency for Research on Cancer (IARC) has classified several microbes as carcinogenic (causing or contributing to the development of cancer in people), including HPV and HBV. These

Table 53.1. Cancer and the causing agents

Infectious Agents	Type of Organism	Associated Cancers
hepatitis B virus (HBV)	virus	hepatocellular carcinoma (a type of liver cancer)
hepatitis C virus (HCV)	virus	hepatocellular carcinoma (a type of liver cancer)
human papillomavirus (HPV) types 16 and 18, as well as other HPV types	virus	cervical cancer; vaginal cancer; vulvar cancer; oropharyngeal cancer (cancers of the base of the tongue, tonsils, or upper throat); anal cancer; penile cancer; squamous cell carcinoma of the skin
Epstein-Barr virus	virus	Burkitt lymphoma; non-Hodgkin lymphoma; Hodgkin lymphoma; nasopharyngeal carcinoma (cancer of the upper part of the throat behind the nose)
Kaposi sarcoma-associated herpesvirus (KSHV), also known as human herpesvirus 8 (HHV8)	virus	Kaposi sarcoma
human T-cell lymphotropic virus type 1 (HTLV1)	virus	adult T-cell leukemia/lymphoma
Helicobacter pylori	bacterium	stomach cancer; mucosa-associated lymphoid tissue (MALT) lymphoma
schistosomes (Schistosoma hematobium)	parasite	bladder cancer
liver flukes (Opisthorchis viverrini)	parasite	cholangiocarcinoma (a type of liver cancer)

infectious agents—bacteria, viruses, and parasites—and the cancer types with which they are most strongly associated are listed in the table below:

How are cancer treatment vaccines designed to work?

Cancer treatment vaccines are designed to treat cancers that have already developed. They are intended to delay or stop cancer cell growth; to cause tumor shrinkage; to prevent cancer from coming back; or to eliminate cancer cells that have not been killed by other forms of treatment.

Developing effective cancer treatment vaccines requires a detailed understanding of how immune system cells and cancer cells interact. The immune system often does not "see" cancer cells as dangerous or foreign, as it generally does with microbes. Therefore, the immune system does not mount a strong attack against the cancer cells.

Several factors may make it difficult for the immune system to target growing cancers for destruction. Most important, cancer cells carry normal self-antigens in addition to specific cancer-associated antigens. Furthermore, cancer cells sometimes undergo genetic changes that may lead to the loss of cancer-associated antigens. Finally, cancer cells can produce chemical messages that suppress anticancer immune responses by killer T cells. As a result, even when the immune system recognizes a growing cancer as a threat, the cancer may still escape a strong attack by the immune system.

Producing effective treatment vaccines has proven much more difficult and challenging than developing cancer preventive vaccines. To be effective, cancer treatment vaccines must achieve two goals. First, like traditional vaccines and cancer preventive vaccines, cancer treatment vaccines must stimulate specific immune responses against the correct target. Second, the immune responses must be powerful enough to overcome the barriers that cancer cells use to protect themselves from attack by B cells and killer T cells. Recent advances in understanding how cancer cells escape recognition and attack by the immune system are now giving researchers the knowledge required to design cancer treatment vaccines that can accomplish both goals.

Has the FDA approved any cancer treatment vaccines?

In April 2010, the FDA approved the first cancer treatment vaccine. This vaccine, sipuleucel-T (Provenge®, manufactured by Dendreon), is approved for use in some men with metastatic prostate. It is designed to stimulate an immune response to prostatic acid phosphatase (PAP), an antigen that is found on most prostate cancer cells. In a clinical trial, sipuleucel-T increased the survival of men with a certain type of metastatic prostate cancer by about 4 months.

Unlike some other cancer treatment vaccines under development, sipuleucel-T is customized to each patient. The vaccine is created by isolating immune system cells called antigen-presenting cells (APCs) from a patient's blood through a procedure called leukapheresis. The

APCs are sent to Dendreon, where they are cultured with a protein called PAP-GM-CSF. This protein consists of PAP linked to another protein called granulocyte-macrophage colony-stimulating factor (GM-CSF). The latter protein stimulates the immune system and enhances antigen presentation.

APC cells cultured with PAP-GM-CSF constitute the active component of sipuleucel-T. Each patient's cells are returned to the patient's treating physician and infused into the patient. Patients receive three treatments, usually 2 weeks apart, with each round of treatment requiring the same manufacturing process. Although the precise mechanism of action of sipuleucel-T is not known, it appears that the APCs that have taken up PAP-GM-CSF stimulate T cells of the immune system to kill tumor cells that express PAP.

How are cancer vaccines made?

All cancer preventive vaccines approved by the FDA to date have been made using antigens from microbes that cause or contribute to the development of cancer. These include antigens from HBV and specific types of HPV. These antigens are proteins that help make up the outer surface of the viruses. Because only part of these microbes is used, the resulting vaccines are not infectious and, therefore, cannot cause disease.

Researchers are also creating synthetic versions of antigens in the laboratory for use in cancer preventive vaccines. In doing this, they often modify the chemical structure of the antigens to stimulate immune responses that are stronger than those caused by the original antigens.

Similarly, cancer treatment vaccines are made using antigens from cancer cells or modified versions of them. Antigens that have been used thus far include proteins, carbohydrates (sugars), glycoproteins or glycopeptides (carbohydrate-protein combinations), and gangliosides (carbohydrate-lipid combinations).

Cancer treatment vaccines are also being developed using weakened or killed cancer cells that carry a specific cancer-associated antigen or immune cells that are modified to express such an antigen. These cells can come from a patient himself or herself (called an autologous vaccine, such as sipuleucel-T) or from another patient (called an allogeneic vaccine).

Other types of cancer treatment vaccines are made using molecules of deoxyribonucleic acid (DNA) or ribonucleic acid (RNA) that contain the genetic instructions for cancer-associated antigens. The DNA or

RNA can be injected alone into a patient as a "naked nucleic acid" vaccine, or researchers can insert the DNA or RNA into a harmless virus. After the naked nucleic acid or virus is injected into the body, the DNA or RNA is taken up by cells, which begin to manufacture the tumor-associated antigens. Researchers hope that the cells will make enough of the tumor-associated antigens to stimulate a strong immune response.

Scientists have identified a large number of cancer-associated antigens, several of which are now being used to make experimental cancer treatment vaccines. Some of these antigens are found on or in many or most types of cancer cells. Others are unique to specific cancer types.

Can researchers add ingredients to cancer vaccines to make them work better?

Antigens and other substances are often not strong enough inducers of the immune response to make effective cancer treatment vaccines. Researchers often add extra ingredients, known as adjuvants, to treatment vaccines. These substances serve to boost immune responses that have been set in motion by exposure to antigens or other means. Patients undergoing experimental treatment with a cancer vaccine sometimes receive adjuvants separately from the vaccine itself.

Adjuvants used for cancer vaccines come from many different sources. Some microbes, such as the bacterium Bacillus Calmette-Guérin (BCG) originally used as a vaccine against tuberculosis, can serve as adjuvants. Substances produced by bacteria, such as Detox B, are also frequently used. Biological products derived from nonmicrobial organisms can be used as adjuvants, too. One example is keyhole limpet hemocyanin (KLH), which is a large protein produced by a sea animal. Attaching antigens to KLH has been shown to increase their ability to stimulate immune responses. Even some nonbiological substances, such as an emulsified oil known as montanide ISA-51, can be used as adjuvants.

Natural or synthetic cytokines can also be used as adjuvants. Cytokines are substances that are naturally produced by white blood cells to regulate and fine-tune immune responses. Some cytokines increase the activity of B cells and killer T cells, whereas other cytokines suppress the activities of these cells. Cytokines frequently used in cancer treatment vaccines or given together with them include interleukin 2 (IL2, also known as aldesleukin), interferon alpha (INF-a), and GM-CSF, also known as sargramostim.

Do cancer vaccines have side effects?

Vaccines intended to prevent or treat cancer appear to have safety profiles comparable to those of traditional vaccines. However, the side effects of cancer vaccines can vary among vaccine formulations and from one person to another.

The most commonly reported side effect of cancer vaccines is inflammation at the site of injection, including redness, pain, swelling, warming of the skin, itchiness, and occasionally a rash.

People sometimes experience flu-like symptoms after receiving a cancer vaccine, including fever, chills, weakness, dizziness, nausea or vomiting, muscle ache, fatigue, headache, and occasional breathing difficulties. Blood pressure may also be affected.

Other, more serious health problems have been reported in smaller numbers of people after receiving a cancer vaccine. These problems may or may not have been caused by the vaccine. The reported problems have included asthma, appendicitis, pelvic inflammatory disease, and certain autoimmune diseases, including arthritis and systemic lupus erythematous.

Vaccines, like any other medication affecting the immune system, can cause adverse effects that may prove life threatening. For example, severe hypersensitivity (allergic) reactions to specific vaccine ingredients have occurred following vaccination. However, such severe reactions are quite rare.

Can cancer treatment vaccines be combined with other types of cancer therapy?

Yes. In many of the clinical trials of cancer treatment vaccines that are now under way, vaccines are being given with other forms of cancer therapy. Therapies that have been combined with cancer treatment vaccines include surgery, chemotherapy, radiation therapy, and some forms of targeted therapy, including therapies that are intended to boost immune system responses against cancer.

Several studies have suggested that cancer treatment vaccines may be most effective when given in combination with other forms of cancer therapy. In addition, in some clinical trials, cancer treatment vaccines have appeared to increase the effectiveness of other cancer therapies.

Additional evidence suggests that surgical removal of large tumors may enhance the effectiveness of cancer treatment vaccines. In patients with extensive disease, the immune system may be overwhelmed by the cancer. Surgical removal of the tumor may make it easier for the body to develop an effective immune response.

Researchers are also designing clinical trials to answer questions such as whether a specific cancer treatment vaccine works best when it is administered before chemotherapy, after chemotherapy, or at the same time as chemotherapy. Answers to such questions may not only provide information about how best to use a specific cancer treatment vaccine but also reveal additional basic principles to guide the future development of combination therapies involving vaccines.

Chapter 54

Complementary and Alternative Therapies for Cancer

Chapter Contents

Text in this chapter is excerpted from "Complementary and Alternative Therapies (PDQ®)," National Cancer Institute at the National Institutes of Health (NIH), April 2, 2015.

Overview

Complementary and alternative medicine (CAM) includes a wide variety of therapies, botanicals, nutritional products, and practices. These forms of treatment are used in addition to (complementary) or instead of (alternative) standard treatments. The 2007 National Health Interview Survey reported that about 4 out of 10 adults use a CAM therapy, naming natural products and deep breathing exercises as the most commonly used treatments.

One large survey reported on the use of complementary therapies in cancer survivors. The therapies used most often were prayer and spiritual practice, relaxation, faith and spiritual healing, and nutritional supplements and vitamins. CAM therapies are used often by children with cancer, both in and outside clinical trials. CAM therapies have been used to manage side effects caused by cancer or cancer treatment.

Section 54.1

Acupuncture

What is acupuncture?

Acupuncture applies needles, heat, pressure, and other treatments to certain places on the skin to cause a change in the physical functions of the body. The use of acupuncture is part of traditional Chinese medicine (TCM). TCM is a medical system that has been used for thousands of years to prevent, diagnose, and treat disease.

Acupuncture is based on the belief that qi (vital energy) flows through the body along a network of paths, called meridians. Qi is said to affect a person's spiritual, emotional, mental, and physical condition. According to TCM, qi has two forces, yin and yang. Yin and yang are opposite forces that work together to form a whole. The forces of yin and yang depend on each other and are made from each other in an unending cycle, such as hot and cold, day and night, and health and disease. Nothing is ever all yin or all yang, both exist in all things, including people. Many of the major organs of the body are believed to be yin-yang pairs that must be in balance to be healthy. When a person's yin and yang are not in balance, qi can become blocked. Blocked qi causes pain, illness, or other health problems. TCM uses acupuncture, diet, herbal therapy, meditation, physical exercise, and massage to restore health by unblocking qi and correcting the balance of yin and yang within the person.

Most acupuncturists in the United States practice acupuncture according to the traditions of Chinese medicine. However, there are other types of acupuncture, including some used for medical treatment, that have different theories about meridians and acupoint locations.

What is the history of the discovery and use of acupuncture as a complementary and alternative treatment for cancer?

The oldest known medical book in China (second century BC) describes the use of needles to treat medical problems. The use of the treatment spread to other Asian countries and to other regions of the world, including to Europe by the 1700s. In the United States, acupuncture has been used for about 200 years.

Research on acupuncture began in the United States in 1976. Twenty years later, the US Food and Drug Administration (FDA) approved the acupuncture needle as a medical device. Many illnesses are treated with acupuncture. In cancer treatment, its main use is to control symptoms, including the following:

- Pain.

- Fatigue.

- Nausea and vomiting caused by chemotherapy.

- Weight loss.

- Anxiety.

- Depression.

- Insomnia.

- Poor appetite.

- Dry mouth.

- Hot flashes.

- Nerve problems.

- Constipation and diarrhea.

Acupuncture is usually used as an addition to conventional (standard) therapy for cancer patients.

What is the theory behind the claim that acupuncture is useful in treating cancer?

According to TCM, qi can be unblocked by using acupuncture at certain places on the skin, called acupoints. Acupoints are places where the meridians come to the surface of the body. There are more than 360 acupoints on the human body, with specific acupoints for each condition being treated.

What physical effects may acupuncture have when used in cancer patients?

Acupuncture may cause physical responses in nerve cells, the pituitary gland, and parts of the brain. These responses can cause the body to release proteins, hormones, and brain chemicals that control a number of body functions. It is proposed that, in this way, acupuncture affects blood pressure and body temperature, boosts immune system activity, and causes the body's natural painkillers, such as endorphins, to be released.

How is acupuncture administered?

The acupuncture method most well-known uses needles. Disposable, stainless steel needles that are slightly thicker than a human hair are inserted into the skin at acupoints. The acupuncture practitioner determines the correct acupoints to use for the problem being treated. The inserted needles may be twirled, moved up and down at different speeds and depths, heated, or charged with a weak electric current. There are other acupuncture methods that do not use needles.

Some acupuncture techniques include the following:

- Electroacupuncture: A procedure in which pulses of weak electrical current are sent through acupuncture needles into acupoints in the skin.

- Trigger point acupuncture: The placing of acupuncture needles in a place on the skin that is away from the painful part of the body. Trigger points have to do with referred pain, pain that is not felt at the site of injury, but is sent along nerves and felt elsewhere in the body.

- Laser acupuncture: The use of a weak laser beam instead of an acupuncture needle to stimulate an acupoint.

- Acupuncture point injection: The use of a syringe and needle to inject drugs, vitamins, herbal extracts, or other fluids into the body at an acupoint.

- Microwave acupuncture: The use of a microwave device attached to an acupuncture needle to deliver microwave radiation to an acupoint.

- Acupressure: A type of massage therapy in which the fingers are used to press on an acupoint. In cancer patients, acupressure has been used to control symptoms such as pain or nausea and vomiting.

- Moxibustion: A type of heat therapy in which an herb is burned above the body to warm a meridian at an acupoint and increase the flow of blood and qi. The herb may be placed directly on the skin, held close to the skin for several minutes, or placed on the tip of an acupuncture needle. Heat lamps may also be used to warm the acupoints.

- Cupping: A procedure in which a rounded glass cup is warmed and placed upside down over an area of the body, making a vacuum that holds the cup to the skin. Cupping is used to increase the flow of blood and qi. It is believed to open up the skin's pores and allow toxins to leave the body.

What do patients feel during acupuncture?

Patients may have a needling feeling during acupuncture, known as de qi sensation, making them feel heaviness, numbness, or tingling.

Have any preclinical (laboratory or animal) studies been conducted using acupuncture?

Scientific studies on the use of acupuncture to treat cancer and side effects of cancer began only recently. Laboratory and animal studies suggest that acupuncture can reduce vomiting caused by chemotherapy and may help the immune system be stronger during chemotherapy. Animal studies support the use of electroacupuncture to relieve cancer pain. Laboratory and animal studies have also looked at how acupuncture works for cancer treatment, such as the role of acupuncture in stimulating immune functions, including increasing blood cell count and enhancing lymphocyte and natural killer cell activity.

1031

Have any clinical trials (research studies with people) of acupuncture been conducted?

In 1997, the National Institutes of Health (NIH) began evaluating the safety and effectiveness of acupuncture as a complementary and alternative therapy.

- **Studies of the effect of acupuncture on the immune system**

  Human studies on the effect of acupuncture on the immune system have been done.

- **Studies of the effect of acupuncture on pain**

  In clinical studies, acupuncture reduced the amount of pain in some cancer patients. In one study, most of the patients treated with acupuncture were able to stop taking drugs for pain relief or to take smaller doses. The findings from these studies are not considered strong, however, because of weaknesses in study design and size. Studies using strict scientific methods are needed to prove how acupuncture affects pain.

- **Studies of the effect of acupuncture on muscle and joint pain from aromatase inhibitors**

  Aromatase inhibitors, a type of hormone therapy for postmenopausal women who have hormone-dependent breast cancer, may cause muscle and joint pain. A randomized study found that true acupuncture was much more effective in relieving joint pain and stiffness than sham (inactive) acupuncture in patients taking aromatase inhibitors.

- **Studies of the effect of acupuncture on nausea and vomiting caused by cancer therapies**

  The strongest evidence of the effect of acupuncture has come from clinical trials on the use of acupuncture to relieve nausea and vomiting. Several types of clinical trials using different acupuncture methods showed acupuncture reduced nausea and vomiting caused by chemotherapy, surgery, and morning sickness. It appears to be more effective in preventing vomiting than in reducing nausea.

  A study of acupuncture, vitamin B6 injections, or both for nausea and vomiting in patients treated with chemotherapy for ovarian cancer found that acupuncture and vitamin B6 together gave more relief from vomiting than acupuncture or vitamin B6 alone.

A study of acupressure for relief of nausea and vomiting was done in women undergoing chemotherapy. The study found that acupressure applied to an acupuncture point with a wristband helped to decrease nausea and vomiting and reduced the amount of medicine the women used for those symptoms.

A study of acupuncture for relief of nausea and vomiting was done in patients undergoing radiation therapy. Patients who received either true acupuncture or sham acupuncture were compared to patients who received standard care. The study found that patients in both the true and sham acupuncture groups developed less nausea and vomiting than those in the standard care group.

- **Studies of the effect of acupuncture on hot flashes in patients treated for cancer**

Hormone therapy may cause hot flashes in women with breast cancer and men with prostate cancer. Some studies have shown that acupuncture may be effective in relieving hot flashes in these patients.

- **Study of the effect of acupuncture on fatigue in patients treated for cancer**

Randomized studies of patients with cancer-related fatigue found that those who had a series of acupuncture treatments had less fatigue compared to those who had acupressure, sham acupressure, or information about managing fatigue.

- **Studies of the effect of acupuncture on xerostomia (dry mouth) in patients treated for cancer**

Clinical trials have been done to study the effect of acupuncture in the treatment and prevention of xerostomia (dry mouth) caused by radiation therapy given to patients with nasopharyngeal carcinoma and head and neck cancer.

Two studies compared acupuncture with standard care for preventing xerostomia in patients being treated with radiation therapy. The studies found that patients treated with acupuncture had fewer symptoms and increased saliva flow.

Compared to standard care, acupuncture markedly improves xerostomia symptoms in patients who have xerostomia after treatment with radiation therapy.

A study on the long-term effects of acupuncture on xerostomia found that patients had notable differences in salivary flow at

6 months compared to before treatment. Patients who received additional acupuncture had increased saliva flow at 3 years compared to patients who did not continue acupuncture treatment.

- **Studies of the effect of acupuncture on other symptoms of cancer and side effects of cancer treatment**

  The aim of most acupuncture clinical observation and clinical trials in cancer patients has been to study the effects of acupuncture on cancer symptoms and side effects caused by cancer treatment, including weight loss, cough, coughing up blood, anxiety, depression, proctitis, speech problems, blocked esophagus, hiccups, and fluid in the arms or legs. Studies have shown that, for many patients, treatment with acupuncture either relieves symptoms or keeps them from getting worse.

Have any side effects or risks been reported from acupuncture?

There have been few complications reported. Problems are caused by using needles that are not sterile (free of germs) and from placing the needle in the wrong place, movement of the patient, or a defect in the needle. Problems include soreness and pain during treatment; feeling tired, lightheaded, or sleepy; and infections. Because chemotherapy and radiation therapy weaken the body's immune system, a strict clean needle method must be used when acupuncture treatment is given to cancer patients. It is important to seek treatment from a qualified acupuncture practitioner who uses a new set of disposable (single-use) needles for each patient.

Is acupuncture approved by the US Food and Drug Administration (FDA) for use as a cancer treatment in the United States?

The FDA approved acupuncture needles for use by licensed practitioners in 1996. The FDA requires that sterile, nontoxic needles be used and that they be labeled for single use by qualified practitioners only.

More than 40 states and the District of Columbia have laws regulating acupuncture practice. The National Certification Commission for Acupuncture and Oriental Medicine (www.nccaom.org) certifies practitioners of acupuncture and traditional Chinese medicine (TCM). Most states require this certification.

Section 54.2

Botanicals / Herbal Products

Black Cohosh

Black cohosh is a North American perennial herb. A substance found in the root of this plant has been used in some cultures to treat a number of medical conditions. Black cohosh has been studied to relieve hot flashes. However, randomized, placebo-controlled clinical trials using this herb have found that black cohosh is no better than a placebo in relieving hot flashes.

Cannabis and Cannabinoids

Cannabis, also known as marijuana, is a plant from Central Asia that is grown in many parts of the world today. In the United States, it is a controlled substance and is classified as a Schedule I agent (a drug with increased potential for abuse and no known medical use). The *Cannabis* plant makes a resin that contains active chemicals called cannabinoids. Cannabinoids cause drug-like effects throughout the body, including the central nervous system and the immune system. Possible benefits of medicinal *Cannabis* for people living with cancer include control of nausea and vomiting, increasing appetite, relieving pain, and improving sleep.

Essiac/Flor Essence

Essiac and Flor Essence are herbal tea mixtures originally developed in Canada. They are marketed worldwide as dietary supplements. Supporters of Essiac and Flor Essence say that these products can help detoxify the body, make the immune system stronger, and fight cancer. There is no evidence in clinical trials that Essiac or Flor Essence can be effective in treating patients with cancer.

Flaxseed

Flaxseed comes from the flax plant. It is a rich source of omega-3 fatty acid, fiber, and a compound called lignin. It is being studied in the prevention of several types of cancer. Flaxseed has also been studied for its effect on hot flashes.

Ginger

Ginger is an herb that is used in cooking and in some cultures to treat medical conditions such as nausea. It can be used fresh, dried and powdered, or as a juice or oil. Ginger has been studied for the relief of nausea and vomiting in cancer patients.

Ginseng

Ginseng is an herb that is used to treat fatigue. It may be taken in capsules of ground ginseng root. Studies of ginseng have been done in patients either during or after their treatment for cancer. Patients who were given ginseng had less fatigue than patients who were given a placebo (inactive substance).

L-carnitine

L-carnitine is a dietary supplement that is thought to be helpful in treating fatigue related to cancer. L-carnitine helps the body make energy and lowers inflammation that may be linked to fatigue.

Milk Thistle

Milk thistle is a plant whose fruit and seeds have been used for more than 2,000 years as a treatment for liver and bile duct disorders. The active substance in milk thistle is silymarin. Laboratory studies show that silymarin stimulates repair of liver tissue and acts as an antioxidant that protects against cell damage. It slows the growth of certain types of cancer cells and may make some types of chemotherapy less toxic and more effective.

Mistletoe Extracts

Mistletoe is a semi parasitic plant that has been used since ancient times to treat many ailments. It is used commonly in Europe, where a variety of different extracts are made and marketed as injectable prescription drugs. The FDA does not allow these injectable drugs to be sold in the United States and they are not approved as a treatment for patients with cancer.

PC-SPES

PC-SPES is a patented mixture of eight herbs. Each herb used in PC-SPES has been reported to have anti-inflammatory, antioxidant, or anticancer properties. PC-SPES was taken off the market because some batches were found to contain prescription medicines in addition to the herbs. The manufacturer is no longer in business and PC-SPES is no longer being made.

St. John's Wort

St. John's wort is a plant with yellow flowers that has been used since ancient times for medical conditions. St. John's wort is sold as an over-the-counter herbal treatment for depression. Studies comparing St. John's wort with standard antidepressant medicines have shown mixed results. St. John's wort may change the way other medicines work, including anticancer medicines.

Selected Vegetables/Sun's Soup

"Selected Vegetables" and "Sun's Soup" are different mixtures of vegetables and herbs that have been studied as treatments for cancer. Dried and frozen forms of Selected Vegetables are sold in the United States as dietary supplements. The vegetables and herbs in Selected Vegetables/Sun's Soup are thought to have substances that block the growth of cancer cells and/or help the body's immune system kill cancer cells. There is limited evidence that Selected Vegetables/Sun's Soup is useful as a treatment for cancer and no randomized or controlled clinical trials have been done.

Section 54.3

Mind-Body Therapies and Massage

Aromatherapy and Essential Oils

Aromatherapy is the use of essential oils from plants (flowers, herbs, or trees) as therapy to improve physical, emotional, and spiritual well-being. Patients with cancer use aromatherapy mainly as supportive care to improve their quality of life, such as lowering stress and anxiety. Aromatherapy may be combined with other complementary treatments (e.g., massage and acupuncture) as well as with standard treatment.

Cognitive-Behavioral Therapy (CBT)

Cognitive-behavioral therapy (CBT) is a type of psychotherapy that helps patients change their behavior by changing the way they think and feel about certain things. CBT may be helpful in treating many side effects of cancer and cancer treatment.

Thinking and behavioral interventions focus on positive thoughts and images instead of negative thoughts and behaviors. Patients may gain a sense of control and develop coping skills to deal with the disease and its symptoms. These interventions also show promise for the treatment of insomnia in patients with cancer.

Relaxation and imagery techniques may be used for short periods of pain or discomfort (e.g., during procedures). Quick, simple techniques are useful when the patient has trouble concentrating due to severe pain, anxiety, fatigue, or nausea.

CBT for may be helpful for depression in patients with cancer. Most counseling or talk therapy programs for depression are offered in both individual and small-group settings. CBT may also help decrease a cancer patient's fatigue by working on cancer-related factors that make fatigue worse.

CBT may be used to treat post-traumatic stress disorder symptoms in patients with cancer. The treatment can focus on solving problems, teaching coping skills, and providing a supportive setting for the patient.

Hypnosis

Hypnosis is a trance-like state that allows a person to be more aware and focused and more open to suggestion. Under hypnosis, the person can concentrate more clearly on a specific thought, feeling, or sensation without becoming distracted.

Manual Lymphedema Therapy

Manual lymphedema therapy is a massage that helps move lymph fluid out of a swollen arm or leg into healthy lymph nodes where it can drain.

Massage

Massage therapy has been studied as part of supportive care in managing cancer-related pain. Massage may help improve relaxation and benefit mood. Massage stimulates the release of substances that relieve pain and give a feeling of well-being and increases blood and lymphatic circulation.

Music Interventions for Pain

Music interventions may help relieve pain and lessen anxiety in some patients. Music therapy and music medicine have been used to relieve pain caused by cancer and by procedures and treatments.

Qigong

Qigong is a form of traditional Chinese medicine that combines movement, meditation, and controlled breathing. Its purpose is to enhance the vital energy or life force that keeps a person's spiritual, emotional, mental, and physical health in balance.

Spirituality

Studies have shown that religious and spiritual values are important to most Americans. Many patients with cancer rely on spiritual or religious beliefs and practices to help them cope with their disease. For healthcare providers, spiritual or religious well-being are sometimes viewed as an aspect of complementary and alternative medicine.

Yoga

Yoga is an ancient system of practices used to balance the mind and body through exercise, meditation (focusing thoughts), and control of breathing and emotions. Yoga is being studied as a way to relieve stress and treat sleep problems in cancer patients.

Section 54.4

Nutritional Therapies

Antioxidants and Cancer Prevention

Antioxidants are substances that may protect cells from the damage caused by unstable molecules known as free radicals. Free radical damage may lead to cancer. Examples of antioxidants include beta-carotene, lycopene, vitamins C, E, and A, and other substances.

There has been some concern about whether antioxidants may make chemotherapy and radiation therapy less effective.

Coenzyme Q10

Coenzyme Q10 is made naturally by the human body. Coenzyme Q10 helps cells produce energy and acts as an antioxidant. Studies show that coenzyme Q10 may boost the immune system and protect the heart from damage caused by certain chemotherapy drugs. No report of a randomized clinical trial using coenzyme Q10 as a treatment for cancer has been published in a peer-reviewed scientific journal.

Dietary Supplements

Many studies suggest that the use of complementary and alternative medicine is common among prostate cancer patients, and the use of vitamins, supplements, and specific foods is frequently reported by these patients.

Gerson Therapy

The Gerson therapy is used by some practitioners as a treatment for cancer based on changes in diet and nutrient intake. An organic vegetarian diet plus nutritional and biological supplements, pancreatic enzymes, and coffee or other types of enemas are the main features of the Gerson therapy. Few clinical studies of the Gerson therapy have been published.

Gonzalez Regimen

The Gonzalez regimen is a cancer treatment that is tailored by the practitioner for each patient and is currently available only to the patients of its developer. It involves taking certain pancreatic enzymes thought to have anticancer activity. The regimen also includes specific diets, vitamin and mineral supplements, extracts of animal organs, and coffee enemas.

Lycopene

Lycopene is a carotenoid (a natural pigment made by plants). It is found in a number of fruits and vegetables, including apricots, guava, and watermelon. The main source of lycopene in the American diet is tomato-based products. Lycopene is thought to have antioxidant activity. Lycopene has been studied for its role in chronic diseases, including cardiovascular disease and cancer.

Melatonin

Melatonin is a hormone made by the pineal gland during the hours of darkness. It plays a major role in the sleep-wake cycle. Clinical studies in renal, breast, colon, lung, and brain cancer suggest that melatonin may make chemotherapy and radiation therapy more effective; however randomized, blinded trials are needed to study these results.

Modified Citrus Pectin

Citrus pectin is found in the peel and pulp of citrus fruits such as oranges, grapefruit, lemons, and limes. Citrus pectin can be modified with high pH and heat so that it can be digested and absorbed by the body. Modified citrus pectin (MCP) may have effects on cancer growth and metastasis. Some research suggests that MCP may be protective against various types of cancer, including colon, lung, and prostate cancer.

Pomegranate

The pomegranate (*Punica granatum L.*) is native to Asia and grown in many parts of the world. Different parts of the pomegranate fruit have bioactive compounds that may support good health, including antioxidants found in the peel. Certain pomegranate extracts have been shown in laboratory studies to slow the growth and spread of prostate cancer cells and to cause cell death.

Probiotics

Probiotics are live microorganisms used as a dietary supplement to help with digestion and normal bowel function. A bacterium found in yogurt called *Lactobacillus acidophilus* is the most common probiotic. The use of probiotics may be recommended in conditions related to diarrhea, gut-barrier dysfunction, and inflammatory response.

Selenium

Selenium is a trace mineral (a nutrient that is essential to humans in tiny amounts). Selenium is found in certain proteins that are active in many body functions, including reproduction and immunity. Selenium is being studied for its role in cancer.

Soy

Soy is from a plant native to Asia that grows beans used in many food products. Soy foods (e.g., soy milk, miso, tofu, and soy flour) contain phytochemicals that may have health benefits. Isoflavones are the most widely researched compounds in soy. Soy is being studied for the prevention of cancer, hot flashes during menopause, and osteoporosis (loss of bone density).

Tea

Tea has long been thought to have health benefits, and many believe it can help lower the risk of cancer. Tea contains polyphenol compounds including catechins, which are antioxidants that help protect cells from damage caused by free radicals.

Some studies suggest that green tea may have a protective effect against cardiovascular disease. There is also evidence that green tea may protect against various forms of cancer.

Vitamin C, High-Dose

Vitamin C (ascorbic acid) is a nutrient that humans must get from food or supplements since it cannot be made in the body. Vitamin C is an antioxidant and helps prevent oxidative stress. It also works with enzymes to play a key role in making collagen. High-dose vitamin C has been studied as a treatment for cancer patients.

Vitamin D

Vitamin D is a nutrient involved in a number of functions that are essential for good health. Skin exposed to sunshine can make Vitamin D. It can also be consumed in the diet, but very few foods naturally contain vitamin D. These foods include fatty fish, fish liver oil, and eggs.

Vitamin E

Vitamin E is a nutrient that the body needs in small amounts to stay healthy and work the way it should. It is fat-soluble (can dissolve in fats and oils) and is found in seeds, nuts, leafy green vegetables, and vegetable oils. Vitamin E boosts the immune system and helps keep blood clots from forming. It also helps prevent cell damage caused by free radicals (unstable molecules in the body). Vitamin E is being studied in the prevention and treatment of some types of cancer. It is a type of antioxidant.

Section 54.5

Pharmacologic Treatments

714-X

714-X is a chemical compound that contains camphor, a natural substance that comes from the wood and bark of the camphor tree. Nitrogen, water, and salts are added to camphor to make 714-X. It is claimed that 714-X protects the immune system and helps the body fight cancer. No peer-reviewed studies of 714-X has been published to show that it is safe or effective in treating cancer.

Antineoplastons

Antineoplastons are drugs made of chemical compounds that are naturally present in the urine and blood. It has been claimed that antineoplaston therapy can be used to stop certain cancer cells from dividing, while healthy cells are not affected.

Cancell/Cantron/Protocel

Cancell/Cantron/Protocel is a liquid that has been made in different forms since the late 1930s. It is also known by the names Sheridan's Formula, Jim's Juice, JS-114, JS-101, 126-F, and the "Cancell-like" products Cantron and Protocel. The exact ingredients of Cancell/ Cantron/Protocel are not known and it is not effective in treating any type of cancer.

Cartilage (Bovine and Shark)

Bovine (cow) cartilage and shark cartilage have been studied as treatments for people with cancer and other medical conditions for more than 30 years. Substances that prevent the body from making the new blood vessels that a tumor needs to grow have been found in bovine cartilage and shark cartilage. However, these substances have not shown an effect on the growth of normal cells or tumor cells.

Hydrazine Sulfate

Hydrazine sulfate is a chemical that has been studied as a treatment for cancer and as a treatment for body wasting (i.e., cachexia) that can develop with this disease. It has been claimed that hydrazine sulfate limits the ability of tumors to take in glucose, which is a type of sugar that tumor cells need to grow.

Laetrile/Amygdalin

Laetrile is another name for the chemical amygdalin, which is found in the pits of many fruits and in numerous plants. Cyanide is thought to be the active anticancer ingredient of laetrile. Laetrile has shown little anticancer activity in animal studies and no anticancer activity in human clinical trials.

Newcastle Disease Virus (NDV)

Newcastle Disease Virus (NDV) is usually thought to be an avian (bird) virus, but it also infects humans. It causes a potentially fatal, noncancerous disease (Newcastle disease) in birds, but causes only minor illness in humans. NDV appears to copy itself much better in human cancer cells than in most normal human cells and may have anticancer effects.

Chapter 55

Cancer Treatment Scams

While health fraud is a cruel form of greed, fraud involving cancer treatments can be particularly heartless—especially because fraudulent information can travel around the Web in an instant.

"Anyone who suffers from cancer, or knows someone who does, understands the fear and desperation that can set in," says Gary Coody, R.Ph., the National Health Fraud Coordinator and a Consumer Safety Officer with the Food and Drug Administration's (FDA) Office of Regulatory Affairs. "There can be a great temptation to jump at anything that appears to offer a chance for a cure."

Medicinal products and devices intended to treat cancer must gain FDA approval before they are marketed. The agency's review process helps ensure that these products are safe and effective.

Nevertheless, it's always possible to find someone or some company hawking bogus cancer "treatments." Such "treatments" come in many forms, including pills, tonics, and creams. "They're frequently offered as natural treatments and 'dietary supplements,'" says Coody. Many of these fraudulent cancer products even appear completely harmless, but may cause indirect harm by delaying or interfering with proven, beneficial treatments.

"Advertisements and other promotional materials touting bogus cancer 'cures' have probably been around as long as the printing press," says Coody. "However, the Internet has compounded the problem by providing the peddlers of these often dangerous products a whole new outlet."

Text in this chapter is excerpted from "Beware of Online Cancer Fraud," U.S. Food and Drug Administration (FDA), October 14, 2014.

Unproven 'Remedies,' False Promises

Coody cites black salves as one of the fake cancer "remedies" that indeed have proven to be harmful. "Although it is illegal to market these salves as a cancer treatment, they are readily available online," he says.

The salves are sold with false promises that they will cure cancer by "drawing out" the disease from beneath the skin. "However, there is no scientific evidence that black salves are effective," says Janet Woodcock, Director of FDA's Center for Drug Evaluation and Research (CDER). "Even worse, black salves can cause direct harm to the patient."

The corrosive, oily salves "essentially burn off layers of the skin and surrounding normal tissue," says Woodcock. "This is not a simple, painless process. There are documented cases of these salves destroying large parts of people's skin and underlying tissue, leaving terrible scars."

Another unproven "remedy" that has been hawked for decades is an herbal regimen known as the Hoxsey Cancer Treatment. "FDA has taken regulatory and enforcement action against this discredited course of therapy beginning in the 1950s," says Coody.

"There is no scientific evidence that it has any value to treat cancer," he adds. "Yet consumers can go online right now and find all sorts of false claims that Hoxsey treatment is effective against the disease."

Red Flags

- Coody says that firms engaged in cancer treatment or prevention fraud often use exaggerated and bogus claims to promote these products. He adds that consumers should recognize the following phrases as red flags:

- "Treats all forms of cancer"

- "Skin cancers disappear"

- "Shrinks malignant tumors"

- "Non-toxic"

- "Doesn't make you sick"

- "Avoid painful surgery, radiotherapy, chemotherapy, or other conventional treatments"

- "Treat Non Melanoma Skin Cancers easily and safely"

"Unproven claims are also found in unverified testimonials, research results, or even in product and website names," says Coody. He offers important points that consumers seeking cancer treatments should keep in mind:

- Always consult with your health care professional before starting a new treatment or adding one to existing therapies. "Some products may interact with your medicines or keep them from working the way they are supposed to," says Coody.

- Understand the difference between fraudulent drug products and what FDA calls "investigational drugs." Investigational drugs undergo clinical testing to determine if they are safe and effective for their intended uses. Fraudulent products, on the other hand, are unapproved and typically have never been clinically tested or reviewed by FDA for safety and effectiveness. Marketing them is a violation of federal law.

"There are legal ways for patients to access investigational drugs," says Coody. "The most common way is by taking part in clinical trials. But patients can also receive investigational drugs outside of clinical trials in some cases."

Agencies Take Action

FDA and the U.S. Federal Trade Commission (FTC), in collaboration with other North American government agencies, have announced a new initiative to prevent these deceptive products from reaching consumers. Coody says that as part of the joint campaign, FDA and FTC have sent approximately 135 warning letters and two advisory letters to firms that market these products online.

The initiative originated not only from consumer complaints, he says, but also from a Web surf for fraudulent cancer products by FDA and members of the Mexico-United States-Canada Health fraud working group (MUCH).

Signs of Health Fraud

All consumers seeking information about any health product or medical treatment should be familiar with the following signs of health fraud:

- Statements that the product is a quick and effective cure-all or a diagnostic tool for a wide variety of ailments.

- Suggestions that a product can treat or cure serious or incurable diseases.

- Claims such as "scientific breakthrough," "miraculous cure," "secret ingredient," and "ancient remedy."

- Impressive-sounding terms, such as "hunger stimulation point" and "thermogenesis" for a weight loss product.

- Claims that the product is safe because it is "natural."

- Undocumented case histories or personal testimonials by consumers or doctors claiming amazing results.

- Claims of limited availability and advance payment requirements.

- Promises of no-risk, money-back guarantees.

- Promises of an "easy" fix for problems like excess weight, hair loss, or impotency.

Part Six

Coping with Cancer

Chapter 56

Cancer Treatment Side Effects

Cancer treatments can cause side effects—problems that occur when treatment affects healthy tissues or organs. Side effects vary from person to person, even among those receiving the same treatment. Some people have very few side effects while others have many. The type of treatment(s) you receive, as well as the amount or frequency of the treatment, your age, and other health conditions you have may also factor into the side effects you may have.

Before you start treatment, ask your health care team what side effects you are likely to have. Learn about steps you can take, as well as supportive care that you will receive, to lessen side effects during and after treatment. Speak up about any side effects you have and changes you notice, so your health care team can treat or help you manage them.

Common side effects caused by cancer treatment include:

Anemia
Appetite Loss
Bleeding and Bruising (Thrombocytopenia)
Constipation
Diarrhea
Edema
Fatigue

Text in this chapter is excerpted from "Side Effects," National Cancer Institute at National Institutes of Health (NIH), April 29, 2015.

Hair Loss (Alopecia)
Infection and Neutropenia
Lymphedema
Memory or Concentration Problems
Mouth and Throat Problems
Nausea and Vomiting
Nerve Problems (Peripheral Neuropathy)
Pain
Sexual and Fertility Problems (Men)
Sexual and Fertility Problems (Women)
Skin and Nail Changes
Sleep Problems
Urinary and Bladder Problems

Anemia

Anemia is a condition that can make you feel very tired, short of breath, and lightheaded. Other signs of anemia may include feeling dizzy or faint, headaches, a fast heartbeat, and/or pale skin.

Cancer treatments, such as chemotherapy and radiation therapy, as well as cancers that affect the bone marrow, can cause anemia. When you are anemic, your body does not have enough red blood cells. Red blood cells are the cells that that carry oxygen from the lungs throughout your body to help it work properly. You will have blood tests to check for anemia. Treatment for anemia is also based on your symptoms and on what is causing the anemia.

Ways to Manage

Here are some steps you can take if you have fatigue caused by anemia:

- **Save your energy and ask for help**. Choose the most important things to do each day. When people offer to help, let them do so. They can take you to the doctor, make meals, or do other things you are too tired to do.

- **Balance rest with activity**. Take short naps during the day, but keep in mind that too much bed rest can make you feel weak. You may feel better if you take short walks or exercise a little every day.

- **Eat and drink well**. Talk with your doctor, nurse, or a registered dietitian to learn what foods and drinks are best for you. You may need to eat foods that are high in protein or iron.

Talking with Your Health Care Team

Prepare for your visit by making a list of questions to ask. Consider adding these questions to your list:

- What is causing the anemia?
- What problems should I call you about?
- What steps can I take to feel better?
- Would medicine, iron pills, a blood transfusion, or other treatments help me?
- Would you give me the name of a registered dietitian who could also give me advice?

Appetite Loss

Cancer treatments may lower your appetite or change the way food tastes or smells. Side effects such as mouth and throat problems, or nausea and vomiting can also make eating difficult. Cancer-related fatigue can also lower your appetite.

Talk with your health care team if you are not hungry or if your find it difficult to eat. Don't wait until you feel weak, have lost too much weight, or are dehydrated, to talk with your doctor or nurse. It's important to eat well, especially during treatment for cancer.

Ways to Manage

Take these steps to get the nutrition you need to stay strong during treatment:

- **Drink plenty of liquids**. Drinking plenty of liquids is important, especially if you have less of an appetite. Losing fluid can lead to dehydration, a dangerous condition. You may become weak or dizzy and have dark yellow urine if you are not drinking enough liquids.

- **Choose healthy and high-nutrient foods**. Eat a little, even if you are not hungry. It may help to have five or six small meals throughout the day instead of three large meals. Most people need to eat a variety of nutrient-dense foods that are high in protein and calories.

- **Be active**. Being active can actually increase your appetite. Your appetite may increase when you take a short walk each day.

Talking with Your Health Care Team

Prepare for your visit by making a list of questions to ask. Consider adding these questions to your list:

- What symptoms or problems should I call you about?
- What steps can I take to feel better?
- What food and drink choices are best for me?
- Do you recommend supplemental nutrition drinks for me?
- Are there vitamins and supplements that I should avoid? Are there any I should take?
- Would you recommend a registered dietitian who could also help me?

Bleeding and Bruising (Thrombocytopenia)

Some cancer treatments, such as chemotherapy and targeted therapy, can increase your risk of bleeding and bruising. These treatments can lower the number of platelets in the blood. Platelets are the cells that help your blood to clot and stop bleeding. When your platelet count is low, you may bruise or bleed a lot or very easily and have tiny purple or red spots on your skin. This condition is called thrombocytopenia. It is important to tell your doctor or nurse if you notice any of these changes.

Call your doctor or nurse if you have more serious problems, such as:

- Bleeding that doesn't stop after a few minutes; bleeding from your mouth, nose, or when you vomit; bleeding from your vagina when you are not having your period (menstruation); urine that is red or pink; stools that are black or bloody; or bleeding during your period that is heavier or lasts longer than normal.
- Head or vision changes such as bad headaches or changes in how well you see, or if you feel confused or very sleepy.

Ways to Manage

Steps to take if you are at increased risk of bleeding and bruising:

- **Avoid certain medicines**. Many over-the-counter medicines contain aspirin or ibuprofen, which can increase your risk of bleeding. When in doubt, be sure to check the label. Get a list of medicines and products from your health care team that you should avoid taking. You may also be advised to limit or avoid alcohol if your platelet count is low.

- **Take extra care to prevent bleeding**. Brush your teeth gently, with a very soft toothbrush. Wear shoes, even when you are inside. Be extra careful when using sharp objects. Use an electric shaver, not a razor. Use lotion and a lip balm to prevent dry, chapped skin and lips. Tell your doctor or nurse if you are constipated or notice bleeding from your rectum.

- **Care for bleeding or bruising**. If you start to bleed, press down firmly on the area with a clean cloth. Keep pressing until the bleeding stops. If you bruise, put ice on the area.

Talking with Your Health Care Team

Prepare for your visit by making a list of questions to ask. Consider adding these questions to your list:

- What steps can I take to prevent bleeding or bruising?

- How long should I wait for the bleeding to stop before I call you or go the emergency room?

- Do I need to limit or avoid things that could increase my risk of bleeding, such as alcohol or sexual activity?

- What medicines, vitamins, or herbs should I avoid? Could I get a list from you of medicines to avoid?

Constipation

Constipation is when you have infrequent bowel movements and stool that may be hard, dry, and difficult to pass. You may also have stomach cramps, bloating, and nausea when you are constipated.

Cancer treatments such as chemotherapy can cause constipation. Certain medicines (such as pain medicines), changes in diet, not drinking enough fluids, and being less active may also cause constipation.

There are steps you can take to prevent constipation. It is easier to prevent constipation than to treat its complications which may include fecal impaction or bowel obstruction.

Ways to Prevent or Treat

Take these steps to prevent or treat constipation:

- **Eat high-fiber foods**. Adding bran to foods such as cereals or smoothies is an easy way to get more fiber in your diet. Ask your health care team how many grams of fiber you should have each day. If you have had an intestinal obstruction or intestinal surgery, you should not eat a high-fiber diet.

- **Drink plenty of liquids**. Most people need to drink at least 8 cups of liquid each day. You may need more based on your treatment, medications you are taking, or other health factors. Drinking warm or hot liquids may also help.

- **Try to be active every day**. Ask your health care team about exercises that you can do. Most people can do light exercise, even in a bed or chair. Other people choose to walk or ride an exercise bike for 15 to 30 minutes each day.

- **Learn about medicine**. Use only medicines and treatments for constipation that are prescribed by your doctor, since some may lead to bleeding, infection, or other harmful side effects in people being treated for cancer. Keep a record of your bowel movements to share with your doctor or nurse.

Talking with Your Health Care Team

Prepare for your visit by making a list of questions to ask. Consider adding these questions to your list:

- What problems should I call you about?

- What information should I keep track of and share with you? (For example, you may be asked to keep track of your bowel movements, meals that you have, and exercise that you do each day.)

- How much liquid should I drink each day?

- What steps can I take to feel better?

- Would you give me the name of a registered dietitian who can tell me about foods that might help?

- Should I take medicine for constipation? If so, what medicine should I take? What medicine should I avoid?

Diarrhea

Diarrhea means having bowel movements that are soft, loose, or watery more often than normal. If diarrhea is severe or lasts a long time, the body does not absorb enough water and nutrients. This can cause you to become dehydrated or malnourished. Cancer treatments, or the cancer itself, may cause diarrhea or make it worse. Some medicines, infections, and stress can also cause diarrhea. Tell your health care team if you have diarrhea.

Diarrhea that leads to dehydration (the loss of too much fluid from the body) and low levels of salt and potassium (important minerals needed by the body) can be life threatening. Call your health care team if you feel dizzy or light headed, have dark yellow urine or are not urinating, or have a fever of 100.5 °F (38 °C) or higher.

Ways to Manage

You may be advised to take steps to prevent complications from diarrhea:

- **Drink plenty of fluid each day**. Most people need to drink 8 to 12 cups of fluid each day. Ask your doctor or nurse how much fluid you should drink each day. For severe diarrhea, only clear liquids or IV (intravenous) fluids may be advised for a short period.

- **Eat small meals that are easy on your stomach**. Eat six to eight small meals throughout the day, instead of three large meals. Foods high in potassium and sodium (minerals you lose when you have diarrhea) are good food choices, for most people. Limit or avoid foods and drinks that can make your diarrhea worse.

- **Check before taking medicine**. Check with your doctor or nurse before taking medicine for diarrhea. Your doctor will prescribe the correct medicine for you.

- **Keep your anal area clean and dry**. Try using warm water and wipes to stay clean. It may help to take warm, shallow baths. These are called sitz baths.

Talking with Your Health Care Team

Prepare for your visit by making a list of questions to ask. Consider adding these questions to your list:

- What is causing the diarrhea?

- What symptoms should I call you about?

1059

- How much liquid should I drink each day?

- Can I speak to a registered dietitian to learn more about foods and drinks that are best for me?

- What medicine or other steps can I take to prevent diarrhea and to decrease rectal pain?

Edema

Edema, a condition in which fluid builds up in your body's tissues, may be caused by some types of chemotherapy, certain cancers, and conditions not related to cancer.

Signs of edema may include:

- swelling in your feet, ankles, and legs

- swelling in your hands and arms

- swelling in your face or abdomen

- skin that is puffy, shiny, or looks slightly dented after being pressed

- shortness of breath, a cough, or irregular heartbeat

Tell your health care team if you notice swelling. Your doctor or nurse will determine what is causing your symptoms, advise you on steps to take, and may prescribe medicine.

Some problems related to edema are serious. Call your doctor or nurse if you feel short of breath, have a heartbeat that seems different or is not regular, have sudden swelling or swelling that is getting worse or is moving up your arms or legs, you gain weight quickly, or you don't urinate at all or urinate only a little.

Ways to Prevent or Lessen Edema

Steps you can take to prevent or lessen edema-related swelling include:

Get comfortable. Wear loose clothing and shoes that are not too tight. When you sit or lie down, raise your feet with a stool or pillows. Avoid crossing your legs when you sit. Talk with your health care team about wearing special stockings, sleeves, or gloves that help with circulation if your swelling is severe.

Exercise. Moving the part of your body with edema can help. Your doctor may give you specific exercises, including walking, to improve circulation. However, you may be advised not to stand or walk too much at one time.

Limit salt (sodium) in your diet. Avoid foods such as chips, bacon, ham, and canned soup. Check food labels for the sodium content. Don't add salt or soy sauce to your food.

Take your medicine. If your doctor prescribes a medicine called a diuretic, take it exactly as instructed. The medicine will help move the extra fluid and salt out of your body.

Talking with Your Health Care Team

Prepare for your visit by making a list of questions to ask. Consider adding these questions to your list:

- Are my medications or treatment likely to increase my risk of developing edema?
- Are there steps I can take to prevent edema?
- What symptoms or problems should I call you about?
- What steps can I take to feel better if I notice swelling?
- Are there foods, drinks, or activities I should avoid?

Fatigue

Fatigue is a common side effect of many cancer treatments, including chemotherapy, radiation therapy, biological therapy, bone marrow transplant, and surgery. Conditions such as anemia, as well as pain, medications, and emotions, can also cause or worsen f atigue.

People often describe cancer-related fatigue as feeling extremely tired, weak, heavy, run down, and having no energy. Resting does not always help with cancer-related fatigue. Cancer-related fatigue is one of the most difficult side effects for many people to cope with.

Tell your health care team if you feel extremely tired and are not able to do your normal activities or are very tired even after resting or sleeping. There are many causes of fatigue. Keeping track of your levels of energy throughout the day will help your doctor to assess your fatigue. Write down how fatigue affects your daily activities and what makes the fatigue better or worse.

Ways to Manage

You may be advised to take these and other steps to feel better:

- **Make a plan that balances rest and activity**. Choose activities that are relaxing for you. Many people choose to listen to music, read, meditate, practice guided imagery, or spend time with people they enjoy. Relaxing can help you save your energy and lower stress. Light exercise may also be advised by your doctor to give you more energy and help you feel better.

- **Plan time to rest**. If you are tired, take short naps of less than 1 hour during the day. However, too much sleep during the day can make it difficult to sleep at night. Choose the activities that are most important to you and do them when you have the most energy. Ask for help with important tasks such as making meals or driving.

- **Eat and drink well**. Meet with a registered dietitian to learn about foods and drinks that can increase your level of energy. Foods high in protein and calories will help you keep up your strength. Some people find it easier to eat many small meals throughout the day instead of three big meals. Stay well hydrated. Limit your intake of caffeine and alcohol.

- **Meet with a specialist**. It may help to meet with a counselor, psychologist, or psychiatrist. These experts help people to cope with difficult thoughts and feelings. Lowering stress may give you more energy. Since pain that is not controlled can also be major source of fatigue, it may help to meet with a pain or palliative care specialist..

Talking with Your Health Care Team

Prepare for your visit by making a list of questions to ask. Consider adding these questions to your list:

- What is most likely causing my fatigue?

- What should I keep track of and share so we can develop a plan to help me feel better?

- What types of exercise (and how much) do you recommend for me?

- How much rest should I have during the day? How much sleep should I get at night?

- What food and drinks are best for me?

- Are there treatments or medicines that could help me feel better?

Hair Loss (Alopecia)

Some types of chemotherapy cause the hair on your head and other parts of your body to fall out. Radiation therapy can also cause hair loss on the part of the body that is being treated. Hair loss is called alopecia. Talk with your health care team to learn if the cancer treatment you will be receiving causes hair loss. Your doctor or nurse will share strategies that have help others, including those listed below.

Ways to Manage

Talk with your health care team about ways to manage before and after hair loss:

- **Treat your hair gently**. You may want to use a hairbrush with soft bristles or a wide-tooth comb. Do not use hair dryers, irons, or products such as gels or clips that may hurt your scalp. Wash your hair with a mild shampoo. Wash it less often and be very gentle. Pat it dry with a soft towel.

- **You have choices**. Some people choose to cut their hair short to make it easier to deal with when it starts to fall out. Others choose to shave their head. If you choose to shave your head, use an electric shaver so you won't cut yourself. If you plan to buy a wig, get one while you still have hair so you can match it to the color of your hair. If you find wigs to be itchy and hot, try wearing a comfortable scarf or turban.

- **Protect and care for your scalp**. Use sunscreen or wear a hat when you are outside. Choose a comfortable scarf or hat that you enjoy and that keeps your head warm. If your scalp itches or feels tender, using lotions and conditioners can help it feel better.

- **Talk about your feelings**. Many people feel angry, depressed, or embarrassed about hair loss. It can help to share these feelings with someone who understands. Some people find it helpful to talk with other people who have lost their hair during cancer treatment. Talking openly and honestly with your children and close family members can also help you all. Tell them that you expect to lose your hair during treatment.

Ways to Care for Your Hair When It Grows Back

- **Be gentle**. When your hair starts to grow back, you will want to be gentle with it. Avoid too much brushing, curling, and blow-drying. You may not want to wash your hair as frequently.

- **After chemotherapy**. Hair often grows back in 2 to 3 months after treatment has ended. Your hair will be very fine when it starts to grow back. Sometimes your new hair can be curlier or straighter—or even a different color. In time, it may go back to how it was before treatment.

- **After radiation therapy**. Hair often grows back in 3 to 6 months after treatment has ended. If you received a very high dose of radiation your hair may grow back thinner or not at all on the part of your body that received radiation.

Talking with Your Health Care Team

Prepare for your visit by making a list of questions to ask. Consider adding these questions to your list:

- Is treatment likely to cause my hair to fall out?

- How should I protect and care for my head? Are there products that you recommend? Ones I should avoid?

- Where can I get a wig or hairpiece?

- What support groups could I meet with that might help?

- When will my hair grow back?

Infection and Neutropenia

An infection is the invasion and growth of germs in the body, such as bacteria, viruses, yeast, or other fungi. An infection can begin anywhere in the body, may spread throughout the body, and can cause one or more of these signs:

- fever of 100.5 °F (38 °C) or higher or chills

- cough or sore throat

- diarrhea

- ear pain, headache or sinus pain, or a stiff or sore neck

- skin rash

- sores or white coating in your mouth or on your tongue

- swelling or redness, especially where a catheter enters your body

- urine that is bloody or cloudy, or pain when you urinate

Call your health care team if you have signs of an infection. Infections during cancer treatment can be life threatening and require urgent medical attention. Be sure to talk with your doctor or nurse before taking medicine—even aspirin, acetaminophen (such as Tylenol®), or ibuprofen (such as Advil®) for a fever. These medicines can lower a fever but may also mask or hide signs of a more serious problem.

Some types of cancer and treatments such as chemotherapy may increase your risk of infection. This is because they lower the number of white blood cells, the cells that help your body to fight infection. During chemotherapy, there will be times in your treatment cycle when the number of white blood cells (called neutrophils) is particularly low and you are at increased risk of infection. Stress, poor nutrition, and not enough sleep can also weaken the immune system, making infection more likely.

You will have blood tests to check for neutropenia (a condition in which there is a low number of neutrophils). Medicine may sometimes be given to help prevent infection or to increase the number of white blood cells.

Ways to Prevent Infection

Your health care team will talk with you about these and other ways to prevent infection:

- **Wash your hands often and well**. Use soap and warm water to wash your hands well, especially before eating. Have people around you wash their hands well too.

- **Stay extra clean**. If you have a catheter, keep the area around it clean and dry. Clean your teeth well and check your mouth for sores or other signs of an infection each day. If you get a scrape or cut, clean it well. Let your doctor or nurse know if your bottom is sore or bleeds, as this could increase your risk of infection.

- **Avoid germs**. Stay away from people who are sick or have a cold. Avoid crowds and people who have just had a live vaccine, such as one for chicken pox, polio, or measles. Follow food safety guidelines; make sure the meat, fish, and eggs you eat are well cooked. Keep hot foods hot and cold foods cold. You may be advised to eat only fruits and vegetables that can be peeled, or to wash all raw fruits and vegetables very well.

Talking with Your Health Care Team

Prepare for your visit by making a list of questions to ask. Consider adding these questions to your list:

- Am I at increased risk of infection during treatment? When am I at increased risk?
- What steps should I take to prevent infection?
- What signs of infection should I look for?
- Which signs signal that I need urgent medical care at the emergency room? Which should I call you about?

Lymphedema

Lymphedema is a condition in which the lymph fluid does not drain properly. It may build up in the tissues and causes swelling. This can happen when part of the lymph system is damaged or blocked, such as during surgery to remove lymph nodes, or radiation therapy. Cancers that block lymph vessels can also cause lymphedema.

Lymphedema usually affects an arm or leg, but it can also affect other parts of the body, such as the head and neck. You may notice symptoms of lymphedema at the part of your body where you had surgery or received radiation therapy. Swelling usually develops slowly, over time. It may develop during treatment or it may start years after treatment.

At first, lymphedema in an arm or leg may cause symptoms such as:

- swelling and a heavy or achy feeling in your arms or legs that may spread to your fingers and toes
- a dent when you press on the swollen area
- swelling that is soft to the touch and is usually not painful at first

Lymphedema that is not controlled may cause:

- more swelling, weakness, and difficulty moving your arm or leg
- itchy, red, warm skin, and sometimes a rash

- wounds that don't heal, and an increased risk of skin infections that may cause pain, redness, and swelling
- thickening or hardening of the skin
- tight feeling in the skin; pressing on the swollen area does not leave a dent
- hair loss

Lymphedema in the head or neck may cause:

- swelling and a tight uncomfortable feeling on your face, neck, or under your chin
- difficulty moving your head or neck

Tell your health care team as soon as you notice symptoms. Early treatment may prevent or reduce the severity of problems caused by lymphedema.

Ways to Manage

Steps you may be advised to take to prevent lymphedema or to keep it from getting worse:

- **Protect your skin**. Use lotion to avoid dry skin. Use sunscreen. Wear plastic gloves with cotton lining when working in order to prevent scratches, cuts, or burns. Keep your feet clean and dry. Keep your nails clean and short to prevent ingrown nails and infection. Avoid tight shoes and tight jewelry.
- **Exercise**. Work to keep body fluids moving, especially in places where lymphedema has developed. Start with gentle exercises that help you to move and contract your muscles. Ask your doctor or nurse what exercises are best for you.
- **Manual lymph drainage**. See a trained specialist (a certified lymphedema therapist) to receive a type of therapeutic massage called manual lymph drainage. Therapeutic massage works best to lower lymphedema when given early, before symptoms progress.

Ways to Treat

Your doctor or nurse may advise you to take these and other steps to treat lymphedema:

- **Wear compression garments or bandages**. Wear special garments, such as sleeves, stockings, bras, compression shorts, gloves, bandages, and face or neck compression wear. Some garments are meant to be worn during the day, while others are to be worn at night.

- **Other practices**. Your health care team may advise you to use compression devices (special pumps that apply pressure periodically) or have laser therapy or other treatments.

Talking with Your Health Care Team

Prepare for your visit by making a list of questions to ask. Consider adding these questions to your list:

- What can I do to prevent these problems?
- What symptoms should I call you about?
- What steps can I take to feel better?
- Would you recommend that I see a certified lymphedema therapist?
- If lymphedema advances, what special garments should I wear during the day? During the night?

Memory or Concentration Problems

Whether you have memory or concentration problems (sometimes described as a mental fog or chemo brain) depends on the type of treatment you receive, your age, and other health-related factors. Cancer treatments such as chemotherapy may cause difficulty with thinking, concentrating, or remembering things. So can some types of biological therapies and radiation therapy to the brain.

These cognitive problems may start during or after cancer treatment. Some people notice very small changes, such as a bit more difficulty remembering things, whereas others have much greater memory or concentration problems.

Your doctor will assess your symptoms and advise you about ways to manage or treat these problems. Treating conditions such as poor nutrition, anxiety, depression, fatigue, and insomnia may also help.

Ways to Manage

It's important for you or a family member to tell your health care team if you have difficulty remembering things, thinking, or concentrating. Here are some steps you can take to manage minor memory or concentration problems:

- **Plan your day**. Do things that need the most concentration at the time of day when you feel best. Get extra rest and plenty of sleep at night. If you need to rest during the day, short naps of less than 1 hour are best. Long naps can make it more difficult to sleep at night. Keep a daily routine.

- **Exercise your body and mind**. Exercise can help to decrease stress and help you to feel more alert. Exercise releases endorphins, also known as "feel-good chemicals,"which give people a feeling of well-being. Ask what light physical exercises may be helpful for you. Mind–body practices such as meditation or mental exercises such as puzzles or games also help some people.

- **Get help to remember things**. Write down and keep a list handy of important information. Use a daily planner, recorder, or other electronic device to help you remember important activities. Make a list of important names and phone numbers. Keep it in one place so it's easy to find.

Talking with Your Health Care Team

It's important for you or a family member to talk with your doctor or nurse about any memory or cognitive changes you may have. Prepare for your visit by making a list of questions to ask. Consider adding these questions to your list:

- Am I at increased risk of cognitive problems based on the treatment I am receiving?

- When might these problems start to occur? How long might they last?

- Are there steps I can take to decrease these problems?

- What symptoms or other problems should I, or a family member, call you about?

- Could I meet with a social worker to get ideas about additional support and resources?

- Are there specialists who could assess, treat, or advise me on these problems (such as neuropsychologists, occupational therapists, vocational therapists, and others)?

Mouth and Throat Problems

Cancer treatments may cause dental, mouth, and throat problems. Radiation therapy to the head and neck may harm the salivary glands and tissues in your mouth and/or make it hard to chew and swallow safely. Some types of chemotherapy and biological therapy can also harm cells in your mouth, throat, and lips. Drugs used to treat cancer and certain bone problems may also cause oral complications.

Mouth and throat problems may include:

- changes in taste (dysgeusia) or smell
- dry mouth (xerostomia)
- infections and mouth sores
- pain or swelling in your mouth (oral mucositis)
- sensitivity to hot or cold foods
- swallowing problems (dysphagia)
- tooth decay (cavities)

Mouth problems are more serious if they interfere with eating and drinking because they can lead to dehydration and/or malnutrition. It's important to call your doctor or nurse if you have pain in your mouth, lips, or throat that makes it difficult to eat, drink, or sleep or if you have a fever of 100.5 °F (38 °C) or higher.

Ways to Prevent Mouth and Dental Problems

Your doctor or nurse may advise you to take these and other steps:

- **Get a dental check-up before starting treatment.** Before you start treatment, visit your dentist for a cleaning and check-up. Tell the dentist about your cancer treatment and try to get any dental work completed before starting treatment.

- **Check and clean your mouth daily.** Check your mouth every day for sores or white spots. Tell your doctor or nurse as soon as you notice any changes, such as pain or sensitivity. Rinse your mouth throughout the day with a solution of warm water, baking soda, and salt. Ask your nurse to write down the mouth rinse recipe that is recommended for you. Gently brush your teeth, gums, and tongue after each meal and before going to bed at night. Use a very soft toothbrush or cotton swabs. If you are at risk of bleeding, ask if you should floss.

Ways to Manage

Your health care team may suggest that you take these and other steps to manage these problems:

- **For a sore mouth or throat:** Choose foods that are soft, wet, and easy to swallow. Soften dry foods with gravy, sauce, or other liquids. Use a blender to make milkshakes or blend your food to make it easier to swallow. Ask about pain medicine, such as lozenges or sprays that numb your mouth and make eating less painful. Avoid foods and drinks that can irritate your mouth; foods that are crunchy, salty, spicy, or sugary; and alcoholic drinks. Don't smoke or use tobacco products.

- **For a dry mouth:** Drink plenty of liquids because a dry mouth can increase the risk of tooth decay and mouth infections. Keep water handy and sip it often to keep your mouth wet. Suck on ice chips or sugar-free hard candy, have frozen desserts, or chew sugar-free gum. Use a lip balm. Ask about medicines such as saliva substitutes that can coat, protect, and moisten your mouth and throat. Acupuncture may also help with dry mouth.

- **For changes to your sense of taste:** Foods may seem to have no taste or may not taste the way they used to or food may not have much taste at all. Radiation therapy may cause a change in sweet, sour, bitter, and salty tastes. Chemotherapy drugs may cause an unpleasant chemical or metallic taste in your mouth. If you have taste changes it may help to try different foods to find ones that taste best to you. Trying cold foods may also help. Here are some more tips to consider:

- If food tastes bland, marinate foods to improve their flavor or add spices to foods.
  - If red meat tastes strange, switch to other high-protein foods such as chicken, eggs, fish, peanut butter, turkey, beans, or dairy products.
  - If foods taste salty, bitter, or acidic, try sweetening them.
  - If foods taste metallic, switch to plastic utensils and non-metal cooking dishes.

1071

- If you have a bad taste in your mouth, try sugar-free lemon drops, gum, or mints.

Talking with Your Health Care Team

Prepare for your visit by making a list of questions to ask. Consider adding these questions to your list:

- When might these problems start to occur? How long might they last?
- What steps can I take to feel better?
- What medicines can help?
- What symptoms or problems should I call the doctor about?
- What pain medicine and/or mouthwashes could help me?
- Would you recommend a registered dietitian who I could see to learn about good food choices?
- For people receiving radiation therapy to the head and neck: Should I take supplements such as zinc, to help my sense of taste come back after treatment?

Nausea and Vomiting

Nausea is when you feel sick to your stomach, as if you are going to throw up. Vomiting is when you throw up. There are different types of nausea and vomiting caused by cancer treatment, including anticipatory, acute, and delayed nausea and vomiting. Controlling nausea and vomiting will help you to feel better and prevent more serious problems such as malnutrition and dehydration.

Your doctor or nurse will determine what is causing your symptoms and advise you on ways to prevent them. Medicines called anti-nausea drugs or antiemetics are effective in preventing or reducing many types of nausea and vomiting. The medicine is taken at specific times to prevent and/or control symptoms of nausea and vomiting. There are also practical steps you may be advised to take to feel better, including those listed below.

Ways to Manage

You may be advised to take these steps to feel better:

- **Take an anti-nausea medicine.** Talk with your doctor or nurse to learn when to take your medicine. Most people need to take an anti-nausea medicine even on days when they feel well. Tell your doctor or nurse if the medicine doesn't help. There are different kinds of medicine and one may work better than another for you.

- **Drink plenty of water and fluids.** Drinking will help to prevent dehydration, a serious problem that happens when your body loses too much fluid and you are not drinking enough. Try to sip on water, fruit juices, ginger ale, tea, and/or sports drinks throughout the day.

- **Avoid certain foods.** Don't eat greasy, fried, sweet, or spicy foods if you feel sick after eating them. If the smell of food bothers you, ask others to make your food. Try cold foods that do not have strong smells, or let food cool down before you eat it.

- **Try these tips on treatment days.** Some people find that it helps to eat a small snack before treatment. Others avoid eating or drinking right before or after treatment because it makes them feel sick. After treatment, wait at least 1 hour before you eat or drink.

- **Learn about complementary medicine practices that may help.** Acupuncture relieves nausea and/or vomiting cause by chemotherapy in some people. Deep breathing, guided imagery, hypnosis, and other relaxation techniques (such as listening to music, reading a book, or meditating) also help some people.

Talking with Your Health Care Team

Prepare for your visit by making a list of questions to ask. Consider adding these questions to your list:

- What symptoms or problems should I call you about?

- What medicine could help me? When should I take this medicine?

- How much liquid should I drink each day? What should I do if I throw up?

- What foods would be easy on my stomach? What foods should I avoid?

- Could I meet with a registered dietitian to learn more?

- What specialists could I see to learn about acupuncture and other practices that could help to lower my symptoms?

Nerve Problems (Peripheral Neuropathy)

Some cancer treatments cause peripheral neuropathy, a result of damage to the peripheral nerves. These nerves carry information from the brain to other parts of the body. Side effects depend on which peripheral nerves (sensory, motor, or autonomic) are affected.

Damage to sensory nerves (nerves that help you feel pain, heat, cold, and pressure) can cause:

- tingling, numbness, or a pins-and-needles feeling in your feet and hands that may spread to your legs and arms

- inability to feel a hot or cold sensation, such as a hot stove

- inability to feel pain, such as from a cut or sore on your foot

Damage to motor nerves (nerves that help your muscles to move) can cause:

- weak or achy muscles. You may lose your balance or trip easily. It may also be difficult to button shirts or open jars.

- muscles that twitch and cramp or muscle wasting (if you don't use your muscles regularly).

- swallowing or breathing difficulties (if your chest or throat muscles are affected)

Damage to autonomic nerves (nerves that control functions such as blood pressure, digestion, heart rate, temperature, and urination) can cause:

- digestive changes such as constipation or diarrhea

- dizzy or faint feeling, due to low blood pressure

- sexual problems; men may be unable to get an erection and women may not reach orgasm

- sweating problems (either too much or too little sweating)

- urination problems, such as leaking urine or difficulty emptying your bladder

If you start to notice any of the problems listed above, talk with your doctor or nurse. Getting these problems diagnosed and treated early is the best way to control them, prevent further damage, and to reduce pain and other complications.

Ways to Prevent or Manage Problems Related to Nerve Changes

You may be advised to take these steps:

- **Prevent falls.** Have someone help you prevent falls around the house. Move rugs out of your path so you will not trip on them. Put rails on the walls and in the bathroom, so you can hold on to them and balance yourself. Put bathmats in the shower or tub. Wear sturdy shoes with soft soles. Get up slowly after sitting or lying down, especially if you feel dizzy.

- **Take extra care in the kitchen and shower.** Use potholders in the kitchen to protect your hands from burns. Be careful when handling knives or sharp objects. Ask someone to check the water temperature, to make sure it's not too hot.

- **Protect your hands and feet.** Wear shoes, both inside and outside. Check your arms, legs, and feet for cuts or scratches every day. When it's cold, wear warm clothes to protect your hands and feet.

- **Ask for help and slow down.** Let people help you with difficult tasks. Slow down and give yourself more time to do things.

- **Ask about pain medicine and integrative medicine practices.** You may be prescribed pain medicine. Sometimes practices such as acupuncture, massage, physical therapy, yoga, and others may also be advised to lower pain. Talk with your health care team to learn what is advised for you.

Talking with Your Health Care Team

Prepare for your visit by making a list of questions to ask. Consider adding these questions to your list:

- What symptoms or problems might I have? Which ones should I call you about?

- When will these problems start? How long might they last?

- What medicine, treatments, and integrative medicine practices could help me to feel better?

- What steps can I take to feel better? What precautions should I take to stay safe?

- Could you refer me to a specialist who could give me additional advice?

Pain

Cancer itself and the side effects of cancer treatment can sometimes cause pain. Pain is not something that you have to "put up with." Controlling pain is an important part of your cancer treatment plan. Pain can suppress the immune system, increase the time it takes your body to heal, interfere with sleep, and affect your mood.

Talk with your health care team about pain, especially if:

- the pain isn't getting better or going away with pain medicine
- the pain comes on quickly
- the pain makes it hard to eat, sleep, or perform your normal activities
- you feel new pain
- you have side effects from the pain medicine such as sleepiness, nausea, or constipation

Your doctor will work with you to develop a pain control plan that is based on your description of the pain. Taking pain medicine is an important part of the plan. Your doctor will talk with you about using drugs to control pain and prescribe medicine (including opioids and nonopioid medicines) to treat the pain.

Ways to Treat or Lessen Pain

Here are some steps you can take, as you work with your health care team to prevent, treat, or lessen pain:

- **Keep track of your pain levels.** Each day, write about any pain you feel. Writing down answers to the questions below will help you describe the pain to your doctor or nurse.
  - What part of your body feels painful?
  - What does the pain feel like (is it sharp, burning, shooting, or throbbing) and where do you feel the pain?
  - When does the pain start? How long does the pain last?
  - What activities (such as eating, sleeping, or other activities) does pain interfere with?
  - What makes the pain feel better or worse? For example, do ice packs, heating pads, or exercises help? Does pain

medicine help? How much do you take? How often do you take it?

- How bad is the pain, on a scale of 1 to 10, where "10" is the most pain and "1" is the least pain?

- **Take the prescribed pain medicine.** Take the right amount of medicine at the right time. Do not wait until your pain gets too bad before taking pain medicine. Waiting to take your medicine could make it take longer for the pain to go away or increase the amount of medicine needed to lower pain. Do not stop taking the pain medicine unless your doctor advises you to. Tell your doctor or nurse if the medicine no longer lowers the pain, or if you are in pain, but it's not yet time to take the pain medicine.

- **Meet with a pain specialist.** Specialists who treat pain often work together as part of a pain or palliative care team. These specialists may include a neurologist, surgeon, physiatrist, psychiatrist, psychologist, or pharmacist. Talk with your health care team to find a pain specialist.

- **Ask about integrative medicine.** Treatments such as acupuncture, biofeedback, hypnosis, massage therapy and physical therapy may also be used to treat pain.

Talking with Your Health Care Team

Prepare for your visit by making a list of questions to ask. Consider adding these questions to your list:

- What problems or levels of pain should I call you about?
- What is most likely causing the pain?
- What can I do to lessen the pain?
- What medicine should I take? If the pain doesn't go away, how much more medicine can I take, and when can I take it?
- What are the side effects of this pain medicine? How long will they last?
- Is there a pain specialist I could meet with to get more support to lower my pain?

Sexual and Fertility Problems (Men)

Many cancer treatments and some types of cancer can cause sexual and fertility-related side effects. Whether you have these problems depends on the type of treatment(s) you receive, your age at time of treatment, and how long it has been since you had treatment.

It is important to learn how the treatment recommended for you may affect your fertility before you start treatment. Many men also find it helpful to talk with their doctor or nurse about sexual problems they may have during treatment. Learning about these issues will help you make decisions that are best for you.

Treatments That May Cause Sexual and Fertility Problems

- Radiation therapy to the pelvic area (such as to the anus, bladder, penis, or prostate) may make it difficult to get or keep an erection. It may also cause infertility, which may be temporary or permanent. Some men notice that changes in sexual function occur slowly over the period of about a year. Smoking, heart disease, high blood pressure, and diabetes can make some problems worse.

- Hormone therapy may cause mood changes, decreased sexual desire, erectile dysfunction, and trouble reaching orgasm.

- Some types of chemotherapy may cause low testosterone levels and lower your sexual desire. Chemotherapy may also cause infertility, which may be temporary or permanent.

- Surgery for penile, rectal, prostate, testicular, and other pelvic cancers may affect sexual function and fertility.

- Other side effects of cancer and its treatment, such as fatigue and anxiety, can also lower your interest in sexual activity.

Learn What to Expect

Before starting treatment talk with your health care team to learn what to expect based on the type of treatment you will be receiving. Get answers to questions about:

- **Sexual activity.** Ask your doctor or nurse if it is okay for you to be sexually active during your treatment period. Most men can, but you will want to confirm this with your doctor or nurse.

- **Infertility.** Ask if your treatment could affect your fertility or make you infertile. If you would like to have children after treatment, talk with your doctor or nurse before you start treatment. Learn ahead of time about your options, such as sperm banking.

Procedures such as testicular sperm extraction, testicular tissue freezing and testicular tissue cryopreservation (for young boys) are available. Talk with your doctor or a fertility specialist to learn more about these procedures and other that may be available through a clinical trial.

- **Birth control.** It is important to prevent pregnancy during treatment and for some time after treatment. Ask your doctor or nurse about different methods of birth control to choose one that may be best for you and your partner.

- **Condom use.** If you receive chemotherapy you will most likely be advised to use a condom during intercourse, even if your partner is on birth control or cannot have children. This is because your semen may have traces of the chemotherapy drugs.

Talking with Your Health Care Team

Prepare for your visit by making a list of questions to ask. Consider adding these questions to your list:

Sexual and Sexuality-Related Questions

- What problems or changes might I have during or after treatment?

- How long might these problems last? Will any of these problems be permanent?

- How can these problems be treated or managed?

- Could you give me the name of a specialist who I can talk with to learn more?

- What precautions do I need to take during treatment? For example, do I need to use a condom?

- Is there a support group for men that you would recommend for me?

Fertility-Related Questions

- Will the treatment I receive make me infertile (unable to have children in the future)?

- What are all of my options now if I would like to have children in the future?

- Could you give me the name of a fertility specialist who I can talk with to learn more?

- After treatment, how long should I use some method of birth control?

Sexual and Fertility Problems (Women)

Many cancer treatments and some types of cancer can cause sexual and fertility-related side effects. Whether or not you have these problems depends on the type of treatment(s) you receive, your age at time of treatment, and the length of time since treatment.

It is important to get information about how the treatment recommended for you may affect your fertility before you start treatment. Many women also find it helpful to talk with their doctor or nurse about sexual problems they may have during treatment. Learning about these issues will help you make decisions that are best for you.

Treatments That May Cause Sexual and Fertility Problems

- Some types of chemotherapy may cause symptoms of early menopause (hot flashes, vaginal dryness, irregular or no periods, and feeling irritable) or lead to vaginal infections. It may also cause temporary or permanent infertility.

- Hormone therapy can stop or slow the growth of certain cancers, such as breast cancer. However, lower hormone levels can cause problems (hot flashes, vaginal discharge or pain, and trouble reaching orgasm). These problems are more likely in women over the age of 45.

- Radiation therapy to the pelvic area (vagina, uterus, or ovaries) can cause:

  - infertility

  - symptoms of menopause (hot flashes, vaginal dryness, and no periods)

  - pain or discomfort during sex

  - increased risk of birth defects; use a method of birth control to avoid pregnancy

  - vaginal stenosis (less elastic, narrow, shorter vagina)

  - vaginal itching, burning, or dryness

  - vaginal atrophy (weak vaginal muscles and thin vaginal wall)

- Surgery for cancers of the uterus, bladder, vulvar, endometrium, cervix, or ovaries may cause sexual and infertility-related side effects, depending on the size and location of the tumor.

- Other side effects of cancer and its treatment, such as fatigue and anxiety, can also lower your interest in sexual activity.

What to Expect

Before starting treatment talk with your health care team to learn what to expect, based on the type of treatment you will be receiving. Get answers to questions about:

- **Infertility.** Ask if treatment could lower your fertility or make you infertile. If you would like to have children after treatment, talk with your doctor or nurse before you start treatment. Learn ahead of time about options such as embryo banking, ovarian tissue banking, ovarian transposition, and clinical trials for egg banking. Talk with your doctor or a fertility specialist to learn more about these procedures and others that may be available through a clinical trial.

- **Pregnancy.** It is important to prevent pregnancy during treatment and for some time after treatment. Ask your doctor or nurse about different methods of birth control, to choose one that may be best for you and your partner.

- **Sexual activity.** Ask your doctor or nurse if it is okay for you to be sexually active during your treatment period. Most women can be sexually active, but you will want to confirm this with your health care team.

Talking with Your Health Care Team

Prepare for your visit by making a list of questions. Consider adding these questions to your list:

Sexual and Sexuality-Related Questions

- What problems or changes might I have during treatment?
- How long might these problems last? Will any be permanent?
- Is there treatment for these problems?
- Would you give me the name of a specialist that I could meet with?
- Is there a support group for women that you would recommend?

Fertility-Related Questions

- Will my fertility be affected by the treatment I receive?

- What are all of my options now if I would like to have children in the future?

- Could you give me the name of a fertility specialist who I can talk with to learn more?

- After treatment, how long should I use birth control?

Skin and Nail Changes

Cancer treatments may cause a range of skin and nail changes. Talk with your health care team to learn whether or not you will have these changes, based on the treatment you are receiving.

- Radiation therapy can cause the skin on the part of your body receiving radiation therapy to become dry and peel, itch (called pruritus), and turn red or darker. It may look sunburned or tan and be swollen or puffy.

- Chemotherapy may damage fast growing skin and nail cells. This can cause problems such as skin that is dry, itchy, red, and/or that peels. Some people may develop a rash or sun sensitivity, causing you to sunburn easily. Nail changes may include dark, yellow, or cracked nails and/or cuticles that are red and hurt. Chemotherapy in people who have received radiation therapy in the past can cause skin to become red, blister, peel, or hurt on the part of the body that received radiation therapy; this is called radiation recall.

- Biological therapy may cause itching (pruritus).

- Targeted therapy may cause a dry skin, a rash, and nail problems.

These skin problems are more serious and need urgent medical attention:

- Sudden or severe itching, a rash, or hives during chemotherapy. These may be signs of an allergic reaction.

- Sores on the part of your body where you are receiving treatment that become painful, wet, and/or infected. This is called a moist reaction and may happen in areas where the skin folds, such as around your ears, breast, or bottom.

Your doctor or nurse will talk with about possible skin and nail changes and advise you on ways to treat or prevent them.

Ways to Manage

Depending on what treatment you are receiving, you may be advised to take these steps to protect your skin, prevent infection, and reduce itching:

- **Use only recommended skin products.** Use mild soaps that are gentle on your skin. Ask your nurse to recommend specific lotions and creams. Ask when and how often to use them. Ask what skin products to avoid. For example, you may be advised to not use powders or antiperspirants before radiation therapy.

- **Protect your skin.** Ask about lotions or antibiotics for dry, itchy, infected or swollen skin. Don't use heating pads, ice packs, or bandages on the area receiving radiation therapy. Shave less often and use an electric razor or stop shaving if your skin is sore. Wear sunscreen and lip balm or a loose-fitting long-sleeved shirt, pants, and a hat with a wide brim when outdoors.

- **Prevent or treat dry, itchy skin (pruritus).** Your doctor will work to assess the cause of pruritus. There are also steps you can take to feel better. Avoid products with alcohol or perfume, which can dry or irritate your skin. Take short showers or baths in luke-warm, not hot, water. Put on lotion after drying off from a shower, while your skin is still slightly damp. Keep your home cool and humid. Eat a healthy diet and drink plenty of fluids to help keep your skin moist and healthy. Applying a cool washcloth or ice to the affected area may also help. Acupuncture also helps some people.

- **Prevent or treat minor nail problems.** Keep your nails clean and cut short. Wear gloves when you wash the dishes, work in the garden, or clean the house. Check with your nurse about products that can help your nails.

If your skin hurts in the area where you get treatment, tell your doctor or nurse. Your skin might have a moist reaction. Most often this happens in areas where the skin folds, such as behind the ears or under the breasts. It can lead to an infection if not properly treated. Ask your doctor or nurse how to care for these areas.

Talking with Your Health Care Team

Prepare for your visit by making a list of questions to ask. Consider adding these questions to your list:

- What symptoms or problems should I call you about?

- What steps can I take to feel better?

- What brands of soap and lotion are best for me to use? What products can help my nails stay healthy?

- What skin and nail products should I avoid?

- When will these problems go away?

Sleep Problems

Sleeping well is important for your physical and mental health. A good night's sleep not only helps you to think clearly, it also lowers your blood pressure, helps your appetite, and strengthens your immune system.

However, sleep problems are common among people being treated for cancer. Studies show that as many as half of all patients have sleep-related problems. These problems may be caused by the side effects of treatment, medicine, long hospital stays, or stress.

Talk with your health care team if you have difficulty sleeping, so you can get help you need. Sleep problems that go on for a long time may increase the risk of anxiety or depression. Your doctor will do an assessment, which may include a polysomnogram (recordings taken during sleep that show brain waves, breathing rate, and others activities such as heart rate) to correctly diagnose and treat sleep problems. Assessments may be repeated from time to time, since sleeping problems may change over time.

Ways to Manage

There are steps that you and your health care team can take to help you sleep well again.

- **Tell your doctor about problems that interfere with sleep.** Getting treatment to lower side effects such as pain or bladder or gastrointestinal problems may help you sleep better.

- **Cognitive behavioral therapy (CBT) and relaxation therapy may help.** Practicing these therapies can help you to relax. For example, a CBT therapist can help you learn to change negative thoughts and beliefs about sleep into positive ones. Strategies such as muscle relaxation, guided imagery, and self-hypnosis may also help you.

- **Set good bedtime habits**. Go to bed only when sleepy, in a quiet and dark room, and in a comfortable bed. If you do not fall asleep, get out of bed and return to bed when you are sleepy. Stop watching television or using other electrical devices a couple of hours before going to bed. Don't drink or eat a lot before bedtime. While it's important to keep active during the day with regular exercise, exercising a few hours before bedtime may make sleep more difficult.

- **Sleep medicine may be prescribed.** Your doctor may prescribe sleep medicine, for a short period if other strategies don't work. The sleep medicine prescribed will depend on your specific problem (such as trouble falling asleep or trouble staying asleep) as well as other medicines you are taking.

Talking with Your Health Care Team

Prepare for your visit by making a list of questions to ask. Consider adding these questions to your list:

- Why am I having trouble sleeping?

- What problems should I call you about?

- What steps can I take to sleep better?

- Would you recommend a sleep therapist who could help with the problems I am having?

- Would sleep medicine be advised for me?

Urinary and Bladder Problems

Some cancer treatments, such as those listed below, may cause the urinary and bladder problems:

- Radiation therapy to the pelvis (including reproductive organs, the bladder, colon and rectum) can irritate the bladder and urinary tract. These problems often start several weeks after radiation therapy begins and go away several weeks after treatment has been completed.

- Some types of chemotherapy and biological therapy can also affect or damage cells in the bladder and kidneys.

- Surgery to remove the prostate (prostatectomy), bladder cancer surgery, and surgery to remove a woman's uterus, the tissue on the sides of the uterus, the cervix, and the top part of the vagina (radical hysterectomy) can also cause urinary problems. These types of surgery may also increase the risk of a urinary tract infection.

Symptoms of a Urinary Problem

Talk with your doctor or nurse to learn what symptoms you may experience and ask which ones to call about. Some urinary or bladder changes may be normal, such as changes to the color or smell of your urine caused by some types of chemotherapy. Your health care team will determine what is causing your symptoms and will advise on steps to take to feel better.

Irritation of the bladder lining (radiation cystitis):

- pain or a burning feeling when you before or after you urinate
- blood in your urine
- trouble starting to urinate
- trouble emptying your bladder completely
- feeling that you need to urinate urgently or frequently
- leaking a little urine when you sneeze or cough
- bladder spasms, cramps, or discomfort in the pelvic area

Urinary tract infection (UTI):

- pain or a burning feeling when you urinate
- urine that is cloudy or red
- a fever of 100.5 °F (38 °C) or higher, chills, and fatigue
- pain in your back or abdomen
- difficulty urinating or not being able to urinate

In people being treated for cancer, a UTI can turn into a serious condition that needs immediate medical care. Antibiotics will be prescribed if you have a bacterial infection.

Symptoms that may occur after surgery:

- leaking urine (incontinence)
- trouble emptying your bladder completely

Ways to Prevent or Manage

Here are some steps you may be advised to take to feel better and to prevent problems:

- **Have plenty of liquids.** Drink plenty of liquids. Most people need to drink at least 8 cups of fluid each day, so that urine is light yellow or clear. You'll want to stay away from things that can make bladder problems worse. These include caffeine, drinks with alcohol, spicy foods, and tobacco products.

- **Prevent urinary tract infections.** Your doctor or nurse will talk with you about ways to lower your chances of getting a urinary tract infection. These may include going to the bathroom often, wearing cotton underwear and loose fitting pants, learning about safe and sanitary practices for catheterization, taking showers instead of baths, and checking with your nurse before using products such as creams or lotions near your genital area.

Talking with Your Health Care Team

Prepare for your visit by making a list of questions to ask. Consider adding these questions to your list:

- What symptoms or problems should I call you about?
- What steps can I take to feel better?
- How much should I drink each day? What liquids are best for me?
- Are there certain drinks or foods that I should avoid?

Chapter 57

Cardiopulmonary Syndromes

Cardiopulmonary Syndrome Overview

Cardiopulmonary syndromes are conditions of the heart and lung that may be caused by cancer or by other health problems. Five cardiopulmonary syndromes that may be caused by cancer are covered in this chapter:

- Dyspnea (shortness of breath).
- Chronic cough.
- Malignant pleural effusion (extra fluid around the lungs).
- Malignant pericardial effusion (extra fluid in the sac around the heart).
- Superior vena cava syndrome (a blocked superior vena cava, the large vein that takes blood back to the heart).

Dyspnea During Advanced Cancer

Many conditions can cause dyspnea.

Dyspnea is the feeling of difficult or uncomfortable breathing or of not getting enough air. It also may be called shortness of breath,

Text in this chapter is excerpted from "Cardiopulmonary Syndromes," National Cancer Institute at the National Institutes of Health (NIH), February 13, 2015.

breathlessness, or air hunger. In cancer patients, causes of dyspnea include the following:

- Effects related to the tumor:

  - The tumor blocks the airways in the chest and lung or the vein that carries blood through the chest to the heart.

  - The tumor causes extra fluid to build up in the space between the thin layer of tissue covering the lung and the thin layer of tissue covering the chest wall (pleural effusion), between the sac that covers the heart and the heart (pericardial effusion), or in the abdominal cavity (ascites).

  - Carcinomatous lymphangitis (inflammation of the lymph vessels).

  - Chest infections. Some cancer treatments may increase the risk of an infection, such as pneumonia.

  - Blood clots or tumor cells break loose and block a blood vessel in the lungs.

  - Paralysis of part of the diaphragm (a muscle used for breathing).

  - Breathing muscles get weaker.

- Effects related to treatment:

  - Damage to the lung caused by radiation therapy or chemotherapy.

  - Weakened heart muscle caused by chemotherapy.

- Conditions that are not related to cancer:

  - Chronic obstructive pulmonary disease (COPD), such as chronic bronchitis or emphysema.

  - Bronchospasm. The muscles in the airways contract and cause spasms.

  - A weak diaphragm.

  - Congestive heart failure.

  - Anemia.

- Conditions with no known physical cause, such as anxiety.

A diagnosis of the cause of dyspnea helps to plan treatment.

Diagnostic tests and procedures include the following:

- Physical exam and history
- Functional assessment
- Chest x-ray
- CT scan (CAT scan)
- Complete blood count
- Oxygen saturation test
- Maximum inspiratory pressure (MIP test)

It may be possible to treat the cause of dyspnea.

Treatment may include the following:

- Chemotherapy
- Lasertherapy for tumors inside large airways
- Cauterization of tumors inside large airways
- malignant pleural effusion
- malignant pericardial effusion
- ascites
- stent placement
- Medicine: Steroid drugs, Antibiotics, Anticoagulants, Diurectics
- Blood transfusion

Treatment of dyspnea depends on the cause of it.

The treatment of dyspnea depends on its cause, as follows:

If the dyspnea is caused by:	Then the treatment may be:
Tumor blocking the large or small airways in the chest or lung	Radiation therapy
	Chemotherapy, for tumors that usually respond quickly to this treatment.

If the dyspnea is caused by:	Then the treatment may be:
	Laser surgery to remove the tumor.
	Cauterization of tumors.
Pleural effusion	Removal of the extra fluid around the lung using a needle or chest drain.
Pericardial effusion	Removal of the extra fluid around the heart using a needle.
Ascites	Removal of the extra fluid in the abdominal cavity using a needle.
Carcinomatous lymphangitis	Steroid therapy
	Chemotherapy, for tumors that usually respond quickly to this treatment.
Superior vena cava syndrome	Chemotherapy, for tumors that usually respond quickly to this treatment.
	Radiation therapy
	Surgery to place a stent in the superior vena cava to keep it open.
Chest infections	Antibiotics.
	Breathing treatments.
Blood clots	Anticoagulants.
Bronchospasms or chronic obstructive pulmonary disease	Bronchodilators.
	Inhaled steroids.
Heart failure	Diuretics and other heart medicines.
Anemia	Blood transfusion

Treatment may be to control the signs and symptoms of dyspnea.

Treatment to control the signs and symptoms of dyspnea may include the following:

- Oxygen therapy: Patients who cannot get enough oxygen from the air may be given extra oxygen to inhale from a tank. Devices that increase the amount of oxygen already in the air may also be prescribed.

- Medicines: Opioids, such as morphine, may lessen physical and mental distress and exhaustion and the feeling that the patient cannot take in enough air. Other drugs may be used to treat dyspnea that is related to panic disorder or severe anxiety.

- Supportive care:
  - Breathing methods, such as breathing with the lips pursed (almost closed).
  - Using a fan to blow cold air across the cheek.
  - Meditation.
  - Relaxation training.
  - Biofeedback.
  - Talk therapy to relieve anxiety.

Chronic Coughing

Chronic coughing may cause much physical distress.

Chronic cough may cause severe pain, trouble sleeping, dyspnea, or fatigue. The causes of chronic coughing are almost the same as the causes of dyspnea.

It may be possible to treat the cause of chronic coughing.

Treatments may include:

- Radiation therapy for a tumor that is blocking the airway.
- Placement of an expandable stent (tube) to close a fistula caused by esophageal cancer.
- Draining the fluid of a pleural effusion.
- Corticosteroids for lymphangitic carcinomatosis.

Medicines may be used to control chronic coughing.

Medicines may include:

- Medicines to suppress the cough, including opioids.
- Medicine that breaks down mucus.
- An inhaled drug for chronic coughing related to lung cancer.

Malignant Pleural Effusion

Pleural effusion is extra fluid around the lungs.

The pleural cavity is the space between the pleura (thin layer of tissue) that covers the outer surface of each lung and lines the inner wall of the chest cavity. Pleural tissue usually makes a small amount of fluid that helps the lungs move smoothly in the chest while a person is breathing. A pleural effusion is extra fluid in the pleural cavity. The fluid presses on the lungs and makes it hard to breathe.

Pleural effusion may be caused by cancer, cancer treatment, or other conditions.

A pleural effusion may be malignant (caused by cancer) or nonmalignant (caused by a condition that is not cancer). Malignant pleural effusion is a common problem for patients who have certain cancers. Lung cancer, breast cancer, lymphoma, and leukemia cause most malignant effusions. An effusion also may be caused by cancer treatment, such as radiation therapy or chemotherapy. Some cancer patients have conditions such as congestive heart failure, pneumonia, blood clot in the lung, or poor nutrition that may lead to a pleural effusion.

A diagnosis of the cause of pleural effusion is important in planning treatment.

These and other signs and symptoms may be caused by a pleural effusion. Talk to your doctor if you have any of the following problems:

- Dyspnea (shortness of breath).
- Cough.
- An uncomfortable feeling or pain in the chest.

Treatment for a malignant pleural effusion is different from treatment for a nonmalignant effusion, so the right diagnosis is important. Diagnostic tests include the following:

- Chest x-ray
- CT scan
- Thoracentesis
- Biopsy

The type of cancer, previous treatment for cancer, and the patient's wishes also are important in planning treatment.

Treatment may be to control signs and symptoms of pleural effusion and improve quality of life.

A malignant pleural effusion often occurs in cancer that is advanced, cannot be removed by surgery, or continues to grow or spread during treatment. It is also common during the last few weeks of life. The goal of treatment is usually palliative, to relieve signs and symptoms and improve quality of life.

Treatment of the signs and symptoms of malignant pleural effusion includes the following:

- Thoracentesis
- Indwelling pleural catheter (IPC)
- Pleurodesis
- Surgery

Malignant Pericardial Effusion

Pericardial effusion is extra fluid around the heart.

Pericardial effusion is extra fluid inside the sac that surrounds the heart. The extra fluid causes pressure on the heart, which stops it from pumping blood normally. Lymph vessels may also be blocked, which often causes bacterial or viral infections. If fluid builds up quickly, a condition called cardiac tamponade may occur. In cardiac tamponade, the heart cannot pump enough blood to the rest of the body. This is life-threatening and must be treated right away.

Pericardial effusion may be caused by cancer or other conditions.

A pericardial effusion may be malignant (caused by cancer) or non-malignant (caused by a condition that is not cancer). A malignant effusion is common in certain types of cancer. Lung cancer, breast cancer, melanoma, lymphoma, and leukemia cause most malignant effusions. An effusion also may be caused by cancer treatment, such as radiation therapy or chemotherapy.

Signs and symptoms of pericardial effusion include dyspnea (shortness of breath) and anxiety.

At first, a pericardial effusion may not cause any signs or symptoms. These and other signs and symptoms may be caused by a pericardial effusion or by other conditions. Check with your doctor if you have any of the following:

- Dyspnea (shortness of breath).
- Cough.
- Trouble breathing while lying flat.
- Chest pain.
- Fast heart beat or breathing.
- Feeling faint.
- Swelling in the upper abdomen.
- Extreme tiredness or weakness.
- Being anxious.

Pericardial effusion usually occurs in advanced cancer or in the last few weeks of life. During these times, it may be more important to relieve the symptoms than to diagnose the condition. However, in some cases, the following tests and procedures may be used to diagnose pericardial effusion:

- Chest x-ray
- Echocardiography
- Electrocardiogram
- Pericardiocentesis

Treatment may be to control the symptoms of pericardial effusion and improve quality of life.

The goal of treatment is usually palliative, to relieve symptoms and improve quality of life. A large malignant pericardial effusion is controlled by draining the fluid.

Treatment options include the following:

- Pericardiocentesis
- Pericardial sclerosis

- Pericardiotomy
- Pericardiectomy
- Balloon pericardiostomy

Superior Vena Cava Syndrome

Superior vena cava syndrome (SVCS) is a group of signs and symptoms that occur when the superior vena cava is partly blocked.

The superior vena cava is a major vein that leads to the heart. The heart is divided into four parts. The right and left atrium make up the top parts of the heart and the right and left ventricle make up the bottom parts of the heart. The right atrium of the heart receives blood from two major veins:

- The superior vena cava returns blood from the upper body to the heart.
- The inferior vena cava returns blood from the lower body to the heart.

Different conditions can slow the flow of blood through the superior vena cava. These include a tumor in the chest, nearby lymph nodes that are swollen (from cancer), or a blood clot in the superior vena cava. The vein may become completely blocked. Sometimes, smaller veins in the area become larger and take over for the superior vena cava if it is blocked, but this takes time. Superior vena cava syndrome (SVCS) is the group of signs and symptoms that occur when this vein is partly blocked.

SVCS is usually caused by cancer.

Superior vena cava syndrome (SVCS) is usually caused by cancer. In adults, SVCS is most common in the following types of cancer:

- Lung cancer.
- Non-Hodgkin lymphoma (NHL).

Less common causes of SVCS include:

- A blood clot that forms during the use of an intravenous catheter (flexible tube used to put fluids into or take blood out of a vein) in the superior vena cava. A clot may also be caused by pacemaker wires.

- Infection or cancer in the chest that causes affected tissues to become thick and hard.

- Other cancers, including metastatic breast cancer, metastatic germ cell tumors, colon cancer, esophageal cancer, Kaposi sarcoma, Hodgkin lymphoma, thymus cancer, and thyroid cancer.

- Behcet syndrome (a disease of the immune system).

- Sarcoidosis (a disease of the lymph nodes that acts like tuberculosis).

Common signs and symptoms of SVCS include breathing problems and coughing.

The signs and symptoms of SVCS are more severe if the vein becomes blocked quickly. This is because the other veins in the area do not have time to widen and take over the blood flow that cannot pass through the superior vena cava.

The most common signs are:

- Trouble breathing.

- Coughing.

- Swelling in the face, neck, upper body, or arms.

- Less common signs and symptoms include the following:

- Hoarse voice.

- Trouble swallowing or talking.

- Coughing up blood.

- Swollen veins in the chest or neck.

- Chest pain.

- Reddish skin color.

Tests are done to find and diagnose the blockage.

The following tests may be done to diagnose SVCS and find the blockage:

- Chest x-ray

- CT scan

- Venography
- MRI
- Ultrasound

It is important to find out the cause of SVCS before starting treatment. The type of cancer can affect the type of treatment needed. Unless the airway is blocked or the brain is swelling, waiting to start treatment while a diagnosis is made usually causes no problem in adults. If doctors think lung cancer is causing the problem, a sputum sample may be taken and a biopsy may be done.

Treatment for SVCS caused by cancer depends on the cause, signs and symptoms, and prognosis.

Treatment for SCVS caused by cancer depends on the following:

- The type of cancer.
- The cause of the blockage.
- How severe the signs and symptoms are.
- The prognosis (chance of recovery).
- Whether treatment is meant to cure, control, or relieve the signs and symptoms of cancer.
- The patient's wishes.

Treatments include watchful waiting, chemotherapy, radiation therapy, thrombolysis, stent placement, and surgery.

- **Watchful waiting**

  Watchful waiting is closely monitoring a patient's condition without giving any treatment unless signs or symptoms appear or change. A patient who has good blood flow through smaller veins in the area and mild symptoms may not need treatment.

  The following may be used to relieve signs or symptoms and keep the patient comfortable:

  - Keeping the upper body raised higher than the lower body.
  - Corticosteroids (drugs that reduce swelling).

- Diuretics (drugs that make excess fluid pass from the body in urine). Patients taking diuretics are closely watched because these drugs can cause dehydration (loss of too much fluid from the body).

- **Chemotherapy**
  Chemotherapy is the usual treatment for tumors that respond to anticancer drugs, including small cell lung cancer and lymphoma. Chemotherapy stops the growth of cancer cells, either by killing the cells or by stopping them from dividing. When chemotherapy is taken by mouth or injected into a vein or muscle, the drugs enter the bloodstream and can reach cancer cells throughout the body (systemic chemotherapy). When chemotherapy is placed directly into the cerebrospinal fluid, an organ, or a body cavity such as the abdomen, the drugs mainly affect cancer cells in those areas (regional chemotherapy). The way the chemotherapy is given depends on the type and stage of the cancer being treated.

- **Radiation therapy**

  If the blockage of the superior vena cava is caused by a tumor that does not usually respond to chemotherapy, radiation therapy may be given. Radiation therapy is a cancer treatment that uses high-energy x-rays or other types of radiation to kill cancer cells. External radiation therapy uses a machine outside the body to send radiation toward the cancer. The way the radiation therapy is given depends on the type and stage of the cancer being treated.

- **Thrombolysis**

  SVCS may occur when a thrombus (blood clot) forms in a partly blocked vein. Thrombolysis is a way to break up and remove blood clots. This may done by a thrombectomy. Thrombectomy is surgery to remove the blood clot or the use of a device inserted into the vein to remove the blood clot. This may be done with or without the use of drugs to break up the clot.

- **Stent placement**

  If the superior vena cava is partly blocked by the tumor, an expandable stent (tube) may be placed inside the superior vena cava to help keep it open and allow blood to pass through. This helps most patients. Drugs to keep more blood clots from forming may also be used.

- **Surgery**

  Surgery to bypass (go around) the blocked part of the vein is sometimes used for cancer patients, but is used more often for patients who do not have cancer.

Palliative care may be given to relieve signs and symptoms in patients with SVCS.

Superior vena cava syndrome is serious and the signs and symptoms can be upsetting for the patient and family. It is important that patients and family members ask questions about superior vena cava syndrome and how to treat it. This can help relieve anxiety about signs and symptoms such as swelling, trouble swallowing, coughing, and hoarseness.

Patients with advanced cancer sometimes decide not to have any serious treatment. Palliative treatment can help keep patients comfortable by relieving signs and symptoms to improve their quality of life.

Superior Vena Cava Syndrome in Children

Superior vena cava syndrome in a child is a serious medical emergency because the child's windpipe can become blocked.

Superior vena cava syndrome (SVCS) in children can be life-threatening. This is because the trachea (windpipe) can quickly become blocked. In adults, the windpipe is fairly stiff, but in children, it is softer and can more easily be squeezed shut. Also, a child's windpipe is narrower, so any amount of swelling can cause breathing problems. Squeezing of the trachea is called superior mediastinal syndrome (SMS). Because SVCS and SMS usually happen together in children, the two syndromes are considered to be the same.

The most common symptoms of SVCS in children are a lot like those in adults.

Common signs and symptoms include the following:

- Coughing.
- Hoarseness.
- Trouble breathing.
- Chest pain.

There are other less common but more serious signs and symptoms:

- Fainting.
- Anxiety.
- Confusion.
- Headache.
- Vision problems.
- A feeling of fullness in the ears.

The causes, diagnosis, and treatment of SVCS in children are not the same as in adults.

The most common cause of SVCS in children is non-Hodgkin lymphoma.

SVCS in children is rare. The most common cause is non-Hodgkin lymphoma. As in adults, SVCS may also be caused by a blood clot that forms during use of an intravenous catheter (flexible tube used to put fluids into or take blood out of a vein) in the superior vena cava.

SVCS in children may be diagnosed and treated before a diagnosis of cancer is made.

A physical exam, chest x-ray, and medical history are usually all that are needed to diagnose superior vena cava syndrome in children. Even if doctors think cancer is causing SVCS, a biopsy may not be done. This is because the lungs and heart of a child with SVCS may not be able to handle the anesthesia needed. Other imaging tests may be done to help find out if anesthesia can be safely used. In most cases, treatment will begin before a diagnosis of cancer is made.

The following treatments may be used for SVCS in children:

- **Radiation therapy**

  Radiation therapy is usually used to treat a tumor that is blocking the vein. After radiation therapy, there may be more trouble breathing because swelling narrows the windpipe. A drug to reduce swelling may be given.

- **Drugs**

  Anticancer drugs, steroids, or other drugs may be used.

- **Surgery**

  This may include surgery to bypass (go around) the blocked part of the vein or to place a stent (thin tube) to open the vein.

Chapter 58

Nutrition in Cancer Care

Overview of Nutrition in Cancer Care

Nutrition is a process in which food is taken in and used by the body for growth, to keep the body healthy, and to replace tissue. Good nutrition is important for good health. Eating the right kinds of foods before, during, and after cancer treatment can help the patient feel better and stay stronger. A healthy diet includes eating and drinking enough of the foods and liquids that have the important nutrients (vitamins, minerals, protein, carbohydrates, fat, and water) the body needs.

When the body does not get or cannot absorb the nutrients needed for health, it causes a condition called malnutrition or malnourishment.

This chapter is about nutrition in adults with cancer.

Healthy eating habits are important during cancer treatment.

Nutrition therapy is used to help cancer patients get the nutrients they need to keep up their body weight and strength, keep body tissue healthy, and fight infection. Eating habits that are good for cancer patients can be very different from the usual healthy eating guidelines.

Healthy eating habits and good nutrition can help patients deal with the effects of cancer and its treatment. Some cancer treatments

---

Text in this chapter is excerpted from "Nutrition In Cancer Care," National Cancer Institute at the National Institutes of Health (NIH), December 5, 2014.

work better when the patient is well nourished and gets enough calories and protein in the diet. Patients who are well nourished may have a better prognosis (chance of recovery) and quality of life.

Cancer can change the way the body uses food.

Some tumors make chemicals that change the way the body uses certain nutrients. The body's use of protein, carbohydrates, and fat may be affected, especially by tumors of the stomach or intestines. A patient may seem to be eating enough, but the body may not be able to absorb all the nutrients from the food.

Cancer and cancer treatments may affect nutrition.

For many patients, the effects of cancer and cancer treatments make it hard to eat well. Cancer treatments that affect nutrition include:

- Surgery.
- Chemotherapy.
- Radiation therapy.
- Immunotherapy.
- Stem cell transplant.

When the head, neck, esophagus, stomach, or intestines are affected by the cancer treatment, it is very hard to take in enough nutrients to stay healthy.

The side effects of cancer and cancer treatment that can affect eating include:

- Anorexia (loss of appetite).
- Mouth sores.
- Dry mouth.
- Trouble swallowing.
- Nausea.
- Vomiting.
- Diarrhea.
- Constipation.
- Pain.

- Depression.

- Anxiety.

Cancer and cancer treatments may affect taste, smell, appetite, and the ability to eat enough food or absorb the nutrients from food. This can cause malnutrition (a condition caused by a lack of key nutrients). Malnutrition can cause the patient to be weak, tired, and unable to fight infections or get through cancer treatment. Malnutrition may be made worse if the cancer grows or spreads. Eating too little protein and calories is a very common problem for cancer patients. Having enough protein and calories is important for healing, fighting infection, and having enough energy.

Anorexia and cachexia are common causes of malnutrition in cancer patients.

Anorexia (the loss of appetite or desire to eat) is a common symptom in people with cancer. Anorexia may occur early in the disease or later, if the cancer grows or spreads. Some patients already have anorexia when they are diagnosed with cancer. Almost all patients who have advanced cancer will have anorexia. Anorexia is the most common cause of malnutrition in cancer patients.

Cachexia is a condition marked by a loss of appetite, weight loss, muscle loss, and general weakness. It is common in patients with tumors of the lung, pancreas, and upper gastrointestinal tract. It is important to watch for and treat cachexia early in cancer treatment because it is hard to correct.

Cancer patients may have anorexia and cachexia at the same time. Weight loss can be caused by eating fewer calories, using more calories, or both.

It is important to treat weight loss caused by cancer and its treatment.

It is important that cancer symptoms and side effects that affect eating and cause weight loss are treated early. Both nutrition therapy and medicine can help the patient stay at a healthy weight. Medicine may be used for the following:

- To help increase appetite.

- To help digest food.

- To help the muscles of the stomach and intestines contract (to keep food moving along).

- To prevent or treat nausea and vomiting.

- To prevent or treat diarrhea.

- To prevent or treat constipation.

- To prevent and treat mouth problems (such as dry mouth, infection, pain, and sores).

- To prevent and treat pain.

Nutrition Therapy in Cancer Care

Screening and assessment are done before cancer treatment begins, and assessment continues during treatment.

Screening is used to look for nutrition risks in a patient who has no symptoms. This can help find out if the patient is likely to become malnourished, so that steps can be taken to prevent it.

Assessment checks the nutritional health of the patient and helps to decide if nutrition therapy is needed to correct a problem.

Screening and assessment may include questions about the following:

- Weight changes over the past year.

- Changes in the amount and type of food eaten compared to what is usual for the patient.

- Problems that have affected eating, such as loss of appetite, nausea, vomiting, diarrhea, constipation, mouth sores, dry mouth, changes in taste and smell, or pain.

- Ability to walk and do other activities of daily living (dressing, getting into or out of a bed or chair, taking a bath or shower, and using the toilet).

A physical exam is also done to check the body for general health and signs of disease. The doctor will look for loss of weight, fat, and muscle, and for fluid buildup in the body.

Finding and treating nutrition problems early may improve the patient's prognosis (chance of recovery).

Early nutrition screening and assessment help find problems that may affect how well the patient's body can deal with the effects of cancer treatment. Patients who are underweight or malnourished may not be able to get through treatment as well as a well-nourished patient. Finding and treating nutrition problems early can help the patient gain weight or prevent weight loss, decrease problems with the treatment, and help recovery.

A healthcare team of nutrition specialists will continue to watch for nutrition problems.

A nutrition support team will check the patient's nutritional health often during cancer treatment and recovery. The team may include the following specialists:

- Physician.

- Nurse.

- Registered dietitian.

- Social worker.

- Psychologist.

A patient whose religion doesn't allow eating certain foods may want to talk with a religious advisor about allowing those foods during cancer treatment and recovery.

There are three main goals of nutrition therapy for cancer patients in active treatment and recovery.

The main goals of nutrition therapy for patients in active treatment and recovery are to provide nutrients that are missing, maintain nutritional health, and prevent problems. The health care team will use nutrition therapy to do the following:

- Prevent or treat nutrition problems, including preventing muscle and bone loss.

- Decrease side effects of cancer treatment and problems that affect nutrition.

- Keep up the patient's strength and energy.

- Help the immune system fight infection.

- Help the body recover and heal.

- Keep up or improve the patient's quality of life.

Good nutrition continues to be important for patients who are in remission or whose cancer has been cured.

The goal of nutrition therapy for patients who have advanced cancer is to help with the patient's quality of life.

The goals of nutrition therapy for patients who have advanced cancer include the following:

- Control side effects.
- Lower the risk of infection.
- Keep up strength and energy.
- Improve or maintain quality of life.

Types of Nutrition Care

Nutrition support gives nutrition to patients who cannot eat or digest normally.

It is best to take in food by mouth whenever possible. Some patients may not be able to take in enough food by mouth because of problems from cancer or cancer treatment. Medicine to increase appetite may be used.

Nutrition support for patients who cannot eat can be given in different ways.

A patient who is not able to take in enough food by mouth may be fed using enteral nutrition (through a tube inserted into the stomach or intestines) or parenteral nutrition (infused into the bloodstream). The nutrients are given in liquid formulas that have water, protein, fats, carbohydrates, vitamins, and/or minerals.

Nutrition support can improve a patient's quality of life during cancer treatment, but there are harms that should be considered before making the decision to use it. The patient and health care providers should discuss the harms and benefits of each type of nutrition support.

Enteral Nutrition

Enteral nutrition is also called tube feeding.

Enteral nutrition is giving the patient nutrients in liquid form (formula) through a tube that is placed into the stomach or small intestine. The following types of feeding tubes may be used:

- A nasogastric tube is inserted through the nose and down the throat into the stomach or small intestine. This kind of tube is used when enteral nutrition is only needed for a few weeks.

- A gastrostomy tube is inserted into the stomach or a jejunostomy tube is inserted into the small intestine through an opening made on the outside of the abdomen. This kind of tube is usually used for long-term enteral feeding or for patients who cannot use a tube in the nose and throat.

The type of formula used is based on the specific needs of the patient. There are formulas for patients who have special health conditions, such as diabetes. Formula may be given through the tube as a constant drip (continuous feeding) or 1 to 2 cups of formula can be given 3 to 6 times a day (bolus feeding).

Enteral nutrition is sometimes used when the patient is able to eat small amounts by mouth, but cannot eat enough for health. Nutrients given through a tube feeding add the calories and nutrients needed for health.

Enteral nutrition may continue after the patient leaves the hospital.

If enteral nutrition is to be part of the patient's care after leaving the hospital, the patient and care giver will be trained to do the nutrition support care at home.

Parenteral Nutrition

Parenteral nutrition carries nutrients directly into the blood stream.

Parenteral nutrition is used when the patient cannot take food by mouth or by enteral feeding. Parenteral feeding does not use the stomach or intestines to digest food. Nutrients are given to the patient directly into the blood, through a catheter (thin tube) inserted into a vein. These nutrients include proteins, fats, vitamins, and minerals.

Parenteral nutrition is used only in patients who need nutrition support for five days or more.

The catheter may be placed into a vein in the chest or in the arm.

A central venous catheter is placed beneath the skin and into a large vein in the upper chest. The catheter is put in place by a surgeon. This type of catheter is used for long-term parenteral feeding.

A peripheral venous catheter is placed into a vein in the arm. A peripheral venous catheter is put in place by trained medical staff. This type of catheter is usually used for short-term parenteral feeding.

The patient is checked often for infection or bleeding at the place where the catheter enters the body.

Parenteral nutrition support may continue after the patient leaves the hospital.

If parenteral nutrition is to be part of the patient's care after leaving the hospital, the patient and caregiver will be trained to do the nutrition support care at home.

Ending parenteral nutrition support must be done under medical supervision.

Going off parenteral nutrition support needs to be done slowly and is supervised by a medical team. The parenteral feedings are decreased by small amounts over time until they can be stopped, or as the patient is changed over to enteral or oral feeding.

Effects of Cancer Treatment on Nutrition

Surgery and Nutrition

Surgery increases the body's need for nutrients and energy.

The body needs extra energy and nutrients to heal wounds, fight infection, and recover from surgery. If the patient is malnourished before surgery, it may cause problems during recovery, such as poor healing or infection. For these patients, nutrition care may begin before surgery.

Surgery to the head, neck, esophagus, stomach, or intestines may affect nutrition.

Most cancer patients are treated with surgery. Surgery that removes all or part of certain organs can affect a patient's ability to eat and digest food. The following are nutrition problems caused by specific types of surgery:

- Surgery to the head and neck may cause problems with:
  - Chewing.
  - Swallowing.
  - Tasting or smelling food.

- Making saliva.

- Seeing.

- Surgery that affects the esophagus, stomach, or intestines may keep these organs from working as they should to digest food and absorb nutrients.

All of these can affect the patient's ability to eat normally. Emotional stress about the surgery itself also may affect appetite.

Nutrition therapy can help relieve nutrition problems caused by surgery.

Nutrition therapy can relieve or decrease the side effects of surgery and help cancer patients get the nutrients they need. Nutrition therapy may include the following:

- Nutritional supplement drinks.

- Enteral nutrition (feeding liquid through a tube into the stomach or intestines).

- Parenteral nutrition (feeding through a catheter into the bloodstream).

- Medicines to increase appetite.

It is common for patients to have pain, tiredness, and/or loss of appetite after surgery. For a short time, some patients may not be able to eat what they usually do because of these symptoms. Following certain tips about food may help. These include:

- Stay away from carbonated drinks (such as sodas) and foods that cause gas, such as:
  - Beans.
  - Peas.
  - Broccoli.
  - Cabbage.
  - Brussels sprouts.
  - Green peppers.
  - Radishes.
  - Cucumbers.

- Increase calories by frying foods and using gravies, mayonnaise, and salad dressings. Supplements high in calories and protein can also be used.

- Choose high-protein and high-calorie foods to increase energy and help wounds heal. Good choices include:
  - Eggs.
  - Cheese.
  - Whole milk.
  - Ice cream.
  - Nuts.
  - Peanut butter.
  - Meat.
  - Poultry.
  - Fish.
- If constipation is a problem, increase fiber by small amounts and drink lots of water. Good sources of fiber include:
  - Whole-grain cereals (such as oatmeal and bran).
  - Beans.
  - Vegetables.
  - Fruit.
  - Whole-grain breads.

Chemotherapy and Nutrition

Chemotherapy affects cells all through the body.

Chemotherapy affects fast-growing cells and is used to treat cancer because cancer cells grow and divide quickly. Healthy cells that normally grow and divide quickly may also be killed. These include cells in the mouth, digestive tract, and hair follicles.

Chemotherapy may affect nutrition.

Chemotherapy may cause side effects that cause problems with eating and digestion. When more than one anticancer drug is given, more side effects may occur or they may be more severe. The following side effects are common:

- Loss of appetite.
- Inflammation and sores in the mouth.
- Changes in the way food tastes.

- Feeling full after only a small amount of food.
- Nausea.
- Vomiting.
- Diarrhea.
- Constipation.

Nutrition therapy can help relieve nutrition problems caused by chemotherapy.

Patients who have side effects from chemotherapy may not be able to eat normally and get all the nutrients they need to restore healthy blood counts between treatments. Nutrition therapy can help relieve these side effects, help patients recover from chemotherapy, prevent delays in treatment, prevent weight loss, and maintain general health. Nutrition therapy may include the following:

- Nutrition supplement drinks between meals.
- Enteral nutrition (tube feedings).
- Changes in the diet, such as eating small meals throughout the day.

Radiation Therapy and Nutrition

Radiation therapy can affect cancer cells and healthy cells in the treatment area.

Radiation therapy can kill cancer cells and healthy cells in the treatment area. The amount of damage depends on the following:

- The part of the body that is treated.
- The total dose of radiation and how it is given.

Radiation therapy may affect nutrition.

Radiation therapy to any part of the digestive system often has side effects that cause nutrition problems. Most of the side effects begin a few weeks after radiation therapy begins and go away a few weeks after it is finished. Some side effects can continue for months or years after treatment ends.

The following are some of the more common side effects:

- For radiation therapy to the head and neck
  - Loss of appetite.
  - Changes in the way food tastes.

- Pain when swallowing.

- Dry mouth or thick saliva.

- Sore mouth and gums.

- Narrowing of the upper esophagus, which can cause choking, breathing, and swallowing problems.

- For radiation therapy to the chest

  - Infection of the esophagus.

  - Trouble swallowing.

  - Esophageal reflux (a backward flow of the stomach contents into the esophagus).

  - For radiation therapy to the abdomen or pelvis

  - Diarrhea.

  - Nausea.

  - Vomiting.

  - Inflamed intestines or rectum.

  - A decrease in the amount of nutrients absorbed by the intestines.

Radiation therapy may also cause tiredness, which can lead to a decrease in appetite.

Nutrition therapy can help relieve the nutrition problems caused by radiation therapy.

Nutrition therapy during radiation treatment can help the patient get enough protein and calories to get through treatment, prevent weight loss, help wound and skin healing, and maintain general health. Nutrition therapy may include the following:

- Nutritional supplement drinks between meals.

- Enteral nutrition (tube feedings).

- Changes in the diet, such as eating small meals throughout the day.

Patients who receive high-dose radiation therapy to prepare for a bone marrow transplant may have many nutrition problems and should see a dietitian for nutrition support.

Biologic Therapy and Nutrition

Biologic therapy may affect nutrition.

The side effects of biologic therapy are different for each patient and each type of biologic agent. The following nutrition problems are common:

- Fever.

- Nausea.

- Vomiting.

- Diarrhea.

- Loss of appetite.

- Tiredness.

- Weight gain.

Nutrition therapy can help relieve nutrition problems caused by biologic therapy.

The side effects of biologic therapy can cause weight loss and malnutrition if they are not treated. Nutrition therapy can help patients receiving biologic therapy get the nutrients they need to get through treatment, prevent weight loss, and maintain general health.

Stem Cell Transplant and Nutrition

Stem cell transplant patients have special nutrition needs.

Chemotherapy, radiation therapy, and medicines used for a stem cell transplant may cause side effects that keep a patient from eating and digesting food as usual. Common side effects include the following:

- Changes in the way food tastes.

- Dry mouth or thick saliva.

- Mouth and throat sores.

- Nausea.

- Vomiting.

- Diarrhea.

- Constipation.

- Weight loss and loss of appetite.

- Weight gain.

Nutrition therapy is very important for patients who have a stem cell transplant.

Transplant patients have a very high risk of infection. High doses of chemotherapy or radiation therapy decrease the number of white blood cells, which fight infection. It is especially important that transplant patients avoid getting infections.

Patients who have a transplant need plenty of protein and calories to get through and recover from the treatment, prevent weight loss, fight infection, and maintain general health. It is also important to avoid infection from bacteria in food. Nutrition therapy during transplant treatment may include the following:

- A diet of cooked and processed foods only, because raw vegetables and fresh fruit may carry harmful bacteria.

- Guidelines on safe food handling.

- A specific diet based on the type of transplant and the part of the body affected by cancer.

- Parenteral nutrition (feeding through the bloodstream) during the first few weeks after the transplant, to give the patient the calories, protein, vitamins, minerals, and fluids they need to recover.

Treatment of Symptoms

When side effects of cancer or cancer treatment affect normal eating, changes can be made to help the patient get the nutrients needed. Medicines may be given to increase appetite. Eating foods that are high in calories, protein, vitamins, and minerals is usually best. Meals should be planned to meet the patient's nutrition needs and tastes in food. The following are some of the more common symptoms caused by cancer and cancer treatment and ways to treat or control them.

Anorexia

Anorexia (the loss of appetite or desire to eat) is one of the most common problems for cancer patients. Eating in a calm, comfortable place and getting regular exercise may improve appetite. The following may help cancer patients who have a loss of appetite:

- Eat small high-protein and high-calorie meals every 1-2 hours instead of three large meals. The following are high-calorie, high-protein food choices:

- Cheese and crackers.

- Muffins.

- Puddings.

- Nutritional supplements.

- Milkshakes.

- Yogurt.

- Ice cream.

- Powdered milk added to foods such as pudding, milkshakes, or any recipe using milk.

- Finger foods (handy for snacking) such as deviled eggs, deviled ham on crackers, or cream cheese or peanut butter on crackers or celery.

- Chocolate.

- Add extra calories and protein to food by using butter, skim milk powder, honey, or brown sugar.

- Drink liquid supplements (special drinks that have nutrients), soups, milk, juices, shakes, and smoothies, if eating solid food is a problem.

- Eat breakfasts that have one third of the calories and protein needed for the day.

- Eat snacks that have plenty of calories and protein.

- Eat foods that smell good. Strong odors can be avoided in the following ways:

  - Use boiling bags or microwave steaming bags.

  - Cook outdoors on the grill.

  - Use a kitchen fan when cooking.

  - Serve cold food instead of hot (since odors are in the rising steam).

  - Take off any food covers to release the odors before going into a patient's room.

  - Use a small fan to blow food odors away from patients.

  - Order take-out food.

- Try new foods and new recipes, flavorings, spices, and foods with a different texture or thickness. Food likes and dislikes may change from day to day.

- Plan menus ahead of time and get help preparing meals.

- Make and store small amounts of favorite foods so they are ready to eat when hungry.

Taste Changes

Changes in how foods taste may be caused by radiation treatment, dental problems, mouth sores and infections, or some medicines. Many cancer patients who receive chemotherapy notice a bitter taste or other changes in their sense of taste. A sudden dislike for certain foods may occur. This can cause a loss of appetite, weight loss, and a decreased quality of life. Some or all of a normal sense of taste may return, but it may take up to a year after treatment ends. The following may help cancer patients who have taste changes:

- Eat small meals and healthy snacks several times a day.

- Eat meals when hungry rather than at set mealtimes.

- Eat favorite foods and try new foods when feeling best.

- Eat poultry, fish, eggs, and cheese instead of red meat.

- Eat citrus fruits (oranges, tangerines, lemons, grapefruit) unless mouth sores are present.

- Add spices and sauces to foods.

- Eat meat with something sweet, such as cranberry sauce, jelly, or applesauce.

- Find nonmeat, high-protein recipes in a vegetarian or Chinese cookbook.

- Use sugar-free lemon drops, gum, or mints if there is a metallic or bitter taste in the mouth.

- Rinse mouth with water before eating.

- Eat with family and friends.

- Have others prepare the meal.

- Use plastic utensils if foods have a metal taste.

Taking zinc sulfate tablets during radiation therapy to the head and neck may help a normal sense of taste come back faster after treatment.

Dry Mouth

Dry mouth is often caused by radiation therapy to the head and neck and by certain medicines. Dry mouth may affect speech, taste, and the ability to swallow or to use dentures or braces. There is also an increased risk of cavities and gum disease because less saliva is made to wash the teeth and gums.

The main treatment for dry mouth is drinking plenty of liquids. Other ways to help relieve dry mouth include the following:

- Keep water handy at all times to moisten the mouth.

- Eat moist foods with extra sauces, gravies, butter, or margarine.

- Eat foods and drinks that are very sweet or tart (to increase saliva).

- Eat ice chips or frozen desserts (such as frozen grapes and ice pops).

- Drink fruit nectar instead of juice.

- Suck on hard candy or chew gum.

- Use a straw to drink liquids.

- Clean teeth (including dentures) and rinse mouth at least four times a day (after eating and at bedtime). Don't use mouth rinses that contain alcohol.

Mouth Sores and Infections

Mouth sores can be caused by chemotherapy and radiation therapy. These treatments affect fast-growing cells, such as cancer cells. Normal cells inside the mouth also grow quickly and may be damaged by these cancer treatments. Mouth sores can be painful and become infected or bleed and make it hard to eat. By choosing certain foods and taking good care of their mouths, patients can usually make eating easier. The following can help patients who have mouth sores and infections:

- Eat soft foods that are easy to chew and swallow, such as the following:

- Soft fruits, including bananas, applesauce, and watermelon.

- Peach, pear, and apricot nectars.

- Cottage cheese.

- Mashed potatoes.

- Macaroni and cheese.

- Custards and puddings.

- Gelatin.

- Milkshakes.

- Scrambled eggs.

- Oatmeal or other cooked cereals.

- Stay away from the following:

  - Citrus fruits and juices, (such as oranges, tangerines, lemons, and grapefruit).

  - Spicy or salty foods.

  - Rough, coarse, or dry foods, including raw vegetables, granola, toast, and crackers.

- Use a blender to make vegetables (such as potatoes, peas, and carrots) and meats smooth.

- Add gravy, broth, or sauces to food.

- Drink high-calorie, high-protein drinks in addition to meals.

- Cook foods until soft and tender.

- Eat foods cold or at room temperature. Hot and warm foods can irritate a tender mouth.

- Cut foods into small pieces.

- Use a straw to drink liquids.

- Numb the mouth with ice chips or flavored ice pops before eating.

- Clean teeth (including dentures) and rinse mouth at least four times a day (after eating and at bedtime).

Nausea

Nausea caused by cancer treatment can affect the amount and kinds of food eaten. The following may help cancer patients control nausea:

- Eat before cancer treatments.

- Rinse out the mouth before and after eating.

- Eat foods that are bland, soft, and easy-to-digest, rather than heavy meals. Eat small meals several times a day.

- Eat dry foods such as crackers, bread sticks, or toast throughout the day.

- Slowly sip fluids throughout the day.

- Suck on hard candies such as peppermints or lemon drops if the mouth has a bad taste.

- Stay away from foods that are likely to cause nausea. For some patients, this includes spicy foods, greasy foods, and foods that have strong odors.

- Sit up or lie with the upper body raised for one hour after eating.

- Don't eat in a room that has cooking odors or that is very warm. Keep the living space at a comfortable temperature with plenty of fresh air.

Diarrhea

Diarrhea may be caused by cancer treatments, surgery on the stomach or intestines, or by emotional stress. Long-term diarrhea may lead to dehydration (lack of water in the body) or low levels of salt and potassium, which are important minerals needed by the body.

The following may help cancer patients control diarrhea:

- Eat broth, soups, bananas, and canned fruits to help replace salt and potassium lost by diarrhea. Sports drinks can also help.

- Drink plenty of fluids during the day. Liquids at room temperature may cause fewer problems than hot or cold liquids.

- Drink at least one cup of liquid after each loose bowel movement.
  - Stay away from the following:

- Greasy foods, hot or cold liquids, or caffeine.

- High-fiber foods—especially dried beans and cruciferous vegetables (such as broccoli, cauliflower, and cabbage).

- Milk and milk products, until the cause of the diarrhea is known.

- Foods and beverages that cause gas (such as peas, lentils, cruciferous vegetables, chewing gum, and soda).

- Sugar-free candies or gum made with sorbitol (sugar alcohol).

Low White Blood Cell Counts and Infections

A low white blood cell count may be caused by radiation therapy, chemotherapy, or the cancer itself. Patients who have a low white blood cell count have an increased risk of infection. The following may help cancer patients prevent infections when white blood cell counts are low:

- Stay away from:

  - Raw eggs or raw fish.

  - Old, moldy, or damaged fruits and vegetables.

  - Food sold in open bins or containers.

  - Salad bars and buffets when eating out.

  - Wash hands often to prevent the spread of bacteria.

  - Thaw foods in the refrigerator or microwave. Never thaw foods at room temperature. Cook foods immediately after thawing.

  - Keep hot foods hot and cold foods cold.

  - Cook all meat, poultry, and fish until well done.

  - Refrigerate all leftovers within 2 hours of cooking and eat them within 24 hours.

  - Buy foods packed as single servings, to avoid leftovers.

  - Do not buy or eat food that is out of date.

  - Do not buy or eat food in cans that are swollen, dented, or damaged.

  - Dehydration (Lack of Fluid)

The body needs plenty of water to replace the fluids lost every day. Nausea, vomiting, and pain may keep the patient from drinking and eating enough to get the amount of water the body needs. Long-term diarrhea causes a loss of fluid from the body. One of the first signs of dehydration (lack of water in the body) is feeling very tired. The following may help cancer patients prevent dehydration:

- Drink 8 to 12 cups of liquids a day. This can be water, juice, milk, or foods that have a lot of liquid in them, such as ice pops, flavored ices, and gelatins.

- Stay away from drinks that have caffeine in them, such as sodas, coffee, and tea (both hot and cold).

- Take a water bottle whenever leaving home. It is important to drink even if not thirsty.

- Drink most liquids between meals.

- Use medicines that help prevent and treat nausea and vomiting.

Constipation

It is very common for cancer patients to have constipation (fewer than three bowel movements a week). Constipation may be caused by the following:

- Too little water or fiber in the diet.

- Not being active.

- Cancer treatment, such as chemotherapy.

- Certain medicines used to treat the side effects of chemotherapy, such as nausea and pain.

Preventing and treating constipation is a part of cancer care.

To prevent constipation:

- Eat more fiber-containing foods. Twenty-five to 35 grams of fiber a day is best. Food labels show the amount of fiber in a serving. (Some sources of fiber are listed below.) Add a little more fiber each day and drink plenty of fluids at the same time to keep the fiber moving through the intestines.

- Drink 8 to 12 cups of fluid each day. Water, prune juice, warm juices, lemonade, and teas without caffeine can be very helpful.

- Take walks and exercise regularly. Wear shoes made for exercise.

- To treat constipation:

- Continue to eat high-fiber foods and drink plenty of fluids. Try adding wheat bran to the diet; begin with 2 heaping tablespoons each day for 3 days, then increase by 1 tablespoon each day until constipation is relieved. Do not take more than 6 tablespoons a day.

- Stay physically active.

- Use over-the-counter constipation treatments, if needed. These include:

  - Bulk-forming products (such as Citrucel, Metamucil, Fiberall, and Fiber-Lax).

  - Stimulants (such as Dulcolax and Senokot).

  - Stool softeners (such as Colace and Surfak).

  - Osmotics (such as milk of magnesia).

- Cottonseed and aerosol enemas can also help. Do not use lubricants such as mineral oil because they may keep the body from using important nutrients the way it should.

Good food sources of fiber include the following:

- Legumes (beans and lentils).

- Vegetables.

- Cold cereals (whole grain or bran).

- Hot cereals.

- Fruit.

- Whole-grain breads.

Nutrition in Advanced Cancer

Palliative care helps relieve symptoms that bother the patient and helps improve the patient's quality of life.

The goal of palliative care is to improve the quality of life of patients who have a serious or life-threatening disease. Palliative care is meant to prevent or treat symptoms, side effects, and psychological, social, and spiritual problems caused by a disease or its treatment.

Palliative care for patients with advanced cancer includes nutrition therapy and / or drug therapy.

Nutrition needs are different for patients with advanced cancer.

It is common for patients with advanced cancer to want less food. Patients usually prefer soft foods and clear liquids. Those who have problems swallowing may do better with thick liquids than with thin liquids. Patients often do not feel much hunger at all and may need very little food.

In patients with advanced cancer, most foods are allowed. During this time, eating can be focused on pleasure rather than getting enough nutrients. Patients usually cannot eat enough of any food that might cause a problem. However, some patients may need to stay on a special diet. For example, patients with cancer that affects the abdomen may need a soft diet to keep the bowel from getting blocked.

The benefits and harms of nutrition support are different for each patient.

Answering the following questions may help to make decisions about using nutrition support:

- What are the wishes and needs of the patient and family?

- Will the patient's quality of life be improved?

- Do the possible benefits outweigh the risks and costs?

- Is there an advance directive? An advance directive is a legal document that states the treatment or care a person wishes to receive or not receive if he or she becomes unable to make medical decisions. One type of advance directive is a living will.

Cancer patients and their caregivers have the right to make informed decisions. The healthcare team and a registered dietitian can explain the benefits and risks of using nutrition support for patients with advanced cancer. In most cases, there are more harms than benefits, especially with parenteral nutrition support. However, for someone who still has good quality of life but is unable to get enough food and water by mouth, enteral feedings may be best. The benefits and risks of enteral nutrition during advanced cancer include the following:

Benefits

- May make the patient more alert.

- May be a comfort to the family.

- May relieve nausea.

- May make the patient feel more hopeful.

Harms

- Surgery may be needed to place a tube through the abdomen.

- May increase the amount of saliva in the mouth and throat. This may cause choking or pneumonia.

- May cause diarrhea or constipation.

- May cause nausea.

- May cause infection.

- Makes patient care harder for caregiver.

Food and Drug Interactions

Some foods do not mix safely with certain drugs.

Cancer patients may be treated with a number of drugs. Taking certain foods and drugs together may decrease or change how well the drugs work or cause life-threatening side effects. The following table lists some of the food and drug interactions that may occur with certain anticancer drugs:

Brand Name	Generic Name	Food Interactions
Targretin	Bexarotene	Grapefruit juice may increase the drug's effects.
Folex Rheumatrex	Methotrexate	Alcohol may cause liver damage.
Mithracin	Plicamycin	Supplements of calcium and vitamin D may decrease the drug's effect.

Brand Name	Generic Name	Food Interactions
Matulane	Procarbazine	Alcohol may cause headache, trouble breathing, flushed skin, nausea, or vomiting, Caffeine may raise blood pressure.
Temodar	Temozolomide	Food may slow or decrease the drug's effect.

Talk with your doctor about possible food and drug interactions.

Some herbal supplements do not mix safely with certain drugs or foods.

Taking some herbal supplements with certain foods and drugs may change how well cancer treatment works or cause life-threatening side effects. Talk with your doctor about how herbal supplements may affect your cancer treatment.

Nutrition and Lifestyle in Cancer Survivors

Cancer survivors have special nutrition needs.

Everyone needs a healthy diet and exercise for good health and to help prevent disease. Cancer survivors have special health needs, especially because of the risks of late effects and the cancer coming back. Studies have shown that a healthy diet helps to prevent late effects such as obesity, heart disease, and metabolic syndrome. Researchers are also studying whether certain diet and exercise habits in cancer survivors can keep cancer from coming back or keep new cancers from forming.

Healthy diet and lifestyle habits can improve the quality of life for cancer survivors.

Surveys show that many cancer survivors do not follow cancer prevention guidelines and have lifestyle behaviors that may increase their risk for late effects or make late effects worse. Education programs can help cancer survivors learn how to make behavior changes that keep them healthier. Programs that cover diet, exercise, and stress management are more likely to help cancer survivors make lasting changes.

The effects of diet and lifestyle on cancer continue to be studied.

Nutrition in Cancer Prevention

Following certain dietary guidelines may help prevent cancer.

The American Cancer Society and the American Institute for Cancer Research both have dietary guidelines that may help prevent cancer. Their guidelines are a lot alike and include the following:

- Eat a plant-based diet with a large variety of fruits and vegetables.
- Eat foods low in fat.
- Eat foods low in salt.
- Get to and stay at a healthy weight.
- Be active for 30 minutes on most days of the week.
- Drink few alcoholic drinks or don't drink at all.
- Prepare and store food safely.
- Do not use tobacco in any form.

The effect of soy on breast cancer and breast cancer prevention is being studied.

Study results include the following:

- Some studies show that eating soy may decrease the risk of having breast cancer.
- Taking soy supplements in the form of powders or pills has not been shown to prevent breast cancer.
- Adding soy foods to the diet after being diagnosed with breast cancer has not been shown to keep the breast cancer from coming back.

Soy has substances in it that act like estrogen in the body. Studies were done to find out how soy affects breast cancer in patients who have tumors that need estrogen to grow. Some studies have shown that soy foods are safe for women with breast cancer when eaten in moderate amounts as part of a healthy diet.

If you are a breast cancer survivor be sure to check the most up-to-date information when deciding whether to include soy in your diet.

Chapter 59

Oral Complications of Chemotherapy and Head / Neck Radiation

General Information About Oral Complications

Oral complications are common in cancer patients, especially those with head and neck cancer.

Complications are new medical problems that occur during or after a disease, procedure, or treatment and that make recovery harder. The complications may be side effects of the disease or treatment, or they may have other causes. Oral complications affect the mouth.

Cancer patients have a high risk of oral complications for a number of reasons:

- Chemotherapy and radiation therapy slow or stop the growth of new cells. These cancer treatments slow or stop the growth of fast growing cells, such as cancer cells. Normal cells in the lining of the mouth also grow quickly, so anticancer treatment can stop

Text in this chapter is excerpted from "Oral Complications of Chemotherapy and Head/Neck Radiation," National Cancer Institute at the National Institutes of Health (NIH), April 24, 2014.

them from growing, too. This slows down the ability of oral tissue to repair itself by making new cells.

- Radiation therapy may directly damage and break down oral tissue, salivary glands, and bone.

- Chemotherapy and radiation therapy upset the healthy balance of bacteria in the mouth.

  There are many different kinds of bacteria in the mouth. Some are helpful and some are harmful. Chemotherapy and radiation therapy may cause changes in the lining of the mouth and the salivary glands, which make saliva. This can upset the healthy balance of bacteria. These changes may lead to mouth sores, infections, and tooth decay.

This chapter is about oral complications caused by chemotherapy and radiation therapy.

Preventing and controlling oral complications can help you continue cancer treatment and have a better quality of life.

Sometimes treatment doses need to be decreased or treatment stopped because of oral complications. Preventive care before cancer treatment begins and treating problems as soon as they appear may make oral complications less severe. When there are fewer complications, cancer treatment may work better and you may have a better quality of life.

Patients receiving treatments that affect the head and neck should have their care planned by a team of doctors and specialists.

To manage oral complications, the oncologist will work closely with your dentist and may refer you to other health professionals with special training. These may include the following specialists:

- Oncology nurse.
- Dental specialists.
- Dietitian.
- Speech therapist.
- Social worker.

The goals of oral and dental care are different before, during, and after cancer treatment:

- Before cancer treatment, the goal is to prepare for cancer treatment by treating existing oral problems.

- During cancer treatment, the goals are to prevent oral complications and manage problems that occur.

- After cancer treatment, the goals are to keep teeth and gums healthy and manage any long-term side effects of cancer and its treatment.

The most common oral complications from cancer treatment include the following:

- Oral mucositis (inflamed mucous membranes in the mouth).

- Infection.

- Salivary gland problems.

- Change in taste.

- Pain.

These complications can lead to other problems such as dehydration and malnutrition.

Oral Complications and Their Causes

Cancer treatment can cause mouth and throat problems.

Complications of chemotherapy

Oral complications caused by chemotherapy include the following:

- Inflammation and ulcers of the mucous membranes in the stomach or intestines.

- Easy bleeding in the mouth.

- Nerve damage.

Complications of radiation therapy

Oral complications caused by radiation therapy to the head and neck include the following:

- Fibrosis (growth of fibrous tissue) in the mucous membrane in the mouth.

1133

- Tooth decay and gum disease.

- Breakdown of tissue in the area that receives radiation.

- Breakdown of bone in the area that receives radiation.

- Fibrosis of muscle in the area that receives radiation.

Complications caused by either chemotherapy or radiation therapy

The most common oral complications may be caused by either chemotherapy or radiation therapy. These include the following:

- Inflamed mucous membranes in the mouth.

- Infections in the mouth or that travel through the bloodstream. These can reach and affect cells all over the body.

- Taste changes.

- Dry mouth.

- Pain.

- Changes in dental growth and development in children.

- Malnutrition (not getting enough of the nutrients the body needs to be healthy) caused by being unable to eat.

- Dehydration (not getting the amount of water the body needs to be healthy) caused by being unable to drink.

- Tooth decay and gum disease.

Oral complications may be caused by the treatment itself (directly) or by side effects of the treatment (indirectly).

Radiation therapy can directly damage oral tissue, salivary glands, and bone. Areas treated may scar or waste away. Total-body radiation can cause permanent damage to the salivary glands. This can change the way foods taste and cause dry mouth.

Slow healing and infection are indirect complications of cancer treatment. Both chemotherapy and radiation therapy can stop cells from dividing and slow the healing process in the mouth. Chemotherapy may decrease the number of white blood cells and weaken the immune system (the organs and cells that fight infection and disease). This makes it easier to get an infection.

Complications may be acute (short-term) or chronic (long-lasting).

Acute complications are ones that occur during treatment and then go away. Chemotherapy usually causes acute complications that heal after treatment ends.

Chronic complications are ones that continue or appear months to years after treatment ends. Radiation can cause acute complications but may also cause permanent tissue damage that puts you at a life-long risk of oral complications. The following chronic complications may continue after radiation therapy to the head or neck has ended:

- Dry mouth.
- Tooth decay.
- Infections.
- Taste changes.
- Problems in the mouth and jaw caused by loss of tissue and bone.
- Problems in the mouth and jaw caused by the growth of benign tumors in the skin and muscle.

Oral surgery or other dental work can cause problems in patients who have had radiation therapy to the head or neck. Make sure that your dentist knows your health history and the cancer treatments you received.

Preventing and Treating Oral Complications Before Chemotherapy or Radiation Therapy Begins

Finding and treating oral problems before cancer treatment begins can prevent oral complications or make them less severe.

Problems such as cavities, broken teeth, loose crowns or fillings, and gum disease can get worse or cause problems during cancer treatment. Bacteria live in the mouth and may cause an infection when the immune system is not working well or when white blood cell counts are low. If dental problems are treated before cancer treatments begin, there may be fewer or milder oral complications.

Prevention of oral complications includes a healthy diet, good oral care, and dental checkups.

Ways to prevent oral complications include the following:

- Eat a well-balanced diet. Healthy eating can help the body stand the stress of cancer treatment, help keep up your energy, fight infection, and rebuild tissue.

- Keep your mouth and teeth clean. This helps prevent cavities, mouth sores, and infections.

- Have a complete oral health exam.

Your dentist should be part of your cancer care team. It is important to choose a dentist who has experience treating patients with oral complications of cancer treatment. A checkup of your oral health at least a month before cancer treatment begins usually allows enough time for the mouth to heal if any dental work is needed. The dentist will treat teeth that have a risk of infection or decay. This will help avoid the need for dental treatments during cancer treatment. Preventive care may help lessen dry mouth, which is a common complication of radiation therapy to the head or neck.

A preventive oral health exam will check for the following:

- Mouth sores or infections.

- Tooth decay.

- Gum disease.

- Dentures that do not fit well.

- Problems moving the jaw.

- Problems with the salivary glands.

Patients receiving high-dose chemotherapy, stem cell transplant, or radiation therapy should have an oral care plan in place before treatment begins.

The goal of the oral care plan is to find and treat oral disease that may cause complications during treatment and to continue oral care during treatment and recovery. Different oral complications may occur during the different phases of a transplant. Steps can be taken ahead of time to prevent or lessen how severe these side effects will be.

Oral care during radiation therapy will depend on the following:

- Specific needs of the patient.

- The radiation dose.

- The part of the body treated.

- How long the radiation treatment lasts.

- Specific complications that occur.

It is important that patients who have head or neck cancer stop smoking.

Continuing to smoke tobacco may slow down recovery. It can also increase the risk that the head or neck cancer will recur or that a second cancer will form.

Managing Oral Complications During and After Chemotherapy or Radiation Therapy

Regular Oral Care

Good dental hygiene may help prevent or decrease complications.

It is important to keep a close watch on oral health during cancer treatment. This helps prevent, find, and treat complications as soon as possible. Keeping the mouth, teeth, and gums clean during and after cancer treatment may help decrease complications such as cavities, mouth sores, and infections.

Everyday oral care for cancer patients includes keeping the mouth clean and being gentle with the tissue lining the mouth.

Everyday oral care during chemotherapy and radiation therapy includes the following:

Brushing teeth

- Brush teeth and gums with a soft-bristle brush 2 to 3 times a day for 2 to 3 minutes. Be sure to brush the area where the teeth meet the gums and to rinse often.

- Rinse the toothbrush in hot water every 15 to 30 seconds to soften the bristles, if needed.

- Use a foam brush only if a soft-bristle brush cannot be used. Brush 2 to 3 times a day and use an antibacterial rinse. Rinse often.

- Let the toothbrush air-dry between brushings.

- Use a fluoride toothpaste with a mild taste. Flavoring may irritate the mouth, especially mint flavoring.

- If toothpaste irritates your mouth, brush with a mixture of 1/4 teaspoon of salt added to 1 cup of water.

1137

Rinsing

- Use a rinse every 2 hours to decrease soreness in the mouth. Dissolve 1/4 teaspoon of salt and 1/4 teaspoon of baking soda in 1 quart of water.

- An antibacterial rinse may be used 2 to 4 times a day for gum disease. Rinse for 1 to 2 minutes.

- If dry mouth occurs, rinsing may not be enough to clean the teeth after a meal. Brushing and flossing may be needed.

Flossing

- Floss gently once a day.

Lip care

- Use lip care products, such as cream with lanolin, to prevent drying and cracking.

Denture care

- Brush and rinse dentures every day. Use a soft-bristle tooth-brush or one made for cleaning dentures.

- Clean with a denture cleaner recommended by your dentist.

- Keep dentures moist when not being worn. Place them in water or a denture soaking solution recommended by your dentist. Do not use hot water, which can cause the denture to lose its shape.

Editor's Note: For special oral care during high-dose chemotherapy and stem cell transplant, see the Managing Oral Complications of High-Dose Chemotherapy and/or Stem Cell Transplant section of this chapter.

Oral Mucositis

Oral mucositis is an inflammation of mucous membranes in the mouth.

The terms "oral mucositis" and "stomatitis" are often used in place of each other, but they are different.

- Oral mucositis is an inflammation of mucous membranes in the mouth. It usually appears as red, burn-like sores or as ulcer-like sores in the mouth.

- Stomatitis is an inflammation of mucous membranes and other tissues in the mouth. These include the gums, tongue, roof and floor of the mouth, and the inside of the lips and cheeks.

Mucositis may be caused by either radiation therapy or chemotherapy.

- Mucositis caused by chemotherapy will heal by itself, usually in 2 to 4 weeks if there is no infection.

- Mucositis caused by radiation therapy usually lasts 6 to 8 weeks, depending on how long the treatment was.

- In patients receiving high-dose chemotherapy or chemoradiation for stem cell transplant: Mucositis usually begins 7 to 10 days after treatment begins, and lasts for about 2 weeks after treatment ends.

Swishing ice chips in the mouth for 30 minutes, beginning 5 minutes before patients receive fluorouracil, may help prevent mucositis. Patients who receive high-dose chemotherapy and stem cell transplant may be given medicine to help prevent mucositis or keep it from lasting as long.

Mucositis may cause the following problems:

- Pain.

- Infection.

- Bleeding, in patients receiving chemotherapy. Patients receiving radiation therapy usually do not have bleeding.

- Trouble breathing and eating.

Care of mucositis during chemotherapy and radiation therapy includes cleaning the mouth and relieving pain.

Treatment of mucositis caused by either radiation therapy or chemotherapy is about the same. Treatment depends on your white blood cell count and how severe the mucositis is. The following are ways to treat mucositis during chemotherapy, stem cell transplant, or radiation therapy:

Cleaning the mouth

- Clean your teeth and mouth every 4 hours and at bedtime. Do this more often if the mucositis becomes worse.

- Use a soft-bristle toothbrush.

- Replace your toothbrush often.

- Use lubricating jelly that is water-soluble, to help keep your mouth moist.

- Use mild rinses or plain water. Frequent rinsing removes pieces of food and bacteria from the mouth, prevents crusting of sores, and moistens and soothes sore gums and the lining of the mouth.

- If mouth sores begin to crust over, the following rinse may be used:

  - Three percent hydrogen peroxide mixed with an equal amount of water or saltwater. To make a saltwater mixture, put 1/4 teaspoon of salt in 1 cup of water.

This should not be used for more than 2 days because it will keep mucositis from healing.

Relieving mucositis pain

- Try topical medicines for pain. Rinse your mouth before putting the medicine on the gums or lining of the mouth. Wipe mouth and teeth gently with wet gauze dipped in saltwater to remove pieces of food.

- Painkillers may help when topical medicines do not. Nonsteroidal anti-inflammatory drugs (NSAIDS, aspirin -type painkillers) should not be used by patients receiving chemotherapy because they increase the risk of bleeding.

- Zinc supplements taken during radiation therapy may help treat pain caused by mucositis as well as dermatitis (inflammation of the skin).

- Povidone-iodine mouthwash that does not contain alcohol may help delay or decrease mucositis caused by radiation therapy.

Pain

There can be many causes of oral pain in cancer patients.

A cancer patient's pain may come from the following:

- The cancer.

- Side effects of cancer treatments.

- Other medical conditions not related to the cancer.

Because there can be many causes of oral pain, a careful diagnosis is important. This may include:

- A medical history.

- Physical and dental exams.

- X-rays of the teeth.

Oral pain in cancer patients may be caused by the cancer.

Cancer can cause pain in different ways:

- The tumor presses on nearby areas as it grows and affects nerves and causes inflammation.

- Leukemias and lymphomas, which spread through the body and may affect sensitive areas in the mouth. Multiple myeloma can affect the teeth.

- Brain tumors may cause headaches.

- Cancer may spread to the head and neck from other parts of the body and cause oral pain.

- With some cancers, pain may be felt in parts of the body not near the cancer. This is called referred pain. Tumors of the nose, throat, and lungs can cause referred pain in the mouth or jaw.

Oral pain may be a side effect of treatments.

Oral mucositis is the most common side effect of radiation therapy and chemotherapy. Pain in the mucous membranes often continues for a while even after the mucositis is healed.

Surgery may damage bone, nerves, or tissue and may cause pain. Bisphosphonates, drugs taken to treat bone pain, sometimes cause bone to break down. This is most common after a dental procedure such as having a tooth pulled.

Patients who have transplants may develop graft-versus-host-disease (GVHD). This can cause inflammation of the mucous membranes and joint pain.

Certain anticancer drugs can cause oral pain.

If an anticancer drug is causing pain, stopping the drug usually stops the pain. Because there may be many causes of oral pain during cancer treatment, a careful diagnosis is important. This may include a medical history, physical and dental exams, and x-rays of the teeth.

Some patients may have sensitive teeth weeks or months after chemotherapy has ended. Fluoride treatments or toothpaste for sensitive teeth may relieve the discomfort.

Teeth grinding may cause pain in the teeth or jaw muscles.

Pain in the teeth or jaw muscles may occur in patients who grind their teeth or clench their jaws, often because of stress or not being able to sleep. Treatment may include muscle relaxers, drugs to treat anxiety, physical therapy (moist heat, massage, and stretching), and mouth guards to wear while sleeping.

Pain control helps improve the patient's quality of life.

Oral and facial pain can affect eating, talking, and many other activities that involve the head, neck, mouth, and throat. Most patients with head and neck cancers have pain. The doctor may ask the patient to rate the pain using a rating system. This may be on a scale from 0 to 10, with 10 being the worst. The level of pain felt is affected by many different things. It's important for patients to talk with their doctors about pain.

Pain that is not controlled can affect all areas of the patient's life. Pain may cause feelings of anxiety and depression, and may prevent the patient from working or enjoying everyday life with friends and family. Pain may also slow the recovery from cancer or lead to new physical problems. Controlling cancer pain can help the patient enjoy normal routines and a better quality of life.

For oral mucositis pain, topical treatments are usually used.

Other pain medicines may be also be used. Sometimes, more than one pain medicine is needed. Muscle relaxers and medicines for anxiety or depression or to prevent seizures may help some patients. For severe pain, opioids may be prescribed.

Non-drug treatments may also help, including the following:

- Physical therapy.
- TENS (transcutaneous electrical nerve stimulation).
- Applying cold or heat.
- Hypnosis.
- Acupuncture.
- Distraction.
- Relaxation therapy or imagery.
- Cognitive behavioral therapy.

- Music or drama therapy.
- Counseling.

Infection

Damage to the lining of the mouth and a weakened immune system make it easier for infection to occur.

Oral mucositis breaks down the lining of the mouth, which lets bacteria and viruses get into the blood. When the immune system is weakened by chemotherapy, even good bacteria in the mouth can cause infections. Germs picked up from the hospital or other places may also cause infections.

As the white blood cell count gets lower, infections may occur more often and become more serious. Patients who have low white blood cell counts for a long time have a higher risk of serious infections. Dry mouth, which is common during radiation therapy to the head and neck, may also raise the risk of infections in the mouth.

Dental care given before chemotherapy and radiation therapy are started can lower the risk of infections in the mouth, teeth, or gums.

Infections may be caused by bacteria, a fungus, or a virus.

Bacterial infections

Treatment of bacterial infections in patients who have gum disease and receive high-dose chemotherapy may include the following:

- Using medicated and peroxide mouth rinses.
- Brushing and flossing.
- Wearing dentures as little as possible.

Fungal infections

The mouth normally contains fungi that can live on or in the oral cavity without causing any problems. However, an overgrowth (too much fungi) in the mouth can be serious and should be treated.

Antibiotics and steroid drugs are often used when a patient receiving chemotherapy has a low white blood cell count. These drugs change the balance of bacteria in the mouth, making it easier for a fungal overgrowth to occur. Also, fungal infections are common in patients treated with radiation therapy. Patients receiving cancer treatment may be given drugs to help prevent fungal infections from occurring.

Candidiasis is a type of fungal infection that is common in patients receiving both chemotherapy and radiation therapy. Symptoms may include a burning pain and taste changes. Treatment of fungal infections in the lining of the mouth only may include mouthwashes and lozenges that contain antifungal drugs. An antifungal rinse should be used to soak dentures and dental devices and to rinse the mouth. Drugs may be used to when rinses and lozenges do not get rid of the fungal infection. Drugs are sometimes used to prevent fungal infections.

Viral infections

Patients receiving chemotherapy, especially those with immune systems weakened by stem cell transplant, have an increased risk of viral infections. Herpesvirus infections and other viruses that are latent (present in the body but not active or causing symptoms) may flare up. Finding and treating the infections early is important. Giving antiviral drugs before treatment starts can lower the risk of viral infections.

Bleeding

Bleeding may occur when anticancer drugs make the blood less able to clot.

High-dose chemotherapy and stem cell transplants can cause a lower-than-normal number of platelets in the blood. This can cause problems with the body's blood clotting process. Bleeding may be mild (small red spots on the lips, soft palate, or bottom of the mouth) or severe, especially at the gum line and from ulcers in the mouth. Areas of gum disease may bleed on their own or when irritated by eating, brushing, or flossing. When platelet counts are very low, blood may ooze from the gums.

Most patients can safely brush and floss while blood counts are low.

Continuing regular oral care will help prevent infections that can make bleeding problems worse. Your dentist or medical doctor can explain how to treat bleeding and safely keep your mouth clean when platelet counts are low.

Treatment for bleeding during chemotherapy may include the following:

- Medicines to reduce blood flow and help clots form.

- Topical products that cover and seal bleeding areas.

- Rinsing with a mixture of saltwater and 3% hydrogen peroxide. (The mixture should have 2 or 3 times the amount of saltwater than hydrogen peroxide.) To make the saltwater mixture, put 1/4 teaspoon of salt in 1 cup of water. This helps clean wounds in the mouth. Rinse carefully so clots are not disturbed.

Dry Mouth

Dry mouth (xerostomia) occurs when the salivary glands don't make enough saliva.

Saliva is made by salivary glands. Saliva is needed for taste, swallowing, and speech. It helps prevent infection and tooth decay by cleaning off the teeth and gums and preventing too much acid in the mouth.

Radiation therapy can damage salivary glands and cause them to make too little saliva. Some types of chemotherapy used for stem cell transplant may also damage salivary glands.

When there is not enough saliva, the mouth gets dry and uncomfortable. This condition is called dry mouth (xerostomia). The risk of tooth decay, gum disease, and infection increases, and your quality of life suffers.

Symptoms of dry mouth include the following:

• Thick, stringy saliva.

• Increased thirst.

• Changes in taste, swallowing, or speech.

• A sore or burning feeling (especially on the tongue).

• Cuts or cracks in the lips or at the corners of the mouth.

• Changes in the surface of the tongue.

• Problems wearing dentures.

Salivary glands usually return to normal after chemotherapy ends.

Dry mouth caused by chemotherapy for stem cell transplant is usually temporary. The salivary glands often recover 2 to 3 months after chemotherapy ends.

Salivary glands may not recover completely after radiation therapy ends.

The amount of saliva made by the salivary glands usually starts to decrease within 1 week after starting radiation therapy to the head or neck. It continues to decrease as treatment goes on. How severe the dryness is depends on the dose of radiation and the number of salivary glands that receive radiation.

Salivary glands may partly recover during the first year after radiation therapy. However, recovery is usually not complete, especially if the salivary glands received direct radiation. Salivary glands that did not receive radiation may start making more saliva to make up for the loss of saliva from the damaged glands.

Careful oral hygiene can help prevent mouth sores, gum disease, and tooth decay caused by dry mouth.

Care of dry mouth may include the following:

- Clean the mouth and teeth at least 4 times a day.
- Floss once a day.
- Brush with a fluoride toothpaste.
- Apply fluoride gel once a day at bedtime, after cleaning the teeth.
- Rinse 4 to 6 times a day with a mixture of salt and baking soda (mix ½ teaspoon salt and ½ teaspoon baking soda in 1 cup of warm water).
- Avoid foods and liquids that have a lot of sugar in them.
- Sip water often to relieve mouth dryness.

A dentist may give the following treatments:

- Rinses to replace minerals in the teeth.
- Rinses to fight infection in the mouth.
- Saliva substitutes or medicines that help the salivary glands make more saliva.
- Fluoride treatments to prevent tooth decay.

Acupuncture may also help relieve dry mouth.

Tooth Decay

Dry mouth and changes in the balance of bacteria in the mouth increase the risk of tooth decay (cavities). Careful oral hygiene and regular care by a dentist can help prevent cavities.

Taste Changes

Changes in taste (dysguesia) are common during chemotherapy and radiation therapy.

Changes in the sense of taste is a common side effect of both chemotherapy and head or neck radiation therapy. Taste changes can be caused by damage to the taste buds, dry mouth, infection, or dental problems. Foods may seem to have no taste or may not taste the way they did before cancer treatment. Radiation may cause a change in sweet, sour, bitter, and salty tastes. Chemotherapy drugs may cause an unpleasant taste.

In most patients receiving chemotherapy and in some patients receiving radiation therapy, taste returns to normal a few months after treatment ends. However, for many radiation therapy patients, the change is permanent. In others, the taste buds may recover 6 to 8 weeks or more after radiation therapy ends. Zinc sulfate supplements may help some patients recover their sense of taste.

Fatigue

Cancer patients who are receiving high-dose chemotherapy or radiation therapy often feel fatigue (a lack of energy). This can be caused by either the cancer or its treatment. Some patients may have problems sleeping. Patients may feel too tired for regular oral care, which may further increase the risk for mouth ulcers, infection, and pain.

Malnutrition

Loss of appetite can lead to malnutrition.

Patients treated for head and neck cancers have a high risk of malnutrition. The cancer itself, poor diet before diagnosis, and complications from surgery, radiation therapy, and chemotherapy can lead to nutrition problems. Patients may lose the desire to eat because of nausea, vomiting, trouble swallowing, sores in the mouth, or dry mouth. When eating causes discomfort or pain, the patient's quality of life and nutritional well-being suffer. The following may help patients with cancer meet their nutrition needs:

- Serve food chopped, ground, or blended, to shorten the amount of time it needs to stay in the mouth before being swallowed.

- Eat between-meal snacks to add calories and nutrients.

- Eat foods high in calories and protein.

- Take supplements to get vitamins, minerals, and calories.

Meeting with a nutrition counselor may help during and after treatment.

Nutrition support may include liquid diets and tube feeding.
Many patients treated for head and neck cancers who receive radiation therapy only are able to eat soft foods. As treatment continues,

most patients will add or switch to high-calorie, high-protein liquids to meet their nutrition needs. Some patients may need to receive the liquids through a tube that is inserted into the stomach or small intestine. Almost all patients who receive chemotherapy and head or neck radiation therapy at the same time will need tube feedings within 3 to 4 weeks. Studies show that patients do better if they begin these feedings at the start of treatment, before weight loss occurs.

Normal eating by mouth can begin again when treatment is finished and the area that received radiation is healed. A team that includes a speech and swallowing therapist can help the patients with the return to normal eating. Tube feedings are decreased as eating by mouth increases, and are stopped when you are able to get enough nutrients by mouth. Although most patients will once again be able to eat solid foods, many will have lasting complications such as taste changes, dry mouth, and trouble swallowing.

Mouth and Jaw Stiffness

Treatment for head and neck cancers may affect the ability to move the jaws, mouth, neck, and tongue. There may be problems with swallowing. Stiffness may be caused by:

- Oral surgery.

- Late effects of radiation therapy. An overgrowth of fibrous tissue (fibrosis) in the skin, mucous membranes, muscle, and joints of the jaw may occur after radiation therapy has ended.

- Stress caused by the cancer and its treatment.

Jaw stiffness may lead to serious health problems, including:

- Malnutrition and weight loss from being unable to eat normally.

- Slower healing and recovery from poor nutrition.

- Dental problems from being unable to clean the teeth and gums well and have dental treatments.

- Weakened jaw muscles from not using them.

- Emotional problems from avoiding social contact with others because of trouble speaking and eating.

The risk of having jaw stiffness from radiation therapy increases with higher doses of radiation and with repeated radiation treatments. The stiffness usually begins around the time the radiation treatments end. It may get worse over time, stay the same, or get somewhat better on its own. Treatment should begin as soon as possible to keep the condition from getting worse or becoming permanent. Treatment may include the following

- Medical devices for the mouth.
- Pain treatments.
- Medicine to relax muscles.
- Jaw exercises.
- Medicine to treat depression.

Swallowing Problems

Pain during swallowing and being unable to swallow (dysphagia) are common in cancer patients before, during, and after treatment.

Swallowing problems are common in patients who have head and neck cancers. Cancer treatment side effects such as oral mucositis, dry mouth, skin damage from radiation, infections, and graft-versus-host-disease (GVHD) may all cause problems with swallowing.

Trouble swallowing increases the risk of other complications.

Other complications can develop from being unable to swallow and these can further decrease the patient's quality of life:

- Pneumonia and other respiratory problems: Patients who have trouble swallowing may aspirate (inhale food or liquids into the lung) when trying to eat or drink. Aspiration can lead to serious conditions, including pneumonia and respiratory failure.

- Poor nutrition: Being unable to swallow normally makes it hard to eat well. Malnutrition occurs when the body doesn't get all the nutrients needed for health. Wounds heal slowly and the body is less able to fight off infections.

- Need for tube feeding: A patient who is not able to take in enough food by mouth may be fed through a tube. The health-care team and a registered dietitian can explain the benefits and risks of tube feeding for patients who have swallowing problems.

- Side effects of pain medicine: Opioids used to treat painful swallowing may cause dry mouth and constipation.

- Emotional problems: Being unable to eat, drink, and speak normally may cause depression and the desire to avoid other people.

Whether radiation therapy will affect swallowing depends on several factors.

The following may affect the risk of swallowing problems after radiation therapy:

- Total dose and schedule of radiation therapy. Higher doses over a shorter time often have more side effects.
- The way the radiation is given. Some types of radiation cause less damage to healthy tissue.
- Whether chemotherapy is given at the same time. The risk of side effects is increased if both are given.
- The patient's genetic makeup.
- Whether the patient is taking any food by mouth or only by tube feeding.
- Whether the patient smokes.
- How well the patient copes with problems.

Swallowing problems sometimes go away after treatment

Some side effects go away within 3 months after the end of treatment, and patients are able to swallow normally again. However, some treatments can cause permanent damage or late effects. Late effects are health problems that occur long after treatment has ended. Conditions that may cause permanent swallowing problems or late effects include:

- Damaged blood vessels.
- Wasting away of tissue in the treated areas.
- Lymphedema (buildup of lymph in the body).
- Overgrowth of fibrous tissue in head or neck areas, which may lead to jaw stiffness.
- Chronic dry mouth.
- Infections.

Swallowing problems are managed by a team of experts.

The oncologist works with other health care experts who specialize in treating head and neck cancers and the oral complications of cancer treatment. These specialists may include the following:

- Speech therapist: A speech therapist can assess how well the patient is swallowing and give the patient swallowing therapy and information to better understand the problem.

- Dietitian: A dietitian can help plan a safe way for the patient to receive the nutrition needed for health while swallowing is a problem.

- Dental specialist: Replace missing teeth and damaged area of the mouth with artificial devices to help swallowing.

- Psychologist: For patients who are having a hard time adjusting to being unable to swallow and eat normally, psychological counseling may help.

Tissue and Bone Loss

Radiation therapy can destroy very small blood vessels within the bone. This can kill bone tissue and lead to bone fractures or infection. Radiation can also kill tissue in the mouth. Ulcers may form, grow, and cause pain, loss of feeling, or infection.

Preventive care can make tissue and bone loss less severe.

The following may help prevent and treat tissue and bone loss:

- Eat a well-balanced diet.

- Wear removable dentures or devices as little as possible.

- Don't smoke.

- Don't drink alcohol.

- Use topical antibiotics.

- Use painkillers as prescribed.

- Surgery to remove dead bone or to rebuild bones of the mouth and jaw.

- Hyperbaric oxygen therapy (a method that uses oxygen under pressure to help wounds heal).

Managing Oral Complications of High-Dose Chemotherapy and/or Stem Cell Transplant

Patients who receive transplants have an increased risk of graft-versus-host disease.

Graft-versus-host disease (GVHD) occurs when your tissue reacts to bone marrow or stem cells that come from a donor. Symptoms of oral GVHD include the following:

- Sores that are red and have ulcers, which appear in the mouth 2 to 3 weeks after the transplant.

- Dry mouth.

- Pain from spices, alcohol, or flavoring (such as mint in toothpaste).

- Swallowing problems.

- A feeling of tightness in the skin or in the lining of the mouth.

- Taste changes.

It's important to have these symptoms treated because they can lead to weight loss or malnutrition. Treatment of oral GVHD may include the following:

- Topical rinses, gels, creams, or powders.

- Antifungal drugs taken by mouth or injection.

- Psoralen and ultraviolet A (PUVA) therapy.

- Drugs that help the salivary glands make more saliva.

- Fluoride treatments.

- Treatments to replace minerals lost from teeth by acids in the mouth.

Oral devices need special care during high-dose chemotherapy and/or stem cell transplant.

The following can help in the care and use of dentures, braces, and other oral devices during high-dose chemotherapy or stem cell transplant:

- Have brackets, wires, and retainers removed before high-dose chemotherapy begins.

- Wear dentures only when eating during the first 3 to 4 weeks after the transplant.

- Brush dentures twice a day and rinsing them well.

- Soak dentures in an antibacterial solution when they are not being worn.

- Clean denture soaking cups and changing denture soaking solution every day.

- Remove dentures or other oral devices when cleaning your mouth.
- Continue your regular oral care 3 or 4 times a day with dentures or other devices out of the mouth.
- If you have mouth sores, avoid using removable oral devices until the sores have healed.

Care of the teeth and gums is important during chemotherapy or stem cell transplant.

Talk to your medical doctor or dentist about the best way to take care of your mouth during high-dose chemotherapy and stem cell transplant. Careful brushing and flossing may help prevent infection of oral tissues. The following may help prevent infection and relieve discomfort of oral in tissues:

- Brush teeth with a soft-bristle brush 2 to 3 times a day. Be sure to brush the area where the teeth meet the gums.
- Rinse the toothbrush in hot water every 15 to 30 seconds to keep the bristles soft.
- Rinse your mouth 3 or 4 times while brushing.
- Avoid rinses that have alcohol in them.
- Use a mild-tasting toothpaste.
- Let the toothbrush air-dry between uses.
- Floss according to your medical doctor's or dentist's directions.
- Clean the mouth after meals.
- Use foam swabs to clean the tongue and roof of the mouth.
- Avoid the following:
  - Foods that are spicy or acidic.
  - "Hard" foods that could irritate or break the skin in your mouth, such as chips.
  - Hot foods and drinks.

Medicines and ice may be used to prevent and treat mucositis from stem cell transplant.

Medicines may be given to help prevent mouth sores or help the mouth heal faster if it is damaged by chemotherapy or radiation therapy. Also, holding ice chips in the mouth during high-dose chemotherapy, may help prevent mouth sores.

Dental treatments may be put off until the patient's immune system returns to normal.

Regular dental treatments, including cleaning and polishing, should wait until the transplant patient's immune system returns to normal. The immune system can take 6 to 12 months to recover after high-dose chemotherapy and stem cell transplant. During this time, the risk of oral complications is high. If dental treatments are needed, antibiotics and supportive care are given.

Supportive care before oral procedures may include giving antibiotics or immunoglobulin G, adjusting steroid doses, and/or platelet transfusion.

Oral Complications in Second Cancers

Cancer survivors who received chemotherapy or a transplant or who underwent radiation therapy are at risk of developing a second cancer later in life. Oral squamous cell cancer is the most common second oral cancer in transplant patients. The lips and tongue are the areas that are affected most often.

Second cancers are more common in patients treated for leukemia or lymphoma, Multiple myeloma patients who received a stem cell transplant using their own stem cells sometimes develop an oral plasmacytoma.

Patients who received a transplant should see a doctor if they have swollen lymph nodes or lumps in soft tissue areas. This could be a sign of a second cancer.

Oral Complications Not Related to Chemotherapy or Radiation Therapy

Certain drugs used to treat cancer and other bone problems are linked to bone loss in the mouth.

Some drugs break down bone tissue in the mouth. This is called osteonecrosis of the jaw (ONJ). ONJ can also cause infection. Symptoms include pain and inflamed lesions in the mouth, where areas of damaged bone may show.

Drugs that may cause ONJ include the following:

- Bisphosphonates: Drugs given to some patients whose cancer has spread to the bones. They are used to decrease pain and the risk of broken bones. Bisphosphonates are also used to treat hypercalcemia (too much calcium in the blood). Bisphosphonates commonly used include zoledronic acid, pamidronate, and alendronate.

- Denosumab: A drug used to prevent or treat certain bone problems. Denosumab is a type of monoclonal antibody.

- Angiogenesis inhibitors: Drugs or substances that keep new blood vessels from forming. In cancer treatment, angiogenesis inhibitors may prevent the growth of new blood vessels that tumors need to grow. Some of the angiogenesis inhibitors that may cause ONJ are bevacizumab, sunitinib, and sorafenib.

It's important for the health care team to know if a patient has been treated with these drugs. Cancer that has spread to the jawbone can look like ONJ. A biopsy may be needed to find out the cause of the ONJ.

ONJ is not a common condition. It occurs more often in patients who receive bisphosphonates or denosumab by injection than in patients who take them by mouth. Taking bisphosphonates, denosumab, or angiogenesis inhibitors increases the risk of ONJ. The risk of ONJ is much greater when angiogenesis inhibitors and bisphosphonates are used together.

The following may also increase the risk of ONJ:

- Having teeth removed.
- Wearing dentures that do not fit well.
- Having multiple myeloma.

Patients with bone metastases may decrease their risk of ONJ by getting screened and treated for dental problems before bisphosphonate or denosumab therapy is started.

Treatment of ONJ usually includes treating the infection and good dental hygiene.

Treatment of ONJ may include the following:

- Removing the infected tissue, which may include bone. Laser surgery may be used.

- Smoothing sharp edges of exposed bone.

- Using antibiotics to fight infection.

- Using medicated mouth rinses.

- Using pain medicine.

During treatment for ONJ, you should continue to brush and floss after meals to keep your mouth very clean. It is best to avoid tobacco use while ONJ is healing.

You and your doctor can decide whether you should stop using medicines that cause ONJ, based on the effect it would have on your general health.

Oral Complications and Social Problems

The social problems related to oral complications can be the hardest problems for cancer patients to cope with. Oral complications affect eating and speaking and may make you unable or unwilling to take part in mealtimes or to dine out. Patients may become frustrated, withdrawn, or depressed, and they may avoid other people. Some drugs that are used to treat depression cannot be used because they can make oral complications worse.

Education, supportive care, and the treatment of symptoms are important for patients who have mouth problems that are related to cancer treatment. Patients are watched closely for pain, ability to cope, and response to treatment. Supportive care from health care providers and family can help the patient cope with cancer and its complications.

Part Seven

Research and Clinical Trials

Chapter 60

Cancer Clinical Trials

What is a clinical study?

A clinical study involves research using human volunteers (also called participants) that is intended to add to medical knowledge. There are two main types of clinical studies: clinical trials (also called interventional studies) and observational studies. ClinicalTrials.gov includes both interventional and observational studies.

Clinical Trials

In a clinical trial, participants receive specific interventions according to the research plan or protocol created by the investigators. These interventions may be medical products, such as drugs or devices; procedures; or changes to participants' behavior, such as diet. Clinical trials may compare a new medical approach to a standard one that is already available, to a placebo that contains no active ingredients, or to no intervention. Some clinical trials compare interventions that are already available to each other. When a new product or approach is being studied, it is not usually known whether it will be helpful, harmful, or no different than available alternatives (including no intervention). The investigators try to determine the safety and efficacy of the intervention by measuring certain outcomes in the participants. For

Text in this chapter is excerpted from "Learn about Clinical Studies," ClinicalTrials.gov, a service of the U.S. National Institutes of Health (NIH), December 2014.

example, investigators may give a drug or treatment to participants who have high blood pressure to see whether their blood pressure decreases.

Clinical trials used in drug development are sometimes described by phase. These phases are defined by the Food and Drug Administration (FDA).

Some people who are not eligible to participate in a clinical trial may be able to get experimental drugs or devices outside of a clinical trial through an Expanded Access Program.

What is "expanded access"?

Expanded access is a means by which manufacturers make investigational new drugs available, under certain circumstances, to treat a patient(s) with a serious disease or condition who cannot participate in a controlled clinical trial.

Most human use of investigational new drugs takes place in controlled clinical trials conducted to assess the safety and efficacy of new drugs. Data from these trials are used to determine whether a drug is safe and effective, and serve as the basis for the drug marketing application. Sometimes, patients do not qualify for these controlled trials because of other health problems, age, or other factors, or are otherwise unable to enroll in such trials (e.g., a patient may not live sufficiently close to a clinical trial site).

For patients who cannot participate in a clinical trial of an investigational drug, but have a serious disease or condition that may benefit from treatment with the drug, FDA regulations enable manufacturers of such drugs to provide those patients access to the drug under certain situations, known as "expanded access." For example, the drug cannot expose patients to unreasonable risks given the severity of the disease to be treated and the patient does not have any other satisfactory therapeutic options (e.g., an approved drug that could be used to treat the patient's disease or condition). The manufacturer must be willing to make the drug available for expanded access use. The primary intent of expanded access is to provide treatment for a patient's disease or condition, rather than to collect data about the study drug.

Observational Studies

In an observational study, investigators assess health outcomes in groups of participants according to a research plan or protocol. Participants may receive interventions (which can include medical products such as drugs or devices) or procedures as part of their routine medical care, but participants are not assigned to specific interventions by the investigator (as in a clinical trial). For example, investigators may observe a group of older adults to learn more about the effects of different lifestyles on cardiac health.

Who conducts clinical Studies?

Every clinical study is led by a principal investigator, who is often a medical doctor. Clinical studies also have a research team that may include doctors, nurses, social workers, and other health care professionals.

Clinical studies can be sponsored, or funded, by pharmaceutical companies, academic medical centers, voluntary groups, and other organizations, in addition to Federal agencies such as the National Institutes of Health, the U.S. Department of Defense, and the U.S. Department of Veterans Affairs. Physicians, health care providers, and other individuals can also sponsor clinical research.

Where are clinical studies conducted?

Clinical studies can take place in many locations, including hospitals, universities, doctors' offices, and community clinics. The location depends on who is conducting the study.

How long does clinical studies last?

The length of a clinical study varies depending on what is being studied. Participants are told how long the study will last before enrolling.

Reasons for conducting clinical studies

In general, clinical studies are designed to add to medical knowledge related to the treatment, diagnosis, and prevention of diseases or conditions. Some common reasons for conducting clinical studies include:

- Evaluating one or more interventions (for example, drugs, medical devices, approaches to surgery or radiation therapy) for treating a disease, syndrome, or condition

- Finding ways to prevent the initial development or recurrence of a disease or condition. These can include medicines, vaccines, or lifestyle changes, among other approaches

- Evaluating one or more interventions aimed at identifying or diagnosing a particular disease or condition

- Examining methods for identifying a condition or the risk factors for that condition

- Exploring and measuring ways to improve the comfort and quality of life through supportive care for people with a chronic illness

Participating in clinical studies

A clinical study is conducted according to a research plan known as the protocol. The protocol is designed to answer specific research questions and to safeguard the health of participants. It contains the following information:

- The reason for conducting the study

- Who may participate in the study (the eligibility criteria)

- The number of participants needed

- The schedule of tests, procedures, or drugs and their dosages

- The length of the study

- What information will be gathered about the participants

Who can participate in a clinical study?

Clinical studies have standards outlining who can participate, called eligibility criteria, which are listed in the protocol. Some research studies seek participants who have the illnesses or conditions that will be studied, other studies are looking for healthy participants, and some studies are limited to a predetermined group of people who are asked by researchers to enroll.

Eligibility. The factors that allow someone to participate in a clinical study are called inclusion criteria, and the factors that disqualify someone from participating are called exclusion criteria. These are based on things such as age, gender, the type and stage of a disease, previous treatment history, and other medical conditions.

How are Participants Protected?

Informed consent is a process in which researchers provide potential and enrolled participants with information about a clinical study. This information helps people decide whether they want to enroll or continue to participate in the study. The informed consent process is intended to protect participants and should provide enough information for a person to understand the risks of, potential benefits of, and alternatives to the study. In addition to the informed consent document, the process may involve recruitment materials, verbal instructions, question-and-answer sessions, and activities to measure participant understanding. In general, a person must sign an informed consent document before joining a study to show that he or she was given information on risks, potential benefits, and alternatives and understands it. Signing the document and providing consent is not a contract. Participants may withdraw from a study at any time, even if the study is not over.

Institutional review boards. Each federally supported or conducted clinical study and each study of a drug, biological product, or medical device regulated by the FDA must be reviewed, approved, and monitored by an institutional review board (IRB). An IRB is made up of physicians, researchers, and members of the community. Its role is to make sure that the study is ethical and that the rights and welfare of participants are protected. This includes making sure that research risks are minimized and are reasonable in relation to any potential benefits, among other things. The IRB also reviews the informed consent document.

In addition to being monitored by an IRB, some clinical studies are also monitored by data monitoring committees (also called data safety and monitoring boards).

Various Federal agencies, including the Office of Human Subjects Research Protection and the FDA, have the authority to determine whether sponsors of certain clinical studies are adequately protecting research participants.

Relationship to Usual Health Care

Typically participants continue to see their usual health care providers while enrolled in a clinical study. While most clinical studies provide participants with medical products or interventions related to the illness or condition being studied, they do not provide extended or complete health care. By having his or her usual health care provider work with the research team, the participant can make sure that the study protocol will not conflict with other medications or treatments being received.

Considerations for Participation

Participating in a clinical study contributes to medical knowledge. The results of these studies can make a difference in the care of future patients by providing information about the benefits and risks of therapeutic, preventative, or diagnostic products or interventions.

Clinical trials provide the basis for the development and marketing of new drugs, biological products, and medical devices. Sometimes, the safety and the effectiveness of the experimental approach or use may not be fully known at the time of the trial. Some trials may provide participants with the prospect of receiving direct medical benefits, while others do not. Most trials involve some risk of harm or injury to the participant, although it may not be greater than the risks related to routine medical care or disease progression. (For trials approved by IRBs, the IRB has decided that the risks of participation have been minimized and are reasonable in relation to anticipated benefits.) Many trials require participants to undergo additional procedures, tests, and assessments based on the study protocol. These will be described in the informed consent document for a particular trial. A potential participant should also discuss these issues with members of the research team and with his or her usual health care provider.

Questions to Ask

Anyone interested in participating in a clinical study should know as much as possible about the study and feel comfortable asking the research team questions about the study, the related procedures, and any expenses. The following questions might be helpful during such a discussion. Many of these questions are specific to clinical trials, but some also apply to observational studies.

- What is being studied?

- Why do researchers believe the intervention being tested might be effective? Why might it not be effective? Has it been tested before?

- What are the possible interventions that I might receive during the trial?

- How will it be determined which interventions I receive (for example, by chance)?
- Who will know which intervention I receive during the trial? Will I know? Will members of the research team know?
- How do the possible risks, side effects, and benefits of this trial compare with those of my current treatment?
- What will I have to do?
- What tests and procedures are involved?
- How often will I have to visit the hospital or clinic?
- Will hospitalization be required?
- How long will the study last?
- Who will pay for my participation?
- Will I be reimbursed for other expenses?
- What type of long-term follow-up care is part of this trial?
- If I benefit from the intervention, will I be allowed to continue receiving it after the trial ends?
- Will results of the study be provided to me?
- Who will oversee my medical care while I am participating in the trial?
- What are my options if I am injured during the study?

Chapter 61

Cancer Clinical Trials at the NIH Clinical Center

What is the National Institutes of Health (NIH) Clinical Center?

The NIH Clinical Center in Bethesda, Maryland, is the research hospital for the NIH, the federal government's principal agency for biomedical research. The NIH Clinical Center is actually made up of two centers: the Warren Grant Magnuson Clinical Center and the Mark O. Hatfield Clinical Research Center. The NIH Clinical Center as a whole promotes translational research—that is, the transformation of scientific laboratory research into applications that benefit patient health and medical care. At the Clinical Center, patient care units are in close proximity to cutting-edge technologies and laboratories doing related research. This "bench-to-bedside" approach facilitates interaction and collaboration among clinicians and researchers.

The NIH Clinical Center is devoted exclusively to clinical investigation. Unlike most facilities, the Clinical Center does not routinely provide standard diagnostic and treatment services. NIH physicians accept patients for clinical trials if the patient has an illness being studied by one or more of the Institutes and the patient meets the

Text in this chapter is excerpted from "Cancer Clinical Trials at the NIH Clinical Center," National Cancer Institute at the National Institutes of Health (NIH), November 25, 2014.

trial's specific medical eligibility requirements (also called eligibility criteria).

What is NCI's Center for Cancer Research?

The mission of NCI's Center for Cancer Research (CCR) is to make breakthrough discoveries in basic and clinical cancer research and develop them into novel therapeutic interventions for adults and children with cancer or HIV. CCR investigators include basic, clinical, and translational scientists who collaborate with each other, with scientists at other NIH Institutes and Centers, and with scientists in academia and industry. The clinical trials conducted by CCR on the NIH campus represent the core of NCI's intramural research program in Bethesda, Maryland.

Why are clinical trials important?

Clinical trials are the way in which new and more effective cancer treatments are discovered and proven. If a new treatment proves effective in a clinical trial, it can become a new standard of care.

Due to progress made through clinical trials, many people with cancer are living longer. However, it is important to recognize that new treatments under study do not always turn out to be more effective than the standard treatment.

What are eligibility criteria?

To enter a clinical trial, each prospective applicant must meet specific requirements, called eligibility criteria. Eligibility criteria are an important part of each clinical trial's protocol or action plan. The criteria vary from study to study and may include age, gender, medical history, and current health status. Treatment studies often require that patients have a particular type and stage of cancer. Eligibility criteria help ensure the participants' safety. For example, some people have other health problems that could be made worse by the treatment being studied. The qualifications also help researchers achieve accurate and meaningful results.

How can health care providers and cancer patients learn about cancer clinical trials at the NIH Clinical Center?

Information about cancer clinical trials being conducted at the NIH Clinical Center is available by phone and online.

- Call the NIH Clinical Center Patient Recruitment and Liaison Office at 1–800–411–1222.

- Visit the Search for CCR Trials at NIH page or use NCI's clinical trials search form to identify clinical trials that may be appropriate for the patient. Review the trial information and contact a member of the research team listed in the trial summary to discuss a screening visit or to request more information.

- Contact one of the clinical research teams that study specific types of cancer at the NIH Clinical Center. Patients who meet medical eligibility requirements may be asked to schedule an appointment at the Clinical Center. During this appointment, patients will learn more about the clinical trial and may be asked to undergo some tests. Before agreeing to take part in the trial, patients need to understand key information about the clinical trial, including details about the treatment, tests, and possible risks and benefits.

The following NCI branches study specific types of cancer at the NIH Clinical Center, provide various types of support and care, and may be contacted directly. Many provide second opinions for patients and their families.

- The Endocrine Oncology Branch conducts preclinical and clinical research and offers consultations for patients with endocrine cancers (thyroid, adrenal, pancreas, and parathyroid). Staff can provide a second opinion for health care providers, patients, and family members. Specialists can either evaluate the patient in person or provide a second opinion after reviewing the patient's medical records and scans. For more information, call 301–496–6457 between 8:00 a.m. and 5:00 p.m. (ET).

- The Experimental Transplantation and Immunology Branch conducts clinical trials of stem cell transplant-based treatments for several types of cancer, including lymphoma, leukemia, and multiple myeloma, as well as for immune deficiency conditions that may become cancer. For more information, call 301–435–1623 between 9:00 a.m. and 5:00 p.m. (ET). A branch member will obtain relevant information by phone, may request medical records, and will discuss open trials for which the patient may be eligible. A screening visit is scheduled if eligibility criteria are met.

- The Immunotherapy Service conducts clinical trials for patients with melanoma. The patient, a family member, or a health care provider can get information about these studies by calling the Immunotherapy Referral Office at 1–866–820–4505 or 301–451–1929 between 8:30 a.m. and 5:30 p.m. (ET). A member of the study team can discuss open studies for which the patient may be eligible. If a patient is thought to be eligible, their health care provider will be asked to send medical records and scans. A screening visit will be scheduled only after all of the information has been received and reviewed. The Immunotherapy Service does not offer consultations or second opinions for patients. The Immunotherapy Service is part of the Surgery Branch.

- Multiple branches conduct medical oncology trials for patients with a variety of cancers, including lymphoma and gastrointestinal, prostate, lung, and women's cancers. These branches are: Lymphoid Malignancies Branch, Genitourinary Malignancies Branch, Urologic Oncology Branch, Thoracic and Gastrointestinal Oncology Branch, and the Women's Malignancies Branch. For more information, call the Medical Oncology Referral Office at 1–866–611–6310 or 301–451–1228 between 9:00 a.m. and 5:00 p.m. (ET). A member of the referral team will discuss open studies for which the patient may be eligible. If a patient is thought to be eligible, the person's health care provider will be asked to send medical records, including scan images and pathology materials. A screening visit will be scheduled after appropriate medical information is received and reviewed. Consultations or second opinions for patients who are not eligible for trials may be provided at the discretion of the investigator.

- The Neuro-Oncology Branch offers clinical trials and consultations for patients with brain tumors. Staff can provide second opinions for health care providers, patients, and family members. Specialists can either evaluate the patient in person or offer a second opinion after reviewing the patient's medical records and scans. To find out more about this service, call 301–594–6767 or 1–866–251–9686 between 9:00 a.m. and 6:00 p.m. (ET).

- The Pediatric Oncology Branch conducts clinical trials for various childhood cancers. To refer children, teenagers, or young adults, the patient's health care provider should call the branch at 301–496–4256 or 1–877–624–4878 between 8:30 a.m. and

5:00 p.m. (ET). The attending physician will discuss the case with the patient's health care provider, determine eligibility for treatment under a clinical protocol, and help arrange the referral. After the patient has been accepted for evaluation, a social worker from the branch will contact the family and provide information about the study, as well as details about travel and lodging.

- The Radiation Oncology Branch designs and conducts pre-clinical and clinical research on the biologic and therapeutic effects of radiation therapy. Clinical trials conducted by this branch involve novel technologies and/or imaging-based approaches to radiation therapy. Computed tomography and magnetic resonance (MR) image fusion are routine components of patients' treatment plans. The Radiation Oncology Branch also provides radiosurgery, intensity-modulated 3-D conformal radiotherapy, real-time dose measurement, brachytherapy, and MR-guided procedures. To find out more about current clinical trials, patients and health care providers can call 301–451–8905 or 301–496–5457 between 8:00 a.m. and 5:00 p.m. (ET).

- The Thoracic and Gastrointestinal Oncology Branch conducts clinical trials for patients with esophageal cancer, lung cancer, pleural mesothelioma, and lung metastases (cancer that spread to the lung). Patients and health care providers may call 301–451–1233 between 6:00 a.m. and 2:30 p.m. (ET) to receive information about available trials and eligibility requirements. Consultations and second opinions may be offered to patients and health care providers. If a patient is interested in participating in a trial, all medical records must be sent to the team. The patient's case will then be reviewed by a physician on staff and a screening visit will be scheduled if the patient is thought to be a likely candidate for the trial.

- The Urologic Oncology Branch offers consultations for patients who have been diagnosed with renal (kidney) or localized prostate or bladder cancer and who have not had surgery. Health care providers and patients may call 301–496–6353 between 7:30 a.m. and 5:00 p.m. (ET). After speaking with a physician on staff, the patient may be asked to come in for a screening visit. Surgery and/or referral to clinical trials will be offered if appropriate.

Can cancer patients who live outside the United States participate in clinical trials at the NIH Clinical Center?

Yes. People from other countries can participate in clinical trials at the NIH Clinical Center if they meet the trial's specific medical eligibility requirements. Due to limitations on resources and funding, however, U.S. citizens and lawful permanent residents have priority for participation in these trials.

International patients planning to travel to the United States for cancer treatment should contact the U.S. Embassy or Consulate in their home country for visa eligibility and application procedures. Participants must pay for their own travel to the United States, and they must have a place to stay while they are in the United States.

How much does it cost to participate in a clinical trial at the NIH Clinical Center?

There is no charge for medical care received at the NIH Clinical Center. Participants will be responsible for costs for travel to their initial screening visits. Once a participant is enrolled in a trial, NCI will pay for transportation for subsequent trial-related visits for participants who do not live in the local area. In addition, these participants will receive a small per diem for food and lodging expenses if they are being treated as outpatients. However, it is important for participants to maintain current health insurance for medical care that is required outside of the trial or that is provided away from the Clinical Center.

Participants who live outside the United States are responsible for all travel costs to the United States, including the initial visit and all subsequent visits.

How are the participant's health, rights, and privacy protected?

Every effort is made to protect and promote the welfare of the participant and to provide the best medical and nursing care possible.

Informed consent is an ongoing process during which information is presented that enables a person to decide voluntarily whether to begin or to continue to participate in a clinical trial. The purpose of the trial, its risks and benefits, the procedures, the schedule, the alternatives to participation, and other important details of the study are explained to the patient. If a person decides to enter a trial, he/she is asked to read, sign, and date an informed consent document. This document contains a summary of the clinical trial and explains the rights of the participant. The participant should be given a copy of the signed document.

All participants at the NIH Clinical Center are protected by the Clinical Center Patients' Bill of Rights. This document ensures that medical records remain private and are not disclosed or released without the participant's consent. In addition, each trial is carefully reviewed for risks and merit by the NCI Institutional Review Board (IRB), which includes doctors, researchers, and community leaders. IRBs check to see that the trial is well designed, legal, and ethical; does not involve unnecessary risks; and includes safeguards for patients. No test or treatment is ever given that is unnecessarily hazardous to the participant. The participant is always free to decline to participate in any aspect of the study at any time. Researchers will stop any trial if unexpected problems arise.

How is the referring health care provider kept informed of patient care and progress during the trial?

NCI and the referring health care provider coordinate patient care. The NCI principal investigator discusses the trial and treatment with the patient's health care provider upon receiving a referral. Once a patient is enrolled in a trial, the investigator will send updates and test results at regular intervals.

NCI encourages health care providers to continue open communication with their patients throughout the clinical trial. Patients are encouraged to share their clinical trial experience with their health care providers. Referring health care providers are welcome to call the NCI research team at any time to discuss patient treatment plans and care.

Chapter 62

Donating Tissues for Cancer Research

What are Biospecimens and Biorepositories

What are biospecimens?

Biospecimens are materials taken from the human body, such as tissue, blood, plasma, and urine that can be used for cancer diagnosis and analysis. When patients have a biopsy, surgery, or other procedure, often a small amount of the specimen removed can be stored and used for later research. Once these samples have been properly processed and stored they are known as human biospecimens.

Doctors and researchers may analyze biospecimens to look for indications of disease in the donor. Biospecimens can confirm whether a disease is present or absent in a particular patient, but they also provide other information that may be useful to the physician or a researcher. Each sample may contain DNA, proteins, and other molecules important for understanding disease progression.

What are biorepositories?

Biorepositories (or biobanks) are "libraries" where biospecimens are stored and made available for scientists to study for clinical or research

Text in this chapter is excerpted from "Patient Corner," Biorepositories and Biospecimen Research Branch—a Division of Cancer Treatment and Diagnosis, National Cancer Institute at the National Institutes of Health (NIH), July 28, 2014.

purposes. These biospecimens are commonly annotated with information about the patient from whom the biospecimen was taken, including data about their medical conditions and background. There are thousands of biorepositories in the United States, which vary widely by size, the type of biospecimens collected, and purpose.

One of the biorepository's highest priorities is protecting the privacy and sanctity of personal and medical information.

Why are Biospecimens Important in Cancer Research

Biospecimens contain an extraordinary amount of biological information, written in the language of cells, genes and proteins. Each biospecimen is also defined by a clinical context - the age, gender, race, diet, and various aspects of the environment the patient has been exposed to during his life. The personal and clinical information comes from interviews at the time the specimen is donated, from medical records patients consent to provide, and from clinical trials that patients volunteer to join. Annotation is the term for this personal and clinical information that labels each biospecimen. The quality of the annotation is as important as the quality of the biospecimen itself.

Researchers can then frame questions that will be answered by looking at hundreds or thousands of samples. For example, they often use the biospecimen to identify the biological characteristics of cancer cells over time, and then correlate those patterns with the clinical picture—how different patients experience progression of the disease.

With unprecedented advances in technology in recent years, scientists are building a greater understanding of how cancer begins and grows in the human body. This is providing a foundation of knowledge and laying the groundwork for "personalized medicine" as scientists begin developing tailored treatments and interventions for cancer patients based on one's molecular features. This personalized approach will mitigate many of the risks associated with treatment under the current trial-and-error method. However, the development of personalized medicine, with benefits of more effective and less toxic individualized therapies, depends heavily upon the availability of high quality biospecimens. Unfortunately, cancer research is currently suffering because of a lack of high quality biospecimens harvested and stored according to standard protocols.

Specifically, human biospecimens are used to:

- Identify (and validate) ways to deliver drugs or agents to specific cells

- Identify how diseases progress and vary

- Group patients, based on their genetic characteristics, as more or less likely to respond to specific drugs

- Group patients, based on biomarkers of their disease, to determine which treatment is most appropriate

- Develop screening tests to detect biomarkers that are associated with certain stages or sub-types of a disease

How can patients help?

Biospecimens are available for medical research only when patients donate tissue while they are undergoing surgery, biopsy, or other medical procedures. Patients, their families and the public can help support research using biospecimens in the following ways:

- Stay Informed

  There is an increasing amount of interest and activity in how biospecimens can help medical researchers. This website, and other professional and policy organizations (http://www.isber. org/), provide information about trends, issues and events that affect biorepository operations. You can ask your surgeon and local hospital for information about biorepositories operating in your region.

- Consider donating a biospecimen

  As a patient scheduled for a biopsy or surgery, you may be asked before the procedure if you would consider donating a biospecimen for research. You will receive a brochure describing how the process works, as well as a consent form to review.

  Donating your biospecimens is entirely voluntary. Whether or not you decide to donate, there will be no impact on the surgical procedure itself. Your specimens cannot be taken until you give written consent (permission), and you will be able to withdraw that permission at any time thereafter.

- Spread the word

  If you know other people who are going to be in a medical position to provide biospecimens, consider telling them what you've learned about the need for donors and steering them to the NIH.gov website.

1177

- Share your thoughts

  Please contact biospecimens@mail.nih.gov with any comments or questions.

Future of Biorepositories

It is now well known that biorepositories are a key resource for large-scale genomic- and proteomic-based research into cancer. Researchers need access to large numbers of high- quality biospecimens that are "annotated" (accompanied by relevant clinical information). The quality of a specimen is determined not only by the physical integrity of the biomolecules within it but by the quality of the specimen-associated information and the ethical, legal and policy parameters that determine the use of the specimen in research.

Due to the need for high quality samples and the use of appropriate sampling procedures for every aspect of the collection and dissemination process, biorepository operations have become highly complex. As a result, the biorepository community is increasingly focused on standardization and harmonization of technical and operational practices, as well as ethical, legal and policy issues.

Part Eight

Trends and Statistics

Chapter 63

Cancer Statistics

Chapter Contents

Section 63.1

Cancer Statistics—An Overview

Text in this section is excerpted from "Cancer Statistics," National
Cancer Institute at the National Institutes of Health (NIH).

Cancer has a major impact on society in the United States and
across the world. Cancer statistics describe what happens in large
groups of people and provide a picture in time of the burden of cancer
on society. Statistics tell us things such as how many people are diagnosed with and die from cancer each year, the number of people who
are currently living after a cancer diagnosis, the average age at diagnosis, and the numbers of people who are still alive at a given time after
diagnosis. They also tell us about differences among groups defined by
age, sex, racial/ethnic group, geographic location, and other categories.

Although statistical trends are usually not directly applicable to
individual patients, they are essential for governments, policy mak-
ers, health professionals, and researchers to understand the impact
of cancer on the population and to develop strategies to address the
challenges that cancer poses to the society at large. Statistical trends
are also important for measuring the success of efforts to control and
manage cancer.

Statistics at a Glance: The Burden of Cancer in the United States

- In 2015, an estimated 1,658,370 new cases of cancer will be diagnosed in the United States and 589,430 people will die from the
  disease.

- The most common cancers in 2015 are projected to be breast
  cancer, lung and bronchus cancer, prostate cancer, colon and rectum cancer, bladder cancer, melanoma of the skin, non-Hodgkin
  lymphoma, thyroid cancer, kidney and renal pelvis cancer, endometrial cancer, leukemia, and pancreatic cancer.

- The number of new cases of cancer (cancer incidence) is 454.8 per
  100,000 men and women per year (based on 2008-2012 cases).

- The number of cancer deaths (cancer mortality) is 171.2 per 100,000 men and women per year (based on 2008-2012 deaths).

- Cancer mortality is higher among men than women (207.9 per 100,000 men and 145.4 per 100,000 women). It is highest in African American men (261.5 per 100,000) and lowest in Asian/Pacific Islander women (91.2 per 100,000). (Based on 2008-2012 deaths.)

- The number of people living beyond a cancer diagnosis reached nearly 14.5 million in 2014 and is expected to rise to almost 19 million by 2024.

- Approximately 39.6 percent of men and women will be diagnosed with cancer at some point during their lifetimes (based on 2010-2012 data).

- In 2014, an estimated 15,780 children and adolescents ages 0 to 19 were diagnosed with cancer and 1,960 died of the disease.

- National expenditures for cancer care in the United States totaled nearly $125 billion in 2010 and could reach $156 billion in 2020.

Statistics at a Glance: The Burden of Cancer Worldwide

- Cancer is among the leading causes of death worldwide. In 2012, there were 14 million new cases and 8.2 million cancer-related deaths worldwide.
- The number of new cancer cases will rise to 22 million within the next two decades.
- More than 60 percent of the world's new cancer cases occur in Africa, Asia, and Central and South America; 70 percent of the world's cancer deaths also occur in these regions.

U.S. Cancer Mortality Trends

The best indicator of progress against cancer is a change in age-adjusted mortality (death) rates, although other measures, such as quality of life, are also important. Incidence is also important, but it is not always straightforward to interpret changes in incidence. For example, if a new screening test detects many cancer cases that would never have caused a problem during someone's life (called overdiagnosis), the incidence of that cancer would appear to increase even though the death rates do not change. But a rise in incidence can also reflect a real increase in disease, as is the case when an increase in exposure to a risk factor causes more cases of cancer. In this scenario the increased incidence would likely lead to a rise in mortality from the cancer.

In the United States, the overall cancer death rate has declined since the early 1990s. The most recent Annual Report to the Nation on the Status of Cancer, published in March 2015, shows that from 2002 to 2011, cancer death rates decreased by:

- 1.8 percent per year among men

- 1.4 percent per year among women

- 2.1 percent per year among children ages 0-14

- 2.3 percent per year among children ages 0-19

Although death rates for many individual cancer types have also declined, rates for a few cancers have stabilized or even increased.

As the overall cancer death rate has declined, the number of cancer survivors has increased. These trends show that progress is being made against the disease, but much work remains. Although rates of smoking, a major cause of cancer, have declined, the U.S. population is aging, and cancer rates increase with age. Obesity, another risk factor for cancer, is also increasing.

Section 63.2

Statistics—Common Cancer Types

This section includes excerpts from "Common Cancer Types ," National Cancer Institute at the National Institutes of Health (NIH), January 26, 2015; and text from "Cancer Stat Fact Sheets," National Cancer Institute at the National Institutes of Health (NIH).

Cancer incidence and mortality statistics reported by the American Cancer Society[1] and other resources were used to create the list. To qualify as a common cancer for the list, the estimated annual incidence for 2015 had to be 40,000 cases or more.

The most common type of cancer on the list is breast cancer, with more than 234,000 new cases expected in the United States in 2015. The next most common cancers are prostate cancer and lung cancer.

Because colon and rectal cancers are often referred to as "colorectal cancers," these two cancer types are combined for the list. For 2015, the estimated number of new cases of colon cancer and rectal cancer are 93,090 and 39,610, respectively, adding to a total of 132,700 new cases of colorectal cancer.

The following table gives the estimated numbers of new cases and deaths for each common cancer type:

Cancer Type	Estimated New Cases	Estimated Deaths
Bladder	74,000	16,000
Breast (Female—Male)	231,840–2350	40,290–440
Colon and Rectal (Combined)	132,700	49,700
Endometrial	54,870	10,170
Kidney (Renal Cell and Renal Pelvis) Cancer	61,560	14,080
Leukemia (All Types)	54,270	24,450
Lung (Including Bronchus)	221,200	158,040
Melanoma	73,870	9,940
Non-Hodgkin Lymphoma	71,850	19,790
Pancreatic	48,960	40,560
Prostate	220,800	27,540
Thyroid	62,450	1,950

References

1. American Cancer Society: Cancer Facts and Figures 2015. Atlanta, Ga: American Cancer Society, 2015. Also available online. Last accessed January 23, 2015.

Statistics at a glance—All types of Cancer

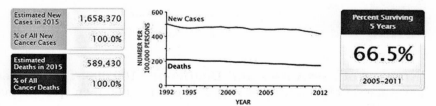

1185

Number of New Cases and Deaths per 100,000: The number of new cases of all cancer sites was 454.8 per 100,000 men and women per year. The number of deaths was 171.2 per 100,000 men and women per year. These rates are age-adjusted and based on 2008-2012 cases and deaths.

Lifetime Risk of Developing Cancer: Approximately 39.6 percent of men and women will be diagnosed with all cancer sites at some point during their lifetime, based on 2010-2012 data.

Prevalence of This Cancer: In 2012, there were an estimated 13,776,251 people living with all cancer sites in the United States.

Statistics at a glance—Anal Cancer

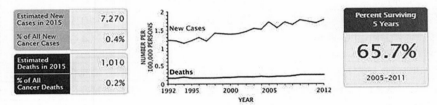

Number of New Cases and Deaths per 100,000: The number of new cases of anal cancer was 1.8 per 100,000 men and women per year. The number of deaths was 0.2 per 100,000 men and women per year. These rates are age-adjusted and based on 2008-2012 cases and deaths.

Lifetime Risk of Developing Cancer: Approximately 0.2 percent of men and women will be diagnosed with anal cancer at some point during their lifetime, based on 2010-2012 data.

Statistics at a glance—Bladder Cancer

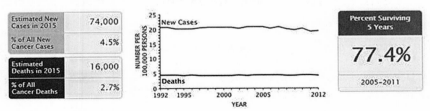

Number of New Cases and Deaths per 100,000: The number of new cases of bladder cancer was 20.3 per 100,000 men and women per year. The number of deaths was 4.4 per 100,000 men and women per year. These rates are age-adjusted and based on 2008-2012 cases and deaths.

Lifetime Risk of Developing Cancer: Approximately 2.4 percent of men and women will be diagnosed with bladder cancer at some point during their lifetime, based on 2010-2012 data.

Prevalence of This Cancer: In 2012, there were an estimated 577,403 people living with bladder cancer in the United States.

Statistics at a glance—Bone and Joint Cancer

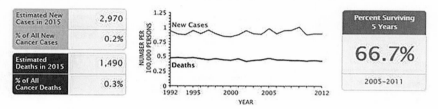

Number of New Cases and Deaths per 100,000: The number of new cases of bone and joint cancer was 0.9 per 100,000 men and women per year. The number of deaths was 0.4 per 100,000 men and women per year. These rates are age-adjusted and based on 2008-2012 cases and deaths.

Lifetime Risk of Developing Cancer: Approximately 0.1 percent of men and women will be diagnosed with bone and joint cancer at some point during their lifetime, based on 2010-2012 data.

Statistics at a glance—Brain and Other Nervous System Cancer

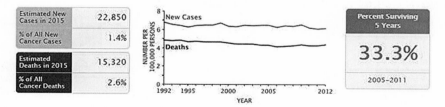

Number of New Cases and Deaths per 100,000: The number of new cases of brain and other nervous system cancer was 6.4 per 100,000 men and women per year. The number of deaths was 4.3 per

100,000 men and women per year. These rates are age-adjusted and based on 2008-2012 cases and deaths.

Lifetime Risk of Developing Cancer: Approximately 0.6 percent of men and women will be diagnosed with brain and other nervous system cancer at some point during their lifetime, based on 2010-2012 data.

Prevalence of This Cancer: In 2012, there were an estimated 148,818 people living with brain and other nervous system cancer in the United States.

Statistics at a glance—Breast Cancer

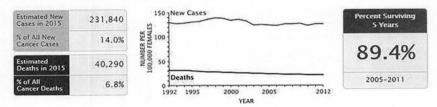

Number of New Cases and Deaths per 100,000: The number of new cases of breast cancer was 124.8 per 100,000 women per year. The number of deaths was 21.9 per 100,000 women per year. These rates are age adjusted and based on 2008-2012 cases and deaths.

Lifetime Risk of Developing Cancer: Approximately 12.3 percent of women will be diagnosed with breast cancer at some point during their lifetime, based on 2010-2012 data.

Prevalence of This Cancer: In 2012, there were an estimated 2,975,314 women living with breast cancer in the United States.

Statistics at a glance—Cervix Uteri Cancer

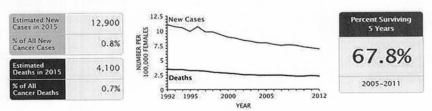

Number of New Cases and Deaths per 100,000: The number of new cases of cervix uteri cancer was 7.7 per 100,000 women per year.

The number of deaths was 2.3 per 100,000 women per year. These rates are age adjusted and based on 2008-2012 cases and deaths.

Lifetime Risk of Developing Cancer: Approximately 0.6 percent of women will be diagnosed with cervix uteri cancer at some point during their lifetime, based on 2010-2012 data.

Prevalence of This Cancer: In 2012, there were an estimated 249,512 women living with cervix uteri cancer in the United States.

Statistics at a glance—Colon and Rectum

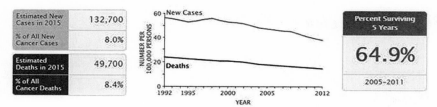

Number of New Cases and Deaths per 100,000: The number of new cases of colon and rectum cancer was 42.4 per 100,000 men and women per year. The number of deaths was 15.5 per 100,000 men and women per year.

These rates are age-adjusted and based on 2008-2012 cases and deaths.

Lifetime Risk of Developing Cancer: Approximately 4.5 percent of men and women will be diagnosed with colon and rectum cancer at some point during their lifetime, based on 2010-2012 data.

Prevalence of This Cancer: In 2012, there were an estimated 1,168,929 people living with colon and rectum cancer in the United States.

Statistics at a glance—Endometrial Cancer

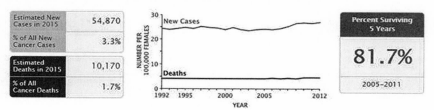

Number of New Cases and Deaths per 100,000: The number of new cases of endometrial cancer was 25.1 per 100,000 women per year. The number of deaths was 4.4 per 100,000 women per year. These rates are age adjusted and based on 2008-2012 cases and deaths.

Lifetime Risk of Developing Cancer: Approximately 2.8 percent of women will be diagnosed with endometrial cancer at some point during their lifetime, based on 2010-2012 data.

Prevalence of This Cancer: In 2012, there were an estimated 621,612 women living with endometrial cancer in the United States.

Statistics at a glance—Esophageal Cancer

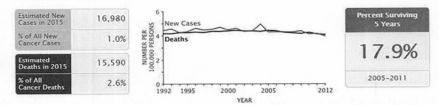

Number of New Cases and Deaths per 100,000: The number of new cases of esophageal cancer was 4.4 per 100,000 men and women per year. The number of deaths was 4.2 per 100,000 men and women per year. These rates are age-adjusted and based on 2008-2012 cases and deaths.

Lifetime Risk of Developing Cancer: Approximately 0.5 percent of men and women will be diagnosed with esophageal cancer at some point during their lifetime, based on 2010-2012 data.

Prevalence of This Cancer: In 2012, there were an estimated 35,781 people living with esophageal cancer in the United States.

Statistics at a glance—Kidney and Renal Pelvis Cancer

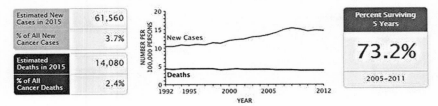

Number of New Cases and Deaths per 100,000: The number of new cases of kidney and renal pelvis cancer was 15.6 per 100,000 men and women per year. The number of deaths was 3.9 per 100,000 men and women per year. These rates are age-adjusted and based on 2008-2012 cases and deaths.

Lifetime Risk of Developing Cancer: Approximately 1.6 percent of men and women will be diagnosed with kidney and renal pelvis cancer at some point during their lifetime, based on 2010-2012 data.

Prevalence of This Cancer: In 2012, there were an estimated 375,925 people living with kidney and renal pelvis cancer in the United States.

Statistics at a glance—Larynx Cancer

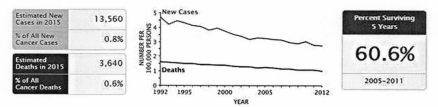

Number of New Cases and Deaths per 100,000: The number of new cases of larynx cancer was 3.2 per 10,000 men and women per year. The number of deaths was 1.1 per 100,000 men and women per year. These rates are a0ge-adjusted and based on 2008-2012 cases and deaths.

Lifetime Risk of Developing Cancer: Approximately 0.4 percent of men and women will be diagnosed with larynx cancer at some point during their lifetime, based on 2010-2012 data.

Prevalence of This Cancer: In 2012, there were an estimated 88,852 people living with larynx cancer in the United States.

Statistics at a glance—Liver and Intraheptic Bile Duct Cancer

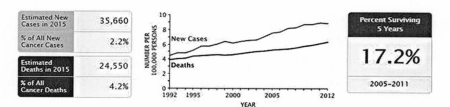

Number of New Cases and Deaths per 100,000: The number of new cases of liver and intrahepatic bile duct cancer was 8.2 per 100,000 men and women per year. The number of deaths was 6.0 per 100,000 men and women per year. These rates are age-adjusted and based on 2008-2012 cases and deaths.

Lifetime Risk of Developing Cancer: Approximately 0.9 percent of men and women will be diagnosed with liver and intrahepatic bile duct cancer at some point during their lifetime, based on 2010-2012 data.

Prevalence of This Cancer: In 2012, there were an estimated 50,734 people living with liver and intrahepatic bile duct cancer in the United States.

Statistics at a glance—Lung and Bronchus Cancer

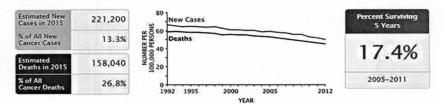

Number of New Cases and Deaths per 100,000: The number of new cases of lung and bronchus cancer was 58.7 per 100,000 men and women per year. The number of deaths was 47.2 per 100,000 men and women per year. These rates are age-adjusted and based on 2008-2012 cases and deaths.

Lifetime Risk of Developing Cancer: Approximately 6.6 percent of men and women will be diagnosed with lung and bronchus cancer at some point during their lifetime, based on 2010-2012 data.

Prevalence of This Cancer: In 2012, there were an estimated 408,808 people living with lung and bronchus cancer in the United States.

Statistics at a glance—Lymphoma (Hodgkin)

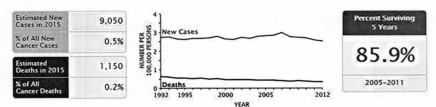

Number of New Cases and Deaths per 100,000: The number of new cases of Hodgkin lymphoma was 2.7 per 100,000 men and women per year. The number of deaths was 0.4 per 100,000 men and women per year. Thesebrates are age-adjusted and based on 2008-2012 cases and deaths.

Lifetime Risk of Developing Cancer: Approximately 0.2 percent of men and women will be diagnosed with Hodgkin lymphoma at some point during their lifetime, based on 2010-2012 data.

Prevalence of This Cancer: In 2012, there were an estimated 189,626 people living with Hodgkin lymphoma in the United States.

Statistics at a glance—Lymphoma (Non-Hodgkin)

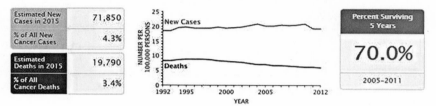

Number of New Cases and Deaths per 100,000: The number of new cases of non-Hodgkin lymphoma was 19.7 per 100,000 men and women per year. The number of deaths was 6.2 per 100,000 men and women per year. These rates are age-adjusted and based on 2008-2012 cases and deaths.

Lifetime Risk of Developing Cancer: Approximately 2.1 percent of men and women will be diagnosed with non-Hodgkin lymphoma at some point during their lifetime, based on 2010-2012 data.

Prevalence of This Cancer: In 2012, there were an estimated 549,625 people living with non-Hodgkin lymphoma in the United States.

Statistics at a glance—Leukemia

Estimated New Cases in 2015	54,270
% of All New Cancer Cases	3.3%
Estimated Deaths in 2015	24,450
% of All Cancer Deaths	4.1%

Percent Surviving 5 Years

58.5%

2005-2011

Number of New Cases and Deaths per 100,000: The number of new cases of leukemia was 13.3 per 100,000 men and women per year. The number of deaths was 7.0 per 100,000 men and women per year. These rates are age-adjusted and based on 2008-2012 cases and deaths.

Lifetime Risk of Developing Cancer: Approximately 1.5 percent of men and women will be diagnosed with leukemia at some point during their lifetime, based on 2010-2012 data.

Prevalence of This Cancer: In 2012, there were an estimated 318,389 people living with leukemia in the United States.

Statistics at a glance—Melanoma of the Skin

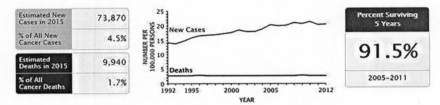

Estimated New Cases in 2015	73,870
% of All New Cancer Cases	4.5%
Estimated Deaths in 2015	9,940
% of All Cancer Deaths	1.7%

Percent Surviving 5 Years: **91.5%** 2005-2011

Number of New Cases and Deaths per 100,000: The number of new cases of melanoma of the skin was 21.6 per 100,000 men and women per year. The number of deaths was 2.7 per 100,000 men and women per year. These rates are age-adjusted and based on 2008-2012 cases and deaths.

Lifetime Risk of Developing Cancer: Approximately 2.1 percent of men and women will be diagnosed with melanoma of the skin at some point during their lifetime, based on 2010-2012 data.

Prevalence of This Cancer: In 2012, there were an estimated 996,587 people living with melanoma of the skin in the United States.

Statistics at a glance—Myeloma

Estimated New Cases in 2015	26,850
% of All New Cancer Cases	1.6%
Estimated Deaths in 2015	11,240
% of All Cancer Deaths	1.9%

Percent Surviving 5 Years: **46.6%** 2005-2011

Number of New Cases and Deaths per 100,000: The number of new cases of myeloma was 6.3 per 100,000 men and women per year. The number of deaths was 3.3 per 100,000 men and women per year. These rates are age adjusted and based on 2008-2012 cases and deaths.

Lifetime Risk of Developing Cancer: Approximately 0.7 percent of men and women will be diagnosed with myeloma at some point during their lifetime, based on 2010-2012 data.

Prevalence of This Cancer: In 2012, there were an estimated 89,658 people living with myeloma in the United States.

Statistics at a glance—Oral cavity and Pharynx Cancer

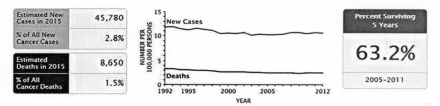

Number of New Cases and Deaths per 100,000: The number of new cases of oral cavity and pharynx cancer was 11.0 per 100,000 men and women per year. The number of deaths was 2.5 per 100,000 men and women per year. These rates are age-adjusted and based on 2008-2012 cases and deaths.

Lifetime Risk of Developing Cancer: Approximately 1.1 percent of men and women will be diagnosed with oral cavity and pharynx cancer at some point during their lifetime, based on 2010-2012 data.

Prevalence of This Cancer: In 2012, there were an estimated 291,108 people living with oral cavity and pharynx cancer in the United States.

Statistics at a glance—Ovary Cancer

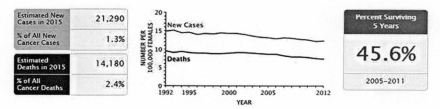

Number of New Cases and Deaths per 100,000: The number of new cases of ovary cancer was 12.1 per 100,000 women per year. The number of deaths was 7.7 per 100,000 women per year. These rates are age-adjusted and based on 2008-2012 cases and deaths.

Lifetime Risk of Developing Cancer: Approximately 1.3 percent of women will be diagnosed with ovary cancer at some point during their lifetime, based on 2010-2012 data.

Prevalence of This Cancer: In 2012, there were an estimated 192,446 women living with ovary cancer in the United States.

Statistics at a glance—Pancreas Cancer

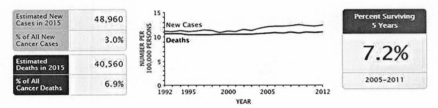

Number of New Cases and Deaths per 100,000: The number of new cases of pancreas cancer was 12.4 per 100,000 men and women per year. The number of deaths was 10.9 per 100,000 men and women per year. These rates are age-adjusted and based on 2008-2012 cases and deaths.

Lifetime Risk of Developing Cancer: Approximately 1.5 percent of men and women will be diagnosed with pancreas cancer at some point during their lifetime, based on 2010-2012 data.

Prevalence of This Cancer: In 2012, there were an estimated 45,702 people living with pancreas cancer in the United States.

Statistics at a glance—Prostate Cancer

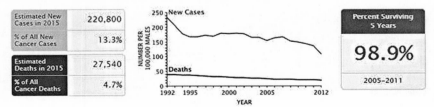

Number of New Cases and Deaths per 100,000: The number of new cases of prostate cancer was 137.9 per 100,000 men per year. The number of deaths was 21.4 per 100,000 men per year. These rates are age-adjusted and based on 2008-2012 cases and deaths.

Lifetime Risk of Developing Cancer: Approximately 14.0 percent of men will be diagnosed with prostate cancer at some point during their lifetime, based on 2010-2012 data.

Prevalence of This Cancer: In 2012, there were an estimated 2,795,592 men living with prostate cancer in the United States.

Statistics at a glance—Small Intestine Cancer

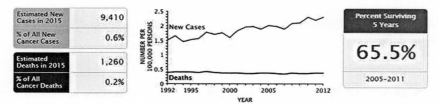

Estimated New Cases in 2015	9,410
% of All New Cancer Cases	0.6%
Estimated Deaths in 2015	1,260
% of All Cancer Deaths	0.2%

Percent Surviving 5 Years: **65.5%** (2005–2011)

Number of New Cases and Deaths per 100,000: The number of new cases of small intestine cancer was 2.2 per 100,000 men and women per year. The number of deaths was 0.4 per 100,000 men and women per year. These rates are age adjusted and based on 2008-2012 cases and deaths.

Lifetime Risk of Developing Cancer: Approximately 0.2 percent of men and women will be diagnosed with small intestine cancer at some point during their lifetime, based on 2010-2012 data.

Statistics at a glance—Stomach Cancer

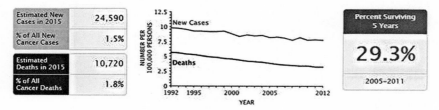

Estimated New Cases in 2015	24,590
% of All New Cancer Cases	1.5%
Estimated Deaths in 2015	10,720
% of All Cancer Deaths	1.8%

Percent Surviving 5 Years: **29.3%** (2005–2011)

Number of New Cases and Deaths per 100,000: The number of new cases of stomach cancer was 7.4 per 100,000 men and women per year. The number of deaths was 3.4 per 100,000 men and women per year. These rates are age-adjusted and based on 2008-2012 cases and deaths.

Lifetime Risk of Developing Cancer: Approximately 0.9 percent of men and women will be diagnosed with stomach cancer at some point during their lifetime, based on 2010-2012 data.

Prevalence of This Cancer: In 2012, there were an estimated 76,829 people living with stomach cancer in the United States.

Statistics at a glance—Testis Cancer

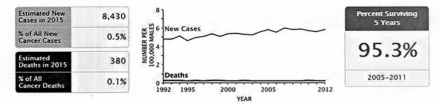

Number of New Cases and Deaths per 100,000: The number of new cases of testis cancer was 5.6 per 100,000 men per year. The number of deaths was 0.3 per 100,000 men per year. These rates are age-adjusted and based on 2008-2012 cases and deaths.

Lifetime Risk of Developing Cancer: Approximately 0.4 percent of men will be diagnosed with testis cancer at some point during their lifetime, based on 2010-2012 data.

Prevalence of This Cancer: In 2012, there were an estimated 233,602 men living with testis cancer in the United States.

Statistics at a glance—Thyroid Cancer

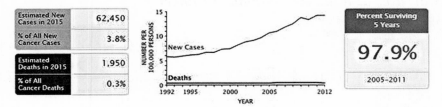

Number of New Cases and Deaths per 100,000: The number of new cases of thyroid cancer was 13.5 per 100,000 men and women per year. The number of deaths was 0.5 per 100,000 men and women per year. These rates are age-adjusted and based on 2008-2012 cases and deaths.

Lifetime Risk of Developing Cancer: Approximately 1.1 percent of men and women will be diagnosed with thyroid cancer at some point during their lifetime, based on 2010-2012 data.

Prevalence of This Cancer: In 2012, there were an estimated 601,789 people living with thyroid cancer in the United States.

Statistics at a glance—Vulvar Cancer

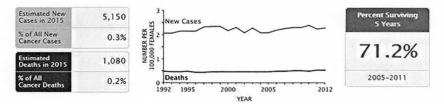

Number of New Cases and Deaths per 100,000: The number of new cases of vulvar cancer was 2.4 per 100,000 women per year. The number of deaths was 0.5 per 100,000 women per year. These rates are age-adjusted and based on 2008-2012 cases and deaths.

Lifetime Risk of Developing Cancer: Approximately 0.3 percent of women will be diagnosed with vulvar cancer at some point during their lifetime, based on 2010-2012 data.

Section 63.3

Statistics—Age, Gender, Ethnicity

Text in this section is excerpted from "Cancer Stat Fact Sheets," National Cancer Institute at the National Institutes of Health (NIH).

Cancer of All Sites

Overall cancer incidence rates are higher among men than women. Among racial/ethnic groups, there are more new cases among African

American men and white women and fewer new cases among Asian/
Pacific Islanders of both sexes. The number of new cases of all cancer
sites was 454.8 per 100,000 men and women per year based on 2008-
2012 cases.

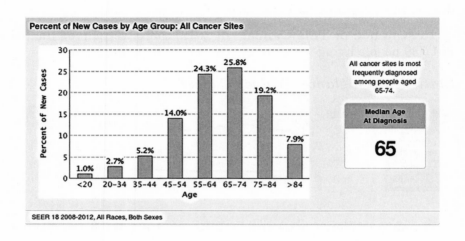

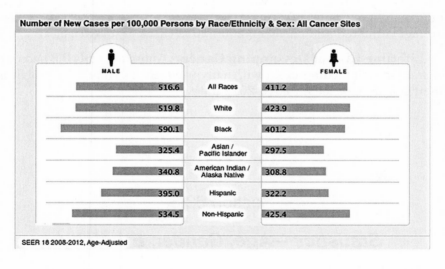

Anal Cancer

Anal cancer is slightly more common in women than men. Infection with human papillomavirus (HPV) has been associated with this cancer. The number of new cases of anal cancer was 1.8 per 100,000 men and women per year based on 2008-2012 cases.

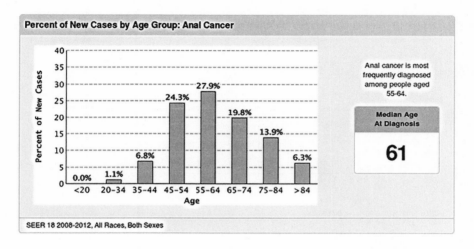

Percent of New Cases by Age Group: Anal Cancer

Anal cancer is most frequently diagnosed among people aged 55-64.

Median Age At Diagnosis

61

SEER 18 2008-2012, All Races, Both Sexes

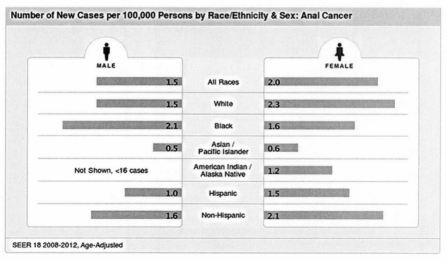

Number of New Cases per 100,000 Persons by Race/Ethnicity & Sex: Anal Cancer

MALE		FEMALE
1.5	All Races	2.0
1.5	White	2.3
2.1	Black	1.6
0.5	Asian / Pacific Islander	0.6
Not Shown, <16 cases	American Indian / Alaska Native	1.2
1.0	Hispanic	1.5
1.6	Non-Hispanic	2.1

SEER 18 2008-2012, Age-Adjusted

Bladder Cancer

Bladder cancer becomes more common with age and is more common in men than women. The number of new cases of bladder cancer was 20.3 per 100,000 men and women per year based on 2008-2012 cases.

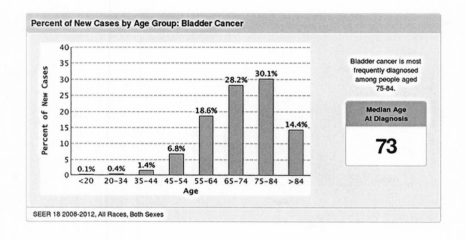

SEER 18 2008-2012, All Races, Both Sexes

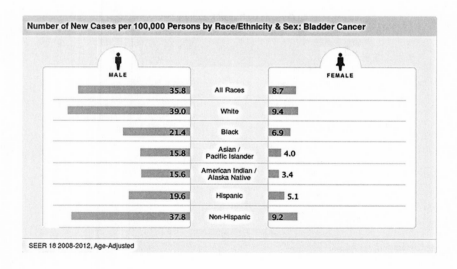

SEER 18 2008-2012, Age-Adjusted

Bone and Joint Cancer

Osteosarcoma is most common in teenagers. Ewing Sarcoma is most common in teenagers and young adults. The number of new cases of bone and joint cancer was 0.9 per 100,000 men and women per year based on 2008-2012 cases.

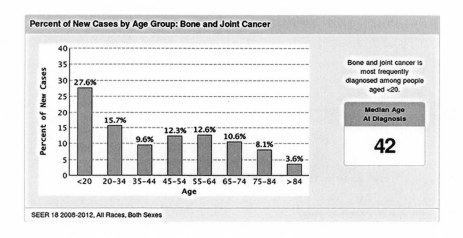

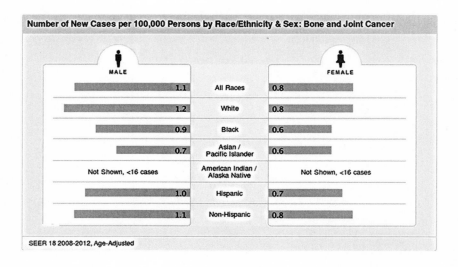

Brain and Other Nervous System Cancer

This cancer is slightly more common in men than women and among those with certain genetic syndromes. The number of new cases of brain and other nervous system cancer was 6.4 per 100,000 men and women per year based on 2008-2012 cases.

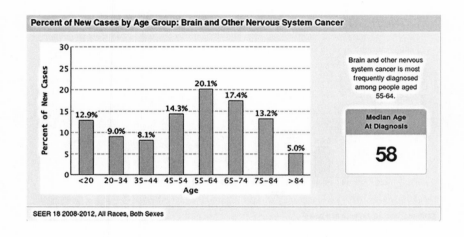

Percent of New Cases by Age Group: Brain and Other Nervous System Cancer

SEER 18 2008-2012, All Races, Both Sexes

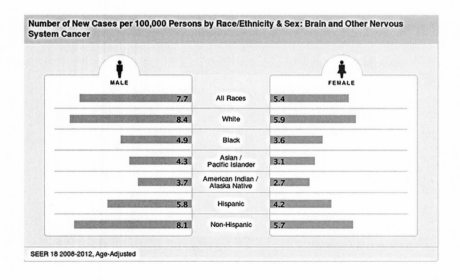

Number of New Cases per 100,000 Persons by Race/Ethnicity & Sex: Brain and Other Nervous System Cancer

SEER 18 2008-2012, Age-Adjusted

Breast Cancer

Female breast cancer is most common in middle-aged and older women. Although rare, men can develop breast cancer as well. The number of new cases of breast cancer was 124.8 per 100,000 women per year based on 2008-2012 cases.

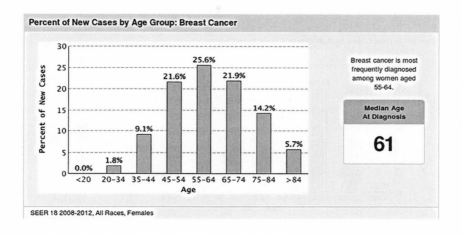

Cervix Uteri Cancer

Infection of the cervix with human papillomavirus (HPV) is the most common cause of cervical cancer, although not all women with HPV infection will develop cervical cancer. The number of new cases of cervix uteri cancer was 7.7 per 100,000 women per year based on 2008-2012 cases.

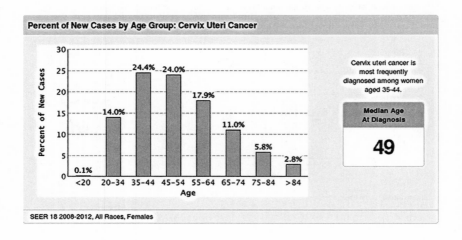

Percent of New Cases by Age Group: Cervix Uteri Cancer

Cervix uteri cancer is most frequently diagnosed among women aged 35-44.

Median Age At Diagnosis

49

SEER 18 2008-2012, All Races, Females

Number of New Cases per 100,000 Persons by Race/Ethnicity: Cervix Uteri Cancer

	MALE		FEMALE
	Sex-Specific Cancer	All Races	7.7
		White	7.7
		Black	9.2
		Asian / Pacific Islander	6.3
		American Indian / Alaska Native	7.5
		Hispanic	9.9
		Non-Hispanic	7.3

SEER 18 2008-2012, Age-Adjusted

Colon and Rectum Cancer

Colorectal cancer is more common in men than women and among those of African American descent. The number of new cases of colon and rectum cancer was 42.4 per 100,000 men and women per year based on 2008-2012 cases.

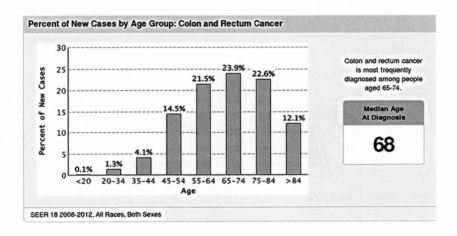

Percent of New Cases by Age Group: Colon and Rectum Cancer

Colon and rectum cancer is most frequently diagnosed among people aged 65-74.

Median Age At Diagnosis

68

SEER 18 2008-2012, All Races, Both Sexes

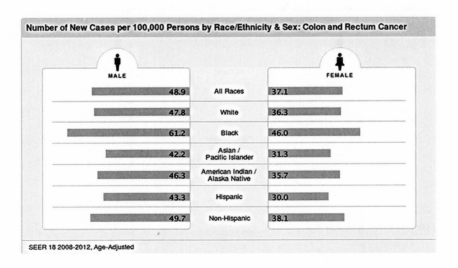

Number of New Cases per 100,000 Persons by Race/Ethnicity & Sex: Colon and Rectum Cancer

	MALE		FEMALE
All Races	48.9		37.1
White	47.8		36.3
Black	61.2		46.0
Asian / Pacific Islander	42.2		31.3
American Indian / Alaska Native	46.3		35.7
Hispanic	43.3		30.0
Non-Hispanic	49.7		38.1

SEER 18 2008-2012, Age-Adjusted

1207

Endometrial Cancer

Most cases of endometrial cancer are diagnosed in women aged 45-74. The number of new cases of endometrial cancer was 25.1 per 100,000 women per year based on 2008-2012 cases.

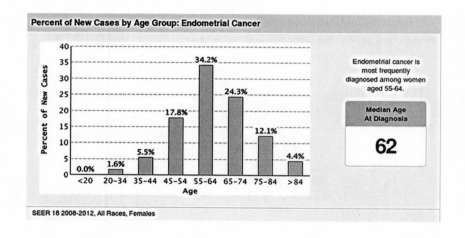

Percent of New Cases by Age Group: Endometrial Cancer

Endometrial cancer is most frequently diagnosed among women aged 55-64.

Median Age At Diagnosis

62

SEER 18 2008-2012, All Races, Females

Number of New Cases per 100,000 Persons by Race/Ethnicity: Endometrial Cancer

	MALE		FEMALE
Sex-Specific Cancer	All Races	25.1	
	White	25.8	
	Black	24.0	
	Asian / Pacific Islander	19.9	
	American Indian / Alaska Native	19.8	
	Hispanic	20.7	
	Non-Hispanic	25.7	

SEER 18 2008-2012, Age-Adjusted

Esophageal Cancer

Esophageal cancer is more common in men than women, and it is associated with older age, heavy alcohol use and tobacco use. The number of new cases of esophageal cancer was 4.4 per 100,000 men and women per year based on 2008-2012 cases.

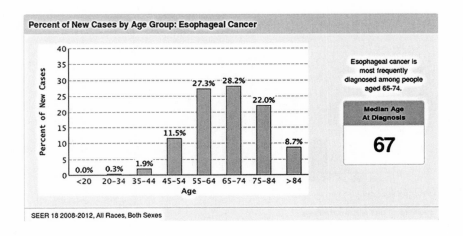

SEER 18 2008-2012, All Races, Both Sexes

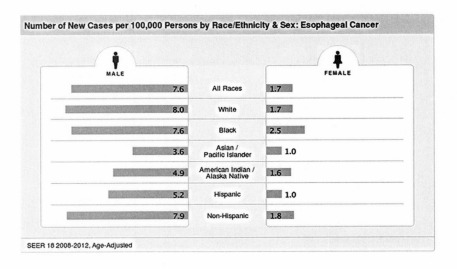

SEER 18 2008-2012, Age-Adjusted

Kidney and Renal Pelvis Cancer

Kidney cancer is more common in men than women and among African Americans and American Indian and Alaska Native populations. The number of new cases of kidney and renal pelvis cancer was 15.6 per 100,000 men and women per year based on 2008-2012 cases.

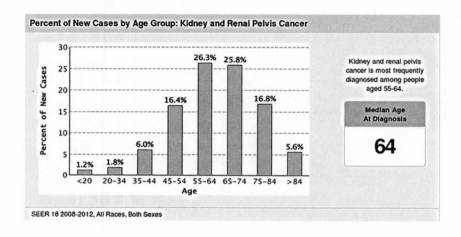

SEER 18 2008-2012, All Races, Both Sexes

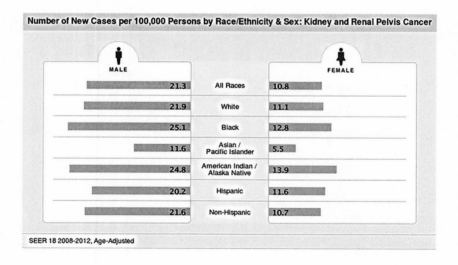

SEER 18 2008-2012, Age-Adjusted

Larynx Cancer

Laryngeal cancer becomes more common with age and is more common in men than in women. Smoking is a major risk factor for this cancer, and reduction smoking rates in recent years has led to a downturn in both incidence and mortality. The number of new cases of larynx cancer was 3.2 per 100,000 men and women per year based on 2008-2012 cases.

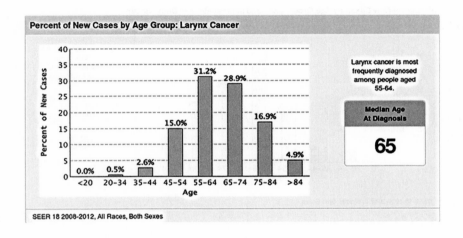

SEER 18 2008-2012, All Races, Both Sexes

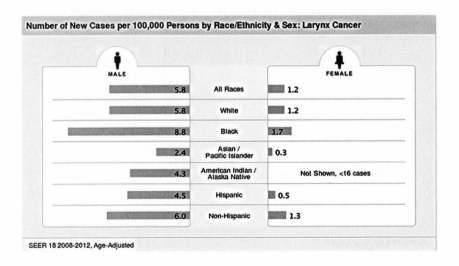

SEER 18 2008-2012, Age-Adjusted

Liver and Intrahepatic Bile Duct Cancer

Liver cancer is more common in men than women, and among Asian/Pacific Islander and American Indian/Alaska Native populations. The number of new cases of liver and intrahepatic bile duct cancer was 8.2 per 100,000 men and women per year based on 2008-2012 cases.

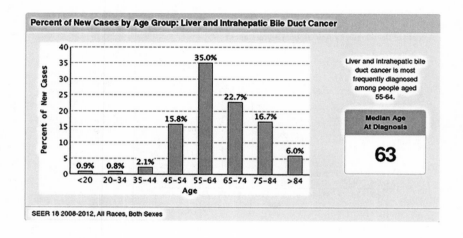

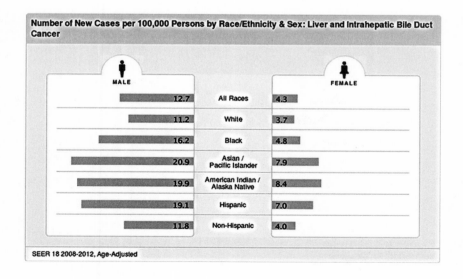

Lung and Bronchus Cancer

Lung cancer is more common in men than women, particularly African American men. Smoking is widely recognized as the leading cause of lung cancer. The number of new cases of lung and bronchus cancer was 58.7 per 100,000 men and women per year based on 2008-2012 cases.

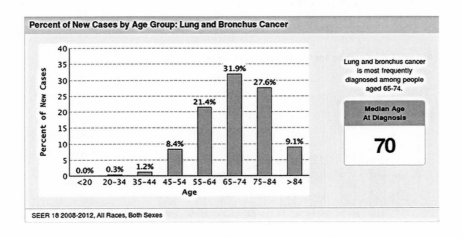

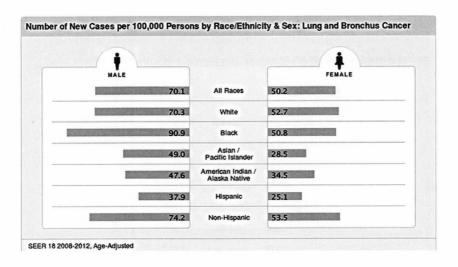

Lymphoma (Hodgkin)

Hodgkin lymphoma is more common among young adults and among men than women. It can occur in both adults and children; however, treatment for adults may be different than treatment for children. Hodgkin lymphoma may also occur in patients who have acquired immunodeficiency syndrome (AIDS); these patients require special treatment. The number of new cases of Hodgkin lymphoma was 2.7 per 100,000 men and women per year based on 2008-2012 cases.

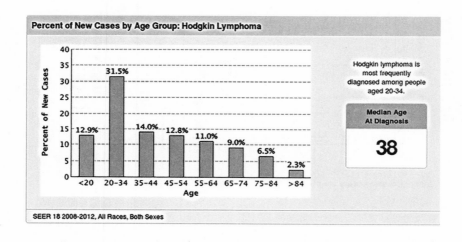

Percent of New Cases by Age Group: Hodgkin Lymphoma

Hodgkin lymphoma is most frequently diagnosed among people aged 20-34.

Median Age At Diagnosis

38

SEER 18 2008-2012, All Races, Both Sexes

Number of New Cases per 100,000 Persons by Race/Ethnicity & Sex: Hodgkin Lymphoma

MALE		FEMALE
3.0	All Races	2.4
3.2	White	2.6
3.0	Black	2.4
1.5	Asian / Pacific Islander	1.2
1.1	American Indian / Alaska Native	1.0
2.6	Hispanic	2.0
3.2	Non-Hispanic	2.6

SEER 18 2008-2012, Age-Adjusted

Lymphoma (Non-Hodgkin)

Non-Hodgkin lymphoma is more common in men than women, and among individuals of Caucasian descent. The number of new cases of non-Hodgkin lymphoma was 19.7 per 100,000 men and women per year based on 2008-2012 cases.

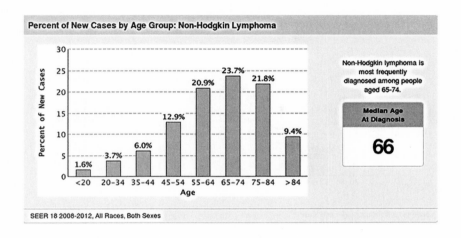

SEER 18 2008-2012, All Races, Both Sexes

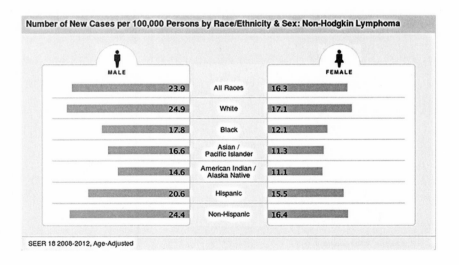

SEER 18 2008-2012, Age-Adjusted

Leukemia

Although leukemia is among the most common childhood cancers, it most often occurs in older adults. Leukemia is slightly more common in men than women. The number of new cases of leukemia was 13.3 per 100,000 men and women per year based on 2008-2012 cases.

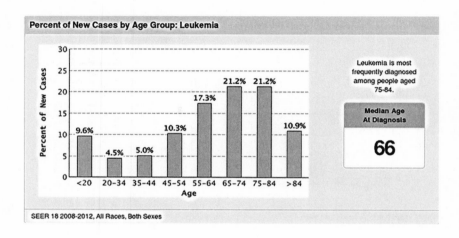

SEER 18 2008-2012, All Races, Both Sexes

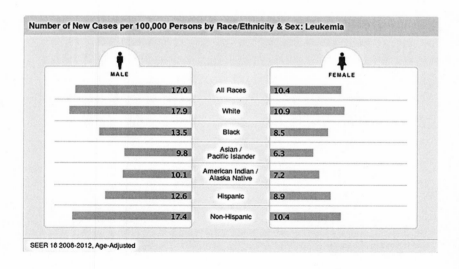

SEER 18 2008-2012, Age-Adjusted

Melanoma of the Skin

Melanoma is more common in men than women and among individuals of fair complexion and those who have been exposed to natural or artificial sunlight (such as tanning beds) over long periods of time. There are more new cases among whites than any other racial/ethnic group. The number of new cases of melanoma of the skin was 21.6 per 100,000 men and women per year based on 2008-2012 cases.

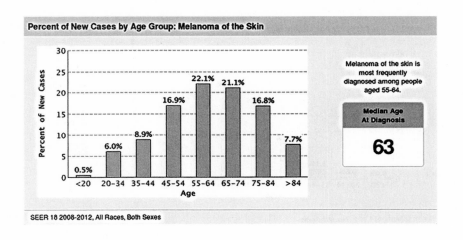

SEER 18 2008-2012, All Races, Both Sexes

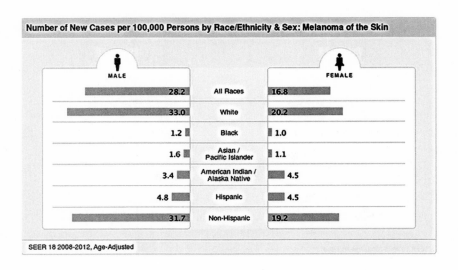

SEER 18 2008-2012, Age-Adjusted

Myeloma

Although a rare disease, myeloma is more common in men than women and among individuals of African American descent. Risk is higher among those with a history of monoclonal gammopathy of undetermined significance (MGUS). The number of new cases of myeloma was 6.3 per 100,000 men and women per year based on 2008-2012 cases.

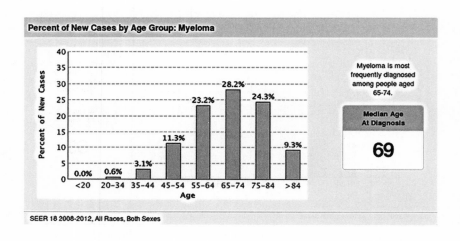

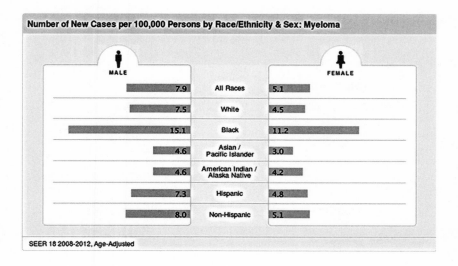

Oral Cavity and Pharynx Cancer

Oral cancer is more common in men than women, among those with a history of tobacco or heavy alcohol use, and individuals infected with human papillomavirus (HPV). The number of new cases of oral cavity and pharynx cancer was 11.0 per 100,000 men and women per year based on 2008-2012 cases.

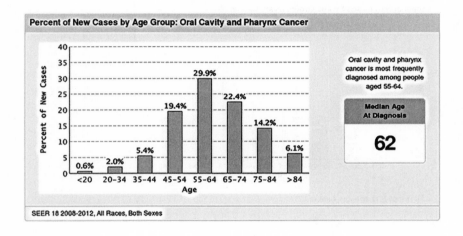

Percent of New Cases by Age Group: Oral Cavity and Pharynx Cancer

Oral cavity and pharynx cancer is most frequently diagnosed among people aged 55-64.

Median Age At Diagnosis: 62

SEER 18 2008-2012, All Races, Both Sexes

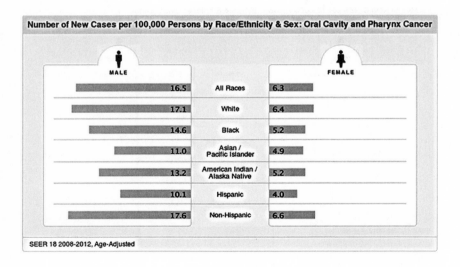

Number of New Cases per 100,000 Persons by Race/Ethnicity & Sex: Oral Cavity and Pharynx Cancer

MALE		FEMALE
16.5	All Races	6.3
17.1	White	6.4
14.6	Black	5.2
11.0	Asian / Pacific Islander	4.9
13.2	American Indian / Alaska Native	5.2
10.1	Hispanic	4.0
17.6	Non-Hispanic	6.6

SEER 18 2008-2012, Age-Adjusted

Ovary Cancer

Ovarian cancer is rare. Women with a family history of ovarian cancer have an increased risk for the disease. The number of new cases of ovary cancer was 12.1 per 100,000 women per year based on 2008-2012 cases.

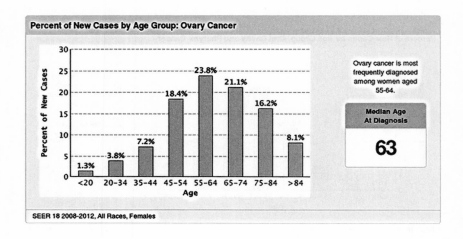

Pancreas Cancer

Pancreatic cancer is more common with increasing age and slightly more common in men than women. The number of new cases of pancreas cancer was 12.4 per 100,000 men and women per year based on 2008-2012 cases.

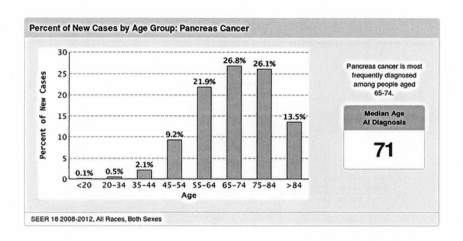

Percent of New Cases by Age Group: Pancreas Cancer

Pancreas cancer is most frequently diagnosed among people aged 65-74.

Median Age At Diagnosis

71

SEER 18 2008-2012, All Races, Both Sexes

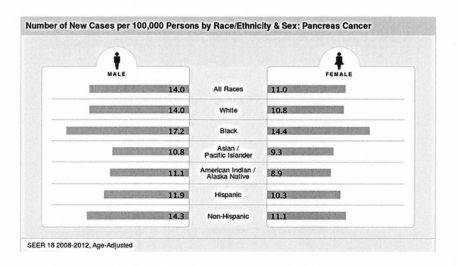

Number of New Cases per 100,000 Persons by Race/Ethnicity & Sex: Pancreas Cancer

	MALE		FEMALE
All Races	14.0		11.0
White	14.0		10.8
Black	17.2		14.4
Asian / Pacific Islander	10.8		9.3
American Indian / Alaska Native	11.1		8.9
Hispanic	11.9		10.3
Non-Hispanic	14.3		11.1

SEER 18 2008-2012, Age-Adjusted

Prostate Cancer

Prostate cancer occurs only in men, and it is more common in older men than younger men. It is more likely to occur in men with a family history of prostate cancer and men of African American descent. The number of new cases of prostate cancer was 137.9 per 100,000 men per year based on 2008-2012 cases.

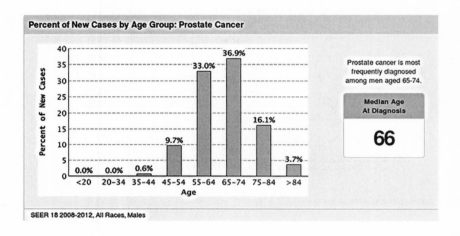

SEER 18 2008-2012, All Races, Males

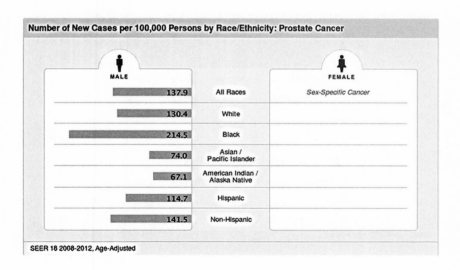

SEER 18 2008-2012, Age-Adjusted

Small Intestine Cancer

Cancer of the small intestine is slightly more common among men than women. Diet and health history can affect the risk of developing this cancer. The number of new cases of small intestine cancer was 2.2 per 100,000 men and women per year based on 2008-2012 cases.

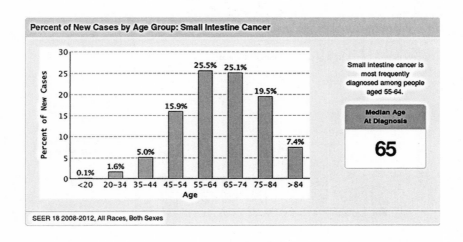

Percent of New Cases by Age Group: Small Intestine Cancer

Small intestine cancer is most frequently diagnosed among people aged 55-64.

Median Age At Diagnosis

65

SEER 18 2008-2012, All Races, Both Sexes

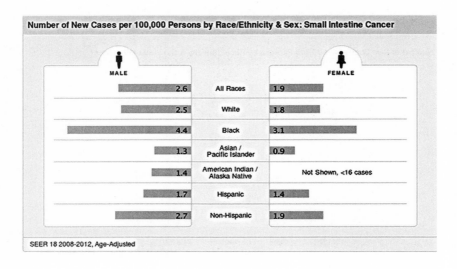

Number of New Cases per 100,000 Persons by Race/Ethnicity & Sex: Small Intestine Cancer

SEER 18 2008-2012, Age-Adjusted

Stomach Cancer

Stomach cancer is more common in men than women and among other races and ethnicities than non-Hispanic whites. Age, diet and stomach disease, including infection with Helicobacter pylori can affect the risk of developing stomach cancer. The number of new cases of stomach cancer was 7.4 per 100,000 men and women per year based on 2008-2012 cases.

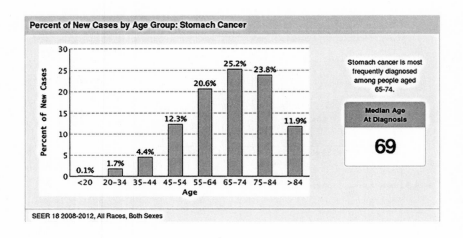

SEER 18 2008-2012, All Races, Both Sexes

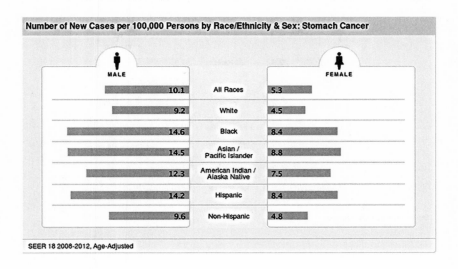

SEER 18 2008-2012, Age-Adjusted

Testis Cancer

Testicular cancer is most common in young adults. The number of new cases of testis cancer was 5.6 per 100,000 men per year based on 2008-2012 cases.

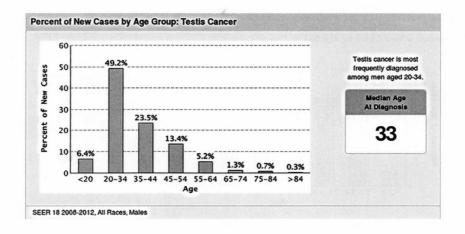

Thyroid Cancer

Thyroid cancer is more common in women than men and among those with a family history of thyroid disease. The number of new cases of thyroid cancer was 13.5 per 100,000 men and women per year based on 2008-2012 cases.

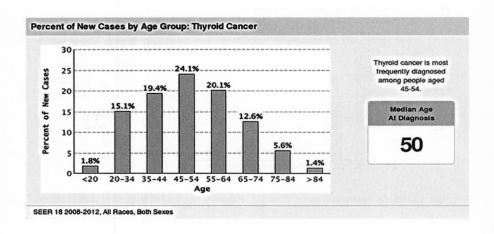

Percent of New Cases by Age Group: Thyroid Cancer

Thyroid cancer is most frequently diagnosed among people aged 45-54.

Median Age At Diagnosis

50

SEER 18 2008-2012, All Races, Both Sexes

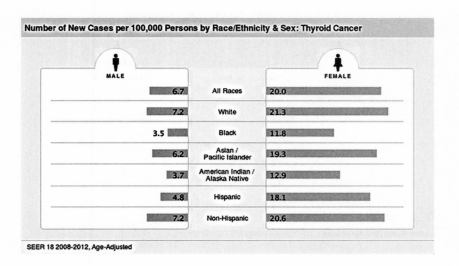

Number of New Cases per 100,000 Persons by Race/Ethnicity & Sex: Thyroid Cancer

	MALE		FEMALE
	6.7	All Races	20.0
	7.2	White	21.3
	3.5	Black	11.8
	6.2	Asian / Pacific Islander	19.3
	3.7	American Indian / Alaska Native	12.9
	4.8	Hispanic	18.1
	7.2	Non-Hispanic	20.6

SEER 18 2008-2012, Age-Adjusted

Vulvar Cancer

Vulvar cancer is rare. It is more common among women with a medical history of vulvar intraepithelial neoplasia, human papillomavirus (HPV) infection, or genital warts. The number of new cases of vulvar cancer was 2.4 per 100,000 women per year based on 2008-2012 cases.

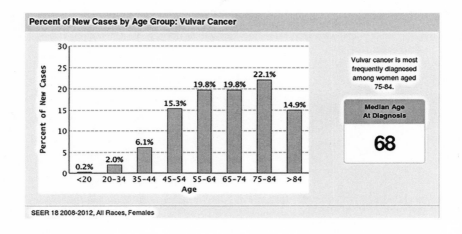

Percent of New Cases by Age Group: Vulvar Cancer

Vulvar cancer is most frequently diagnosed among women aged 75-84.

Median Age At Diagnosis

68

SEER 18 2008-2012, All Races, Females

Number of New Cases per 100,000 Persons by Race/Ethnicity: Vulvar Cancer

	MALE		FEMALE
	Sex-Specific Cancer	All Races	2.4
		White	2.6
		Black	1.8
		Asian / Pacific Islander	0.9
		American Indian / Alaska Native	2.0
		Hispanic	1.7
		Non-Hispanic	2.5

SEER 18 2008-2012, Age-Adjusted

Chapter 64

Cancer Health Disparities

General Disparity Definitions

Cancer Health Disparities

The National Cancer Institute defines cancer health disparities as adverse differences in cancer incidence (new cases), cancer prevalence (all existing cases), morbidity (cancer-related health complications), cancer mortality (deaths), cancer survivorship, and burden of cancer or related health conditions that exist among specific population groups in the United States.

These population groups may be characterized by age, disability, education, ethnicity, gender, geographic location, income, or race. Generally, people who are from low socioeconomic backgrounds (poor, lack health insurance, and are medically underserved with limited or no access to effective health care) often bear a greater burden of disease than the general U.S. population.

Health Disparities

Health disparities are significant differences between one population and another. Below are federal definitions of the term that illustrate the multiple perspectives on health disparities:

Text in this chapter is excerpted from "Cancer Health Disparities," National Cancer Institute at the National Institutes of Health (NIH), February 17, 2015.

The Department of Health and Human Services defines health disparities as differences in health outcomes that are closely linked with social, economic, and environmental disadvantage and are often driven by the social conditions in which individuals live, learn, work, and play.

Healthy People 2020 states that a health disparity is a health difference that is closely linked with social, economic, and/or environmental disadvantage. Health disparities adversely affect groups of people who have systematically experienced greater obstacles to health based on their racial or ethnic group; religion; socioeconomic status; gender; age; mental health; cognitive, sensory, or physical disability; sexual orientation or gender identity; geographic location; or other characteristics historically linked to discrimination or exclusion.

Health Disparity Population

In 2000, United States Public Law 106–525, also known as the "Minority Health and Health Disparities Research and Education Act," which authorized the National Institute on Minority Health and Health Disparities, provided a legal definition of a health disparity population: "A population is a health disparity population if there is a significant disparity in the overall rate of disease incidence, prevalence, morbidity, mortality, or survival rates in the population as compared to the health status of the general population." Minority Health and Health Disparities Research and Education Act United States Public Law 106–525 (2000), p. 2498

Health Disparities Research

The National Institutes of Health defines health disparities research to include basic, clinical, and social sciences studies that focus on identifying, understanding, preventing, diagnosing, and treating health conditions such as diseases, disorders, and other conditions that are unique to, more serious, or more prevalent in health disparity populations.

Health Equity

The Department of Health and Human Services defines health equity as the attainment of the highest level of health for all people. Achieving health equity requires valuing everyone equally with focused and ongoing societal efforts to address avoidable inequalities, historical and contemporary injustices, and the elimination of health and health care disparities.

Health Literacy

The Centers for Disease Control and Prevention defines health literacy as the degree to which an individual has the capacity to obtain, communicate, process, and understand basic health information and services to make appropriate health decisions.

Cancer Disparities by Racial/Ethnic Groups

African Americans

- For all cancers combined, cancer incidence rates between 2007 through 2011 were the highest overall in black men (587.7 per 100,000 men) compared to any other racial or ethnic group. (NCI)

- African Americans have the highest mortality rate of any racial or ethnic group for all cancers combined and for most major cancers. (DHHS Office of Minority Health- OMH)

- For all cancers combined, the death rate is 25 percent higher for African Americans/blacks than for whites. (NCI)

- African American women with cancer have higher death rates despite them having a lower risk of cancer overall (compared to white women). (ACS)

- African American men have lower 5-year cancer survival rates for lung, colon, and pancreatic cancers compared to non-Hispanic white men. (DHHS OMH)

American Indian and Alaska Native

- Cancer is the second leading cause of death among Native Americans over age 45. (NCI)

- While overall cancer mortality rates from 2001 through 2010 decreased by 1.4 percent per year among whites and by 2.1 percent per year among African Americans/blacks, they decreased by only 0.7 percent per year among American Indians and Alaska Natives.(NCI)

- American Indians and Alaska Natives continue to have the poorest 5-year survival rates among all racial and ethnic groups, for all cancers combined. (NCI)

Asian Americans, Native Hawaiians, and other Pacific Islanders

- Asian Americans and Pacific Islanders have the highest incidence rates for both liver and stomach cancers and are twice as likely to die from these cancers as whites.(NCI) This may be caused by a higher prevalence of infections with hepatitis B virus (liver cancer) and the bacterium H. pylori (stomach cancer). (ACS)

- Native Hawaiians/Pacific Islanders are 30 percent more likely to be diagnosed with cancer compared to non-Hispanic whites. (DHHS OMH)

Hispanics / Latinos

- Hispanics and Latinos have the highest rates for cancers associated with infection, such as liver, stomach, and cervical cancers. Higher prevalence of infection with human papillomavirus (cervical cancer), hepatitis B virus (liver cancer), and the bacterium H. pylori (stomach cancer) in immigrant countries of origin contributes to these disparities. (ACS)

- Although Hispanics and Latinos have lower incidence and death rates for the most common cancers than non-Hispanic whites, they are more likely to be diagnosed with advanced stages of disease. (NCI)

Disparities by Cancer Type

Breast

- Where breast cancer rates stabilized between 2002 and 2011 in non-Hispanic white women, rates continue to increase among African American/black women. (JNCI)

- African American/black women are more likely to die from breast cancer despite white women having higher incidence rates for the disease. (NCI)

- African American women are almost 40 percent more likely to die from breast cancer compared to non-Hispanic white women. (DHHS OMH)

- African American women with breast cancer are less likely than white women to survive five years after diagnosis. The survival rate among African American women is 71 percent, compared to 86 percent among whites. (JNCI)

- Recent NCI-supported research indicates that aggressive breast tumors are more common in younger African American/black and Hispanic/Latino women living in low SES areas. This more aggressive form of breast cancer is less responsive to standard cancer treatments and is associated with poorer survival. (NCI)

- Rates for triple-negative breast cancers (HR-/HER2-) were highest among non-Hispanic black women compared with all other racial/ethnic groups with an age-adjusted rate of 27.2 per 100,000 women; a rate 1.9 times higher than the non-Hispanic white rate, 2.3 times higher than the Hispanic rate, and 2.6 times higher than the non-Hispanic API (NHAPI) rate. (JNCI)

- Overall, compared with non-Hispanic white women, African American/black women are screened less frequently for breast cancer, are more likely to have advanced disease when a diagnosis is made, have a poorer prognosis for a given stage of disease, and have less access to medical care. (NCI)

Cervical

- African American/black women are more likely to be diagnosed with cervical cancer compared to white women in the general U.S. population. (NCI)

- Despite recent declines in cervical cancer overall, African American women with cervical cancer have higher mortality rates than women of any other racial or ethnic group in the United States. (NCI)

- Hispanic women are almost twice as likely to have cervical cancer and 1.4 times more likely to die from cervical cancer as compared to non-Hispanic white women. (DHHS OMH)

- The disproportionate burden of cervical cancer in Hispanic/ Latino and African American women is primarily due to a lack of screening. (NCI)

- Among Asian Americans, incidence rates for cervical cancer are almost three times higher in Vietnamese women than in Chinese and Japanese women. (ACS)

Colorectal

- African Americans have higher mortality rates and higher incidence rates of colorectal cancer than all other racial/ethnic groups, except American Indians/Alaska Natives. (NCI)

Kidney

- Kidney cancer incidence and mortality rates are twice as high in men as in women. (NCI)

- American Indians/Alaska Natives have higher kidney cancer incidence and mortality rates than any other racial/ethnic groups in the United States. (NCI)

- American Indian/Alaska Native women are 40 percent more likely to have kidney/renal pelvis cancer than non-Hispanic white women. (DHHS OMH)

Liver

- The incidence rates of liver cancer for Asian American/Pacific Islander men and women are 2.4 and 2.7 times greater, respectively, than those of non-Hispanic white men and women. (DHHS OMH)

- Both Hispanic men and women are twice as likely to be diagnosed with and to die from liver cancer compared to non-Hispanic whites. (DHHS OMH)

Lung

- African American/black men and women have the highest incidence of lung cancer compared to the general U.S. population. (NCI)

- Mortality rates from lung cancer are highest among African American males than other population groups. (NCI)

Multiple Myeloma

- African Americans have approximately twice the incidence and mortality rates of multiple myeloma than the general U.S. population. (NCI)

Pancreatic

- African Americans have higher rates of pancreatic cancer incidence and mortality than any other racial or ethnic group. (NCI)

Prostate

- One in five (20 percent) African American men will be diagnosed with prostate cancer during their lifetime. (ACS)

- African American men have the highest incidence rate for prostate cancer in the U.S. and are more than twice as likely as white men to die of the disease. (NCI)

- Prostate cancer is the second leading cause of cancer-related deaths among African American men. (ACS)

Stomach

- Incidence rates of stomach cancer are highest in American Indians/Alaska Natives, followed by Hispanics/Latinos, Asian Americans/Pacific Islanders, and African Americans. (ACS)

- Mortality rates from stomach cancer are highest in Asian Americans/Pacific Islanders and African Americans, followed by Hispanics/Latinos, American Indians/Alaska Natives, and whites. (NCI)

- African American women are 2.4 times as likely to be diagnosed with stomach cancer, and 2.5 times as likely to die from stomach cancer, compared to non-Hispanic white women. (DHHS OMH)

- Asian/Pacific Islander men are twice as likely to die from stomach cancer compared to the non-Hispanic white population, and Asian/Pacific Islander women are 2.7 times as likely to die from the same disease. (DHHS OMH)

- Hispanic women are 2.2 times more likely to have stomach cancer compared to non-Hispanic white women. (DHHS OMH)

Part Nine

Additional Help and Information

Chapter 65

National Organizations Offering Cancer-Related Services

Air Charity Network
4620 Haygood Rd., Ste. 1
Virginia Beach, VA 23455
800-296-3797
www.aircharitynetwork.org/
info@angel-flight.org

American Cancer Society
250 Williams St.
Atlanta, GA 30303
800-227-2345; Fax: 866-228-4327
www.cancer.org

American Childhood Cancer Organization
10920 Connecticut Ave., Ste. A
Kensington, MD 20895
855-858-2226
www.acco.org
staff@acco.org

Be the Match
3001 BRd.way St., N.E., Ste. 100
Minneapolis, MN 55413-1753
800-627-7692
www.bethematch.org
patientinfo@nmdp.org

Benefits.gov
800-333-4636
www.benefits.gov/

Camp Kesem
P.O. Box 1113
Culver City, CA 90232
260-225-3736
www.campkesem.org
info@campkesem.org

Cancer Care
275 Seventh Ave., 22nd Fl.
New York, NY 10001
800-813-4673
www.cancercare.org
info@cancercare.org

Cancer Financial Assistance Coalition
www.cancerfac.org/

Caritas Internationalis Headquarters
Palazzo San Calisto
Vatican City State, V-00120
www.caritas.org
caritas.internationalis@caritas.va

Catholic Charities USA
2050 Ballenger Ave., Ste. 400
Alexandria, VA 22314
www.catholiccharitiesusa.org
info@catholiccharitiesusa.org

Children's Brain Tumor Foundation
274 Madison Ave., Ste. 1004
New York, NY 22314
866-228-4673
www.cbtf.org
info@cbtf.org

Children's Health Insurance Program
877-543-7669
www.insurekidsnow.gov/
CMSOCHIPRAQuestions@cms.hhs.gov

Chronic Disease Fund
6900 N.Dallas Pkwy, Ste. 200
Plano, TX 75024
877-968-7233
www.cdfund.org/
info@cdfund.org

Cleaning for a Reason Foundation
211 S. Stemmons, Ste. G
Lewisville, TX 75067
877-968-7233
www.cleaningforareason.org

Colorectal Cancer Control Program
4770 Buford Hwy, NE.
Atlanta, GA 30341
800-232-4636; Fax: 888-232-6348
www.cdc.gov/cancer/crccp
cdcinfo@cdc.gov

Colorectal Care Line
421 Butler Farm Rd.
Hampton, VA 23666
866-657-8634
www.colorectalcareline.org
CCL@patientadvocate.org

Co-Pay Relief Program
421 Butler Farm Rd.
Hampton, VA 23666
866-512-3861
www.copays.org

Corporate Angel Network
Westchester County Airport
White Plains, NY 10604
866-328-1313
www.corpangelnetwork.org
info@corpangelnetwork.org

Eldercare Locator
800-677-1116
www.eldercare.gov
eldercarelocator@n4a.org

Fertile Hope
866-965-7205
www.fertilehope.org

Healthcare.gov
200 Independence Ave., SW.
Washington, DC 20201
www.healthcare.gov/

Health Well Foundation
P.O. Box 4133
Gaithersburg, MD 20878
800-675-8416
www.healthwellfoundation.org
info@healthwellfoundation.org

Hill-Burton Program
5600 Fishers Ln.,
Rm. 10-105
Rockville, MD 20857
800-638-0742
www.hrsa.gov

Hospice Education Institute
Three Unity Sq.
Machiasport, ME 04655
800-331-1620
www.hospiceworld.org
hospiceall@aol.com

**International Cancer
Information Service Group**
www.icisg.org
info@icisg.org

Joe's House
505 E.79th St., Ste. 17E
New York, NY 10075
877-563-7468
www.joeshouse.org
info@joeshouse.org

**Leukemia and Lymphoma
Society**
1311 Mamaroneck Ave., Ste. 310
White Plains, NY 10605
800-955-4572
www.lls.org/
infocenter@lls.org

LIVESTRONG
2201 E. Sixth St.
Austin, TX 78702
855-220-7777
www.livestrong.org

**Lymphoma Research
Foundation**
115 Broadway, Ste. 1301
New York, NY 10006
800-500-9976
www.lymphoma.org
helpline@lymphoma.org

Look Good Feel Better
800-395-5665
www.lookgoodfeelbetter.org/

**Look Good Feel Better for
Teens**
800-395-5665
www.lookgoodfeelbetter.org/

**Medicaid (Medical
Assistance)**
7500 Security Blvd.
Baltimore, MD 21244
877-267-2323
www.cms.gov/MedicaidGenInfo/

Medicare
7500 Security Blvd.
Baltimore, MD 21244
800-633-4227; Fax: 877-486-2048
www.medicare.gov

Melanoma International Foundation
250 Mapleflower Rd.
Glenmoore, PA 19343
866-463-6663
www.safefromthesun.org
cpoole@melanomainternational.org

Mesothelioma Applied Research Foundation
1317 King St.
Alexandria, VA 22314
877-363-6376
www.curemeso.org
info@curemeso.org

National Association of Insurance Commissioners
1100 Walnut St., Ste. 1500
Kansas City, MO 64108
866-470-6242
www.naic.org
help@naic.org

National Breast and Cervical Cancer Early Detection Program
4770 Buford Hwy, NE.
Atlanta, GA 30341
800-232-4636
www.cdc.gov/cancer/nbccedp
cdcinfo@cdc.gov

National Cancer Institute (NCI)
Public Inquiries Office
Ste. 300
6116 Executive Blvd.
MSC8322
Bethesda, MD 20892-8322
1-800-4-CANCER
(1-800-422-6237)
www.cancer.gov

National Lymphedema Network
116 New Montgomery St., Ste. 235
San Francisco, CA 94105
800-541-3259
www.lymphnet.org
nln@lymphnet.org

Needy Meds
P.O. Box 219
Gloucester, MA 01931
800-503-6897
www.needymeds.org
info@needymeds.org

Patient Advocate Foundation
421 Butler Farm Rd.
Hampton, VA 23666
800-532-5274
www.patientadvocate.org
help@patientadvocate.org

Planet Cancer (a LIVESTRONG initiative)
855-220-7777
myplanet.planetcancer.org

Ronald McDonald House Charities
One Kroc Dr.
Oak Brook, IL 60523
www.rmhc.org/
info@rmhc.org

Sarcoma Alliance
Number 334
Mill Valley, CA 94941
www.sarcomaalliance.org
info@sarcomaalliance.org

Sisters Network, Inc.
2922 Rosedale St.
Houston, TX 77004
866-781-1808
www.sistersnetworkinc.org
infonet@sistersnetworkinc.org

Social Security Administration
Windsor Park Bldg.
Baltimore, MD 21235
800-772-1213; Fax: 800-325-0778
www.ssa.gov

State Health Insurance Assistance Program
Centers for Medicare & Medicaid Services
Baltimore, MD 21244

State Pharmaceutical Assistance Programs
7700 E.First Pl.
Denver, CO 80230
800-633-4227
www.ncsl.org

The SAMFund for Young Adult Survivors of Cancer
C/o The Nonprofit Center
Boston, MA 02211
866-439-9365
www.thesamfund.org
info@thesamfund.org

Susan G. Komen for the Cure
5005 LBJ Fwy, Ste. 250
Dallas, TX 75244
877-465-6636
www.komen.org

The National Children's Cancer Society
500 N.Broadway, Ste. 1850
St. Louis, MO 63102
800-532-6459
www.thenccs.org/contact
pbeck@children-cancer.org

The Salvation Army International Headquarters
101 Queen Victoria St.
London
EC4V 4EH
United Kingdom
www.salvationarmy.org
websa@salvationarmy.org

The Salvation Army National Headquarters
615 Slaters Ln.
P.O. Box 269
Alexandria, VA 22313
www.salvationarmyusa.org

The Ulman Cancer Fund for Young Adults
6770 Oak Hall Ln., Unit 116
Columbia, MD 21044
888-393-3863
www.ulmanfund.org
info@ulmanfund.org

U.S. Department of Housing and Urban Development
451 Seventh St., SW.
Washington, DC 20410
800-569-4287; Fax: 202-708-1455
www.hud.gov

Union for International Cancer Control
62 Rt. de Frontenex
Geneva 1207
Switzerland
www.uicc.org
info@uicc.org

United Way Worldwide
701 N.Fairfax St.
Alexandria, VA 22314
www.liveunited.org

United Healthcare Children's Foundation
MN012-S286
Minneapolis, MN 55440
www.uhccf.org

Us TOO International, Inc.
2720 S. River Rd., Ste. 112
Des Plaines, IL 60018
800-808-7866
www.ustoo.org
ustoo@ustoo.org

Young Survival Coalition
61 Broadway, Ste. 2235
New York, NY 10006
877-972-1011
www.youngsurvival.org
info@youngsurvival.org
Category: Breast, International,
Advocacy, Educational
Programs, Peer/Buddy
Programs, Support Groups

Chapter 66

Glossary of Terms Related to Cancer

abdominal ultrasound: A procedure used to examine the organs in the abdomen. An ultrasound transducer (probe) is pressed firmly against the skin of the abdomen. High-energy sound waves from the transducer bounce off tissues and create echoes. The echoes are sent to a computer, which makes a picture called a sonogram. Also called transabdominal ultrasound

abdominoperineal resection: Surgery to remove the anus, the rectum, and part of the sigmoid colon through an incision made in the abdomen. The end of the intestine is attached to an opening in the surface of the abdomen and body waste is collected in a disposable bag outside of the body. This opening is called a colostomy. Lymph nodes that contain cancer may also be removed during this operation.

ablation: In medicine, the removal or destruction of a body part or tissue or its function. Ablation may be performed by surgery, hormones, drugs, radio frequency, heat, or other methods.

abnormal: Not normal. An abnormal lesion or growth may be cancer, premalignant (likely to become cancer), or benign (not cancer).

actinic keratosis: A thick, scaly patch of skin that may become cancer. It usually forms on areas exposed to the sun, such as the face, scalp, back of the hands, or chest. It is most common in people with fair skin. Also called senile keratosis and solar keratosis.

active surveillance: Closely watching a patient's condition but not giving treatment unless there are changes in test results. Active surveillance avoids problems that may be caused by treatments such as radiation or surgery. It is used to find early signs that the condition is getting worse. During active surveillance, patients will be given certain exams and tests done on a regular schedule. It is sometimes used in prostate cancer. It is a type of expectant management.

acute: Symptoms or signs that begin and worsen quickly; not chronic.

adenocarcinoma: Cancer that begins in cells that line certain internal organs and that have gland-like (secretory) properties.

adenoma: A tumor that is not cancer. It starts in gland-like cells of the epithelial tissue (thin layer of tissue that covers organs, glands, and other structures within the body).

adjuvant therapy: Additional cancer treatment given after the primary treatment to lower the risk that the cancer will come back. Adjuvant therapy may include chemotherapy, radiation therapy, hormone therapy, targeted therapy, or biological therapy.

antiandrogen: A substance that prevents cells from making or using androgens (hormones that play a role in the formation of male sex characteristics). Antiandrogens may stop some cancer cells from growing. Some antiandrogens are used to treat prostate cancer, and others are being studied for this use. An antiandrogen is a type of hormone antagonist.

advance directive: A legal document that states the treatment or care a person wishes to receive or not receive if he or she becomes unable to make medical decisions (for example, due to being unconscious or in a coma). Some types of advance directives are living wills and do-not-resuscitate (DNR) orders.

advanced cancer: Cancer that has spread to other places in the body and usually cannot be cured or controlled with treatment.

aggressive: In medicine, describes a tumor or disease that forms, grows, or spreads quickly. It may also describe treatment that is more severe or intense than usual.

alopecia: The lack or loss of hair from areas of the body where hair is usually found. Alopecia can be a side effect of some cancer treatments.

anal cancer: Cancer that forms in tissues of the anus. The anus is the opening of the rectum (last part of the large intestine) to the outside of the body.

anaplastic: A term used to describe cancer cells that divide rapidly and have little or no resemblance to normal cells.

angiogenesis inhibitor: A substance that may prevent the formation of blood vessels. In anticancer therapy, an angiogenesis inhibitor may prevent the growth of new blood vessels that tumors need to grow.

angiosarcoma: A type of cancer that begins in the cells that line blood vessels or lymph vessels. Cancer that begins in blood vessels is called hemangiosarcoma. Cancer that begins in lymph vessels is called lymphangiosarcoma.

anorexia: An abnormal loss of the appetite for food. Anorexia can be caused by cancer, AIDS, a mental disorder (anorexia nervosa), or other diseases.

astrocytoma: A tumor that begins in the brain or spinal cord in small, star-shaped cells called astrocytes.

asymptomatic: Having no signs or symptoms of disease.

axillary: Pertaining to the armpit area, including the lymph nodes that are located there.

axillary lymph node: A lymph node in the armpit region that drains lymph from the breast and nearby areas.

Barrett esophagus: A condition in which the cells lining the lower part of the esophagus have changed or been replaced with abnormal cells that could lead to cancer of the esophagus. The backing up of stomach contents (reflux) may irritate the esophagus and, over time, cause Barrett esophagus.

basal cell: A small, round cell found in the lower part (or base) of the epidermis, the outer layer of the skin.

basal cell carcinoma: Cancer that begins in the lower part of the epidermis (the outer layer of the skin). It may appear as a small white or flesh-colored bump that grows slowly and may bleed. Basal cell carcinomas are usually found on areas of the body exposed to the sun. Basal cell carcinomas rarely metastasize (spread) to other parts of the body. They are the most common form of skin cancer.

benign: Not cancerous. Benign tumors may grow larger but do not spread to other parts of the body. Also called nonmalignant.

benign prostatic hyperplasia: A benign (not cancer) condition in which an overgrowth of prostate tissue pushes against the urethra and the bladder, blocking the flow of urine. Also called benign prostatic hypertrophy and BPH.

bile duct cancer: Cancer that forms in a bile duct. A bile duct is a tube that carries bile (fluid made by the liver that helps digest fat) between the liver and gallbladder and the intestine. Bile ducts include the common hepatic, cystic, and common bile ducts. Bile duct cancer may be found inside the liver (intrahepatic) or outside the liver (extrahepatic).

biliary: Having to do with the liver, bile ducts, and/or gallbladder.

biopsy: The removal of cells or tissues for examination by a pathologist. The pathologist may study the tissue under a microscope or perform other tests on the cells or tissue. There are many different types of biopsy procedures. The most common types include: (1) incisional biopsy, in which only a sample of tissue is removed; (2) excisional biopsy, in which an entire lump or suspicious area is removed; and (3) needle biopsy, in which a sample of tissue or fluid is removed with a needle. When a wide needle is used, the procedure is called a core biopsy. When a thin needle is used, the procedure is called a fine-needle aspiration biopsy.

bladder cancer: Cancer that forms in tissues of the bladder (the organ that stores urine). Most bladder cancers are transitional cell carcinomas (cancer that begins in cells that normally make up the inner lining of the bladder). Other types include squamous cell carcinoma (cancer that begins in thin, flat cells) and adenocarcinoma (cancer that begins in cells that make and release mucus and other fluids). The cells that form squamous cell carcinoma and adenocarcinoma develop in the inner lining of the bladder as a result of chronic irritation and inflammation.

bone cancer: Primary bone cancer is cancer that forms in cells of the bone. Some types of primary bone cancer are osteosarcoma, Ewing sarcoma, malignant fibrous histiocytoma, and chondrosarcoma. Secondary bone cancer is cancer that spreads to the bone from another part of the body (such as the prostate, breast, or lung).

brachytherapy: A type of radiation therapy in which radioactive material sealed in needles, seeds, wires, or catheters is placed directly into or near a tumor. Also called implant radiation therapy, internal radiation therapy, and radiation brachytherapy.

brain tumor: The growth of abnormal cells in the tissues of the brain. Brain tumors can be benign (not cancer) or malignant (cancer).

BRCA1: A gene on chromosome 17 that normally helps to suppress cell growth. A person who inherits certain mutations (changes) in a

BRCA1 gene has a higher risk of getting breast, ovarian, prostate, and other types of cancer.

BRCA2: A gene on chromosome 13 that normally helps to suppress cell growth. A person who inherits certain mutations (changes) in a BRCA2 gene has a higher risk of getting breast, ovarian, prostate, and other types of cancer.

breast cancer: Cancer that forms in tissues of the breast, usually the ducts (tubes that carry milk to the nipple) and lobules (glands that make milk). It occurs in both men and women, although male breast cancer is rare.

breast carcinoma in situ: There are two types of breast carcinoma in situ: ductal carcinoma in situ (DCIS) and lobular carcinoma in situ (LCIS). DCIS is a noninvasive condition in which abnormal cells are found in the lining of a breast duct (a tube that carries milk to the nipple). The abnormal cells have not spread outside the duct to other tissues in the breast. In some cases, DCIS may become invasive cancer and spread to other tissues, although it is not known how to predict which lesions will become invasive cancer. LCIS is a condition in which abnormal cells are found in the lobules (small sections of tissue involved with making milk) of the breast. This condition seldom becomes invasive cancer; however, having LCIS in one breast increases the risk of developing breast Also called stage 0 breast carcinoma in situ.

breast-conserving surgery: An operation to remove the breast cancer but not the breast itself. Types of breast-conserving surgery include lumpectomy (removal of the lump), quadrantectomy (removal of one quarter, or quadrant, of the breast), and segmental mastectomy (removal of the cancer as well as some of the breast tissue around the tumor and the lining over the chest muscles below the tumor). Also called breast-sparing surgery.

breast reconstruction: Surgery to rebuild the shape of the breast after a mastectomy.

breast self-exam: An exam by a woman of her breasts to check for lumps or other changes.

bronchoscopy: A procedure that uses a bronchoscope to examine the inside of the trachea, bronchi (air passages that lead to the lungs), and lungs. A bronchoscope is a thin, tube-like instrument with a light and a lens for viewing. It may also have a tool to remove tissue to be checked under a microscope for signs of disease. The bronchoscope is inserted through the nose or mouth. Bronchoscopy may be used to detect cancer or to perform some treatment procedures.

bronchus: A large airway that leads from the trachea (windpipe) to a lung. The plural of bronchus is bronchi.

CA 19-9: A substance released into the bloodstream by both cancer cells and normal cells. Too much CA 19-9 in the blood can be a sign of pancreatic cancer or other types of cancer or conditions. The amount of CA 19-9 in the blood can be used to help keep track of how well cancer treatments are working or if cancer has come back. It is a type of tumor marker.

CA-125: A substance that may be found in high amounts in the blood of patients with certain types of cancer, including ovarian cancer. CA-125 levels may also help monitor how well cancer treatments are working or if cancer has come back. Also called cancer antigen 125.

cachexia: Loss of body weight and muscle mass, and weakness that may occur in patients with cancer, AIDS, or other chronic diseases.

cancer: A term for diseases in which abnormal cells divide without control and can invade nearby tissues. Cancer cells can also spread to other parts of the body through the blood and lymph systems. There are several main types of cancer. Carcinoma is a cancer that begins in the skin or in tissues that line or cover internal organs. Sarcoma is a cancer that begins in bone, cartilage, fat, muscle, blood vessels, or other connective or supportive tissue. Leukemia is a cancer that starts in blood-forming tissue such as the bone marrow, and causes large numbers of abnormal blood cells to be produced and enter the blood. Lymphoma and multiple myeloma are cancers that begin in the cells of the immune system. Central nervous system cancers are cancers that begin in the tissues of the brain and spinal cord. Also called malignancy.

cancer of unknown primary origin: A case in which cancer cells are found in the body, but the place where the cells first started growing (the origin or primary site) cannot be determined. Also called carcinoma of unknown primary and CUP.

carcinoembryonic antigen: A substance that is sometimes found in an increased amount in the blood of people who have certain cancers, other diseases, or who smoke. It is used as a tumor marker for colorectal cancer. Also called CEA.

carcinogen: Any substance that causes cancer.

carcinoid: A slow-growing type of tumor usually found in the gas-tro-intestinal system (most often in the appendix), and sometimes in the lungs or other sites. Carcinoid tumors may spread to the liver or other sites in the body, and they may secrete substances such as serotonin or prostaglandins, causing carcinoid syndrome.

carcinoma: Cancer that begins in the skin or in tissues that line or cover internal organs.

carcinoma in situ: A group of abnormal cells that remain in the place where they first formed. They have not spread. These abnormal cells may become cancer and spread into nearby normal tissue. Also called stage 0 disease.

carcinosarcoma: A malignant tumor that is a mixture of carcinoma (cancer of epithelial tissue, which is skin and tissue that lines or covers the internal organs) and sarcoma (cancer of connective tissue, such as bone, cartilage, and fat).

cervical cancer: Cancer that forms in tissues of the cervix (the organ connecting the uterus and vagina). It is usually a slow-growing cancer that may not have symptoms but can be found with regular Pap tests (a procedure in which cells are scraped from the cervix and looked at under a microscope). Cervical cancer is almost always caused by human papillomavirus (HPV) infection.

cervical intraepithelial neoplasia: Growth of abnormal cells on the surface of the cervix. Numbers from one to three may be used to describe how abnormal the cells are and how much of the cervical tissue is involved.

chemoprevention: The use of drugs, vitamins, or other agents to try to reduce the risk of, or delay the development or recurrence of, cancer.

chemotherapy: Treatment with drugs that kill cancer cells.

cholangiocarcinoma: A rare type of cancer that develops in cells that line the bile ducts in the liver. Cancer that forms where the right and left ducts meet is called Klatskin tumor.

chondrosarcoma: A type of cancer that forms in bone cartilage. It usually starts in the pelvis (between the hip bones), the shoulder, the ribs, or at the ends of the long bones of the arms and legs. A rare type of chondrosarcoma called extraskeletal chondrosarcoma does not form in bone cartilage. Instead, it forms in the soft tissues of the upper part of the arms and legs. Chondrosarcoma can occur at any age but is more common in people older than 40 years. It is a type of bone cancer.

chronic: A disease or condition that persists or progresses over a long period of time.

clinical stage: The stage of cancer (amount or spread of cancer in the body) that is based on tests that are done before surgery. These include physical exams, imaging tests, laboratory tests (such as blood tests), and biopsies.

colon cancer: Cancer that forms in the tissues of the colon (the longest part of the large intestine). Most colon cancers are adenocarcinomas (cancers that begin in cells that make and release mucus and other fluids).

colon polyp: An abnormal growth of tissue in the lining of the bowel. Polyps are a risk factor for colon cancer.

colonoscopy: Examination of the inside of the colon using a colonoscope, inserted into the rectum. A colonoscope is a thin, tube-like instrument with a light and a lens for viewing. It may also have a tool to remove tissue to be checked under a microscope for signs of disease.

colorectal cancer: Cancer that develops in the colon (the longest part of the large intestine) and/or the rectum (the last several inches of the large intestine before the anus).

colostomy: An opening into the colon from the outside of the body. A colostomy provides a new path for waste material to leave the body after part of the colon has been removed.

colposcopy: Examination of the vagina and cervix using a lighted magnifying instrument called a colposcope.

comfort care: Care given to improve the quality of life of patients who have a serious or life-threatening disease. The goal of comfort care is to prevent or treat as early as possible the symptoms of a disease, side effects caused by treatment of a disease, and psychological, social, and spiritual problems related to a disease or its treatment. Also called palliative care, supportive care, and symptom management.

condyloma: A raised growth on the surface of the genitals caused by human papillomavirus (HPV) infection. The HPV in condyloma is very contagious and can be spread by skin-to-skin contact, usually during oral, anal, or genital sex with an infected partner. Also called genital wart.

cone biopsy: Surgery to remove a cone-shaped piece of tissue from the cervix and cervical canal. Cone biopsy may be used to diagnose or treat a cervical condition. Also called conization.

core biopsy: The removal of a tissue sample with a wide needle for examination under a microscope. Also called core needle biopsy.

corpus: The body of the uterus.

cryosurgery: A procedure in which tissue is frozen to destroy abnormal cells. Liquid nitrogen or liquid carbon dioxide is used to freeze the tissue. Also called cryoablation and cryosurgical ablation.

cyst: A sac or capsule in the body. It may be filled with fluid or other material.

cystectomy: Surgery to remove all or part of the bladder (the organ that holds urine) or to remove a cyst (a sac or capsule in the body).

D&C: A procedure to remove tissue from the cervical canal or the inner lining of the uterus. The cervix is dilated (made larger) and a curette (spoon-shaped instrument) is inserted into the uterus to remove tissue. Also called dilatation and curettage and dilation and curettage.

diethylstilbestrol: A synthetic form of the hormone estrogen that was prescribed to pregnant women between about 1940 and 1971 because it was thought to prevent miscarriages. Diethylstilbestrol may increase the risk of uterine, ovarian, or breast cancer in women who took it. It also has been linked to an increased risk of clear cell carcinoma of the vagina or cervix in daughters exposed to diethylstilbestrol before birth. Also called DES.

digital mammography: The use of a computer, rather than x-ray film, to create a picture of the breast.

digital rectal examination: An examination in which a doctor inserts a lubricated, gloved finger into the rectum to feel for abnormalities. Also called DRE.

ductal carcinoma in situ: A noninvasive condition in which abnormal cells are found in the lining of a breast duct. The abnormal cells have not spread outside the duct to other tissues in the breast. In some cases, ductal carcinoma in situ may become invasive cancer and spread to other tissues, although it is not known at this time how to predict which lesions will become invasive. Also called DCIS and intraductal carcinoma.

dysplasia: Cells that look abnormal under a microscope but are not cancer.

early-stage cancer: A term used to describe cancer that is early in its growth, and may not have spread to other parts of the body. What is called early stage may differ between cancer types.

edema: Swelling caused by excess fluid in body tissues.

embryonal tumor: A mass of rapidly growing cells that begins in embryonic (fetal) tissue. Embryonal tumors may be benign or alignant, and include neuroblastomas and Wilms tumors. Also called embryoma.

endocrine cancer: Cancer that occurs in endocrine tissue, the tissue in the body that secretes hormones.

endometrial biopsy: A procedure in which a sample of tissue is taken from the endometrium (inner lining of the uterus) for examination under a microscope. A thin tube is inserted through the cervix into the uterus, and gentle scraping and suction are used to remove the sample.

endometrial cancer: Cancer that forms in the tissue lining the uterus (the small, hollow, pear-shaped organ in a woman's pelvis in which a fetus develops). Most endometrial cancers are adenocarcinomas (cancers that begin in cells that make and release mucus and other fluids).

endoscopy: A procedure that uses an endoscope to examine the inside of the body. An endoscope is a thin, tube-like instrument with a light and a lens for viewing. It may also have a tool to remove tissue to be checked under a microscope for signs of disease.

enucleation: In medicine, the removal of an organ or tumor in such a way that it comes out clean and whole, like a nut from its shell.

ependymoma: A type of brain tumor that begins in cells lining the spinal cord central canal (fluid-filled space down the center) or the ventricles (fluid-filled spaces of the brain). Ependymomas may also form in the choroid plexus (tissue in the ventricles that makes cere brospinal fluid). Also called ependymal tumor.

esophageal cancer: Cancer that forms in tissues lining the esophagus (the muscular tube through which food passes from the throat to the stomach). Two types of esophageal cancer are squamous cell carcinoma (cancer that begins in flat cells lining the esophagus) and adenocarcinoma (cancer that begins in cells that make and release mucus and other fluids).

estrogen receptor: A protein found inside the cells of the female reproductive tissue, some other types of tissue, and some cancer cells. The hormone estrogen will bind to the receptors inside the cells and may cause the cells to grow. Also called ER.

Ewing sarcoma family of tumors: A group of cancers that includes Ewing tumor of bone (ETB or Ewing sarcoma of bone), extraosseous Ewing (EOE) tumors, primitive neuroectoderma tumors (PNET or peripheral neuroepithelioma), and Askin tumors (PNET of the chest wall). These tumors all come from the same type of stem cell. Also called EFTs.

excisional biopsy: A surgical procedure in which an entire lump or suspicious area is removed for diagnosis. The tissue is then examined under a microscope.

extracranial germ cell tumor: A rare cancer that forms in germ cells in the testicle or ovary, or in germ cells that have traveled to areas of the body other than the brain (such as the chest, abdomen, or tailbone). Germ cells are reproductive cells that develop into sperm in males and eggs in females.

extrahepatic bile duct cancer: A rare cancer that forms in the part of the bile duct that is outside the liver. The bile duct is the tube that collects bile from the liver and joins a duct from the gallbladder to form the common bile duct, which carries bile into the small intestine when food is being digested.

extrapleural pneumonectomy: Surgery to remove a diseased lung, part of the pericardium (membrane covering the heart), part of the diaphragm (muscle between the lungs and the abdomen), and part of the parietal pleura (membrane lining the chest). This type of surgery is used most often to treat malignant mesothelioma.

eye cancer: Cancer that forms in tissues of and around the eye. Some of the cancers that may affect the eye include melanoma (a rare cancer that begins in cells that make the pigment melanin in the eye), carcinoma (cancer that begins in tissues that cover structures in the eye), lymphoma (cancer that begins in immune system cells), and retinoblastoma (cancer that begins in the retina and usually occurs in children younger than five years).

false-negative test result: A test result that indicates that a person does not have a specific disease or condition when the person actually does have the disease or condition.

false-positive test result: A test result that indicates that a person has a specific disease or condition when the person actually does not have the disease or condition.

familial cancer: Cancer that occurs in families more often than would be expected by chance. These cancers often occur at an early age, and may indicate the presence of a gene mutation that increases the risk of cancer. They may also be a sign of shared environmental or lifestyle factors.

family medical history: A record of the relationships among family members along with their medical histories. This includes current and past illnesses. A family medical history may show a pattern of certain diseases in a family.

fine-needle aspiration biopsy: The removal of tissue or fluid with a thin needle for examination under a microscope. Also called FNA biopsy.

first-degree relative: The parents, brothers, sisters, or children of an individual.

gallbladder cancer: Cancer that forms in tissues of the gallbladder. The gallbladder is a pear-shaped organ below the liver that collects and stores bile (a fluid made by the liver to digest fat). Gallbladder cancer begins in the innermost layer of tissue and spreads through the outer layers as it grows.

gastric cancer: Cancer that forms in tissues lining the stomach. Also called stomach cancer.

gastrinoma: A tumor that causes overproduction of gastric acid. It usually begins in the duodenum (first part of the small intestine that connects to the stomach) or the islet cells of the pancreas. Rarely, it may also begin in other organs, including the stomach, liver, jejunum (the middle part of the small intestine), biliary tract (organs and ducts that make and store bile), mesentery, or heart. It is a type of neuro-endocrine tumor, and it may metastasize (spread) to the liver and the lymph nodes.

gastrointestinal carcinoid tumor: An indolent (slow-growing) cancer that forms in cells that make hormones in the lining of the gastrointestinal tract (the stomach and intestines). It usually occurs in the appendix (a small fingerlike pouch of the large intestine), small intestine, or rectum. Having gastrointestinal carcinoid tumor increases the risk of forming other cancers of the digestive system.

gastrointestinal stromal tumor: A type of tumor that usually begins in cells in the wall of the gastrointestinal tract. It can be benign or malignant. Also called GIST.

gene therapy: Treatment that alters a gene. In studies of gene therapy for cancer, researchers are trying to improve the body's natural ability to fight the disease or to make the cancer cells more sensitive to other kinds of therapy.

germ cell tumor: A type of tumor that begins in the cells that give rise to sperm or eggs. Germ cell tumors can occur almost anywhere in the body and can be either benign or malignant.

gestational trophoblastic tumor: Any of a group of tumors that develops from trophoblastic cells (cells that help an embryo attach to the uterus and help form the placenta) after fertilization of an egg by a sperm. The two main types of gestational trophoblastic tumors are hydatidiform mole and choriocarcinoma.

glioblastoma: A fast-growing type of central nervous system tumor that forms from glial (supportive) tissue of the brain and spinal cord and has cells that look very different from normal cells. Glioblastoma usually occurs in adults and affects the brain more often than the spinal cord. Also called GBM, glioblastoma multiforme, and grade IV astrocytoma.

grading: A system for classifying cancer cells in terms of how abnormal they appear when examined under a microscope. The objective of a grading system is to provide information about the probable growth rate of the tumor and its tendency to spread. The systems used to grade tumors vary with each type of cancer. Grading plays a role in treatment decisions.

hamartoma: A benign (not cancer) growth made up of an abnormal mixture of cells and tissues normally found in the area of the body where the growth occurs.

Helicobacter pylori: A type of bacterium that causes inflammation and ulcers in the stomach or small intestine. People with H. pylori infections may be more likely to develop cancer in the stomach, including MALT (mucosa-associated lymphoid tissue) lymphoma.

hematologic cancer: A cancer of the blood or bone marrow, such as leukemia or lymphoma.

hepatocellular carcinoma: A type of adenocarcinoma and the most common type of liver tumor.

HER2/neu: A protein involved in normal cell growth. It is found on some types of cancer cells, including breast and ovarian. Cancer cells removed from the body may be tested for the presence of HER2/neu to help decide the best type of treatment. HER2/neu is a type of receptor tyrosine kinase. Also called c-erbB-2, human EGF receptor 2, and human epidermal growth factor receptor 2.

hereditary nonpolyposis colon cancer: An inherited disorder in which affected individuals have a higher-than-normal chance of developing colorectal cancer and certain other types of cancer, often before the age of 50. Also called HNPCC and Lynch syndrome.

high-dose chemotherapy: An intensive drug treatment to kill cancer cells, but that also destroys the bone marrow and can cause other severe side effects. High-dose chemotherapy is usually followed by bone marrow or stem cell transplantation to rebuild the bone marrow.

high-dose radiation: An amount of radiation that is greater than that given in typical radiation therapy. High-dose radiation is precisely directed at the tumor to avoid damaging healthy tissue, and may kill more cancer cells in fewer treatments.

Hodgkin lymphoma: A cancer of the immune system that is marked by the presence of a type of cell called the Reed-Sternberg cell. The two major types of Hodgkin lymphoma are classical Hodgkin lymphoma and nodular lymphocyte-predominant Hodgkin lymphoma. Symptoms include the painless enlargement of lymph nodes, spleen, or other immune tissue. Other symptoms include fever, weight loss, fatigue, or night sweats. Also called Hodgkin disease.

hormone: One of many chemicals made by glands in the body. Hormones circulate in the bloodstream and control the actions of certain cells or organs. Some hormones can also be made in the laboratory.

hormone receptor: A cell protein that binds a specific hormone. The hormone receptor may be on the surface of the cell or inside the cell. Many changes take place in a cell after a hormone binds to its receptor.

hospice: A program that provides special care for people who are near the end of life and for their families, either at home, in freestanding facilities, or within hospitals.

hydatidiform mole: A slow-growing tumor that develops from tropho blastic cells (cells that help an embryo attach to the uterus and help form the placenta) after fertilization of an egg by a sperm. A hydatidiform mole contains many cysts (sacs of fluid). It is usually benign (not cancer) but it may spread to nearby tissues (invasive mole). It may also become a malignant tumor called choriocarcinoma. Hydatidiform mole is the most common type of gestational trophoblastic tumor. Also called molar pregnancy.

hyperfractionated radiation therapy: Radiation treatment in which the total dose of radiation is divided into small doses and treatments are given more than once a day. Also called hyperfractionation and superfractionated radiation therapy.

hypopharyngeal cancer: Cancer that forms in tissues of the hypopharynx (the bottom part of the throat). The most common type is squamous cell carcinoma (cancer that begins in flat cells lining the hypopharynx).

hysterectomy: Surgery to remove the uterus and, sometimes, the cervix. When the uterus and the cervix are removed, it is called a total hysterectomy. When only the uterus is removed, it is called a partial hysterectomy.

idiopathic: Describes a disease of unknown cause.

imaging: In medicine, a process that makes pictures of areas inside the body. Imaging uses methods such as x-rays (high-energy radiation),ultrasound (high-energy sound waves), and radio waves.

immunosuppression: Suppression of the body's immune system and its ability to fight infections and other diseases. Immunosuppression may be deliberately induced with drugs, as in preparation for bone marrow or other organ transplantation, to prevent rejection of the donor tissue. It may also result from certain diseases such as AIDS or lymphoma or from anticancer drugs.

immunotherapy: Treatment to boost or restore the ability of the immune system to fight cancer, infections, and other diseases. Also used to lessen certain side effects that may be caused by some cancer treatments. Agents used in immunotherapy include monoclonal antibodies, growth factors, and vaccines. These agents may also have a direct antitumor effect. Also called biological response modifier therapy, biological therapy, biotherapy, and BRM therapy.

in situ: In its original place. For example, in carcinoma in situ, abnormal cells are found only in the place where they first formed. They have not spread.

in vitro: In the laboratory (outside the body). The opposite of in vivo (in the body).

indolent: A type of cancer that grows slowly.

inflammatory breast cancer: A type of breast cancer in which the breast looks red and swollen and feels warm. The skin of the breast may also show the pitted appearance called peau d'orange (like the skin of an orange). The redness and warmth occur because the cancer cells block the lymph vessels in the skin.

informed consent: A process in which a person is given important facts about a medical procedure or treatment, a clinical trial, or genetic testing before deciding whether or not to participate. It also includes informing the patient when there is new information that may affect his or her decision to continue. Informed consent includes information about the possible risks, benefits, and limits of the procedure, treatment, trial, or genetic testing.

insulinoma: An abnormal mass that grows in the beta cells of the pancreas that make insulin. Insulinomas are usually benign (not cancer). They secrete insulin and are the most common cause of low blood sugar caused by having too much insulin in the body. Also called beta cell neoplasm, beta cell tumor of the pancreas, and pancreatic insulin-producing tumor.

interferon: A biological response modifier (a substance that can improve the body's natural response to infections and other diseases). Interferons interfere with the division of cancer cells and can slow tumor growth. There are several types of interferons, including interferon-alpha, -beta, and -gamma. The body normally produces these substances. They are also made in the laboratory to treat cancer and other diseases.

interleukin: One of a group of related proteins made by leukocytes (white blood cells) and other cells in the body. Interleukins regulate immune responses. Interleukins made in the laboratory are used as biological response modifiers to boost the immune system in cancer therapy. Also called IL.

intraductal carcinoma: A noninvasive condition in which abnormal cells are found in the lining of a breast duct. The abnormal cells have not spread outside the duct to other tissues in the breast. In some cases, intraductal carcinoma may become invasive cancer and spread to other tissues, although it is not known at this time how to predict which lesions will become invasive. Also called DCIS and ductal carcinoma in situ.

islet cell carcinoma: A rare cancer that forms in the islets of Langerhans cells (a type of cell found in the pancreas). Also called pancreatic endocrine cancer.

islet cell tumor: A mass of abnormal cells that forms in the endocrine (hormone-producing) tissues of the pancreas. Islet cell tumors may be benign (not cancer) or malignant (cancer).

invasive cancer: Cancer that has spread beyond the layer of tissue in which it developed and is growing into surrounding, healthy tissues. Also called infiltrating cancer.

investigational: In clinical trials, refers to a drug (including a new drug, dose, combination, or route of administration) or procedure that has undergone basic laboratory testing and received approval from the U.S. Food and Drug Administration (FDA) to be tested in human subjects. A drug or procedure may be approved by the FDA for use in one disease or condition, but be considered investigational in other diseases or conditions. Also called experimental.

jaundice: A condition in which the skin and the whites of the eyes become yellow, urine darkens, and the color of stool becomes lighter than normal. Jaundice occurs when the liver is not working properly or when a bile duct is blocked

Kaposi sarcoma: A type of cancer characterized by the abnormal growth of blood vessels that develop into skin lesions or occur internally.

kidney cancer: Cancer that forms in tissues of the kidneys. Kidney cancer includes renal cell carcinoma (cancer that forms in the lining of very small tubes in the kidney that filter the blood and remove waste products) and renal pelvis carcinoma (cancer that forms in the center of the kidney where urine collects). It also includes Wilms tumor, which is a type of kidney cancer that usually develops in children under the age of five.

Klatskin tumor: Cancer that develops in cells that line the bile ducts in the liver, where the right and left ducts meet. It is a type of cholangiocarcinoma.

Klinefelter syndrome: A genetic disorder in males caused by having one or more extra X chromosomes. Males with this disorder may have larger than normal breasts, a lack of facial and body hair, a rounded body type, and small testicles. They may learn to speak much later than other children and may have difficulty learning to read and write. Klinefelter syndrome increases the risk of developing extragonadal germ cell tumors and breast cancer.

large cell carcinoma: Lung cancer in which the cells are large and look abnormal when viewed under a microscope.

large intestine: The long, tube-like organ that is connected to the small intestine at one end and the anus at the other. The large intestine has four parts: cecum, colon, rectum, and anal canal. Partly digested food moves through the cecum into the colon, where water and some nutrients and electrolytes are removed. The remaining material, solid waste called stool, moves through the colon, is stored in the rectum, and leaves the body through the anal canal and anus.

laryngeal cancer: Cancer that forms in tissues of the larynx (area of the throat that contains the vocal cords and is used for breathing, swallowing, and talking). Most laryngeal cancers are squamous cell carcinomas (cancer that begins in flat cells lining the larynx).

laryngectomy: An operation to remove all or part of the larynx (voicebox).

laser therapy: Treatment that uses intense, narrow beams of light to cut and destroy tissue, such as cancer tissue. Laser therapy may also be used to reduce lymphedema (swelling caused by a buildup of lymph fluid in tissue) after breast cancer surgery.

late effects: Side effects of cancer treatment that appear months or years after treatment has ended. Late effects include physical and mental problems and second cancers.

late-stage cancer: A term used to describe cancer that is far along in its growth, and has spread to the lymph nodes or other places in the body.

leukemia: Cancer that starts in blood-forming tissue such as the bone marrow and causes large numbers of blood cells to be produced and enter the bloodstream.

leukoplakia: An abnormal patch of white tissue that forms on mucous membranes in the mouth and other areas of the body. It may become cancer. Tobacco (smoking and chewing) and alcohol may increase the risk of leukoplakia in the mouth.

liver cancer: Primary liver cancer is cancer that forms in the tissues of the liver. Secondary liver cancer is cancer that spreads to the liver from another part of the body.

liver function test: A blood test to measure the blood levels of certain substances released by the liver. A high or low level of certain substances can be a sign of liver disease.

living will: A type of legal advance directive in which a person describes specific treatment guidelines that are to be followed by healthcare providers if he or she becomes terminally ill and cannot communicate. A living will usually has instructions about whether to use aggressive medical treatment to keep a person alive (such as CPR, artificial nutrition, use of a respirator).

lobe: A portion of an organ, such as the liver, lung, breast, thyroid, or brain.

lobectomy: Surgery to remove a whole lobe (section) of an organ (such as the lungs, liver, brain, or thyroid gland).

lobular carcinoma in situ: A condition in which abnormal cells are found in the lobules of the breast. Lobular carcinoma in situ seldom becomes invasive cancer; however, having it in one breast increases the risk of developing breast cancer in either breast. Also called LCIS.

lobule: A small lobe or a subdivision of a lobe.

local anesthesia: A temporary loss of feeling in one small area of the body caused by special drugs or other substances called anesthetics. The patient stays awake but has no feeling in the area of the body treated with the anesthetic.

local therapy: Treatment that affects cells in the tumor and the area close to it.

localized: Restricted to the site of origin, without evidence of spread.

loop electrosurgical excision procedure: A technique that uses electric current passed through a thin wire loop to remove abnormal tissue. Also called LEEP and loop excision.

low grade: A term used to describe cells that look nearly normal under a microscope. These cells are less likely to grow and spread more quickly than cells in high-grade cancer or in growths that may become cancer.

lower GI series: X-rays of the colon and rectum that are taken after a person is given a barium enema.

lumbar puncture: A procedure in which a thin needle called a spinal needle is put into the lower part of the spinal column to collect cerebrospinal fluid or to give drugs. Also called spinal tap.

lumpectomy: Surgery to remove abnormal tissue or cancer from the breast and a small amount of normal tissue around it. It is a type of breast-sparing surgery.

lung biopsy: The removal of a small piece of lung tissue to be checked by a pathologist for cancer or other diseases. The tissue may be removed using a bronchoscope (a thin, lighted, tube-like instrument that is inserted through the trachea and into the lung). It may also be removed using a fine needle inserted through the chest wall, by surgery guided by a video camera inserted through the chest wall, or by an open biopsy. In an open biopsy, a doctor makes an incision between the ribs, removes a sample of lung tissue, and closes the wound with stitches.

lung cancer: Cancer that forms in tissues of the lung, usually in the cells lining air passages. The two main types are small cell lung cancer and non-small cell lung cancer. These types are diagnosed based on how the cells look under a microscope.

lung function test: A test used to measure how well the lungs work. It measures how much air the lungs can hold and how quickly air is moved into and out of the lungs. It also measures how much oxygen is used and how much carbon dioxide is given off during breathing. A lung function test can be used to diagnose a lung disease and to see how well treatment for the disease is working. Also called PFT and pulmonary function test.

lung metastasis: Cancer that has spread from the original (primary) tumor to the lung.

lymph node: A rounded mass of lymphatic tissue that is surrounded by a capsule of connective tissue. Lymph nodes filter lymph (lymphatic fluid), and they store lymphocytes (white blood cells). They are located along lymphatic vessels. Also called lymph gland.

lymph node dissection: A surgical procedure in which the lymph nodes are removed and a sample of tissue is checked under a microscope for signs of cancer. For a regional lymph node dissection, some of the lymph nodes in the tumor area are removed; for a radical lymph node dissection, most or all of the lymph nodes in the tumor area are removed. Also called lymphadenectomy.

lymphatic system: The tissues and organs that produce, store, and carry white blood cells that fight infections and other diseases. This system includes the bone marrow, spleen, thymus, lymph nodes, and lymphatic vessels (a network of thin tubes that carry lymph and white blood cells). Lymphatic vessels branch, like blood vessels, into all the tissues of the body.

lymphedema: A condition in which extra lymph fluid builds up in tissues and causes swelling. It may occur in an arm or leg if lymph vessels are blocked, damaged, or removed by surgery.

lymphoma: Cancer that begins in cells of the immune system. There are two basic categories of lymphomas. One kind is Hodgkin lymphoma, which is marked by the presence of a type of cell called the Reed-Sternberg cell. The other category is non-Hodgkin lymphomas, which includes a large, diverse group of cancers of immune system cells. Non-Hodgkin lymphomas can be further divided into cancers that have an indolent (slow-growing) course and those that have an aggressive (fast-growing) course. These subtypes behave and respond to treatment differently. Both Hodgkin and non-Hodgkin lymphomas can occur in children and adults, and prognosis and treatment depend on the stage and the type of cancer.

magnetic resonance imaging: A procedure in which radio waves and a powerful magnet linked to a computer are used to create detailed pictures of areas inside the body. These pictures can show the difference between normal and diseased tissue. Magnetic resonance imaging makes better images of organs and soft tissue than other scanning techniques, such as computed tomography (CT) or x-ray. Magnetic resonance imaging is especially useful for imaging the brain, the spine, the soft tissue of joints, and the inside of bones. Also called MRI, NMRI, and nuclear magnetic resonance imaging.

maintenance therapy: Treatment that is given to help keep cancer from coming back after it has disappeared following the initial therapy. It may include treatment with drugs, vaccines, or antibodies that kill cancer cells, and it may be given for a long time.

malignancy: A term for diseases in which abnormal cells divide without control and can invade nearby tissues. Malignant cells can also spread to other parts of the body through the blood and lymph systems. There are several main types of malignancy. Carcinoma is a malignancy that begins in the skin or in tissues that line or cover internal organs. Sarcoma is a malignancy that begins in bone, cartilage, fat, muscle, blood vessels, or other connective or supportive tissue. Leukemia is a malignancy that starts in blood-forming tissue such as the bone marrow, and causes large numbers of abnormal blood cells to be produced and enter the blood. Lymphoma and multiple myeloma are malignancies that begin in the cells of the immune system. Central nervous system cancers are malignancies that begin in the tissues of the brain and spinal cord. Also called cancer.

mammography: The use of film or a computer to create a picture of the breast.

margin: The edge or border of the tissue removed in cancer surgery. The margin is described as negative or clean when the pathologist finds no cancer cells at the edge of the tissue, suggesting that all of the cancer has been removed. The margin is described as positive or involved when the pathologist finds cancer cells at the edge of the tissue, suggesting that all of the cancer has not been removed.

mass: In medicine, a lump in the body. It may be caused by the abnormal growth of cells, a cyst, hormonal changes, or an immune reaction. A mass may be benign (not cancer) or malignant (cancer).

mastectomy: Surgery to remove the breast (or as much of the breast tissue as possible).

medullary thyroid cancer: Cancer that develops in C cells of the thyroid. The C cells make a hormone (calcitonin) that helps maintain a healthy level of calcium in the blood.

medulloblastoma: A malignant brain tumor that begins in the lower part of the brain and that can spread to the spine or to other parts of the body. Medulloblastomas are a type of primitive neuroectodermal tumor (PNET).

melanoma: A form of cancer that begins in melanocytes (cells that make the pigment melanin). It may begin in a mole (skin melanoma),but can also begin in other pigmented tissues, such as in the eye or in the intestines.

meningioma: A type of slow-growing tumor that forms in the meninges (thin layers of tissue that cover and protect the brain and spinal cord). Meningiomas usually occur in adults.

Merkel cell carcinoma: A rare type of cancer that forms on or just beneath the skin, usually in parts of the body that have been exposed to the sun. It is most common in older people and in people with weakened immune systems. Also called Merkel cell cancer, neuroendocrine carcinoma of the skin, and trabecular cancer.

mesothelioma: A benign (not cancer) or malignant (cancer) tumor affecting the lining of the chest or abdomen. Exposure to asbestos particles in the air increases the risk of developing malignant mesothelioma.

metastasis: The spread of cancer from one part of the body to another.A tumor formed by cells that have spread is called a "metastatic tumor" or a "metastasis." The metastatic tumor contains cells that are like those in the original (primary) tumor. The plural form of metastasis is metastases (meh-TAS-tuh-SEEZ).

Mohs surgery: A surgical procedure used to treat skin cancer. Individual layers of cancer tissue are removed and examined under a microscope one at a time until all cancer tissue has been removed.

mole: A benign (not cancer) growth on the skin that is formed by a cluster of melanocytes (cells that make a substance called melanin, which gives color to skin and eyes). A mole is usually dark and may be raised from the skin. Also called nevus.

monoclonal antibody: A type of protein made in the laboratory that can bind to substances in the body, including tumor cells. There are many kinds of monoclonal antibodies. Each monoclonal antibody is made to find one substance. Monoclonal antibodies are being used to treat some types of cancer and are being studied in the treatment of other types. They can be used alone or to carry drugs, toxins, or radioactive materials directly to a tumor.

multiple myeloma: A type of cancer that begins in plasma cells (white blood cells that produce antibodies). Also called Kahler disease, myelomatosis, and plasma cell myeloma.

mutation: Any change in the DNA of a cell. Mutations may be caused by mistakes during cell division, or they may be caused by exposure to DNA-damaging agents in the environment. Mutations can be harmful, beneficial, or have no effect. If they occur in cells that make eggs or sperm, they can be inherited; if mutations occur in other types of cells, they are not inherited. Certain mutations may lead to cancer or other diseases.

myelodysplastic syndromes: A group of diseases in which the bone marrow does not make enough healthy blood cells. Also called preleukemia and smoldering leukemia.

myelogenous: Having to do with, produced by, or resembling the bone marrow. Sometimes used as a synonym for myeloid; for example, acute myeloid leukemia and acute myelogenous leukemia are the same disease.

myeloid: Having to do with or resembling the bone marrow. May also refer to certain types of hematopoietic (blood-forming) cells found in the bone marrow. Sometimes used as a synonym for myelogenous.

myeloma: Cancer that arises in plasma cells, a type of white blood cell.

myeloproliferative disorder: A group of slow growing blood cancers, including chronic myelogenous leukemia, in which large numbers of abnormal red blood cells, white blood cells, or platelets grow and spread in the bone marrow and the peripheral blood.

nasopharyngeal cancer: Cancer that forms in tissues of the nasopharynx (upper part of the throat behind the nose). Most nasopharyngeal cancers are squamous cell carcinomas (cancer that begins in flat cells lining the nasopharynx).

neck dissection: Surgery to remove lymph nodes and other tissues in the neck.

needle biopsy: The removal of tissue or fluid with a needle for examination under a microscope. When a wide needle is used, the procedure is called a core biopsy. When a thin needle is used, the procedure is called a fine-needle aspiration biopsy.

negative axillary lymph node: A lymph node in the armpit that is free of cancer.

neoadjuvant therapy: Treatment given as a first step to shrink a tumor before the main treatment, which is usually surgery, is given. Examples of neoadjuvant therapy include chemotherapy, radiation therapy, and hormone therapy. It is a type of induction therapy.

neoplasm: An abnormal mass of tissue that results when cells divide more than they should or do not die when they should. Neoplasms may be benign (not cancer), or malignant (cancer). Also called tumor.

neuroblastoma: Cancer that arises in immature nerve cells and affects mostly infants and children.

neuroendocrine tumor: A tumor that forms from cells that release hormones in response to a signal from the nervous system. Some examples of neuroendocrine tumors are carcinoid tumors, islet cell tumors, medullary thyroid carcinomas, pheochromocytomas, and neuroendocrine carcinomas of the skin (Merkel cell cancer). These tumors may secrete higher-than-normal amounts of hormones, which can cause many different symptoms.

neuroma: A tumor that arises in nerve cells.

neuropathy: A nerve problem that causes pain, numbness, tingling, swelling, or muscle weakness in different parts of the body. It usually begins in the hands or feet and gets worse over time. Neuropathy may be caused by physical injury, infection, toxic substances, disease (such as cancer, diabetes, kidney failure, or malnutrition), or drugs, including anticancer drugs.

neurofibroma: A benign tumor that develops from the cells and tissues that cover nerves.

nevus: A benign (not cancer) growth on the skin that is formed by a cluster of melanocytes (cells that make a substance called melanin, which gives color to skin and eyes). A nevus is usually dark and may be raised from the skin. Also called mole.

node-negative: Cancer that has not spread to the lymph nodes.

nodule: A growth or lump that may be malignant (cancer) or benign (not cancer).

non-Hodgkin lymphoma: Any of a large group of cancers of lymphocytes (white blood cells). Non-Hodgkin lymphomas can occur at any age and are often marked by lymph nodes that are larger than normal, fever, and weight loss. There are many different types of non-Hodgkin lymphoma. These types can be divided into aggressive (fast-growing) and indolent (slow-growing) types, and they can be formed from either B-cells or T-cells. B-cell non-Hodgkin lymphomas include Burkitt lymphoma, chronic lymphocytic leukemia/small lymphocytic lymphoma (CLL/SLL), diffuse large B-cell lymphoma, follicular lymphoma, immunoblastic large cell lymphoma, precursor B-lymphoblastic lymphoma, and mantle cell lymphoma. T-cell non-Hodgkin lymphomas include mycosis fungoides, anaplastic large cell lymphoma, and pre-cursor T-lymphoblastic lymphoma. Lymphomas that occur after bone marrow or stem cell transplantation are usually B-cell non-Hodgkin lymphomas. Prognosis and treatment depend on the stage and type of disease. Also called NHL.

nonmelanoma skin cancer: Skin cancer that forms in the lower part of the epidermis (the outer layer of the skin) or in squamous cells, but not in melanocytes (skin cells that make pigment).

nonseminoma: A group of testicular cancers that begin in the germ cells (cells that give rise to sperm). Nonseminomas are identified by the type of cell in which they begin and include embryonal carcinoma, teratoma, choriocarcinoma, and yolk sac carcinoma.

non-small cell lung cancer: A group of lung cancers that are named for the kinds of cells found in the cancer and how the cells look under a microscope. The three main types of non-small cell lung cancer are squamous cell carcinoma, large cell carcinoma, and adenocarcinoma. Non-small cell lung cancer is the most common kind of lung cancer.

noninvasive: In medicine, it describes a procedure that does not require inserting an instrument through the skin or into a body opening. In cancer, it describes disease that has not spread outside the tissue in which it began.

nonmalignant: Not cancerous. Nonmalignant tumors may grow larger but do not spread to other parts of the body. Also called benign.

occult primary tumor: Cancer in which the site of the primary (original) tumor cannot be found. Most metastases from occult primary tumors are found in the head and neck.

oncogene: A gene that is a mutated (changed) form of a gene involved in normal cell growth. Oncogenes may cause the growth of cancer cells. Mutations in genes that become oncogenes can be inherited or caused by being exposed to substances in the environment that cause cancer.

oncologist: A doctor who specializes in treating cancer. Some oncologists specialize in a particular type of cancer treatment. For example, a radiation oncologist specializes in treating cancer with radiation.

oral cancer: Cancer that forms in tissues of the oral cavity (the mouth) or the oropharynx (the part of the throat at the back of the mouth).

oral cavity cancer: Cancer that forms in tissues of the oral cavity (the mouth). The tissues of the oral cavity include the lips, the lining inside the cheeks and lips, the front two thirds of the tongue, the upper and lower gums, the floor of the mouth under the tongue, the bony roof of the mouth, and the small area behind the wisdom teeth.

oropharyngeal cancer: Cancer that forms in tissues of the oropharynx (the part of the throat at the back of the mouth, including the soft palate, the base of the tongue, and the tonsils). Most oropharyngeal cancers are squamous cell carcinomas (cancer that begins in flat cells lining the oropharynx).

osteosarcoma: A cancer of the bone that usually affects the large bones of the arm or leg. It occurs most commonly in young people and affects more males than females. Also called osteogenic sarcoma.

ovarian cancer: Cancer that forms in tissues of the ovary (one of a pair of female reproductive glands in which the ova, or eggs, are formed). Most ovarian cancers are either ovarian epithelial carcinomas (cancer that begins in the cells on the surface of the ovary) or malignant germ cell tumors (cancer that begins in egg cells).

p53 gene: A tumor suppressor gene that normally inhibits the growth of tumors. This gene is altered in many types of cancer.

Paget disease of the nipple: A form of breast cancer in which the tumor grows from ducts beneath the nipple onto the surface of the nipple. Symptoms commonly include itching and burning and an eczema-like condition around the nipple, sometimes accompanied by oozing or bleeding.

palliative care: Care given to improve the quality of life of patients who have a serious or life-threatening disease. The goal of palliative care is to prevent or treat as early as possible the symptoms of a disease, side effects caused by treatment of a disease, and psychological, social, and spiritual problems related to a disease or its treatment. Also called comfort care, supportive care, and symptom management.

palliative therapy: Treatment given to relieve the symptoms and reduce the suffering caused by cancer and other life-threatening diseases. Palliative cancer therapies are given together with other cancer treatments, from the time of diagnosis, through treatment, survivorship, recurrent or advanced disease, and at the end of life.

pancreatic cancer: A disease in which malignant (cancer) cells are found in the tissues of the pancreas. Also called exocrine cancer.

pancreatic endocrine cancer: A rare cancer that forms in the islets of Langerhans cells (a type of cell found in the pancreas). Also called islet cell carcinoma.

Pap smear: A procedure in which cells are scraped from the cervix for examination under a microscope. It is used to detect cancer and changes that may lead to cancer. A Pap smear can also show conditions,such as infection or inflammation, that are not cancer. Also called Pap test and Papanicolaou test.

pathologist: A doctor who identifies diseases by studying cells and tissues under a microscope.

pathology report: The description of cells and tissues made by a pathologist based on microscopic evidence, and sometimes used to make a diagnosis of a disease.

pelvic lymphadenectomy: Surgery to remove lymph nodes in the pelvis for examination under a microscope to see if they contain cancer.

penile cancer: A rare cancer that forms in the penis (an external male reproductive organ). Most penile cancers are squamous cell carcinomas (cancer that begins in flat cells lining the penis).

peritoneal cancer: Cancer of the tissue that lines the abdominal wall and covers organs in the abdomen.

Peutz-Jeghers syndrome: A genetic disorder in which polyps form in the intestine and dark spots appear on the mouth and fingers. Having PJS increases the risk of developing gastrointestinal and many other types of cancer. Also called PJS.

pharyngeal cancer: Cancer that forms in tissues of the pharynx (the hollow tube inside the neck that starts behind the nose and ends at the top of the windpipe and esophagus). Pharyngeal cancer includes cancer of the nasopharynx (the upper part of the throat behind the nose), the oropharynx (the middle part of the pharynx), and the hypopharynx (the bottom part of the pharynx). Cancer of the larynx (voice box) may also be included as a type of pharyngeal cancer. Most pharyngeal cancers are squamous cell carcinomas (cancer that begins in thin, flat cells that look like fish scales). Also called throat cancer.

pheochromocytoma: Tumor that forms in the center of the adrenal gland (gland located above the kidney) that causes it to make too much adrenaline. Pheochromocytomas are usually benign (not cancer) but can cause high blood pressure, pounding headaches, heart palpitations, flushing of the face, nausea, and vomiting.

pineoblastoma: A fast growing type of brain tumor that occurs in or around the pineal gland, a tiny organ near the center of the brain.

pineocytoma: A slow growing type of brain tumor that occurs in or around the pineal gland, a tiny organ near the center of the brain.

pituitary tumor: A tumor that forms in the pituitary gland. The pituitary is a pea-sized organ in the center of the brain above the back of the nose. It makes hormones that affect other glands and many body functions, especially growth. Most pituitary tumors are benign (not cancer).

placebo: An inactive substance or treatment that looks the same as, and is given the same way as, an active drug or treatment being tested. The effects of the active drug or treatment are compared to the effects of the placebo.

plasmacytoma: A type of cancer that begins in plasma cells (white blood cells that produce antibodies). A plasmacytoma may turn into multiple myeloma.

polyp: A growth that protrudes from a mucous membrane.

primary tumor: The original tumor.

primitive neuroectodermal tumor: One of a group of cancers that develop from the same type of early cells, and share certain biochemical and genetic features. Some primitive neuroectodermal tumors develop in the brain and central nervous system (CNS-PNET), and others develop in sites outside of the brain such as the limbs, pelvis, and chest wall (peripheral PNET). Also called PNET.

progesterone receptor positive: Describes cells that have a protein to which the hormone progesterone will bind. Cancer cells that are PR+ need progesterone to grow and will usually stop growing when treated with hormones that block progesterone from binding. Also called PR+.

prostate-specific antigen: A protein made by the prostate gland and found in the blood. Prostate-specific antigen blood levels may be higher than normal in men who have prostate cancer, benign prostatic hyperplasia (BPH), or infection or inflammation of the prostate gland. Also called PSA.

proton beam radiation therapy: A type of radiation therapy that uses streams of protons (tiny particles with a positive charge) that come from a special machine. This type of radiation kills tumor cells but does not damage nearby tissues. It is used to treat cancers in the head and neck and in organs such as the brain, eye, lung, spine, and prostate. Proton beam radiation is different from x-ray radiation.

punch biopsy: Removal of a small disk-shaped sample of tissue using a sharp, hollow device. The tissue is then examined under a microscope.

radical local excision: Surgery to remove a tumor and a large amount of normal tissue surrounding it. Nearby lymph nodes may also be removed.

radical lymph node dissection: A surgical procedure to remove most or all of the lymph nodes that drain lymph from the area around a tumor. The lymph nodes are then examined under a microscope to see if cancer cells have spread to them.

radiation therapy: The use of high-energy radiation from x-rays, gamma rays, neutrons, protons, and other sources to kill cancer cells and shrink tumors. Radiation may come from a machine outside the body (external-beam radiation therapy), or it may come from radioactive material placed in the body near cancer cells (internal radiation therapy). Systemic radiation therapy uses a radioactive substance, such as a radiolabeled monoclonal antibody, that travels in the blood to tissues throughout the body. Also called irradiation and radiotherapy.

radioactive iodine: A radioactive form of iodine, often used for imaging tests or to treat an overactive thyroid, thyroid cancer, and certain other cancers. For imaging tests, the patient takes a small dose of radioactive iodine that collects in thyroid cells and certain kinds of tumors and can be detected by a scanner. To treat thyroid cancer, the patient takes a large dose of radioactive iodine, which kills thyroid cells. Radioactive iodine is also used in internal radiation therapy for prostate cancer, intraocular (eye) melanoma, and carcinoid tumors. Radioactive iodine is given by mouth as a liquid or in capsules, by infusion, or sealed in seeds, which are placed in or near the tumor to kill cancer cells.

radiofrequency ablation: A procedure that uses radio waves to heat and destroy abnormal cells. The radio waves travel through electrodes (small devices that carry electricity). Radiofrequency ablation may be used to treat cancer and other conditions.

radiosurgery: A type of external radiation therapy that uses special equipment to position the patient and precisely give a single large dose of radiation to a tumor. It is used to treat brain tumors and other brain disorders that cannot be treated by regular surgery. It is also being studied in the treatment of other types of cancer. Also called radiation surgery, stereotactic radiosurgery, and stereotaxic radiosurgery.

randomized clinical trial: A study in which the participants are assigned by chance to separate groups that compare different treatments; neither the researchers nor the participants can choose which group. Using chance to assign people to groups means that the groups will be similar and that the treatments they receive can be compared objectively. At the time of the trial, it is not known which treatment is best. It is the patient's choice to be in a randomized trial.

recurrent cancer: Cancer that has recurred (come back), usually after a period of time during which the cancer could not be detected. The cancer may come back to the same place as the original (primary) tumor or to another place in the body. Also called recurrence.

Reed-Sternberg cell: A type of cell that appears in people with Hodgkin disease. The number of these cells increases as the disease advances.

remission: A decrease in or disappearance of signs and symptoms of cancer. In partial remission, some, but not all, signs and symptoms of cancer have disappeared. In complete remission, all signs and symptoms of cancer have disappeared, although cancer still may be in the body.

resectable: Able to be removed by surgery.

resection: Surgery to remove tissue or part or all of an organ.

retinoblastoma: Cancer that forms in the tissues of the retina (the light-sensitive layers of nerve tissue at the back of the eye). Retinoblastoma usually occurs in children younger than five years. It may be hereditary or nonhereditary (sporadic).

rhabdomyosarcoma: Cancer that forms in the soft tissues in a type of muscle called striated muscle. Rhabdomyosarcoma can occur anywhere in the body.

risk factor: Something that increases the chance of developing a disease. Some examples of risk factors for cancer are age, a family history of certain cancers, use of tobacco products, being exposed to radiation or certain chemicals, infection with certain viruses or bacteria, and certain genetic changes.

sarcoma: A cancer of the bone, cartilage, fat, muscle, blood vessels, or other connective or supportive tissue.

salpingo-oophorectomy: Surgical removal of the fallopian tubes and ovaries.

secondary cancer: A term that is used to describe either a new primary cancer or cancer that has spread from the place in which it started to other parts of the body.

segmental resection: Surgery to remove part of an organ or gland. It may also be used to remove a tumor and normal tissue around it. In lung cancer surgery, segmental resection refers to removing a section of a lobe of the lung. Also called segmentectomy.

seminoma: A type of cancer of the testicles. Seminomas may spread to the lung, bone, liver, or brain.

sentinel lymph node biopsy: Removal and examination of the sentinel node(s) (the first lymph node(s) to which cancer cells are likely to spread from a primary tumor). To identify the sentinel lymph node(s), the surgeon injects a radioactive substance, blue dye, or both near the tumor. The surgeon then uses a probe to find the sentinel lymph node(s) containing the radioactive substance or looks for the lymph node(s) stained with dye. The surgeon then removes the sentinel node(s) to check for the presence of cancer cells.

shave biopsy: A procedure in which a skin abnormality and a thin layer of surrounding skin are removed with a small blade for examination under a microscope. Stitches are not needed with this procedure.

sigmoidoscopy: Examination of the lower colon using a sigmoidoscope, inserted into the rectum. A sigmoidoscope is a thin, tube-like instrument with a light and a lens for viewing. It may also have a tool to remove tissue to be checked under a microscope for signs of disease. Also called proctosigmoidoscopy.

skin cancer: Cancer that forms in the tissues of the skin. There are several types of skin cancer. Skin cancer that forms in melanocytes (skin cells that make pigment) is called melanoma. Skin cancer that forms in the lower part of the epidermis (the outer layer of the skin) is called basal cell carcinoma. Skin cancer that forms in squamous cells (flat cells that form the surface of the skin) is called squamous cell carcinoma. Skin cancer that forms in neuroendocrine cells (cells that release hormones in response to signals from the nervous system) is called neuroendocrine carcinoma of the skin. Most skin cancers form in older people on parts of the body exposed to the sun or in people who have weakened immune systems.

sleeve resection: Surgery to remove a lung tumor in a lobe of the lung and a part of the main bronchus (airway). The ends of the bronchus are rejoined and any remaining lobes are reattached to the bronchus. This surgery is done to save part of the lung. Also called sleeve lobectomy.

small cell lung cancer: An aggressive (fast-growing) cancer that forms in tissues of the lung and can spread to other parts of the body. The cancer cells look small and oval-shaped when looked at under a microscope.

small intestine cancer: A rare cancer that forms in tissues of the small intestine (the part of the digestive tract between the stomach and the large intestine). The most common type is adenocarcinoma (cancer that begins in cells that make and release mucus and other fluids). Other types of small intestine cancer include sarcoma (cancer that begins in connective or supportive tissue), carcinoid tumor (a slow-growing type of cancer), gastrointestinal stromal tumor (a type of soft tissue sarcoma), and lymphoma (cancer that begins in immune system cells).

soft tissue sarcoma: A cancer that begins in the muscle, fat, fibrous tissue, blood vessels, or other supporting tissue of the body.

solid tumor: An abnormal mass of tissue that usually does not contain cysts or liquid areas. Solid tumors may be benign (not cancer), or malignant (cancer). Different types of solid tumors are named for the type of cells that form them. Examples of solid tumors are sarcomas,carcinomas, and lymphomas. Leukemias (cancers of the blood) generally do not form solid tumors.

sputum cytology: Examination under a microscope of cells found in sputum (mucus and other matter brought up from the lungs by coughing). The test checks for abnormal cells, such as lung cancer cells.

squamous cell carcinoma: Cancer that begins in squamous cells, which are thin, flat cells that look like fish scales. Squamous cells are found in the tissue that forms the surface of the skin, the lining of the hollow organs of the body, and the passages of the respiratory and digestive tracts. Also called epidermoid carcinoma.

stage: The extent of a cancer in the body. Staging is usually based on the size of the tumor, whether lymph nodes contain cancer, and whether the cancer has spread from the original site to other parts of the body.

staging: Performing exams and tests to learn the extent of the cancer within the body, especially whether the disease has spread from the original site to other parts of the body. It is important to know the stage of the disease in order to plan the best treatment.

stem cell transplant: A method of replacing immature blood-forming cells in the bone marrow that have been destroyed by drugs, radiation, or disease. Stem cells are injected into the patient and make healthy blood cells. A stem cell transplant may be autologous (using a patient's own stem cells that were saved before treatment), allogeneic (using stem cells donated by someone who is not an identical twin), or syngeneic (using stem cells donated by an identical twin).

stereotactic biopsy: A biopsy procedure that uses a computer and a three-dimensional scanning device to find a tumor site and guide the removal of tissue for examination under a microscope.

stoma: A surgically created opening from an area inside the body to the outside.

stomach cancer: Cancer that forms in tissues lining the stomach. Also called gastric cancer.

stromal tumor: A tumor that arises in the supporting connective tissue of an organ.

superior vena cava syndrome: A condition in which a tumor presses against the superior vena cava (the large vein that carries blood from the head, neck, arms, and chest to the heart). This pressure blocks blood flow to the heart and may cause coughing, difficulty in breathing, and swelling of the face, neck, and upper arms.

supportive care: Care given to improve the quality of life of patients who have a serious or life-threatening disease. The goal of supportive care is to prevent or treat as early as possible the symptoms of a disease, side effects caused by treatment of a disease, and psychological, social, and spiritual problems related to a disease or its treatment. Also called comfort care, palliative care, and symptom management.

survivorship: In cancer, survivorship covers the physical, psychosocial, and economic issues of cancer, from diagnosis until the end of life. It focuses on the health and life of a person with cancer beyond the diagnosis and treatment phases. Survivorship includes issues related to the ability to get health care and follow-up treatment, late effects of treatment, second cancers, and quality of life. Family members, friends, and caregivers are also part of the survivorship experience.

systemic chemotherapy: Treatment with anticancer drugs that travel through the blood to cells all over the body.

targeted therapy: A type of treatment that uses drugs or other substances, such as monoclonal antibodies, to identify and attack specific cancer cells. Targeted therapy may have fewer side effects than other types of cancer treatments.

teratocarcinoma: A type of germ cell cancer that usually forms in the testes (testicles).

teratoma: A type of germ cell tumor that may contain several different types of tissue, such as hair, muscle, and bone. Teratomas occur most often in the ovaries in women, the testicles in men, and the tailbone in children. Not all teratomas are malignant.

testicular cancer: Cancer that forms in tissues of the testis (one of two egg-shaped glands inside the scrotum that make sperm and male hormones). Testicular cancer usually occurs in young or middle-aged men. Two main types of testicular cancer are seminomas (cancers that grow slowly and are sensitive to radiation therapy) and nonseminomas (different cell types that grow more quickly than seminomas).

thymic carcinoma: A rare type of thymus gland cancer. It usually spreads, has a high risk of recurrence, and has a poor survival rate. Thymic carcinoma is divided into subtypes, depending on the types of cells in which the cancer began. Also called type C thymoma.

thymoma: A tumor of the thymus, an organ that is part of the lyphatic system and is located in the chest, behind the breastbone.

thyroid cancer: Cancer that forms in the thyroid gland (an organ at the base of the throat that makes hormones that help control heart rate, blood pressure, body temperature, and weight). Four main types of thyroid cancer are papillary, follicular, medullary, and anaplastic thyroid cancer. The four types are based on how the cancer cells look under a microscope.

topical chemotherapy: Treatment with anticancer drugs in a lotion or cream applied to the skin.

transperineal biopsy: A procedure in which a sample of tissue is removed from the prostate for examination under a microscope. The sample is removed with a thin needle that is inserted through the skin between the scrotum and rectum and into the prostate.

transplantation: A surgical procedure in which tissue or an organ is transferred from one area of a person's body to another area, or from one person (the donor) to another person (the recipient).

transrectal biopsy: A procedure in which a sample of tissue is removed from the prostate using a thin needle that is inserted through the rectum and into the prostate. Transrectal ultrasound (TRUS) is usually used to guide the needle. The sample is examined under a microscope to see if it contains cancer.

transurethral biopsy: A procedure in which a sample of tissue is removed from the prostate for examination under a microscope. A thin,lighted tube is inserted through the urethra into the prostate, and a small piece of tissue is removed with a cutting loop.

transvaginal ultrasound: A procedure used to examine the vagina, uterus, fallopian tubes, ovaries, and bladder. An instrument is inserted into the vagina that causes sound waves to bounce off organs inside the pelvis. These sound waves create echoes that are sent to a computer, which creates a picture called a sonogram. Also called transvaginal sonography and TVS.

triple-negative breast cancer: Describes breast cancer cells that do not have estrogen receptors, progesterone receptors, or large amounts of HER2/neu protein. Also called ER-negative PR-negative HER2/neu-negative and ER-PR-HER2/neu-.

tumor: An abnormal mass of tissue that results when cells divide more than they should or do not die when they should. Tumors may be benign (not cancer), or malignant (cancer). Also called neoplasm.

tumor debulking: Surgical removal of as much of a tumor as possible. Tumor debulking may increase the chance that chemotherapy or radiation therapy will kill all the tumor cells. It may also be done to relieve symptoms or help the patient live longer.

tumor marker: A substance that may be found in tumor tissue or released from a tumor into the blood or other body fluids. A high level of a tumor marker may mean that a certain type of cancer is in the body. Examples of tumor markers include CA 125 (in ovarian cancer), CA 15-3 (in breast cancer), CEA (in ovarian, lung, breast, pancreas, and gastrointestinal tract cancers), and PSA (in prostate cancer).

tumor necrosis factor: A protein made by white blood cells in response to an antigen (substance that causes the immune system to make a specific immune response) or infection. Tumor necrosis factor can also be made in the laboratory. It may boost a person's immune response, and also may cause necrosis (cell death) of some types of tumor cells. Tumor necrosis factor is being studied in the treatment of some types of cancer. It is a type of cytokine. Also called TNF.

ultrasound: A procedure in which high-energy sound waves are bounced off internal tissues or organs and make echoes. The echo patterns are shown on the screen of an ultrasound machine, forming a picture of body tissues called a sonogram.

unresectable: Unable to be removed with surgery.

upper GI series: A series of x-ray pictures of the esophagus, stomach, and duodenum (the first part of the small intestine). The x-ray pictures are taken after the patient drinks a liquid containing barium sulfate (a form of the silver-white metallic element barium). The barium sulfate coats and outlines the inner walls of the upper gastrointestinal tract so that they can be seen on the x-ray pictures. Also called upper gastrointestinal series.

urethral cancer: A rare cancer that forms in tissues of the urethra (the tube through which urine empties the bladder and leaves the body). Types of urethral cancer include transitional cell carcinoma (cancer that begins in cells that can change shape and stretch without breaking apart), squamous cell carcinoma (cancer that begins in flat cells lining the urethra), and adenocarcinoma (cancer that begins in cells that make and release mucus and other fluids).

vaginal cancer: Cancer that forms in the tissues of the vagina (birth canal). The vagina leads from the cervix (the opening of the uterus) to the outside of the body. The most common type of vaginal cancer is squamous cell carcinoma, which starts in the thin, flat cells lining the vagina. Another type of vaginal cancer is adenocarcinoma, cancer that begins in glandular cells in the lining of the vagina.

virtual colonoscopy: A method to examine the inside of the colon by taking a series of x-rays. A computer is used to make two-dimensional(2-D) and three-dimensional (3-D) pictures of the colon from these x-rays. The pictures can be saved, changed to give better viewing angles, and reviewed after the procedure, even years later. Also called computed tomographic colonography, computed tomography colonography, CT colonography, and CTC.

vulvar cancer: Cancer of the vulva (the external female genital organs, including the clitoris, vaginal lips, and the opening to the vagina).

watchful waiting: Closely watching a patient's condition but not giving treatment unless symptoms appear or change. Watchful waiting is used in conditions that progress slowly, are hard to diagnose, or may get better without treatment. It is also used when the risks of treatment are greater than the possible benefits. During watchful waiting, patients may be given certain tests and exams. Watchful waiting is sometimes used in prostate cancer. It is a type of expectant management.

Waldenström macroglobulinemia: An indolent (slow-growing) type of non-Hodgkin lymphoma marked by abnormal levels of IgM antibodies in the blood and an enlarged liver, spleen, or lymph nodes. Also called lymphoplasmacytic lymphoma.

wedge resection: Surgery to remove a triangle-shaped slice of tissue. It may be used to remove a tumor and a small amount of normal tissue around it.

Whipple procedure: A type of surgery used to treat pancreatic cancer. The head of the pancreas, the duodenum, a portion of the stomach, and other nearby tissues are removed.

wide local excision: Surgery to cut out the cancer and some healthy tissue around it.

wound: A break in the skin or other body tissues caused by injury or surgical incision (cut).

x-ray: A type of high-energy radiation. In low doses, x-rays are used to diagnose diseases by making pictures of the inside of the body. In high doses, x-rays are used to treat cancer.

yttrium: A metal of the rare earth group of elements. A radioactive form of yttrium may be attached to a monoclonal antibody or other molecule that can locate and bind to cancer cells and be used to diagnose or treat some types of cancer.

Index

Index

Page numbers followed by 'n' indicate a footnote. Page numbers in *italics* indicate a table or illustration.

A

1285

ovarian germ cell tumors, described
558–9
"Ovarian Germ Cell Tumors
Treatment" (NIH) 579n
ovarian low malignant, overview
492–8
"Ovarian Low Malignant Potential
Tumors Treatment" (NIH) 492n
overweight, endocrine 760

P

Pacific Islanders, cancer statistics
1232
Paget disease of the nipple, defined
1275
palliative care
childhood superior vena cava
syndrome 1101
defined 1275
described 1126–7
palliative therapy, defined 1275
pancreas
described 359
glucagonoma 386
pancreatic cancer
defined 1275
Helicobacter pylori 109
overview 359–69
statistics 1221
tobacco use 30
"Pancreatic Cancer Treatment" (NIH)
359n
"Pancreatic Neuroendocrine Tumors
(Islet Cell Tumors) Treatment"
(NIH) 370n
pancreatic endocrine cancer, defined
1275
pancreatic endocrine tumor 370
pancreatic neuroendocrine tumor,
overview 370–88
panitumumab 1003
Panretin (alitretinoin) 1003
"Pap and HPV Testing" (NIH) 841n
papillary thyroid cancer 215, 223
Pap smear, defined 1275
Pap tests
cervical cancer screening 842–3
vulvar cancer 546

paracentesis, childhood extracranial
germ cell tumors 563
parietal cell vagotomy, pancreatic
NETs 380
partial hepatectomy
extrahepatic bile duct cancer 346
liver cancer 333
partial hysterectomy, described 489
partial laryngectomy, laryngeal
cancer 197
partial penectomy
urethral cancer 438
penile cancer 457
pathologist, defined 1275
pathology report, defined 1275
Patient Advocate Foundation, contact
1244
"Patient Corner" (NIH) 1175n
pazopanib 1003
PDT *see* photodynamic therapy
pelvic examination
cervical cancer screening 842
diethylstilbestrol 73
pelvic exenteration
cervical cancer 530
childhood rhabdomyosarcoma 624
rectal cancer 416
vaginal cancer 541
vulvar cancer 552
pelvic lymphadenectomy, defined
1276
penectomy
penile cancer 457
urethral cancer 438–9
penile cancer
defined 1276
human papillomavirus infection 451
overview 450–9
"Penile Cancer Treatment" (NIH)
450n
percutaneous ethanol injection, liver
cancer 334
percutaneous transhepatic biliary
drainage, gallbladder cancer 357
percutaneous transhepatic
cholangiography
extrahepatic bile duct cancer 340
gallbladder cancer 352
pancreatic cancer 363

Y

yoga, described 1040
yolk sac tumors 557
Young Survival Coalition, contact
  1247
yttrium, defined 1286

Z

Zevalin (ibritumomab tiuxetan) 1004
Zolinza (vorinostat) 1004